HANDBOOK OF

PEDIATRIC INTENSIVE CARE

THIRD EDITION

HANDBOOK OF
PEDIATRIC INTENSIVE CARE

THIRD EDITION

EDITED BY

MARK C. ROGERS, M.D.

PRESIDENT, PARAMOUNT CAPITAL INCORPORATED
NEW YORK, NEW YORK

MARK A. HELFAER, M.D.
CHIEF, CRITICAL CARE MEDICINE
CHILDREN'S HOSPITAL OF PHILADELPHIA
UNIVERSITY OF PENNSYLVANIA SCHOOL OF MEDICINE
PHILADELPHIA, PENNSYLVANIA

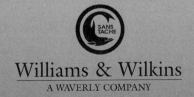

Williams & Wilkins
A WAVERLY COMPANY

BALTIMORE • PHILADELPHIA • LONDON • PARIS • BANGKOK
BUENOS AIRES • HONG KONG • MUNICH • SYDNEY • TOKYO • WROCLAW

Editor: Sharon Zinner
Managing Editor: Tanya Lazar
Marketing Manager: Diane Harnish
Production Editor: June Choe

Copyright © 1999 Williams & Wilkins

351 West Camden Street
Baltimore, Maryland 21201-2436 USA

Rose Tree Corporate Center
1400 North Providence Road
Building II, Suite 5025
Media, Pennsylvania 19063-2043 USA

Printed in the United States of America

First Edition 1989
Second Edition 1995

Library of Congress Cataloging-in-Publication Data

Handbook of pediatric intensive care / edited by Mark C. Rogers, Mark A. Helfaer. — 3rd ed.
    p.   cm.
  Includes index.
  ISBN 0-683-30571-9
  1. Pediatric intensive care—Handbooks, manuals, etc.
  2. Pediatric emergencies—Handbooks, manuals, etc.   I. Rogers, Mark C.   II. Helfaer, Mark A.
  [DNLM: 1. Critical Care—in infancy & childhood handbooks.
  2. Emergencies—in infancy & childhood handbooks.   WS 39 H236 1998]
  RJ370.H36   1998
  618.92'0028—dc21
  DNLM/DLC
  for Library of Congress   98-23780
                                           CIP

The publishers have made every effort to trace the copyright holders for borrowed material. If they have inadvertently overlooked any, they will be pleased to make the necessary arrangements at the first opportunity. Complete citations can be found in the 3rd edition of the Textbook of Pediatric Intensive Care.

To purchase additional copies of this book, call our customer service department at **(800) 638-0672** or fax orders to **(800) 447-8438**. For other book services, including chapter reprints and large quantity sales, ask for the Special Sales department.

Canadian customers should call **(800) 665-1148**, or fax **(800) 665-0103**. For all other calls originating outside of the United States, please call **(410) 528-4223** or fax us at **(410) 528-8550**.

Visit Williams & Wilkins on the Internet: http://www.wwilkins.com or contact our customer service department at **custserv@wwilkins.com**. Williams & Wilkins customer service representatives are available from 8:30 am to 6:00 pm, EST, Monday through Friday, for telephone access.

                                    99 00 01 02 03
                            1 2 3 4 5 6 7 8 9 10

To our families, whose encouragement and support make all of our work possible and rewarding. Elizabeth and Michele have been our traveling companions through life. Bradley, Meredith, Samuel, and Jonathan have allowed us to grow up with them. We are grateful to the joy they all have brought to us.

PREFACE

This book is the third edition of the *Handbook of Pediatric Intensive Care*. It represents the balance between the clinical didactic approach needed in a handbook and the physiologic approach we use in the *Textbook of Pediatric Intensive Care,* but which we feel is also needed in making sophisticated clinical decisions.

As the specialty continues to evolve, we will continue to update the diseases with which the intensivist should be familiar as well as the diagnostic and treatment points which we continue to discuss as current and even in stages of development.

As the resident training shifts from inpatient to outpatient, the responsibility of caring for the sickest of children will fall into the scope of practice of the best trained and qualified individuals. These inpatient doctors, "The Hospitalists," will be best trained in the field of pediatric critical care. It is for these individuals that this *Handbook* is best suited.

MARK C. ROGERS
MARK A. HELFAER

CONTRIBUTORS

Alice D. Ackerman, M.D., F.A.A.P., F.C.C.M.
Department of Pediatrics
University of Maryland School of Medicine
Baltimore, Maryland

Elizabeth M. Allen, M.D.
Division of Pediatric Critical Care
University of Utah School of Medicine
Primary Children's Medical Center
Salt Lake City, Utah

John H. Arnold, M.D.
Multidisciplinary Intensive Care Unit
Children's Hospital
Boston, Massachusetts

Jolene D. Bean, M.D.
Scott & White Hospital
Department of Anesthesiology
Temple, Texas

Frank E. Berkowitz, M.B., B.Ch., F.C.P. (PAED) (SA)
Department of Pediatrics
Emory University School of Medicine
Atlanta, Georgia

Ivor D. Berkowitz, M.B., B.Ch.
Department of Anesthesiology, Critical Care Medicine & Pediatrics
The Johns Hopkins Hospital
Baltimore, Maryland

Mark L. Bernstein, M.D.
Department of Hematology
Montreal Children's Hospital
Montreal, Quebec

Richard S. Boyer, M.D.
Department of Pediatric Radiology
University of Utah
Salt Lake City, Utah

Susan L. Bratton, M.D.
Department of Anesthesia and Critical Care
Children's Hospital and Medical Center
Seattle, Washington

Douglas Brockmeyer, M.D.
Division of Pediatric Neurosurgery
University of Utah
Primary Children's Medical Center
Salt Lake City, Utah

G. Patricia Cantwell, M.D.
Medical Training & Simulation Laboratory
University of Miami School of Medicine
Miami, Florida

W. Bruce Cherny, M.D.
Division of Pediatric Neurosurgery
University of Utah
Primary Children's Medical Center
Salt Lake City, Utah

David Christensen, M.D.
Department of Pediatrics/PICU
Loma Linda University Medical Center
Loma Linda, California

Reginald J. Davis, M.D.
Department of Neurosurgery
Greater Baltimore Medical Center
Baltimore, Maryland

Steve Davis, M.D.
Pediatric Intensive Care
The Cleveland Clinic Foundation
Cleveland, Ohio

J. Michael Dean, M.D.
University of Utah
Primary Children's Medical Center
Salt Lake City, Utah

Jayant K. Deshpande, M.D.
Department of Pediatric Critical Care Medicine
Vanderbilt University Medical Center
Nashville, Tennessee

Robert Englander, M.D.
Department of Pediatrics, Division of Critical Care
University of Maryland School of Medicine
Baltimore, Maryland

James C. Fackler, M.D.
Department of Anesthesia and Critical Care Medicine
The Johns Hopkins Hospital
Baltimore, Maryland

John J. Farley, M.D.
Department of Pediatric Immunology
University of Maryland School of Medicine
Baltimore, Maryland

Andrew L. Goldberg, M.D.
Allegheny General Hospital
Medical College of Pennsylvania
Pittsburgh, Pennsylvania

John B. Gordon, M.D., C.M., F.R.C.P.(C)
Pediatric Intensive Care
University of Wisconsin
Milwaukee, Wisconsin

Mary Jo Grant, M.S., P.N.P., C.C.R.N.
Pediatric Intensive Care Unit
Primary Children's Medical Center
Salt Lake City, Utah

Matthew M. Hand, D.O.
Division of Nephrology
Children's Hospital
Boston, Massachusetts

William E. Harmon, M.D.
Division of Nephrology
Children's Hospital Boston
Boston, Massachusetts

Mark A. Helfaer, M.D.
Pediatric Critical Care
Children's Hospital of Philadelphia
University of Pennsylvania School of Medicine
Philadelphia, Pennsylvania

Daniel S. Kohane, M.D., Ph.D.
Department of Anesthesia
Children's Hospital
Boston, Massachusetts

Isaac S. Kohane, M.D., Ph.D.
Division of Endocrinology
Children's Hospital
Boston, Massachusetts

John W. Kuluz, M.D.
Division of Critical Care Medicine
Department of Pediatrics
University of Miami School of Medicine
Miami, Florida

Gitte Y. Larsen, M.D.
Division of Pediatric Critical Care
Doernbecher Hospital OHSU
Portland, Oregon

Erica Liebelt, M.D.
Yale-New Haven Hospital
New Haven, Connecticut

Lynn D. Martin, M.D.
Department of Anesthesiology and Critical Care Medicine
University of Washington School of Medicine
Children's Hospital and Medical Center
Seattle, Washington

Gwenn E. McLaughlin, M.D.
Department of Pediatrics
University of Miami School of Medicine
Miami, Florida

Michael E. McManus, M.D.
Department of Anesthesia and Pediatrics
Children's Hospital
Boston, Massachusetts

Andrew M. Munster, M.D.
Departments of Surgery and Plastic Surgery
The Francis Scott Key Medical Center
Baltimore, Maryland

Joshua P. Needleman, M.D.
Pediatric Pulmonology
St. Christopher's Hospital for Children
Philadelphia, Pennsylvania

Charles Newton, M.B., Ch.B., M.D., M.R.C.P. (UK)
Johns Hopkins University Medical School
Baltimore, Maryland

David G. Nichols, M.D.
Department of Anesthesia and Critical Care Medicine
The Johns Hopkins Hospital
Baltimore, Maryland

Jay A. Perman, M.D.
Department of Pediatrics
Medical College of Virginia
Richmond, Virginia

W. Bradley Poss, M.D.
Department of Pediatrics
Naval Medical Center
San Diego, California

Elizabeth L. Rogers, M.D.
Primary Care
VA Connecticut Healthcare System
West Haven, Connecticut

Mark C. Rogers, M.D.
Paramount Capital, Incorporated
New York, New York

Mark E. Rowin, M.D.
Children's Medical Center
Dayton, Ohio

Charles L. Schleien, M.D.
Department of Pediatrics
University of Miami School of Medicine
Miami, Florida

Scott R. Schulman, M.D.
Division of Pediatric Cardiac Anesthesia and Critical Care Medicine
Duke University Medical Center
Durham, North Carolina

Nancy A. Setzer, M.D.
University of Florida College of Medicine
Gainesville, Florida

Donald H. Shaffner, M.D.
Departments of Anesthesiology and Critical Care Medicine
The Johns Hopkins University Hospital
Baltimore, Maryland

Robert M. Spear, M.D.
Departments of Anesthesiology and Critical Care Medicine
Children's Hospital and Health Center
San Diego, California

Ellen A. Spurrier, M.D.
Nemours Cardiac Center
Wilmington, Delaware

Vera Fan Tait, M.D.
Department of Pediatrics and Pediatric Neurology
Primary Children's Medical Center
University of Utah
Salt Lake City, Utah

Robert C. Tasker, M.D., B.S., M.R.C.P. (UK)
Cambridge University School of Clinical Medicine
Addenbrokes Hospital
Cambridge, England

Joseph R. Tobin, M.D.
Department of Anesthesia
Bowman Grey School of Medicine
Winston-Salem, North Carolina

Randall L. Tressler, M.D.
Department of Pediatrics
University of Maryland School of Medicine
Baltimore, Maryland

Andreas Tzakis, M.D.
Department of Surgery
University of Miami Medical School
Miami, Florida

Donald D. Vernon, M.D.
Primary Children's Medical Center
Salt Lake City, Utah

Peter E. Vink, M.D.
Department of Pediatrics
University of Maryland School of Medicine
Baltimore, Maryland

L. Kyle Walker, M.D.
Pediatric Intensive Care
Children's Hospital
National Medical Center
Washington, D.C.

Randall C. Wetzel, M.D., B.S., F.C.C.M.
Division of Pediatric Anesthesia and Critical Care
Children's Hospital of Los Angeles
Los Angeles, California

Rodney E. Willoughby, M.D.
Department of Pediatrics
Johns Hopkins School of Medicine
Baltimore, Maryland

Alan Woolf, M.D., M.P.H.
Department of Pediatrics
Massachusetts Poison Control Center
Boston, Massachusetts

Myron Yaster, M.D.
Department of Anesthesia and Critical Care Medicine
The Johns Hopkins Hospital
Baltimore, Maryland

Aaron L. Zuckerberg, M.D., F.A.A.P.
Department of Pediatrics
Sinai Hospital
Baltimore, Maryland

CONTENTS

1.

Cardiopulmonary Resuscitation

Charles L. Schleien, John W. Kuluz, Donald H. Shaffner,
and Mark C. Rogers

Cardiopulmonary arrest is the final common pathway for many life-threatening diseases. Although cardiopulmonary resuscitation (CPR) was once thought to be a miracle cure for patients suffering a cardiac arrest, outcome studies indicate otherwise. These studies show that the survival rate after CPR is less than 50%, and, in many cases, even less than 15%.

ETIOLOGY OF CARDIOPULMONARY ARREST

The etiology of cardiopulmonary arrest in children is different from that in adults. Eisenberg et al. reviewed the causes of cardiac arrest in 119 patients younger than 18 years of age. The most common presentation was associated with sudden infant death syndrome (32%). The second most common cause was drowning (22%), followed by other respiratory causes (9%), congenital cardiac problems (4%), neurological problems (4%), cancer (3%), other cardiac causes (3%), drug overdose (3%), smoke inhalation (2%), anaphylaxis (2%), and endocrinopathies (2%). Forty-five percent of the patients were less than 1 year of age; 64% were less than 3 years of age.

Beginning Steps of CPR
Establishing Unresponsiveness

Unresponsiveness is established by gently shaking, tapping, and shouting at the child. The bystander or physician should then provide approximately 1 minute of basic life support before activating emergency medical services. Care should be taken not to aggravate a spinal cord injury or over-jostle a head-injured patient.

If the patient is unresponsive, the rescuer should determine the absence of adequate ventilation and circulation immediately. If ventilation alone is absent or inadequate, opening the airway, rescue breathing, or both may be all that is necessary. If the circulation is inadequate, the rescuer should initiate artificial circulation.

Opening the Airway

Methods for opening the airway of an unconscious patient are directed at relieving obstruction, which is usually caused by the tongue. Because the tongue is attached to the mandible, moving the mandible forward will lift the tongue away from the back of the throat, thus clearing the airway. If there is enough tone in the muscles of the jaw, tilting the head back will cause the mandible to move forward and open the airway. In the absence of sufficient muscular tone, which is common in an unconscious patient, a head tilt alone may be insufficient to open the airway. Frequently, the tongue occludes the airway during an active inspiration when negative pressure is generated. The mandible may then need active physical support, including the head-tilt/chin-lift method or jaw thrust to provide a sufficient airway (Fig. 1.1).

Head Tilt/Chin Lift This maneuver is used to open the patient's airway unless neck trauma is suspected. The rescuer's hand is placed on the patient's forehead and with gentle backward pressure the head is brought into the sniffing position. Overextension, especially in the infant, may result in airway obstruction.

For additional assistance in opening the airway, the rescuer performs the head-tilt/chin-lift method by placing the fingertips of one hand under the mandible near the protuberance of the chin, bringing the chin forward, and supporting the jaw, which results in tilting the head back. Care should be taken not to compress the soft tissues of the chin, which might obstruct the patient's airway, especially in the infant. The rescuer's other hand continues to press on the patient's forehead in order to tilt the head back. The

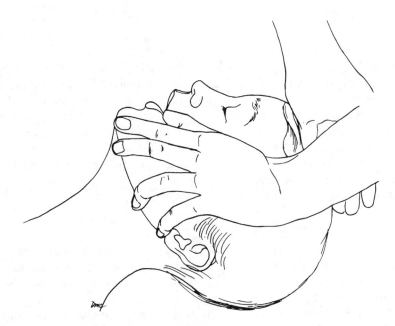

Figure 1.1. Head-tilt/chin-lift airway position. The rescuer places one hand on the patient's forehead, with his or her other hand supporting the angle of the patient's mandible while pulling the chin upward.

chin is lifted so that the teeth are nearly brought together, but without completely closing the mouth. Only rarely should the thumb be used when lifting the chin, and then only to slightly depress the lower lip so that the mouth remains partially open.

Jaw Thrust This maneuver offers additional forward movement of the jaw if the head tilt/chin lift is unsuccessful in opening the airway. The rescuer grabs the angles of the mandible and lifts with both hands, one on each side, displacing the mandible forward while tilting his or her head backward. If the patient's lips close, the lower lip is retracted by the rescuer's thumbs. Jaw thrust without head tilt is the safest technique to open the airway of the patient with a suspected neck injury, because it is accomplished without extending the neck. The head should be carefully supported without turning it from side to side or extending it. If this maneuver is unsuccessful, the rescuer may extend the head slightly and make another attempt to ventilate.

An infant or child who is struggling to breathe but is acyanotic and has an adequate airway is best treated by immediate transportation to a hospital or by assessment in the present hospital by the most experienced person trained in airway management. If the infant or child is unconscious, is cyanotic, or is experiencing bradycardia, the airway should be opened.

Establishing Breathlessness

After the airway is opened, the rescuer should again check whether the patient is breathing effectively, which is accomplished by placing the ear over the victim's mouth and nose, and viewing the patient's chest and abdomen. If the chest and abdomen fall, and the rescuer feels air from the mouth and nose and hears air during exhalation, then the patient is ventilating. If the patient has respiratory efforts without air exhalation, then the airway is obstructed. Frequently, opening the airway and maintaining airway support is all that the patient needs in order to breathe effectively. If the patient is not ventilating, rescue breathing is begun. If after opening the patient's airway, the patient is gasping or struggling to breathe, the decision to begin rescue breathing depends on the presence or absence of cyanosis.

Initiating Rescue Breathing

Rescue breathing is initiated once breathlessness is established. In the infant, the rescuer makes a tight seal covering the infant's mouth and nose with his mouth (Fig. 1.2). The older child's nose is pinched and his or her mouth is covered by the rescuer (Fig. 1.3).

Rate of Breathing When an airtight seal has been established, two slow breaths are delivered, 1.0 to 1.5 seconds per breath with a pause between. An appropriate tidal volume is one that allows the patient's chest to rise and fall. Patency of the airway should be ascertained if air does not enter freely. An obstruction should be suspected if, after adjusting support, the

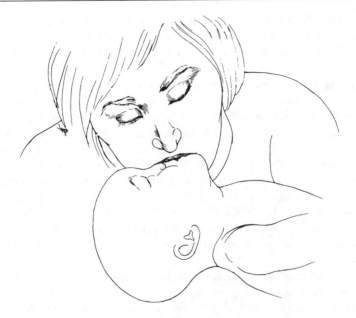

Figure 1.2. Artificial ventilation in infants. The rescuer places the patient's head in sniffing position and places his or her mouth over both the mouth and nose, making a tight seal.

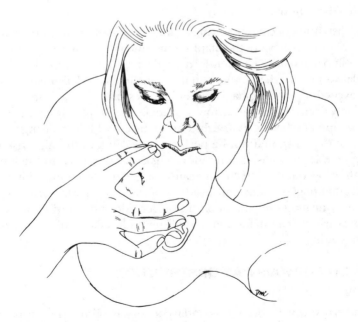

Figure 1.3. Mouth-to-mouth ventilation. The rescuer places the patient's head in the sniffing position, pinches off the nose, takes a deep breath, and exhales into the patient's mouth.

chest still does not rise. During one- or two-rescuer CPR, one breath is administered at the end of every fifth compression. If breathing is absent but a pulse is present, breathing should be provided at a rate of 20 breaths per minute.

Types of Artificial Ventilation Mouth-to-nose ventilation, which is more effective than mouth-to-mouth ventilation in some situations, is recommended when it is impossible to ventilate through the mouth (e.g., because of facial injury or anatomic abnormality, or difficulty achieving a tight seal around the mouth). The rescuer maintains the head tilt while lifting the patient's mandible to close the mouth. During exhalation, it may be necessary to open the patient's mouth or separate the lips to allow the air to escape.

Mouth-to-stoma artificial ventilation is used when a patient has a tracheostomy in place. If a leak exists through the mouth or nose during this maneuver, the rescuer should seal the mouth and nose with his or her hand. This problem usually does not occur if the tracheostomy tube has an inflatable cuff.

Cricoid Pressure To prevent regurgitation and possible aspiration during resuscitation, backward pressure is applied on the patient's cricoid cartilage against the cervical vertebra. Pressure is released when the rescuer confirms successful placement of an endotracheal tube by auscultation of bilateral breath sounds.

Gastric Distention

Gastric distention occurring during artificial ventilation interferes with ventilation because it elevates the diaphragm, which results in a decreased lung volume. It occurs more frequently in children and is minimized by limiting the tidal volume to that amount that raises the chest. This maneuver may avoid exceeding the esophageal opening pressure. Gastric distention also commonly occurs when the airway is partially or completely obstructed.

Attempts at relieving gastric distention during CPR by exerting pressure on the abdomen should not be performed because of the high risk of inducing emesis and causing aspiration of gastric contents into the lungs. If ventilation becomes ineffective because of gastric distention, the rescuer should attempt gastric decompression by using an orogastric or nasogastric tube, or by turning the patient on his or her side and applying pressure to the epigastrium. The maneuver should be undertaken only in the out-of-hospital setting.

FOREIGN BODY AIRWAY OBSTRUCTION
Infants

Cardiac arrest usually occurs secondary to airway obstruction in pediatric patients.

Foreign Body versus Infection

Airway obstruction is most commonly caused by an infectious or allergic process that causes swelling of the airway, or by a foreign body. Differentiating between airway obstruction as a result of a foreign body and that resulting from infection is important. If infection is present, maneuvers to dislodge a foreign body are dangerous and may result in an inappropriate delay in transporting or treating the patient.

A foreign body may cause partial or complete obstruction of the airway. The acyanotic patient with adequate air exchange should be allowed and encouraged to continue to cough and breathe spontaneously without interference.

Clinical signs of poor air exchange include:

- an inefficient cough
- increased respiratory difficulty with retractions
- nasal flaring
- increased work of breathing
- high-pitched noises during inhalation
- stridor
- cyanosis of the lips, nails, and skin

Techniques to Relieve Obstruction

Relief of airway obstruction by a foreign body depends on the age of the patient. In the infant less than 1 year of age, a combination of back blows and chest thrusts is performed (Table 1.1). Abdominal thrusts are not recommended in this age group because of the potential danger of injury to the abdominal organs, especially the liver.

An infant with a foreign body airway obstruction is straddled over the arm of the rescuer with the infant's head lower than his or her trunk. The infant's head is supported with the rescuer's hand around the infant's jaw and chest. When support is adequate, the rescuer delivers five back blows rapidly with the heel of the hand between the shoulder blades (Fig. 1.4). The infant is then turned, with the back placed on the rescuer's thigh, head lower than the body. Five chest thrusts are delivered in the same manner as external chest compressions are performed (using the two-finger or three-finger method) at a slower rate (see Fig. 1.4).

Table 1.1
Foreign Body Airway Obstruction

Infant	Chest thrusts (5 times)
	Back blows (5 times)
Child	Heimlich maneuver (5 times)
Adult	Heimlich maneuver (5 times)

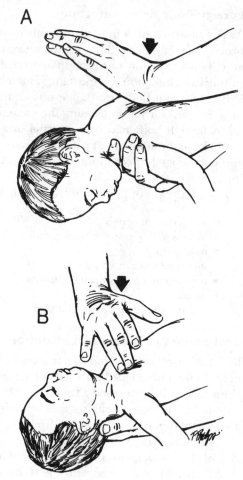

Figure 1.4. Relief of foreign body obstruction in infants. (A) Backblows. (B) Chest thrusts. (From Schleien CL. Cardiopulmonary resuscitation. In: Nichols DG, Yaster M, Lappe DG, Buck JR, eds. The golden hour handbook of advanced pediatric life support. St Louis: Mosby-Year Book, 1991:113.)

If the child is too large to straddle the rescuer's forearm, the rescuer should kneel on the floor and place the child across the thighs, keeping the head lower than the trunk. With greater force than that used in the infant, five back blows are delivered. With the head and back supported, the child is then rolled onto the floor and five chest thrusts are given.

Back blows are recommended because they produce an artificial cough, which increases pressure in the distally blocked respiratory passages and may partially or completely dislodge the foreign body. Back blows can, however, cause upward acceleration of the neck and upper back of more than three times the force of gravity, causing propulsion of a supraglottic foreign body toward the glottis and converting a partial airway obstruction into a complete airway blockage.

Assessing Efficacy

After exercising maneuvers to relieve an airway obstruction, the airway is opened by the head-tilt/chin-lift method. If spontaneous breathing is absent, rescue breathing is performed. If the chest does not rise, and after repositioning of the head the airway is still obstructed, the maneuvers to relieve a foreign body obstruction are repeated.

Children and Adults

Heimlich Maneuver

The Heimlich maneuver, a series of subdiaphragmatic manual thrusts, has become the primary method of relieving foreign body obstruction of the airway. Manual thrusts to the upper abdomen force air out of the lungs, creating an artificial cough. The rescuer stands behind the patient and wraps his or her hands around the patient's waist, grasping one fist with the other hand and placing the thumb side of this fist against the patient's abdomen between the waist and the rib cage. To avoid injury, the rescuer's hands should never be placed on the xiphoid process or on the lower margins of the rib cage. The rescuer then presses his or her fist five times into the patient's abdomen with a quick inward and upward thrust (Fig. 1.5).

To perform this maneuver on an unconscious or supine patient, the rescuer should face the patient kneeling astride his or her hips. With one of the rescuer's hands on top of the other, the rescuer applies manual thrusts as described above. Manual thrusts may be self-administered by forcing the clasped hand into the substernal region.

Chest versus Abdominal Thrusts

Chest thrusts rather than abdominal thrusts are now recommended only for adults and children in special circumstances (e.g., late pregnancy, marked obesity). Chest thrusts are applied by the rescuer as he or she stands behind the patient, with his or her arms directly under the patient's axillae and encircling the patient's chest. The rescuer places the thumb side of his or her fist into the mid-sternal area of the patient, avoiding the xiphoid process or the margins of the rib cage. The rescuer grabs his or her fist with his or her other hand and applies four backward thrusts. Each thrust is administered with the intention of relieving the airway obstruction without necessarily completing the full series.

Abdominal and chest thrusts may cause complications to internal organs, such as rupture or laceration of abdominal or thoracic viscera. In addition, regurgitation of gastric contents may occur as a result of an abdominal thrust.

During an abdominal thrust, one liter of air is expelled with an average pressure at the proximal airway of 31 mm Hg. Back blows may actually be su-

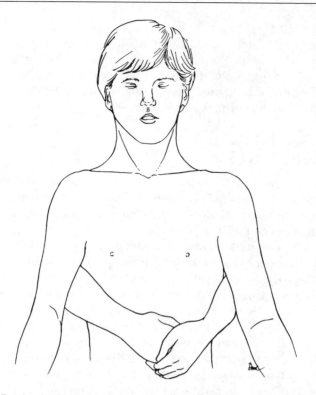

Figure 1.5. Foreign body obstruction—manual thrusts with the patient standing and the rescuer behind the patient. The rescuer places hands and clasps them in the midabdominal area below the xiphoid and exerts a rapid inward thrust on the patient's abdomen.

perior in generating a higher airway pressure. Centrifugation has been used in children with foreign body airway obstruction to achieve the same effect.

Finger Sweeps

Blind finger sweeps are generally avoided in infants and children, as they may force a foreign body deeper into the airway. In the unconscious adult patient, the finger sweep is performed by grasping the patient's tongue and mandible between the thumb and fingers and lifting. Inserting the index finger of the free hand down along the inside of the patient's cheek and deeply into the throat down to the base of the tongue may relieve the obstruction. A hooking action should be used to dislodge the foreign body. Care should be taken not to force the foreign body deeper into the airway. The finger sweep should not be used in the conscious patient. If a foreign body is visualized it may be removed with the use of a Kelly clamp or Magill forceps.

Cricothyrotomy

Indications and Advantages Emergency cricothyrotomy may be the last access to a patient's airway when the intensivist is unable to intubate the trachea. Factors that lead to this inability to intubate are listed in Table 1.2.

Cricothyrotomy was designed to deliver oxygen to the patient without concern for adequate ventilation. Using wall oxygen (50 psi) and a gas flow of 500 mL/sec, this technique can maintain adequate blood gas values in patients with normally compliant lungs. Oxygen delivery through a catheter has been used in arrested pediatric patients.

When percutaneous transtracheal jet ventilation was compared with endotracheal high frequency jet ventilation and IPPB, oxygenation was adequate with both techniques. Although ventilation was inadequate with transtracheal jet ventilation, adequate oxygenation was achieved with 100% oxygen.

Advantages to the use of cricothyrotomy include its ease of placement in adult patients, the requirement of equipment that is readily available to the intensivist, the capability of continuing cardiac massage during placement of a tracheal catheter, and the ability to suction the pharynx if needed. In addition, the use of jet ventilation in this manner has the capability of dislodging a foreign body in the trachea by increasing intrapulmonary pressure.

Technique A 14-gauge or 16-gauge angiocatheter (18-gauge in smaller children) is passed through the cricothyroid membrane, which is located between the inferior edge of the thyroid cartilage and the upper edge of

Table 1.2
Causes of Difficult Airway

Foreign body obstruction
Trauma:
• larynx
• trachea
• facial structures
Edema of upper airway:
• infection (i.e., epiglottitis, croup)
• burn
• allergic reaction
Tumor:
• oropharynx or nasopharynx
• larynx
• extrinsic compression of trachea
Cervical spine injury (patient in halo)
Anatomic abnormality:
• macroglossia (mucopolysaccharidoses, hypothryoidism)
• micrognathia (Pierre-Robin syndrome, Treacher-Collins syndrome)
• midface hypoplasia (Apert syndrome, Goldenhar syndrome)
• short/rigid neck (patient in halo, rheumatoid arthritis, Klippel-Feil syndrome)

the cricoid cartilage. The rescuer stabilizes the larynx with his or her fingers while palpating the cricothyroid membrane. The angiocatheter is placed at a caudad angle (approximately 30° from the skin) in the midline of the neck and into the trachea to avoid injury to the larynx. The rescuer performs this action while aspirating gently on an attached syringe to determine when the angiocatheter has entered the trachea successfully. After air is aspirated, the plastic catheter is advanced into the trachea. The connector from a 3.0 endotracheal tube fits snugly onto the angiocatheter (Fig. 1.6). Alternatively, the barrel of a 3 mL syringe will also fit into the angiocath, which can then be attached to a 7.0 mm endotracheal tube con-

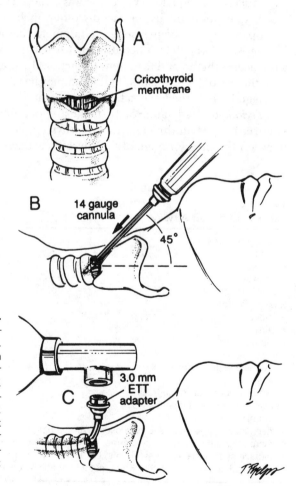

Figure 1.6. Cricothyrotomy. (A) Anatomical view. (B) Insertion of 14-gauge IV cannula. (C) Bag attached to 3.0 mm endotracheal tube adapter connected to an IV cannula. (From Yaster M. Airway management. In: Nichols DG, Yaster M, Lappe DG, Buck JR, eds. The golden hour handbook of advanced pediatric life support. St. Louis: Mosby-Year Book, 1991:46.)

nector. This setup allows an ambu bag or other source of oxygen to be attached. This attachment should be readily available on an arrest crash cart (Table 1.3).

Complications Complications of cricothyrotomy include:

- Difficulty in palpating landmarks in infants and young children
- Formation of a false passage
- Subcutaneous or mediastinal emphysema
- Injury to vascular, neural, or pulmonary structures of the neck
- Infection
- Fistula formation
- Laryngeal edema

BASIC LIFE SUPPORT—CIRCULATION
Assessing Pulse

After the patient's airway has been opened adequately and two breaths have been delivered, it must be determined whether breathing alone has stopped or whether cardiac arrest has occurred simultaneously. Absence of a pulse in the large arteries of an unconscious victim who is not breathing defines a cardiac arrest.

Carotid Pulse

As in an adult, the pulse of a child can be felt over the carotid artery. While maintaining the head tilt, the carotid pulse is palpated between the tracheal cartilage and the neck muscles. The artery should be palpated gently to maintain the pulsation.

Palpation of the carotid pulse provides ready accessibility to the pulse while performing artificial ventilation without the need to remove any of the patient's clothing. In addition, the carotid arteries can frequently be felt when peripheral pulses, such as the radial artery, are no longer palpable when the patient is in the shock state (Fig. 1.7).

Table 1.3
Cricothyrotomy Set-Up

Infants	18-gauge intravenous cannula
	3.0 mm endotracheal tube connector
	Ambu bag
Other Child	14- or 16-gauge intravenous cannula
	3 mL syringe barrel
	7.0 mm endotracheal tube connector
	Ambu bag

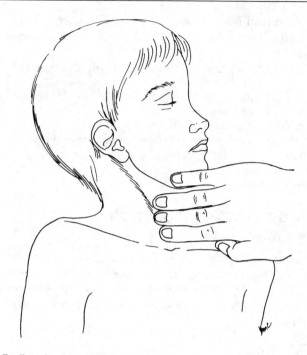

Figure 1.7. Feeling the carotid pulse. The fingers are placed laterally into the groove between the trachea and the sternocleidomastoid muscle.

Brachial Pulse

The rescuer should palpate the brachial pulse in infants for the presence or absence of cardiac arrest. Palpation of the carotid pulse in an infant is difficult because of the infant's short, fat neck. In addition, precordial activity in an infant is unreliable, because it represents an impulse rather than a pulse. Some infants with good cardiac activity may have a quiet precordium, which can lead to the erroneous diagnosis of cardiac arrest.

The brachial pulse can be located on the inside of the patient's upper arm midway between the elbow and shoulder by pressing lightly toward the humerus (Fig. 1.8).

Need for Chest Compression

When there is a pulse but no effective ventilation, then only breathing has arrested. In this case, rescue breathing should be continued. Absence or questionable presence of a pulse is the indication for starting artificial circulation by means of external chest compression. Chest compression should never be performed without rescue breathing.

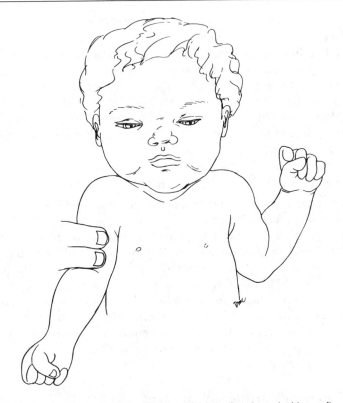

Figure 1.8. Feeling the brachial pulse. The brachial pulse is palpated with two fingers along the medial aspect of the upper arm above the antecubital region.

Chest Compression—Children and Adults

Positioning

The patient must be supine on a firm surface (e.g., hard board the full width of the bed, the ground, or the floor). It is imperative that the patient's head be above the level of his or her heart.

The rescuer should be positioned close to the patient's side. The rescuer locates, with the middle and index fingers, the lower margin of the patient's rib cage on the side next to the rescuer. The rescuer runs his or her fingers along the rib cage to the notch where the ribs join the sternum in the center of the lower part of the chest. One finger is then left on that notch and the other finger is placed next to the first finger on the lower level of the sternum. The location of the xiphoid process is irrelevant with this technique.

The heel of the rescuer's hand closest to the patient's head is then placed next to the index finger of the first hand. This maneuver locates the notch on the long axis of the sternum and keeps the force of compression on the sternum and decreases the chance of a rib fracture. The first hand is then placed on top of the other hand so that the heels of both hands are parallel. The fingers are directed away from the rescuer and may be extended or interlaced but must be kept off the chest.

The rescuer may also grasp the wrist of the hand on the chest with the other hand. This technique is useful for rescuers with arthritic problems of the hand or wrist. The rescuer's elbows are then straightened with the rescuer's shoulders directly over his or her hands so that the thrust for chest compression is straight down.

Technique and Rate of Compression

In a normal-sized child, the sternum should be depressed 1 to 1½ inches and ½ to 2 inches in adults. Between compressions, the rescuer should release pressure completely to allow the return of blood to the chest. The time allowed for release should be equal to the time required for compression. Compressions should be uninterrupted, regular, and smooth. The hands of the rescuer should not be lifted off the patient's chest or changed in position because correct hand position may be lost in that instance. The compression rate should be 100/min. Periodically, the pulse should be palpated to ensure effectiveness of chest compressions or to confirm the return of a spontaneous pulse. This should be performed after 1 minute of CPR and every few minutes thereafter.

Coordination with Artificial Ventilation

In one-rescuer CPR, both artificial ventilation and circulation are performed using a 15:2 chest compression:ventilation ratio at a rate of 80 to 100 compressions/min. After four cycles of compressions are delivered, the patient should be reevaluated for return of breathing and pulse.

Chest Compression—Infants

Positioning

The recommended area of chest compression is one finger width below the intersection of the patient's intermammary line and sternum (Table 1.4). Two techniques to perform external chest compressions in the infant include placement of two or three fingers on the sternum (Fig. 1.9) or to encircle the infant's chest, forming a rigid surface on the back, using the thumbs to deliver compressions (Fig. 1.10). The encircling method may generate higher arterial and coronary perfusion pressures.

Technique and Rate of Compression

The infant's sternum should be compressed approximately 20% of the anteroposterior width of the chest, ½ to 1 inch in the infant. When the infant

Table 1.4
Chest Compressions in Infants and Children

	Compressions/ Method	Hand Position	Sternal Depression (Inches)	Compressions/ Min
Infant	Encircling or two finger	One finger breadth below inter-mammary line	0.5–1	≥100
Toddler	One hand	Lower third of sternum	1–1½	100
Large child	Two hands	Lower third of sternum	1½–2	100

becomes large enough so that three fingers cannot adequately depress the sternum or that the rescuer's hands cannot reach around the infant's chest, the heel of one hand should be used. As in the adult, the rescuer's fingers should be kept off the chest. If the patient is large enough to require the heel of the hand for compression, the depth of the compression is increased to 1 to 1½ inches (Fig. 1.11).

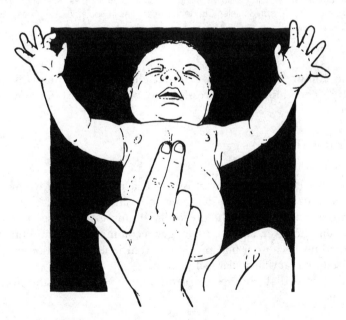

Figure 1.9. Two-finger method of external chest compression in infants. The rescuer places two fingers on the sternum, one finger width below the line intersecting the nipples, and compresses ½ to 1 inch at a rate of 100 compressions/min. Ventilation is not shown for the sake of clarity. (From Schleien CL. Recent advances in pediatric CPR. Anesthesiol Rep 1988;1:6.)

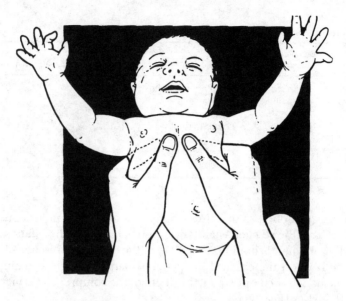

Figure 1.10. Encircling method of external chest compression in infants. Place thumbs over sternum one finger width below the line intersecting the nipples. Rescuer clasps hands behind infant's back. (From Schleien CL. Recent advances in pediatric CPR. Anesthesiol Rep 1988;1:6.)

The compression rate for external chest CPR in infants is at least 100/min. The ratio of compressions to breaths is 5:1 for one or two rescuers.

Precordial Thump

Limited Use

The precordial thump can convert asystole to a life-sustaining rhythm and can restore a sinus rhythm when delivered soon after the onset of ventricular tachycardia or fibrillation. The precordial thump is rarely used in the pediatric patient, however, and it is no longer recommended as a routine procedure in adults because it may precipitate ventricular fibrillation or asystole when used to treat ventricular tachycardia.

The precordial thump is recommended only in the following situations:

1. When a patient is being monitored by an electrocardiogram (ECG), the precordial thump may be administered after recognition of ventricular tachycardia or ventricular fibrillation.
2. When the patient is monitored, the precordial thump may be administered im-

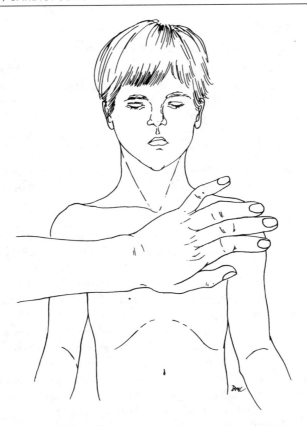

Figure 1.11. External chest compression in the young child. The heel of the rescuer's hand is placed two finger widths above the bottom of the sternum for compression. In the older child, the two-hand compression method is used as it is in adults.

mediately after the onset of asystole caused by heart block, where repetitive thumps produce QRS complexes and an associated pulse, and may thus sustain the circulation until a pacemaker can be inserted. If an effective cardiac output is not maintained, CPR should be initiated.

Technique

A sharp, quick, single blow is delivered over the midportion of the patient's sternum, with the bottom of the rescuer's fist starting from 20 to 30 cm above the patient's chest. After thumping is performed by the rescuer, the ECG and pulse should be checked immediately. If there is ventricular fibrillation or ventricular tachycardia without a pulse, countershock is performed as soon as possible and CPR is begun.

ADVANCED CPR

Vascular Access and Fluid Administration

A key aspect of successful CPR is early establishment of an intravascular line for administering fluids and medications. If rapid establishment of IV access is technically difficult, such as in a chubby, clamped-down infant, intraosseous or endotracheal access are alternatives.

IV Access

Central venous access is preferable to peripheral venous or other modes of fluid and drug administration. A significant delay can occur in the circulation time of drugs administered from a peripheral site compared to a central site during CPR.

Infants and Young Children In children less than 5 years old, a brief attempt should be made to start a peripheral IV line. If no access is achieved after 90 seconds, then an intraosseous needle should be placed for vascular access. A large peripheral vein such as the antecubital vein could be used. Attempts at either the jugular or subclavian vein frequently interfere with bag-mask ventilation during CPR.

When additional assistance is present, then attempts at central venous cannulation should be attempted. Possible approaches to the circulation via the central venous system include the internal and external jugular vein, subclavian vein, femoral vein, saphenous vein via cutdown, or axillary veins. External and internal jugular or subclavian venous cannulation are more easily performed once the trachea is intubated (Table 1.5).

Older Children Peripheral venous access generally is easier to attain in this population than in younger patients. If peripheral IV placement fails, then a saphenous venous cutdown or other central venous line should be placed. The placement of an intraosseous needle in the older child is difficult because of the thick bony cortex.

Table 1.5
Intravenous Access

Children	(younger than 5 years old)
	First attempt—peripheral line (including antecubital vein)
	After 90 seconds (if unsuccessful)—intraosseous line
	Later: saphenous vein cutdown or central line placement—(femoral, subclavian, external or internal jugular vein)
Children	(older than 5 years old)
	First attempt—peripheral line
	Second attempt—saphenous vein cutdown or central line placement

Intraosseous Access

Recommended Use All medications and fluids, including whole blood, used during CPR have been given by the intraosseous route. This technique should be considered a temporary measure during emergencies when other vascular sites are not available. In the young child this route should be used after approximately 90 seconds of attempting peripheral venous access.

Technique A standard 16-gauge or 18-gauge needle, spinal needle with stylet, or bone marrow needle, is inserted into the anterior surface of the tibia, 1 to 3 cm below the tibial tuberosity. The needle is directed in a 90° angle to the medial surface of the tibia or in a slightly inferior position to avoid the epiphyseal plate (Fig. 1.12).

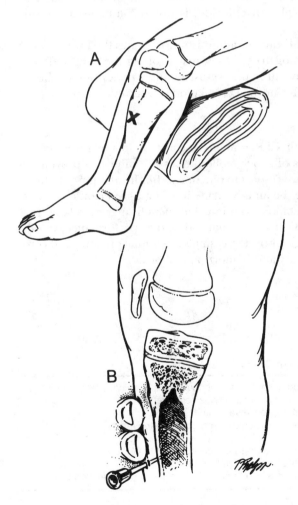

Figure 1.12. Intraosseous needle placement. (A) Insert the needle at a level of tibial tubercle on the medial portion of the tibia. (B) The needle is aimed caudally and laterally. (From Schleien CL. Cardiopulmonary resuscitation. In: Nichols DG, Yaster M, Lappe DG, Buck JR, eds. The golden hour handbook of advanced pediatric life support. St Louis: Mosby-Year Book, 1991:121.)

Infusion is successful if the needle is in the marrow cavity, which is indicated by the needle standing upright without support. The needle loses its upright position if it has slipped into the subcutaneous tissue. In addition, there is loss of resistance after the needle passes through the bony cortex of the tibia. At times, bone marrow can be aspirated into a syringe connected to the needle. Free flow of the drug or fluid infusion without significant subcutaneous infiltration also should be demonstrated.

Endotracheal Access

When rapid establishment of an IV line during CPR is difficult, as in the obese patient, infant, or small child, drugs can be given through the endotracheal tube (Table 1.6). The use of ionized medications, such as sodium bicarbonate or calcium chloride, is not recommended by this route.

With the endotracheal route of administration comes the formation of an intrapulmonary depot of drug, which may prolong the drug's effects. This prolongation could result in post-resuscitation hypertension or the recurrence of fibrillation after normal circulation is restored.

Types of Fluids

Fluid management during CPR remains a constant in the resuscitation process. As in other types of shock, colloid does not offer any proven advantage over crystalloid with respect to outcome. After head injury and hemorrhagic shock, there may be an advantage in using a hypertonic solution instead of an isotonic crystalloid solution. This benefit may be related to a combination of volume expansion, enhanced cardiac performance, vasodilation of systemic arterioles, or by decreasing intracranial pressure and cerebral edema after head injury and hemorrhagic shock.

Table 1.6
Endotracheal Administration of Drugs

Epinephrine	Recommended dose: 10 times intravenous (IV) or intraosseous (IO) dose
	Absorption and physiologic effects compare to IV route
	Peak level and may be lower than IO route
Atropine	Absorption and physiologic effects compare to IV route
Naloxone	
Lidocaine	Absorption and physiologic effects compare to IV route
	Peak level may be lower than IO route
	Inconsistent in obtaining therapeutic levels in humans during CPR

Clinical Assessment During CPR

Basic Physical Evaluation

Clinical monitoring (Table 1.7) and physical assessment (Table 1.8) of the patient during CPR is similar to that used in other clinical situations.

Cardiovascular Function

Hemodynamics The effects of volume expansion and drugs on arterial blood pressure is critical. Aortic diastolic pressure relates directly to adequacy of coronary perfusion during CPR. In addition, establishing an arterial line allows frequent blood sampling, particularly for measurement of arterial pH, $PaCO_2$, PaO_2, and base excess. An arterial line may be placed into the radial artery by percutaneous placement or cutdown, the femoral artery by the Seldinger technique, the axillary artery, dorsalis pedis, or posterior tibial artery. The state of oxygen delivery can also be determined by transcutaneous monitoring of PO_2 or by pulse oximetry. Pulse oximetry may be used during CPR to determine not only the oxygen saturation but also the level of cardiac output, as reflected in the plethysmograph.

Cardiopulmonary Status Vital organ function should be assessed repeatedly during and after CPR. The 12-lead ECG is an integral part of the monitoring protocol during CPR because it can reflect the adequacy of myocardial blood flow, reveal metabolic imbalances that could affect the resuscitation, and show electrical disturbances that require rapid changes in therapy. Cardiac output is often too low to be measured during CPR; however, end-tidal CO_2 concentration has been shown to correlate well with pulmonary blood flow and, thus, cardiac output. Disposable colorimetric $P_{ET}CO_2$ analyzers can reliably differentiate between a tracheal and esophageal intubation in infants and children. End-tidal CO_2 has been correlated with the coronary perfusion pressure, which is the critical parameter for resuscitation of the heart. With epinephrine administration, the end-tidal CO_2 may not be an accurate

Table 1.7
Clinical Monitoring During CPR

Basic physical examination
Electrocardiogram (ECG)
Noninvasive BP
End-tidal CO_2
Arterial pressure (when line is obtained)
Central venous pressure (when line is obtained)
Pulse oximeter
Temperature
Electroencephalogram (if available)
Evoked potentials (experimental)

Table 1.8
Patient Assessment During CPR

Inspection
    Chest excursion
    Depth of compression
    Position of rescuer's hands
Palpation
    Establish pulselessness
    Peripheral pulses
    Landmarks (central line placement)
Auscultation
    Breath sounds
    Heart sounds

indicator of blood flow as it may result in increased intrapulmonary shunting. A low $P_{ET}CO_2$ (<1%) may also be related to airway obstruction, tension pneumothorax, pericardial tamponade, pulmonary embolism, or hypothermia.

Body Temperature

Temperature should be monitored routinely during CPR because it may vary widely during resuscitation or at presentation to the hospital. The resuscitation of the patient with hypothermia as the cause of cardiac arrest must be continued until the patient's core temperature has risen above 35°. Repeated measurements of core body temperature should be made at several sites (i.e., rectum, bladder, esophagus, axillary artery, tympanic membrane) to avoid misleading temperature readings from a single site, which might be affected by the alterations in regional blood flow during CPR. Use of a glass bulb thermometer allows measurement of temperature to much more precise levels.

The patient's temperature can affect the success of resuscitation, the short-term neurologic status, and the eventual neurologic outcome. External rewarming should be performed carefully to avoid overheating the patient when spontaneous circulation has been restored. The therapeutic use of hypothermia may be applied later to improve outcome from resuscitation.

Adjuncts for Airway and Ventilation

Oxygen

In patients in cardiac arrest, numerous factors contribute to hypoxemia and inadequate oxygen delivery to tissues. One hundred percent oxygen must be administered as soon as possible in a cardiac arrest situation. Oxygen toxicity occurs during prolonged mechanical ventilatory support using high oxygen concentrations, but short-term use of 100% oxygen is not considered harmful and is necessary until adequate arterial oxygenation can be ascertained.

Suction

A portable suction unit fitted with a large bore, nonkinking suction tubing, and a tonsil suction tip to provide vacuum and flow adequate for oropharyngeal suction should be available. In the emergency room, two suction devices should be available at the bedside. In addition, this setting should be equipped with appropriate-sized suction catheters for the endotracheal tube or tracheostomy, a nonbreakable collection bottle, and a supply of sterile water for clearing tubes and catheters.

Airway

Oropharyngeal airways should only be used when the patient is unconscious. When introduced into the conscious or stuporous patient, laryngospasm or vomiting may result.

In the hospital setting, and more frequently in the public setting, ventilation is performed using a mask with a bag-valve-mask system. The mask should be tight-fitting and reach from the midportion of the bridge of the nose to the protuberance of the chin without extending over the end of the chin. A variety of mask sizes should always be available.

Endotracheal Intubation

Endotracheal intubation is the preferred technique for acquiring access to the airway and requires skilled, experienced personnel.

Indications The endotracheal tube protects the airway from gastric contents, keeps the trachea patent, and delivers high concentrations of oxygen to the lungs. In an emergency situation, the trachea is intubated by the oral route. Equipment necessary for emergency tracheal intubation is listed in Table 1.9.

Technique The patient should be preoxygenated three to four breaths of 100% oxygen. Cardiac compressions should not be interrupted for more than 15 seconds during the tracheal intubation procedure. During emergency tracheal intubation, cricoid pressure should be administered at the point that anesthetic drugs are given or during the CPR procedure if the patient is unconscious.

Laryngeal Mask Airway

The laryngeal mask airway is a recently developed device that can manage the airway of infants and children. There is a cuff that seals the perimeter of the larynx) and a wide bore tube that connects to an ambu bag or anesthesia circuit. The device has been used successfully during CPR.

Table 1.9
Required Equipment for Emergency Endotracheal Intubation

Two laryngoscopes with functioning bulbs
Variety of laryngoscope blades (straight blades preferable for children)
Assortment of endotracheal tubes (uncuffed tubes for children < 8 years)
Syringe for cuff inflation
Variety of oral airways
Stylet
Tonsil suction catheter with adequate suction
Tape
Benzoin
Kelly clamp or Magill forceps for foreign body extraction

Special Resuscitation Situations

When initiating CPR, assurances of neck stabilization are essential when trauma (e.g., as in diving accidents) is possible.

Hypothermia

Physical Findings Hypothermia is an internal core temperature of 35°C (95°F) or less. Severe hypothermia exists when the core temperature falls below 32°C. At this body temperature, sinus bradycardia usually intervenes, leading to T wave inversion, prolongation of the QT interval, acute elevation of the QRS-ST segment junction, and ultimately leading to ventricular ectopy and ventricular fibrillation. Even when bradycardia is present, peripheral pulses may be difficult to detect because of severe peripheral vasoconstriction. The neurologic examination may be consistent with clinical brain death as a result of the marked depression of cerebral blood flow and cerebral metabolism that exist under this condition. Thus, hypothermic patients who appear to be dead should be resuscitated aggressively.

Populations at Risk Hypothermia occurs most commonly in three specific groups of patients: accident victims, chronically ill patients, and acutely ill patients. Accident victims, particularly the very old, the very young, near-drowning patients, and those suffering an accident coincident with inebriation comprise the first group. Infants are particularly prone to hypothermia because of their large surface area relative to volume, which allows more rapid heat loss, less subcutaneous tissue, and thinner skin than exist in the older child or adult, and the inability to shiver to produce heat.

The second group consists of patients with chronic illness including those suffering hypothyroidism, pituitary insufficiency, Addison's disease, pancreatitis, stroke, and cirrhosis.

The third group consists of patients with acute illness, including shock, some intoxications, sepsis, hypoglycemia, acute respiratory failure, and congestive heart failure. In addition, a person who suffers cardiac arrest while he or she is normothermic will quickly begin to cool, especially when in a cold environment. If the arrest was unwitnessed, rescuers will not know if the arrest was because of hypothermia or if hypothermia was a sequel to the arrest.

Emergency Management If the hypothermic patient is not breathing, rescue breathing should be initiated (Table 1.10). Chest compressions are indicated in the pulseless, unmonitored patient. ECG monitoring is critical because of the difficulty in palpating a peripheral pulse.

During transport, further heat loss should be prevented by removing the patient's wet clothing and by insulating the patient and adding heat by external means if available (e.g., warmed, humidified oxygen; warmed IV fluids; a radiant warmer).

In the emergency department, invasive measures to rewarm the patient include endotracheal intubation and assisted ventilation with heated and humidified gases, peritoneal lavage with warm dialysate, thoracotomy and irrigation of the mediastinum with warmed fluids, and extracorporeal blood warming with partial bypass.

If ventricular fibrillation is detected, three shocks should be delivered. Defibrillation is typically impossible until the patient is warmed to a temperature of 32°C. If CPR is initiated, it should be continued until the patient has remained unresponsive to CPR efforts despite being rewarmed to a temperature greater than 32°C. The use of central venous or pulmonary artery lines during rewarming is discouraged because of the possible induction of ventricular fibrillation.

Table 1.10
Treatment of Hypothermic Arrest

Begin CPR
Transport to warm environment
Begin monitoring (including core temperature)
External rewarming
    Remove wet clothes
    Wrap patient in warm blankets
    Radiant warmer
    Warmed humidified O_2
    Warmed intravenous (IV) fluids
Convective warming (for temperature <32°C)
    Intubation-ventilation with warmed, humidified O_2
    Gastric irrigation with warmed saline
    Thoracotomy and cardiac irrigation with warmed saline
    Cardiopulmonary bypass
If asystole or ventricular fibrillation occur
    Continue CPR until either
        Temperature >32°C and there is no improvement
        or
        Adequate blood pressure and rhythm are reached

When the resuscitation effort is successful, the patient's blood pressure, ECG, central venous pressure, temperature, arterial blood gases, electrolytes, and glucose levels should be monitored.

Electric Shock

Electric shock injuries are the result of current on cell membranes and vascular smooth muscle, and the production of heat energy as it is converted from electrical energy. Factors that determine the severity of electric shock include: voltage, magnitude of energy, resistance of skin, type of current, duration of current, and the pathway taken through the body.

After electrocution, the rescuer ensures he or she is not in danger of electric shock, then initiates basic life support techniques. Smoldering clothing should be removed from the patient to prevent further thermal damage. Endotracheal intubation should be performed early if any soft tissue swelling of the patient's face is present because facial or airway swelling worsens rapidly. Arrhythmias should be treated as described previously. Hypovolemia is common, so rapid intravenous (IV) fluid administration is indicated to treat shock, correct ongoing fluid losses, and maintain a diuresis to avoid renal shutdown as a result of myoglobinuria secondary to tissue breakdown.

Lightning Strike

Lightning strike, which causes 200 to 300 fatalities per year in the United States, has a 30% mortality rate and a 70% rate of significant morbidity. The primary cause of death from lightning strike is cardiac arrest associated with ventricular fibrillation or asystole, which occurs when a massive direct current countershock depolarizes the entire myocardium. Sinus rhythm may return spontaneously, although concomitant respiratory arrest as a result of thoracic muscle spasm or suppression of the brainstem respiratory center may cause a cardiac arrest secondary to hypoxia.

After a lightning strike, triage for multiple victims is reversed from the usual triage procedure. Highest priority should be given to patients in respiratory or cardiac arrest with usual basic and advance life support measures. This procedure is used because most patients who die from lightning strikes are those who suffer an immediate cardiac or respiratory arrest. Patients who do not have a cardiac arrest typically have an excellent chance of recovery.

PHARMACOLOGY
Adrenergic Agonists

The α-adrenergic agonist receptor action of epinephrine is responsible for successful resuscitation (Table 1.11). The correct dose of epinephrine dur-

Table 1.11
α- versus β-Adrenergic Agonist Effects

α-*adrenergic effects*
    Vasoconstrict peripheral vessels
    Maintain aortic diastolic pressure
    Improve coronary blood flow
    No metabolic stimulatory effect
β-*adrenergic effects*
    Vasodilate peripheral vessels
    Decrease aortic diastolic pressure
    Increase cellular metabolic rate
    Positive inotrope
    Increase intensity of ventricular fibrillation
    Increase heart rate and/or arrhythmias following resuscitation

ing CPR, however, remains controversial. Clinical studies have not demonstrated any effect of higher doses of epinephrine on short-term or long-term survival after cardiac arrest.

The differences in the results of these studies account for the ambivalence in recommendations from the 1992 American Heart Association Standards and Guidelines for CPR and ECC. To treat a pulseless arrest in children, the first IV or intraosseous (IO) dose is 0.01 mg/kg. All endotracheal doses are 10 times this dose or 0.1 mg/kg; second and subsequent IV/intraosseous/endotracheal doses are 0.1 mg/kg administered every 3 to 5 minutes during arrest. The present guidelines recommend shortening the epinephrine dosing interval for adult patients from 5 minutes to 3 to 5 minutes. Higher doses of epinephrine are neither recommended nor discouraged. An intermediate dose of 2 to 5 mg intravenously, escalating doses from 1 to 3 to 5 mg, and a high dose of 0.1 mg/kg intravenously are all possible regimens in adults.

Sodium Bicarbonate

Clinical Effects

The use of this drug during CPR remains controversial because of its potential side effects (Table 1.12) and the paucity of evidence to show that either laboratory animals or humans actually benefit from its receipt in this setting.

Dosage

When the $PaCO_2$ and pH are known, the dose of bicarbonate to correct the pH to 7.40 can be calculated using the following formula:

$$0.3 \times \text{weight (kg)} \times \text{base deficit} = \text{mEq bicarbonate}$$

Table 1.12
Adverse Effects of Sodium Bicarbonate

Hypercapnia
Hypernatremia
Hyperosmolality
Paradoxical intracellular acidosis
Decrease myocardial contractility
Leftward shift of oxyhemoglobin dissociation curve, decreasing release of oxygen from
  hemoglobin

Because of the possible side effects of bicarbonate and the large arterial-venous CO_2 gradient that develops during CPR, we recommend giving half the dose based on a volume of distribution of 0.6. If blood gases are not available, the initial dose is 1 mEq/kg followed by 0.5 mEq/kg every 10 minutes of ongoing arrest. Again, the importance of alveolar ventilation cannot be overemphasized, as well as the need for repeated arterial blood gas analysis.

Calcium

Clinical Application

The recommendations for the use of calcium during CPR have been restricted to a few specific situations (Table 1.13) based on the possibility that exogenously administered calcium may worsen ischemia-reperfusion injury.

Calcium should be given slowly through a large-bore, free-flowing IV line, preferably a central venous line. Severe tissue necrosis occurs when calcium infiltrates into subcutaneous tissue. When administered too rapidly, calcium may cause severe bradycardia, heart block, or ventricular standstill.

Table 1.13
Indications and Recommended Dosage for Calcium Administration

Indications
  Hypocalcemia
  Hyperkalemia
  Hypermagnesemia
  Calcium channel blocker overdose
Dosage
  Calcium chloride
    Pediatric dose: 20 mg/kg
    Adult dose: 200 mg, or 2 mL of 10% solution
  Calcium gluconate (as effective as calcium chloride in raising ionized calcium
    concentration during CPR)
  Standard dose: 30 to 100 mg/kg (maximum dose of 2 g in pediatric patients)

Conditions Predisposing to Hypocalcemia

Conditions predisposing to low total body calcium stores include hypoparathyroidism, Di George Syndrome, renal failure, pancreatitis, and long-term use of loop diuretics. Ionized calcium concentration can be low in the presence of a normal total calcium. This situation can occur with severe alkalosis during iatrogenic hyperventilation and after the use of alkalinizing agents. Ionized hypocalcemia also occurs after massive or rapid transfusion of citrated blood products, although the degree of the resultant hypocalcemia depends on the rate of administration, the total dose, and the hepatic and renal function of the patient. Administration of 2 mL/kg/min of citrated whole blood causes a significant decrease in ionized calcium concentration in anesthetized patients.

Atropine

This parasympatholytic agent blocks cholinergic stimulation of the muscarinic receptors of the heart, which usually results in an increase in the sinus rate and shortening of atrioventricular node conduction time. Atropine may activate latent ectopic pacemakers. Atropine has little effect on systemic vascular resistance, myocardial perfusion pressure, or myocardial contractility.

Clinical Application

Atropine is indicated in those situations listed in Table 1.14. In children who present in cardiac arrest, sinus bradycardia or asystole is commonly the initial rhythm, and atropine, therefore, is useful as a first-line drug. Atropine

Table 1.14
Indications and Recommended Dosage for Atropine Administration

Indications
  Bradycardia
  Heart block (second or third degree)
  Slow idioventricular rhythm
  Asystole
  Pulseless electrical activity
Dosage
  Pediatric dose: 0.02 mg/kg
    Minimum: 0.2 mg[a]
    Maximum: 2.0 mg
Adult dose: 0.5 mg IV q 5 minutes, to a maximum of 2.0 mg[b]
For asystole: 1.0 mg IV, repeated after 5 minutes if asystole persists

[a]Minimum dose is used because of the occurrence of paradoxical bradycardia resulting from a central stimulating effect on the medullary vagal nuclei.

[b]Full vagal blockade usually is obtained with a dose of 2.0 mg.

is typically used in clinical conditions associated with excessive parasympathetic tone.

Atropine may be given by any route including IV, endotracheal, intraosseous, intramuscular, or subcutaneous. Its onset of action occurs within 30 seconds and its peak effect occurs between 1 and 2 minutes after an IV dose.

Undesirable Effects

Tachycardia, which increases myocardial oxygen consumption and can lead to ventricular fibrillation, is common after large doses of atropine. As a result, atropine should be used in the lowest dose possible to increase the heart rate in patients after myocardial infarction or ischemia with persistent bradycardia. In patients with pulmonary or systemic outflow tract obstruction or idiopathic hypertrophic subaortic stenosis, tachycardia can decrease ventricular filling and lower cardiac output.

Glucose

The administration of glucose during CPR should be restricted to patients with documented hypoglycemia because of the possible detrimental effects of hyperglycemia on the brain during ischemia.

Oxygen

Patients in cardiac arrest or low cardiac output states should receive 100% oxygen as soon as possible, regardless of the etiology of the arrest. Oxygen increases arterial oxygen tension, hemoglobin saturation, and arterial oxygen content if ventilation is maintained. A higher PaO_2 lowers pulmonary vascular resistance and decreases the right ventricular stroke work index. One hundred percent oxygen should not be withheld from patients in cardiac arrest who have bronchopulmonary dysplasia or chronic obstructive pulmonary disease.

THERAPY FOR VENTRICULAR FIBRILLATION (TABLE 1.15)

Electric Countershock

Indications

Electric countershock is the treatment of choice for ventricular fibrillation and ventricular tachycardia when a pulse is not present or when the patient is comatose as a result of arrhythmia. Drug treatment by itself cannot be relied on to terminate ventricular fibrillation in these instances. Antiarrhythmic agents such as lidocaine are known cardiac depressants and may transform ventricular fibrillation into intractable asystole.

Table 1.15
Algorithm for Treatment of Ventricular Fibrillation

Begin CPR (Airway, Breathing, Circulation)
|
1st defibrillate	(2 J/kg)	
|		
2nd defibrillate	(4 J/kg)	
|		
3rd defibrillate	(4 J/kg)	
|		
1st epinephrine	(10 µg/kg)IV/IO 100 µg/kg-ETT	Subsequent doses of epinephrine every
|		
1st lidocaine	(1 mg/kg) IV/IO/ETT	3–5 mins: 100 µg/kg- IV/IO/ETT
|		
4th defibrillate	(4 J/kg)	
|		
2nd epinephrine	(see sidebar)	
|		
2nd lidocaine	(1 mg/kg)	
|		
1st bretylium	(5 mg/kg)	
|		
5th defibrillate	(4 J/kg)	
|		
2nd bretylium	(10 mg/kg)	

Physiologic Effects

High-voltage electric shock, when properly applied, sends more than 2 amperes through the heart. Ventricular fibrillation is terminated by simultaneously depolarizing and causing a sustained contraction of the entire myocardium, which allows return of spontaneous coordinated cardiac contractions, assuming the myocardium is well oxygenated and the acid-base status is normal.

Dosage and Delivery

Modern day defibrillators deliver only direct current (DC) shocks. Alternating current (AC) countershock is no longer used because it is hazardous to both the patient and the operator. Furthermore, DC defibrillators are portable, while AC defibrillators depend on wall current. The type of wave form of current may influence the amount of energy needed to defibrillate the heart. Most defibrillators use a dampened sine wave form although some use a trapezoidal wave form.

Higher energy levels cause a greater amount of myocardial damage. Moreover, as the energy dose increases, the incidence of postdefibrillation arrhythmias increases. Frequent, concentrated high-density electrical currents can damage the myocardium, decrease the likelihood of successful defibrillation, and lead to postdefibrillation arrhythmias. These arrhythmias are thought to be associated with prolonged depolarization of the myocardial cell membrane, which increases with the intensity of the stimulus and provides an ideal setting for re-entrant arrhythmias. High dose defibrillation causes a transient electromechanical deformation of the cell membrane. After humans have received synchronized defibrillation, the frequency of arrhythmias and the amount of ST segment displacement are directly related to the energy level used. Two low-energy shocks may cause more damage than a single shock of identical total energy; therefore, an adequate energy level should be used. However, in another study, myocardial damage was greater when one dose was given compared to the same total energy delivered in two doses.

In the majority of adult cases, energy levels of 100 to 300 J are successful when shocks are delivered with minimal delay.

Clinical Aspects of Pediatric Defibrillation

If the duration of ventricular fibrillation is less than 2 minutes, then a defibrillatory attempt should be administered as soon as possible. If ventricular fibrillation has been present for longer than 2 minutes or for an undetermined period of time, then basic life support should be initiated for at least 2 minutes before attempting defibrillation to improve myocardial oxygenation and acid-base status.

Use of Paddles

The interface between the paddle and the patient's chest wall can be an electrode cream, paste, saline, soap, or moist gauze pads. The electrode cream produces lower impedance than the paste. Electric current follows the path of least resistance, so care should be taken that the substance from one paddle does not touch that of the other paddle. This is especially important in infants, where the distance between paddles is short. If the gel is continuous between paddles, a short circuit is created, and an insufficient amount of current will cross the heart.

If the chest is already opened, internal paddles may be applied directly to the heart (i.e., open-chest defibrillation). These paddles should have a diameter of 6 cm for adults, 4 cm for children, and 2 cm for infants. Handles should be insulated. Saline-soaked pads or gauze should be placed between the paddles and the heart. The physician places one electrode behind the patient's left ventricle and the other over the right ventricle on the anterior surface of the heart. The dosage used should begin at 5 J in infants and 20 J in adults.

Defibrillatory Attempts

For the first attempt, 200 to 300 J delivered energy should be administered to adults and 2 J to children (Table 1.15). If this attempt is unsuccessful, a second and third attempt are made immediately, using the same energy dose in adults and 4 J in children. If these attempts are unsuccessful, then basic life support is continued, epinephrine is administered, and sodium bicarbonate is given if metabolic acidosis is documented or if the duration of cardiac arrest warrants its administration (Table 1.16). A fourth defibrillatory attempt is then made at a setting that does not exceed 360 J of delivered energy or 4 J in children. If ventricular fibrillation recurs frequently, lidocaine, bretylium, or procainamide may be used (Table 1.18; see Table 1.15).

Pulseless Electrical Activity

Pulseless electrical activity (PEA), formerly known as electromechanical dissociation, is defined as organized ECG activity, excluding ventricular tachycardia and fibrillation, without clinical evidence of a palpable pulse or myocardial contractions. It may occur spontaneously after cardiac arrest or as an intervening rhythm associated with treatment for cardiac arrest. The etiology of PEA is divided into primary (cardiac) and secondary (noncardiac) causes (Table 1.19).

Primary PEA, which is associated with cardiac arrest, responds poorly to therapy. Drugs used for primary PEA include epinephrine, atropine, calcium, and sodium bicarbonate. In secondary PEA, intervention is directed at the underlying disorder and usually results in a successful resuscitation. When the cause of PEA is unknown and the patient does not respond to medical intervention, the physician should consider delivering a fluid bolus and inserting needles into the patient's pleural and pericardial spaces.

OPEN-CHEST CPR

The use of open-chest cardiac massage has generally been replaced by closed-chest CPR. Compared to closed-chest CPR, open-chest CPR generates higher cardiac output and vital organ blood flow. During open-chest

Table 1.16
Defibrillation

	Dose– 1st Attempt	Dose– 2nd Attempt	Dose– 3rd and Subsequent	Paddle Size	
				External	Internal
Infant	2 J/kg	4 J/kg	4 J/kg	4.5 cm	2 cm
Child	2 J/kg	4 J/kg	4 J/kg	8 cm	4 cm
Adult	200 J	200 J	400 J	13 cm	6 cm

Table 1.17
Reevaluation if Defibrillation Is Unsuccessful

Oxygenation
Ventilation
Acid-base status
Mechanical problem
  Pneumothorax
  Inadequate paddle/chest wall interface
  Excessive distance between paddles
  Inadequate paddle pressure on chest
  Poor paddle position

CPR there is much less elevation of intrathoracic, right atrial, or intracranial pressure. This results in higher coronary and cerebral perfusion pressure and higher myocardial and cerebral blood flow (Table 1.20).

TRANSCUTANEOUS CARDIAC PACING

Transcutaneous cardiac pacing (TCP) is used as a method of noninvasive pacing of the ventricles for a relatively short period. Emergency cardiac pacing is successful in resuscitation only if it is initiated soon after the onset of the arrest. In the absence of in situ pacing wires or an indwelling transvenous or esophageal pacing catheter, transcutaneous cardiac pacing is the preferred method for temporary electrical cardiac pacing. The 1992 American Heart Association's ACLS guidelines recommends early use of an external pacemaker in patients with symptomatic bradycardia and suggested its use for patients in asystole.

Indications

TCP is indicated for patients whose primary problem is impulse formation or conduction, with preserved myocardial function. TCP is most effective in patients with sinus bradycardia or high-grade atrio-ventricular (AV) block with slow ventricular response who also have a stroke volume sufficient to generate a pulse.

At this time, TCP is not indicated for patients in prolonged arrest, as this most likely would result in electrical but not mechanical cardiac capture and may delay or interfere with other resuscitative efforts.

Equipment and Technique

TCP involves placing two stimulating electrodes on the patient's thorax, one placed anteriorly at the left sternal border and the other posteriorly just below the left scapula. Smaller pediatric electrodes are available for infants and

Table 1.18
Characteristics of Lidocaine and Bretylium

	Lidocaine	Bretylium
Chemical Structure	Aromatic 2–6 xylidine coupled to diethylglycine	Bromobenzyl quaternary ammonia compound
Metabolism	Liver 10% unchanged in urine	>90% unchanged in urine
Electrophysiology	↓ Automaticity of pacemaker tissue ↑ Ventricular fibrillatory threshold ↓ Action potential duration in ventricle ↑ Effective refractory period of ventricle AV node—no effect	Initial release of norepinephrine followed by a blockade of release of norepinephrine ↑ Action potential duration in ventricle ↑ Effective refractory period in ventricle ↑ Ventricle fibrillatory threshold
Clinical Antiarrhythmic Effects	Frequent ventricular premature beats (VPB) (>6/min) Coupled VPBs Multiform tachycardia Ventricular tachycardia Prophylaxis during cardiac catheterization Prophylaxis following resuscitation Atrial or AV junctional arrhythmias Recurrent ventricular fibrillation after cardioversion	Treat ventricular tachycardia and fibrillation when first line treatment fails
Half-life	~90 min	~10 hours
Dosage	1 mg/kg bolus, IV If arrhythmia recurs, administer second bolus; decrease dose if there is coexisting decrease in cardiac output or hepatic disease	5–10 mg/kg IV by rapid bolus for ventricular fibrillation, or diluted 500 mg in ≥50 mL fluid over 10 min Quick onset of action; may be delayed 10–15 min
Side Effects	CNS—seizures, psychosis, drowsiness, tinnitus, paresthesias, disorientation, muscle twitching, agitation, respiratory arrest CV—slight decrease in cardiac function in patients with preexisting heart disease; conversion of 2° heart block to complete heart block; severe sinus bradycardia with large IV doses	Nausea and vomiting Initial increase in blood pressure and heart rate followed by a decrease in blood pressure Increased sensitivity to dopamine, epinephrine, and nonrepinephrine Parotid swelling

continued

Table 1.18
Characteristics of Lidocaine and Bretylium

	Lidocaine	Bretylium	
Drug Interactions	Phenobarbital 　↑ lidocaine metabolism Isoniazid 　↓ lidocaine metabolism Chloramphenicol 　↓ lidocaine metabolism Propranolol 　↑ serum lidocaine 　concentration Isoproterenol 　↓ serum lidocaine 　concentration	Dopamine Norepinephrine Epinephrine	Exaggerated response after bretylium administration

children; adult-size electrodes can be used in children over 15 kg. ECG leads should be connected to the pacemaker, and the demand or asynchronous mode selected and an age-appropriate heart rate used. The stimulus output should be set at zero when the pacemaker is turned on and then increased gradually until electrical capture is seen on the monitor. The output required for hemodynamically unstable rhythms is higher than that for hemodynamically stable rhythms in children in whom the mean stimulus required for capture was between 51 and 65 mA. After electrical capture is achieved, the physician must ascertain whether effective arterial pulses have been generated. If pulses are not adequate, other resuscitative efforts should be employed.

Complications

The most serious complication of TCP is the induction of ventricular arrhythmias. Fortunately, this is rare and may be prevented by pacing only in the demand mode. Mild transient erythema beneath the electrodes is common. Skeletal muscle contraction can be minimized by using large electrodes,

Table 1.19
Causes of Pulseless Electrical Activity

Cardiac—Primary
　Depletion of myocardial energy stores
Noncardiac—Secondary
　Hypovolemia
　Pericardial tamponade
　Tension pneumothorax
　Pulmonary embolism

Table 1.20
Open-chest CPR—Indications

Operating Room
Cardiac arrest secondary to:
  Cardiac tamponade
  Critical aortic stenosis
  Hypothermia
  Ruptured aortic aneurysm
  Chest already opened during surgery
Nonoperating Room
  Penetrating chest trauma
  Crushed chest injury
  Anatomic chest wall abnormalities
  Failure of closed-chest CPR

a 40 ms pulse duration, and the smallest stimulus required for capture. Sedatives or analgesics may be necessary in the awake patient. If defibrillation or cardioversion is necessary, the physician must allow a distance of 2 to 3 cm between the electrode and paddles to prevent arcing of the current.

SUPRAVENTRICULAR TACHYCARDIA

Supraventricular tachycardia (SVT) is a common arrhythmia that may be associated with severe circulatory compromise or even cardiac arrest. Therapy for this arrhythmia should be based on the child's hemodynamic status.

Moderate to Severe Circulatory Compromise

Cardioversion

SVT associated with poor circulation, including poor peripheral perfusion, hypotension, or a depressed level of consciousness, should be treated immediately with synchronized cardioversion beginning at a dose of 0.5 J. If IV access is available, adenosine can be used as cardioversion is being prepared; however, cardioversion should not be delayed while IV access is being achieved.

Adenosine Therapy

Adenosine is the medical treatment of choice for SVT. The underlying mechanism in children is usually a re-entry circuit involving the AV node. Adenosine is an endogenous nucleoside that causes a temporary block in the AV node and interrupts this re-entry circuit. It is rapidly and highly effective with minimal side effects. It has been used during general anesthesia, open heart surgery, and in the intensive care unit.

The initial dose is 0.1 mg/kg given as a rapid IV bolus. Central venous administration is preferable because the drug is rapidly metabolized by red blood cell adenosine deaminase and thus has a half-life of only 10 seconds; higher doses may be necessary when the drug is given peripherally. If there is no interruption in the re-entry circuit, successive doses should be doubled, up to a maximum single dose of 12 mg until the arrhythmia is broken. In neonates, a smaller initial dose of 0.05 mg/kg is given and increased by 0.05 mg/kg/dose until termination of the arrhythmia up to a maximum of 0.25 mg/kg.

Absence of Circulatory Compromise

When SVT appears without any circulatory compromise, conversion of the arrhythmia may be first attempted with a vagal maneuver such as ice water to the face. If ineffective, then adenosine should be used as the first line drug. Digoxin is often ineffective and may have substantial side effects. Verapamil should be avoided in infants because of its association with congestive heart failure and cardiac arrest as a result of its negative inotropic effects. Its use in older children is also discouraged. Other therapies include β-adrenergic blockers, edrophonium, and β-agonists. If SVT persists despite medical therapy, and the patient progresses to circulatory instability, electrical cardioversion should proceed immediately.

SIMULTANEOUS COMPRESSION-VENTILATION CPR

Simultaneous compression-ventilation CPR (SCV-CPR) augments conventional CPR by increasing the thoracic pump mechanism contribution to blood flow. Delivering ventilation simultaneously with every compression, instead of after every fifth compression, increases intrathoracic pressure and augments blood flow produced by closed-chest CPR.

COMPLICATIONS OF CPR

CPR can adversely affect every organ system in the resuscitated patient and is associated with complications in the rescuer as well (Table 1.21).

INDICATIONS FOR TERMINATION OF RESUSCITATION
Decision to Undertake CPR

CPR should be performed on patients unless a specific order not to resuscitate is on the medical record or communication with a physician familiar with the patient's medical history has occurred. The decision to forego CPR is predicated by the following concerns: possible outcome of the resuscitative attempt based on the patient's medical history; potential quality of life; legal rights of the patient, including living wills and advanced directives (in

Table 1.21
Complications of CPR

CNS	↑ Intracranial Pressure ↓ Cerebral Perfusion Pressure
Neck:	Endotracheal tube placement in esophagus Esophageal tear Trauma to hyoid bone Trauma to thyroid cartilage
Thorax:	Rib fracture Sternal fracture Hemopericardium Ventricular contusion Cardiac laceration Cardiac rupture Pulmonary edema
Abdomen:	Gastric distention Liver rupture Splenic rupture Pneumoperitoneum Aspiration
Vascular:	Fat emboli Bone marrow emboli Disseminated intravascular coagulopathy (DIC) Thrombosis
Electrolytes:	Hypokalemia Hyperkalemia Hypocalcemia Hypomagnesemia
Rescuer associated:	Infection (bacteria, TB, HIV, hepatitis) Physical stress

adults); patient rights regarding their understanding of the disease process; treatment options; risks and benefits of therapy; and prognosis.

Decision to Terminate CPR

The decision to terminate efforts to resuscitate is based on a number of factors. Further history gathering during the resuscitative effort may affect the decision to continue with CPR. In addition, the severity of anatomic or metabolic derangements and other coexisting factors such as age, duration of CPR, and presenting cardiac rhythm will help the physician determine the course of CPR.

Neither absence of neurologic function nor brain death should be used as a criterion to cease CPR efforts. The former is unreliable as a prognostic sign, and the latter is not a valid diagnosis during the CPR effort; only after

cardiovascular function is reestablished should neurologic status be determined in order to consider withdrawal of life support.

Rigid criteria to stop CPR efforts have been advocated by some, but the
uncertainties regarding etiology, duration of arrest, metabolic and biochemical aberrations, and young age all play a role in determining the eventual course of the resuscitation effort.

2.

Airway Management

Aaron L. Zuckerberg and David G. Nichols

Oral intubation requires establishing a line of vision from the incisor teeth to the larynx (Fig. 2.1). This path has three axes: the oral axis, the pharyngeal axis, and the laryngeal axis (Fig. 2.2). Normally the oral axis is perpendicular to the laryngeal axis, and the pharyngeal axis forms a 45-degree angle with the laryngeal axis. Positioning of the patient with modest neck flexion (i.e., the "sniffing position") and atlanto-occipital joint extension superimposes these axes. A cushion or folded towel placed under the occiput will adequately flex the neck. Failure to position the patient correctly is a common error and frequently results in an unnecessarily difficult or impossible intubation.

The line of vision necessary for intubation requires deflection of the tongue and soft tissues out of the oro-pharyngeal-laryngeal path. These structures are displaced into a potential space, defined by the anterior and lateral rami of the mandible and the hyoid bone. Alteration in the anatomic structures of this area, such as in the mandibular dysplasias, will decrease the space

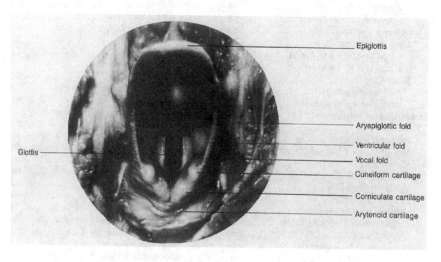

Figure 2.1. Anatomy of the larynx. (From Barash PG, Cullen BF, Stoelting RK. Clinical Anesthesia, 2nd edition. NY: J. B. Lippincott, 1989:544.)

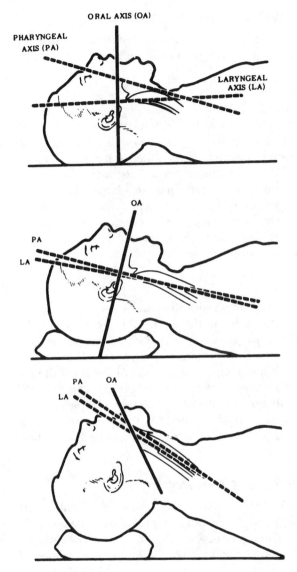

Figure 2.2. The three airway axes. With proper head extension and neck flexion, these axes are superimposed to establish the necessary line of vision. (From Berry FA. Anesthetic management of difficult and routine pediatric patients, 2nd edition. NY: Churchill Livingstone, 1990:172.)

in which the soft tissue can be displaced with the laryngoscope and make laryngoscopy and intubation difficult. An increase in the amount of soft tissue in the tongue, floor of the mouth, or submandibular space has the same effect (e.g., mucopolysaccharidoses). Although neuromuscular blockade will maximize the potential displacement space, no amount of drug will relax bony abnormalities or tense tissue infiltration from either mass or edema.

DEVELOPMENTAL AIRWAY CONSIDERATIONS

The infant's airway differs in many respects from that of the adult. The differences that are critical for airway management are outlined in Table 2.1.

Subglottic Region

Maturational differences also are evident in the subglottic region. The narrowest portion of the infant's airway is at the level of the cricoid ring, producing a funnel shape in the laryngeal complex. In contrast, the narrowest aspect of the adult larynx is the opening between the vocal cords, resulting in a cylindrical shape (Fig. 2.3). This difference affects the size of the endotracheal tube that will fit into the younger patient's larynx. In children less than 8 years of age, an endotracheal tube may pass through the vocal cords but be unable to traverse the region of the cricoid ring. An excessively large endotracheal tube compresses the tracheal mucosa, which may lead to subglottic edema and postextubation croup.

Tracheal Length

The length of the trachea also changes with the child's development. The distance from the glottis to the carina in the newborn is 4 cm. During the first 12 months of life, the trachea grows to 7 cm. A child's trachea is 8 cm long. By adulthood, the trachea is 12 cm long.

In some patients, precise midtracheal positioning of the tip of the endotracheal tube may be difficult (e.g., tracheo-esophageal fistula). After deliberate endobronchial intubation, the endotracheal tube is withdrawn until bilateral breath sounds are just appreciated. At this point the tube is withdrawn an additional 2 cm. The endotracheal tube will be midtracheal in virtually all situations.

RECOGNIZING THE DIFFICULT AIRWAY

The ability to recognize a difficult airway is imperative in individuals responsible for airway management. In the adult population, moderately difficult intubations are relatively common, occurring in 1 to 18% of patients. A definite failure of intubation occurs in 0.35% of adults. Ten percent of

Table 2.1
Distinctive Characteristics of the Infant Airway

- Relatively large tongue
- Higher position of the larynx (C3–4 vs. C4–5)
- Laryngeal configuration
- A protuberant occiput

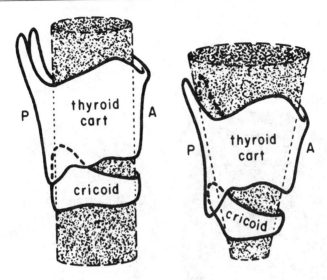

Figure 2.3. The infant's larynx is funnel shaped as compared with the adult's cylindrical larynx. (From Cote CJ, Ryan JF, Todres DI. A practice of anesthesia for infants and children. Philadelphia: WB Saunders, 1993:61.)

these patients could not be ventilated or intubated. In the absence of an obvious airway abnormality or specific syndrome, most difficult airways can be recognized by performing these three maneuvers:

- Examination of the oropharynx
- Evaluation of range of motion at the atlanto-occipital joint
- Measurement of the potential displacement area

The Oropharyngeal Examination

With the patient's mouth open to the widest extent and with maximal tongue protrusion, the range of motion at the temporo-mandibular joint and the size of the tongue relative to the size of the oral cavity are documented. Mallampati classified the degree of airway difficulty based on the ability to visualize the faucial pillars, soft palate, and uvula (Fig. 2.4). Intubation is successful in >99% of patients with a class I airway, in which all three structures are visualized. Patients with a class IV airway, in which none of the pharyngeal structures are visible, suffer a failed intubation 1 to 4% of the time. A highly arched palate also increases the difficulty of intubation.

Atlanto-occipital Joint Extension

Reduction in the range of motion at the atlanto-occipital joint affects the ability to establish a line of sight to the glottic structures. Normally, 35 degrees of

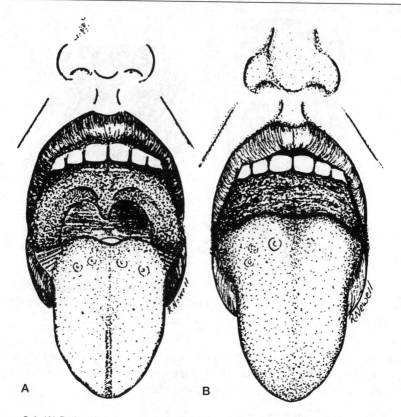

Figure 2.4. (A) Patient in whom the tonsillar pillars, soft palate, and uvula are visualized. A class 1 airway. (B) Patient in whom none of the pharyngeal structures are visualized. A class IV airway. (From Mallampati et al. A clinical sign to predict difficult tracheal intubation: a prospective study. Canadian Anesthetists Society Journal 1985; 32(4):429–434.)

extension is possible. Excessive reduction in this range of motion will lead to increasing difficulties with laryngoscopy.

The Potential Displacement Area

The mandibular space is important. If the thyromental distance is short, then the pharyngeal axis will make a more acute angle with the laryngeal axis and it will be more difficult for atlanto-occipital extension to superimpose the three airway axes into a line of sight.

In the adult with atlanto-occipital extension, a thyromental distance of 6 cm is associated with an easy laryngoscopy. If the mandibular space is small, the tongue and soft tissues must be compressed into a much smaller compartment, which makes laryngoscopy much more difficult.

In a child, if two fingers can be placed between the anterior ramus of the mandible and the hyoid bone, the potential displacement area is adequate.

For a normal airway, with the head in a neutral position, the minimum distance from the hyoid to the mentum is 3 cm (i.e., two finger breadths) in adults and 1.5 cm in infants. The result of a decreased displacement space is an increased difficulty in visualizing the glottis, or the "anterior larynx." The larynx is not truly anterior, but because the laryngoscopy remains in a posterior position, the larynx appears to be anterior to the line of vision.

These three tests, used in combination, have a 100% predictive value in recognizing the difficult airway in adults.

Not all patients with difficult airways can be managed by bag-mask ventilation. Edema, inflammatory or infiltrative processes, or localized lesions in the hypopharyngeal-supraglottic region can increase resistance to airflow through the upper airway. The greater the resistance to airflow, the greater the driving force needed to maintain the required tidal volume. During spontaneous respiration, a larger negative pressure must be generated, which will increase the tendency for the upper airway to collapse.

THE DIFFICULT PEDIATRIC AIRWAY

Airway symptoms or anatomic features usually point to the child with a difficult airway. Nevertheless, in some children, a difficult airway is appreciated only at the time of intubation. For this reason, every intensive care unit must both practice recognition and establish a management strategy for the difficult airway. The syndromes associated with airway difficulties may be categorized by the principal airway anomaly.

Micrognathia

Micrognathia (i.e., abnormal smallness of the jaws) is the most difficult of the airway abnormalities, primarily because of its effects on the insertion of the tongue, the soft tissues, and the suspension of the larynx. These structures lie more cephalad in relation to the mandible and often are perceived as "very anterior." Visualization of the glottis can be extremely difficult, if not impossible, in this situation. Classic examples of micrognathia include the Pierre Robin and Treacher Collins syndromes.

Cervical Spine Abnormalities

Cervical spine abnormalities limit the establishment of the line of sight to the glottis structures. Goldenhar and Klippel-Fiel syndromes exemplify congenital conditions associated with cervical spine abnormalities. Disease processes with significant cervical spine abnormalities include juvenile rheumatoid arthritis and neuromuscular scolioses. Atlanto-occipital instability represents a different form of cervical spine abnormality and is most

commonly considered in patients with trisomy 21. Atlanto-occipital instability is assumed in neck trauma.

Macroglossia and Glossoptosis

Macroglossia and glossoptosis affect visualization of the larynx. Macroglossia
is an enlargement of the tongue and is seen in patients with Beckwith-
Wiedemann syndrome and trisomy 21. Glossoptosis is the downward and backward displacement of the tongue that is commonly seen in achondroplasia.

Infiltration of the Soft Tissues

Infiltration of the soft tissues in the potential displacement area will affect
laryngoscopy. Not only will visualization be difficult, but severe anatomic
distortion of the laryngeal complex should be expected. Examples of this
anatomic distortion include submandibular masses (e.g., cystic hygroma),
edema and cellulitic involvement secondary to oropharyngeal processes
(e.g., Ludwig's angina), and epiglottitis. Epidermolysis bullosa should be included in this category because 25% of patients with epidermolysis bullosa
have difficult oral intubations that require alternative approaches such as
blind nasal or fiberoptic intubations.

The Morbidly Obese Patient

The morbidly obese patient has a short thick neck with a limited range of
motion and a large tongue. Excessive chest wall soft tissue further complicates laryngoscopy and physical obstruction to airway instrumentation.

Mucopolysaccharidoses and Musculoskeletal Syndromes

Children with mucopolysaccharidoses and musculoskeletal syndromes have
a high overall incidence of difficult or failed intubation. Children with
Hurler's syndrome are the most difficult, with a failed intubation rate of
23%. Arthrogryposis multiplex congenita (AMC) is a rare musculoskeletal
disorder defined by multiple fixed joints in the upper and lower extremities
(Fig. 2.5). Abnormalities resulting from AMC that have an impact on airway
management can include: micrognathia; a high arched palate; and an
omega-shaped epiglottis, but otherwise normal larynx, and trachea. Acha-
lasia and multiple aspiration pneumonias can further complicate the clinical management of this disorder.

BASIC AIRWAY MANAGEMENT
Airway Patency

Airway patency is maintained with proper head positioning and secretion
removal. The tongue is the principal cause of airway obstruction in most

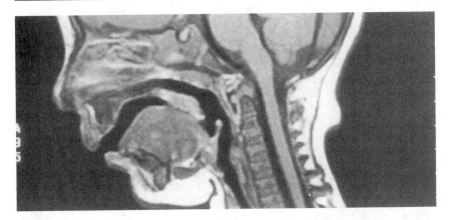

Figure 2.5. Magnetic resonance image of a patient with arthrogryposis multiplex congenita demonstrating the marked micrognathia and high arched palate. The age-appropriate characteristic subglottic narrowing is seen well in this image.

situations. With atlanto-occipital extension, the space between the base of the tongue and the posterior pharynx is increased. Airway patency is frequently re-established with a chin lift and jaw thrust. Airway adjuncts such as an oropharyngeal airway or a nasopharyngeal airway function by further separating the tongue from the soft tissues of the posterior pharynx (Fig. 2.6).

The complications of airway trauma, worsening airway obstruction, laryngospasm, and epistaxis frequently are related to the selection of an inappropriately sized airway. Nasopharyngeal instrumentation is contraindicated in patients with basilar skull fractures and cerebrospinal fluid leaks and in patients who are anticoagulated.

Oxygen Delivery

Once airway patency is assured, oxygen can be administered through a variety of devices. The exact concentration of oxygen administered to the patient depends on the oxygen flow rate, as well as the patient's minute ventilation and inspiratory flow rate, which will dictate the amount of diluent room air inspired. Because oxygen therapy is titrated to the adequacy of the patient's oxygen saturation or oxygen tension, the exact FiO_2 is unimportant. When determining the patient's alveolar-arterial (Aa) pressure difference or PaO_2/FiO_2 index, however, precise delivery of oxygen concentration is desired. In these circumstances, the preferred delivery device is a non-rebreathing oxygen mask attached to a venturi system or a gas blender.

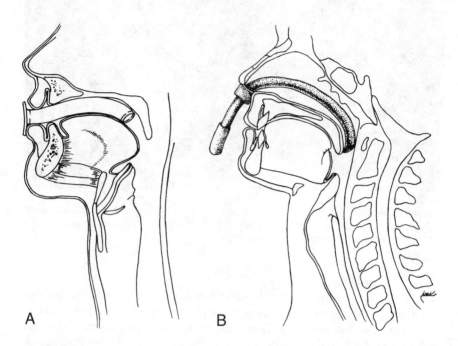

Figure 2.6. (A) An oropharyngeal airway should be placed that follows the curve of the tongue, with the tip of the airway aimed toward the larynx. (B) A soft nasopharyngeal airway is placed in line with the nose to follow the natural curve of the nasal cavity.

Positive Pressure Ventilation

The Full Stomach Quagmire

All acutely injured patients are considered to have full stomachs until proven otherwise. Patients with full stomachs (i.e., gastric residual volume in excess of 0.4 mL/kg and a pH less than 2.5) are at risk of acid aspiration during positive pressure ventilation and induction of anesthesia before intubation. Children appear to be at least as susceptible to regurgitation and aspiration as adults (Table 2.2).

Pediatric anesthesiologists often can delay a procedure to allow for adequate gastric emptying and for gastroprophylactic drugs to take effect. Such delay is inconceivable in a patient with status asthmaticus, epiglottitis, or a central nervous system injury.

Aspiration Pneumonitis

Aspiration pneumonitis is the result of inhalation of acidic fluid, which leads to damage of the pulmonary capillary endothelium and inhibition of surfac-

Table 2.2
Factors That Contribute to the Child's Increased Risk of Pulmonary Aspiration

- Excessive aerophagia during crying
- Strenuous diaphragmatic activity during airway obstruction
- A shorter esophagus
- A smaller hydrostatic gradient between the stomach and the larynx

tant production. Bronchospasm and acute pulmonary vasoconstriction may develop. Atelectasis, interstitial pulmonary edema, and significant hypoxemia follow. Changes in the chest radiograph occur 6 to 12 hours after the injury.

Aspiration syndrome is responsible for 19% of all deaths attributed to anesthesia; therefore, it is appropriate that pediatric intensivists adopt the tenets of the anesthetic approach to the patient with a full stomach (Table 2.3).

Applying Cricoid Pressure

All children encountered in a critical setting, specifically those who receive a nondepolarizing muscle relaxant to facilitate intubation, should receive bag-mask ventilation through applied cricoid pressure to prevent regurgitation of stomach contents. The absolute minimum amount of positive inspiratory pressure sufficient to cause chest wall excursion should be used. Cricoid pressure is removed only after the restoration of the patient's airway reflexes or placement of endotracheal intubation, which is confirmed by bilateral breath sounds and end-tidal CO_2 demonstration.

Equipment and Technique

When the patient exhibits inadequate breathing, the resuscitator should establish airway patency. Positive pressure breaths can be given by mouth-mask-mouth ventilation or by bag-mask ventilation.

Mask Placement

A secure mask fit is necessary to ventilate the patient reliably. The resuscitator should hold the mask firmly on the child's face with 90% of the effort directed toward bringing the face into the mask and only 10% directed toward pushing the mask down on the child's face.

Table 2.3
Approach to the Patient with a Full Stomach

- Decompress the stomach if possible (in the awake patient).
- Denitrogenate and preoxygenate to minimize the ensuing oxygen desaturation.
- Minimize the period of time between the onset of apnea and ideal intubating conditions (The Rapid Sequence).
- Minimize the amount of air entering the stomach during bag-mask ventilation.

Large Children and Adults The resuscitator uses the thumb and index finger for downward pressure on the mask. The remainder of the fingers are placed on the ramus of the mandible to position the neck and bring the face into the mask.

Small Children and Infants Finger misplacement on smaller children leads to inadvertent compression of the submandibular soft tissues and airway obstruction. Infants are particularly susceptible to this iatrogenic airway obstruction, so the resuscitator uses the thumb and index finger to completely encircle the stem of the mask while the middle finger lies along the mandible, extending from the midposition on the left side of the mandible to the midposition of the right. The middle finger is used to provide the necessary chin lift and head position. The remaining two fingers are extended, but not touching any part of the infant's face. The other hand is used to squeeze the bag. Mask repositioning, additional padding, and, on occasion, two hands on the mask are necessary to compensate for abnormalities in mandibular contour and mask leaks.

Ventilating Bags

Two types of ventilating bags are available for use in infants and children: self-inflating bags and anesthesia-type bags.

Self-Inflating Bags Self-inflating bags are easy to use because they do not require an optimal mask seal to function. Self-inflating bags, however, will continue to fill even when disconnected from an oxygen source. Two types of self-inflating bags are the Puritan manual resuscitator (PMR) and the Laerdal resuscitator bag. Both of these bags allow for oxygen administration during spontaneous ventilation. The PMR bag can supply an FiO_2 of 1.0 using a high-flow oxygen source. The Laerdal bag can deliver a 100% FiO_2 only if a reservoir bag is used.

Anesthesia Bag Systems These systems identify an immediate disconnection from the oxygen source and are lightweight. They have no inspiratory valves and allow spontaneous inspiration. Because these systems require an optimal mask seal, they are more difficult for the inexperienced resuscitator to use. A Mapelson D and modified Mapelson C circuit are useful in the pediatric intensive care unit (PICU) and transport setting.

In light of the almost universal use of pulse oximetry and the variable experience among professionals who respond to pediatric airway emergencies, the staff in most institutions uses a self-inflating bag.

ENDOTRACHEAL INTUBATION

The indications for endotracheal intubation are respiratory failure, airway protection, and the relief of airway obstruction. The equipment necessary for endotracheal intubation is listed in Table 2.4.

Table 2.4
Equipment Needed for the "Rapid Sequence Intubation"

- Large suction catheter "Yankauer" and reliable suction
- Bag and mask
- Oxygen source
- Ventilation system
- Endotracheal tubes
- Laryngoscopes and handles
- Oropharyngeal airways
- Tongue blade
- Tape
- Stylet
- Expired carbon dioxide detection device

Technique

Patient Positioning

The resuscitator places the infant's head in a neutral position. For the older child, if the head is extended at the atlanto-occipital joint and the occiput is elevated to the sniffing position, the oropharyngolaryngeal axes are aligned (Fig. 2.7). Extension of the child's head without elevation of the occiput rotates the larynx anteriorly (Fig. 2.8). The child's mouth is opened by pressure on the mandible. The resuscitator holds the laryngoscope in the left hand, inserting it into the right side of the child's mouth with the tongue on the left side of the blade. The child's tongue is moved to the left side of the mouth as the laryngoscope is moved to the midline. The blade is then advanced slowly over the tongue.

Combined

PH-LTR axis

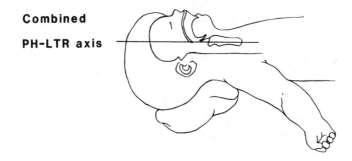

Figure 2.7. Placement of the head in sniffing position aligns the pharyngeal and laryngotracheal axes (combined PH-LTR axis).

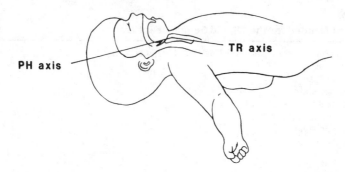

Figure 2.8. Without elevation of the occiput, neck extension results in a separate plane for the tracheal axis (TR) and pharyngeal axis (PH).

Straight versus Curved Blades

The choice of blade is largely dictated by the age of the patient and the preference and experience of the physician (Fig. 2.9). Straight blades usually are used in infants, small children, and patients with "anterior" laryngeal placement. It is easier to lift the base of the tongue and fix an infant's epiglottis with a straight blade. The channel of the straight blade is the intubator's visual path, not the endotracheal tube insertion guide.

Curved blades are used primarily in children older than 2 to 3 years of age. The advantages of a curved blade include a large flange that provides better control of the tongue and less perceived need to exert leverage on

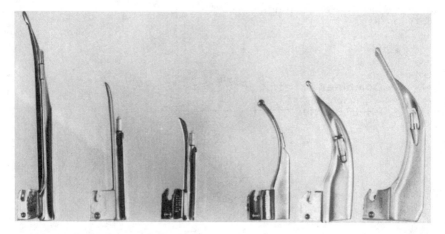

Figure 2.9. Straight and curved laryngoscope blades are available in varying sizes suitable for children.

the child's upper teeth, which results in less potential dental damage and more available oropharyngeal space.

Visualization of the Glottis

A straight blade's (e.g., Miller, Wisconsin, Wis-Hippel) tip is moved under the laryngeal side of the epiglottis. With an upward pull along the axis of the handle, the epiglottis and the base of the tongue are raised to expose the glottis (Fig. 2.10). If the larynx is not easily visualized, external pressure on the larynx may help bring the glottis into view. If the blade has been advanced too deeply into the esophagus, the blade is withdrawn until the glottis is visualized. With a curved blade (e.g., Macintosh), the laryngoscope blade is advanced from the right side of the mouth into the valleculae. With an upward pull along the axis of the laryngoscope handle, the glottis is visualized. The tongue is more easily controlled with the curved blade.

Common errors to avoid are:

1. Exerting leverage on the patient's upper incisors instead of lifting the axis of the laryngoscope handle at a 45-degree angle, thus pulling the tongue away from the upper incisors.
2. Allowing the tongue to slip back into the path of vision when it protrudes over the right side of the laryngoscope blade.
3. Trapping the lips between the laryngoscope blade and the teeth.

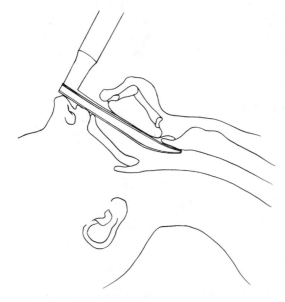

Figure 2.10. The tip of the laryngoscope straight blade is placed under the laryngeal side of the epiglottis.

The endotracheal tube is advanced from the right side of the mouth with the curve aimed anteriorly.

Tube Type and Size

Polyvinylchloride tubes, which are inert, soft, and molded at body temperature to the shape of the airway, are recommended. These tubes have either one or three markings at the distal end to guide appropriate depth of placement. The appropriate endotracheal tube size can be estimated by the size of the child's little finger or by the equation:

$$16 + \text{age (yrs)} \div 4$$

Age is a more reliable determinant of endotracheal tube size than is height (Table 2.5). In children with congenital anomalies, a half-size smaller endotracheal tube usually is appropriate. A variety of tube sizes should be available at the time of intubation, including the appropriate size, a size larger, and a size smaller.

Verifying Tube Size

The appropriate size endotracheal tube is important, because a very small tube will decrease the cross-sectional area of the airway and result in an increased resistance to both flow and work of breathing. With a stethoscope placed on the anterior neck overlying the trachea and an aneroid manometer connected to the breathing system, the inspiratory pressure at which the gas "leaks" around the endotracheal tube can be monitored. If testing is performed with a neutral head position in the presence of a neuromuscular blockade, the leak can be measured reliably. The leak pressure may be an indicator of fit between the endotracheal tube and the size of the trachea.

Table 2.5
Suggested Endotracheal Tube Size

Age	Internal Diameter (ID)
Premature infant	2.5–3.0
Newborn	3.0
Newborn–6 month	3.5
6 m–12 m	3.5–4.0
12 m–2 y	4.0–4.5
3–4 y	4.5–5.0
5–6 y	5.0–5.5
7–8 y	5.5–6.0
9–10 y	6.0–6.5
11–12 y	6.5–7.0
13–14 y	7.0–7.5

It is recommended that the leak be less than 20 to 25 cm H_2O to reduce post-extubation stridor.

Depth of Insertion

The appropriate distance for endotracheal tube insertion also varies with age. By convention, the distance is recorded as the position of the endotracheal tube at the gum or incisor. Insertion nomograms have been devised to estimate the appropriate length for tracheal intubation. In addition to age, weight has been used: 7 cm for the 1 kg infant, 8 cm for the 2 kg infant, and 9 cm for the 3 kg infant. For children over 3 years of age the formula for depth of insertion to the incisors is:

$$\text{Depth of insertion (cm)} = (\text{age} \div) + 12$$

A rule of thumb is that the depth of insertion equals three times the size (i.e., internal diameter) of the endotracheal tube. The patient's head position will affect endotracheal tube position. With neck flexion, the tip of the tube moves closer to the carina, possibly causing an endobronchial intubation. Neck extension results in withdrawal of the tube toward the glottis. The change in the position of the tube mimics the change in position of the patient's nose.

The intubator should watch as the tracheal tube passes through the vocal cords to ensure endotracheal placement. The endotracheal tube should be positioned so that the single line, the middle line, or the cuff is just below the level of the vocal cords.

Common errors to avoid at this stage are:

1. Poor visualization of the glottic structures before endotracheal tube placement.
2. Poor visualization of passage of the endotracheal tube because of inadequate tongue displacement to the left.

Confirmation of Placement

Endotracheal intubation must be confirmed. The detection of expired carbon dioxide with a capnograph or mass spectrometer is the most reliable evidence of tracheal rather than esophageal intubation. Traditional confirmatory findings, such as mist in the tube, auscultation of bilaterally equal breath sounds, and the absence of air entry during epigastrium auscultation, can be misleading. Midtracheal position is then confirmed by auscultation of bilateral breath sounds, palpation of the tube tip at the suprasternal notch, chest radiography, or bronchoscopy.

Cuffed versus Uncuffed Tubes

Cuffed tubes are usually used for children more than 8 years of age. Traditionally, endotracheal tubes used in infants and young children are uncuffed because of concern for the development of subglottic damage. Because the narrow segment of the infant's airway lumen is the cricoid ring, any excessive pressure in this area was thought to result in postextubation stridor. An air leak of 15 to 25 cm H_2O has been suggested as a sign of a safe endotracheal tube fit. Many practitioners are reevaluating this practice now that high volume–low pressure cuffs are available.

Cuffed endotracheal tubes should be considered in children with marked alterations in pulmonary compliance, such as acute respiratory distress syndrome. The cuff should be inflated to the minimal pressure required to seal an air leak and allow effective ventilation. Cuff filling is confirmed by distention of the pilot balloon. Cuff pressure should be monitored; it is recommended to keep the pressure less than 20 mm Hg.

Use of Stylet

A stylet is used to change the position of the tip of the tube for patients with anatomic abnormalities. Fortunately, the stylet is only rarely necessary because trauma to the airway can occur with improper use of the tool itself or from stiffening the tube. The stylet is usually necessitated by poor technique rather than airway abnormalities. The intubator must be certain that the stylet does not protrude from the end of the endotracheal tube and is well lubricated to ensure easy removal once the tube is in place.

Pharmacologic Management

The flaccid child in cardiopulmonary arrest requires no pharmacologic intervention. Bag-mask ventilation through cricoid pressure, laryngoscopy, and intubation are usually accomplished without difficulty. Conversely, a combative child with a rapidly declining neurologic status resulting from head trauma requires a rapid, smooth anesthesia induction and intubation that limits the intracranial pressure response and the risks of pulmonary aspiration. Before committing to a specific technique, the intensivist must assess the child's airway anatomy and intravascular status.

Common problems associated with endotracheal intubation are:

1. Underappreciation of airway anomalies.
2. Underappreciation of the hemodynamic derangement of the patient and the further deleterious effects the pharmacologic agents will have.
3. Underappreciation of the risk of pulmonary aspiration.

The airway must be secured in the safest manner possible. Intubation can be accomplished under three conditions: awake, sedated, and anesthetized. There are situations in which, even in the most experienced of hands, the safest technique is that in which the patient is intubated awake and without drugs.

Awake Intubation

There are no absolute indications for "awake" (i.e., no pharmacologic adjuncts) intubation of the trachea, with the exception of the patient in cardiopulmonary arrest. The intensivist must weigh the risks of a biting, struggling child who will recall intubation against the benefits of maintaining a spontaneously breathing child with a protected airway in the event intubation is difficult. An awake intubation is often necessary in patients with airway anomalies, upper gastrointestinal hemorrhage, cervical spine abnormalities, and facial trauma. Patients who are already hypoxemic may not tolerate even the shortest apneic period and therefore are excellent candidates for an awake intubation.

Sedated Intubation

A carefully titrated sedation is a useful approach to the patient with an uncertain airway or who has lung disease with a moderate O_2 requirement. The goal is to increase the patient's cooperation and ease of intubation without excessively depressing the patient's airway reflexes and spontaneous respiratory drive. This technique is usually more successful in older children than in infants, in whom this "perfect" plan of sedation may be difficult to achieve.

Agents and Dosages

Drugs and dosing guidelines used for sedated intubation are found in Table 2.6. Benzodiazepines provide amnesia and some sedation for laryngoscopy. The initial recommended dose should be decreased by 50 to 75% in the setting of hypovolemia or poor cardiac function. When the cardiovascular effects of the drug have been determined, additional drugs may be given, titrating to the desired sedation plane.

Ketamine Ketamine is a dissociative anesthetic with minimal respiratory effects. Ketamine rarely causes apnea and leaves the laryngeal reflexes intact. It also relieves coughing and laryngospasm and has bronchodilatory properties. Ketamine is a potent sialogogue and requires the coadministration of a

Table 2.6
Dosing Guidelines for Induction Agents

Sodium pentothal	4–6 mg/kg IV 2–3 mg/kg IV if unstable
Ketamine	2 mg/kg IV
Lidocaine	1.5 mg/kg IV
Midazolam	0.05–0.1 mg/kg IV
Diazepam	0.1–0.2 mg/kg IV

muscarinic antagonist (e.g., atropine or glycopyrrolate) to decrease airway secretions. It has indirect sympathomimetic properties and, as a result, will preserve blood pressure and cardiac output in acutely hypovolemic patients. However, in the setting of a prolonged shock state with endogenous catecholamine depletion, ketamine is a primary myocardial depressant and peripheral vasodilator. Ketamine does increase elecroencephalogram activity and intracranial pressure; therefore, it is contraindicated in patients with intracranial pathology. Coadministration of a small amount of benzodiazepine has been effective in decreasing the hallucinations seen with ketamine administration.

Anesthetized Intubation

Complete pharmacologic control with an anesthetic intubation represents optimal intubating conditions, providing amnesia, sedation, and muscle paralysis and blunting the various physiologic responses to intubation that may exacerbate an underlying pathophysiologic process. Airway safety, however, should not be jeopardized for the sake of pharmacologic intervention.

A child with severe head trauma and intracranial hypertension is an optimal candidate for an anesthetized intubation. Laryngoscopy and endotracheal intubation are extremely potent intracranial hypertensive stimuli. Unblunted in a patient with poor intracranial compliance, this response can severely compromise cerebral perfusion and worsen the ultimate neurologic outcome.

The components of an anesthetic induction include a hypnotic such as thiopental or ketamine, a neuromuscular blocker, and drugs to modulate the physiologic responses to intubation. The latter group of drugs is dictated by the child's coexisting disease: bronchodilators for asthma, beta blockade for essential hypertension, lidocaine for intracranial hypertension, or sodium nitroprusside for an intracerebral aneurysm. Because virtually all patients requiring airway management in the pediatric intensive care setting are at significant risk for pulmonary aspiration of gastric contents, this approach is summarized in the rapid sequence intubation section.

Neuromuscular Blockade

Neuromuscular blockade facilitates laryngoscopy, endotracheal intubation, and controlled ventilation; however, muscle relaxants are contraindicated if there is any doubt about the success of endotracheal intubation. Loss of airway reflexes and spontaneous respiration is disastrous, especially when bag-mask ventilation is unreliable. The use of neuromuscular blockade in acute airway management, therefore, include an adequate airway assessment and the use of short onset, short duration drugs to minimize such problems in the event intubation is unsuccessful.

Succinylcholine

Beneficial Physiologic Effects Succinylcholine, the only depolarizing neuromuscular blocking agent available, has many of the characteristics of an ideal muscle relaxant: quick onset, superb intubating conditions, and brief duration of action. Complete airway relaxation is achieved within 30 to 60 seconds. Rapid redistribution away from the neuromuscular junction results in a short duration of action (i.e., 3 to 5 minutes).

Nonparalytic Effects Because of a myriad of nonparalytic effects, many of which are exaggerated in the pediatric population (e.g., nodal rhythms, sinus bradycardia), succinylcholine is contraindicated in some patients (Table 2.7). These side effects have led many practitioners to avoid succinylcholine use in children; nevertheless, in the appropriate patient, when immediate airway control is necessary, succinylcholine has no peer.

Deleterious Effects

Hyperkalemia In normal patients, succinylcholine increases plasma levels of potassium by 0.3 to 0.5 mEq/liter, reaching a peak at 5 minutes. Life-threatening levels of hyperkalemia, as high as 13 mEq/L, have been reported when succinylcholine has been given to patients with progressive neurologic disease, spinal cord injury, cerebrovascular accidents, and recent burn or major muscle trauma. Although the data would suggest that the susceptibility of burn and trauma patients to this hyperkalemic response exists only between 7 and 60 days, our practice is to avoid succinylcholine from 72 hours after the injury to 6 months to 1 year. Cerebral palsy is not a contraindication to succinylcholine. Prolonged severe intraabdominal infections ($\geq$1 week) have also been associated with a hyperkalemic response to succinylcholine administration.

Increased Intracranial, Intragastric, and Intraocular Pressures These effects are related to the intensity of muscle fasciculations. Pretreatment with

Table 2.7
Contraindications to Succinylcholine

Hyperkalemia K > 5.5 mEq/L
Burn 3 days–6 months after injury
Trauma 3 days—1 year after injury
Paraplegia 3 days—1 year after injury
Duchenne's Muscular Dystrophy
Myotonic Dystrophy
Amyotrophic Lateral Sclerosis
Multiple Sclerosis
Friedrich Ataxia
Guillain-Barré syndrome
Parkinson disease
Progressive neuromuscular diseases

a small dose (i.e., 10% of intubating dose) of a nondepolarizing muscle relaxant prevents muscle fasciculations by partially blocking depolarization by succinylcholine. Children have a much lower increase in intragastric pressure after succinylcholine administration than adults.

Malignant Hyperthermia Succinylcholine, especially with the coadministration of a halogenated vapor anesthetic such as halothane, is a trigger agent for malignant hyperthermia, which is characterized by increased CO_2 production and oxygen consumption. Fever, tachycardia, tachypnea, acidosis, hyperkalemia, ventricular dysrhythmias, and rhabdomyolysis result. The mortality rate in fulminant malignant hyperthermia is 10%. Malignant hyperthermia is autosomal dominant in humans, and most cases seem to affect children and young adults. In addition to a positive family history, Duchenne muscular dystrophy and the uncommon myopathies of central core disease, myotonia congenita, and King-Denborough syndrome are thought to be risk factors for the development of malignant hyperthermia.

Masseter Spasm Occasionally, a patient may develop masseter spasm (i.e., a tight jaw) after the administration of succinylcholine. Masseter spasm may be the only initial manifestation of a malignant hyperthermic response. The incidence of masseter spasm in otherwise healthy children is 0.06%. Evaluation of these patients suggests that about 50% are at risk for the development of malignant hyperthermia. Often premature attempts at laryngoscopy before the drug has taken effect will be mistaken as masseter spasm.

Mivacurium

This short-acting nondepolarizing blocker is metabolized rapidly by plasma cholinesterase (i.e., at 70% of the rate of succinylcholine). After a dose of 0.25 to 0.3 mg/kg, mivacurium provides positive intubation conditions within 90 seconds that last about 10 minutes. Complete spontaneous recovery of neuromuscular function occurs by 13 minutes. If a "priming dose" of 0.02 mg/kg is administered 2 minutes before intubation, the onset of action is decreased to 75 seconds, but the duration is increased to 15 to 20 minutes. Similarly, rocuronium may produce paralysis within 60 to 75 seconds if given in high doses (0.6–1.0 mg/kg). When mivacurium is administered in large doses ($\geq$ 0.3 mg/kg) or by rapid injection, histamine release can produce cutaneous flushing and a transient decrease in blood pressure.

RAPID SEQUENCE INTUBATION

The majority of pediatric patients who require intubation are at risk for pulmonary aspiration. Scenarios in which patients are considered to have a full stomach are listed in Table 2.8.

Intubation in these patients is accomplished under "awake" conditions to preserve pharyngolaryngeal reflexes as described previously or by a rapid

Table 2.8
Risk Factors for Pulmonary Aspiration Syndrome

- Recent oral intake
- Delayed gastric emptying from pain, ascites, peritonitis, diabetes mellitus
- Swallowed blood from orofacial trauma
- Increased intraabdominal pressure from abdominal mass
- Abnormal lower esophageal tone: pregnancy, connective tissue diseases
- Gastroesophageal reflux
- Altered level of consciousness

sequence infusion of medications and using cricoid pressure. "Rapid sequence" refers to the brief period of time between infusion of medicines, loss of airway reflexes, and ideal intubating conditions. The risk of passive regurgitation of gastric contents can be reduced significantly with the application of cricoid pressure, which occludes the esophagus.

Personnel and Equipment

Strict adherence to all the steps in the rapid sequence induction, as well as a running intravenous line and the availability of an assistant, are mandatory. All equipment must be within an arm's reach and checked (again) just before the induction. Two suction setups must be available and set to maximal settings. A pulse oximeter is invaluable during a rapid sequence intubation.

Technique

During a rapid sequence intubation, the patient is preoxygenated and actually denitrogenated for 2 to 3 minutes, breathing 100% oxygen through a tight-fitting mask. The patient's head is placed in the optimal sniffing position. The assistant applies cricoid pressure. A defasciculating dose of a nondepolarizer may be administered; it is our practice to use a defasciculating dose only in patients with intracranial hypertension or a ruptured globe. If there is any question regarding the intravascular status of the child, a bolus of isotonic fluid is administered at this time. An assistant then administers the medications listed. If rapid oxygen desaturation occurs while awaiting for complete relaxation, **gentle** bag-mask ventilation through cricoid may be used.

When adequate relaxation is achieved, laryngoscopy and intubation are performed. Cricoid pressure is released only after a successful endotracheal intubation is confirmed by the presence of expired CO_2 gas and bilateral breath sounds. A nasogastric or orogastric tube should be placed at this point to decompress the stomach.

Options After Unsuccessful Intubation

Bag-Mask Ventilation

If intubation is unsuccessful, but bag-mask ventilation and oxygenation (pulse oximeter $\geq$ 90%) are effective, the intensivist can reevaluate the patient's airway position and need for alternative laryngoscopic blades and determine why intubation was unsuccessful. The use of short-acting agents affords the ability to perform bag-mask ventilation until the patient's spontaneous respirations resume.

Establish Artificial Airway

If bag-mask ventilation is difficult and the patient is desaturating rapidly, the intensivist may need to establish an emergent airway by needle cricothyrotomy.

Pharmacologic Intervention

Short-acting barbiturates produce a rapid loss of consciousness. They provide suitable amnesia for intubation although myocardial depression and hypotension may result if the patient is hypovolemic or has poor myocardial function. Thiopental lowers both cerebral blood flow and the cerebral metabolic rate for oxygen ($CMRO_2$) and, therefore, is a useful agent for intubation of patients with elevated intracranial pressure.

Reversal of Neuromuscular Blockade

Reversal of nondepolarizing neuromuscular blocking agents is faster if fewer receptors are blocked when reversal agents are given. Agents suitable for reversal include the anticholinesterase drugs neostigmine (0.07 mg/kg, maximum 5 mg) or pyridostigmine (0.2 mg/kg, maximum 10 mg). In addition, an anticholinergic drug, such as atropine (0.02 mg/kg) or glycopyrrolate (0.01 mg/kg,) is given to prevent the muscarinic effects of anticholinesterase agents. The maximum dose given at one time is usually 1 mg for atropine and 10 mg for pyridostigmine.

Antagonism of neuromuscular blockade is more likely to be successful if some return of neuromuscular function is evident in spontaneous movement or movement elicited by a nerve stimulator before injection of reversal agents. Measures of adequate antagonism include:

- Sustained tetanus during nerve stimulation at 50 Hz
- Inspiratory force greater than -25 cm H_2O
- Flexion of arms and legs
- Ability to lift the head for 5 seconds

Neuromuscular block may be prolonged by hypothermia; magnesium, which prohibits prejunctional release of acetylcholine; the streptomycin/neomycin group of antibiotics, which inhibit prejunctional release of acetylcholine and decrease the postjunctional sensitivity to acetylcholine; and polymyxin, tetracycline, and lincomycin antibiotics by an unknown action.

Nasotracheal Intubation

Indications and Contraindications

Nasotracheal intubation provides a more secure airway for a critically ill patient and may be more comfortable. The tape is less prone to disturbance from oral secretions, and the tube is less susceptible to damage and to becoming dislodged. Nevertheless, nasotracheal tube placement is less time efficient and is a technically more difficult skill.

Contraindications to this type of intubation include:

- Fracture of the cribriform plate with cerebrospinal fluid leak, because of the risk of infection and meningitis or intracranial passage of the tube
- Bleeding disorders or the use of anticoagulants, because of the risk of active hemorrhage necessitating nasal packing
- Deformity of the nose, which obstructs passage of the tube

Technique

Nasotracheal intubation can be accomplished using direct laryngoscopy to visualize the glottis and allow the tube to be guided under direct vision. The tube is advanced by pushing at the nasal end and directing the tip with intubating forceps. The forceps should be used only for directing and not for pushing the tube through the vocal cords.

Complications

Placement of a nasotracheal tube is associated with epistaxis, trauma to the adenoids, pressure necrosis of the nares, trauma to the mucosa, posterior dissection of the posterior pharyngeal wall at the area of the sphenoid prominence, obstruction of the Eustachian tube, and possible otitis media or maxillary sinusitis if long-term intubation is used. The overall complication rate from nasotracheal intubation is 8%. Nasal deformities secondary to nasotracheal intubation are more common in very low birth–weight infants (less than 1000 g) and with prolonged intubation of longer than 5 days' duration.

Special Situations Requiring Intubation

The Child with an Open Globe Injury

With penetrating injuries to the eye, vitreous humor can leak from the open globe if intraocular pressure increases, as may occur with coughing, struggling during laryngoscopy, or intubation. It is imperative, therefore, that laryngoscopy and intubation are performed under ideal pharmacologic control.

In the absence of a full stomach and the risks of pulmonary aspiration syndrome, a recommended sequence for intubation would include preoxygenation with 100% oxygen, followed by thiopental and mivacurium (Table 2.9). The ocular hypertensive response to laryngoscopy and intubation may be blunted by using lidocaine 1.5–2.0 mg/kg intravenously.

When the child has a "full stomach," a rapid sequence induction, with either succinylcholine or mivacurium (0.25–0.3 mg/kg) is used. The increase in intraocular pressure associated with succinylcholine appears to be mitigated by adequate doses of an anesthetic agent and a defasciculating dose of a nondepolarizer.

The Child with Elevated Intracranial Pressure

Children with head injuries frequently require establishment of an artificial airway to protect them from aspiration if the level of consciousness is decreased or if their protective cough and gag reflexes are decreased. In children with intracranial hypertension, elective intubation and controlled ventilation are necessary to control arterial PO_2 and PCO_2. Intubation may be difficult. Cervical spine or facial injuries may be present. It is important to evaluate the mouth for loose teeth, blood, and debris and to avoid manipulation of the cervical spine until radiographic evaluation has been completed. If intubation is necessary before that time, axial in-line traction should be applied to stabilize the neck.

Laryngoscopy and intubation have been associated with an increase in intracranial pressure, even in the anesthetized patient. Awake intubation in a conscious or semiconscious child may aggravate an already elevated intracranial pressure with struggling and coughing. Nasotracheal intubation may be contraindicated if basilar skull fracture or nasopharyngeal bleeding is present. If the child has a normal hemodynamic status, sedation and relaxation can be achieved with thiopental and either mivacurium or succinylcholine after pretreatment with a defasciculating dose of a nondepolarizing muscle relaxant (i.e., pancuronium 0.01 mg/kg intravenously) (see Table 2.9). If hypovolemia is present or vital signs are unstable, a smaller dose of thiopental (1–2 mg/kg intravenously) is sufficient. Intravenous lidocaine at 1.5 mg/kg may be used to prevent elevations of intracranial pressure that occur with laryngoscopy and intubation. If the airway anatomy is obscured by orofacial trauma or difficulty with laryngoscopy is anticipated, fiberoptic intubation, a retrograde catheter, or a cricothyrotomy airway as described in the section on the difficult airway may be required.

The Child with Hypovolemia

Determining Intravascular Status Children with airway embarrassment frequently have coexisting hemodynamic instability either from hypo-

Table 2.9
Drugs for Rapid Sequence Induction

Defasciculating dose:	Pancuronium 0.01 mg/kg	
Induction agent:		
Isovolemic	Thiopental	5–7 mg/kg
Head trauma	Thiopental	5–7 mg/kg
Hypovolemia + head trauma	Thiopental	2–3 mg/kg
Asthma	Ketamine	2 mg/kg
Hypovolemia	Ketamine	2 mg/kg
Shock	Ketamine	0.5–1 mg/kg

volemia or cardiac dysfunction secondary to traumatic injury. The intravascular status of the child can be rapidly assessed by performing a "tilt test." While monitoring heart rate and blood pressure, reposition the patient successively in the Trendelenburg, neutral, and then reverse Trendelenburg positions. If the heart rate increase is greater than 10 to 15 beats per minute, hypovolemia is reasonably assured. If possible, fluid therapy to replenish the intravascular volume should be started immediately, coincident with efforts to establish a secure airway.

Pharmacologic Approach Preoxygenation with 100% oxygen is important in patients with hypovolemia and marginal cardiac output. The minimal doses of drugs should be used to achieve adequate intubation conditions without precipitating cardiovascular collapse. If hypovolemia has not been adequately corrected, ketamine followed by a muscle relaxant would be the technique of choice. In the presence of a full stomach as a result of recent oral intake, swallowed blood, ascites, or increased abdominal pressure from intraabdominal bleeding, a rapid sequence technique using cricoid pressure should be used. *Nevertheless, there are certain instances in which the child is so unstable that the only safe approach is to intubate the child without pharmacologic adjuncts.* Care should be taken to avoid the cardiovascular collapse that can be precipitated by the use of excessive airway pressures in the hypovolemic patient.

The Child with Epiglottitis

Acute epiglottitis is a life-threatening acute inflammation of the entire supraglottic region with an extremely rapid clinical course.

Clinical Presentation Typically, the affected child is well until hours before the onset of fever, stridor, and a very painful dysphagia. The child often assumes the classic tripod position: sitting up and forward with the mouth open, drooling. Although some data suggest that the patient with epiglottitis is most likely to be between 2 and 4 years of age, up to 33% of patients may be less than 2 years of age.

Prevalence With licensure of the first polysaccharide-protein conjugate vaccines, the prevalence of epiglottitis has decreased dramatically. Nevertheless, many cases are still attributable to Haemophilus Influenzae type B, as well as *Staphylococcus aureus, Klebsiella,* or *Candida albicans.* Of those children infected with Haemophilus Influenzae type B, 50% have not been immunized.

Case Management Care of a child suspected of having acute epiglottitis is best managed in a collaborative fashion by an experienced otolaryngologist, anesthesiologist, and pediatric intensivist. Radiography plays no role in the evaluation of a patient with epiglottitis, and the value of miniflexible nasopharyngoscopy in the emergency department of these patients remains unclear.

Establishment of an Airway The child is maintained in a calm atmosphere and upright position during evaluation and transported to the operating room as soon as possible. Laying the child down to do unnecessary procedures may result in complete and irreversible airway obstruction. Oxygen administration and pulse-oximetry monitoring are sufficient until the child arrives in the operating room accompanied by all the resources needed to establish a surgical airway should airway obstruction occur.

Anesthetic Technique The type of anesthetic technique used depends on the clinical experience of the physicians in attendance. The most experienced individuals available should direct the management of these difficult cases. The principal considerations in the approach to these patients are outlined in Table 2.10.

The child's anatomy may be so distorted from inflammation and edema that the glottic structures will be unidentifiable. If the child is breathing spontaneously, air bubbles during exhalation will define the glottis, and an endotracheal tube can be introduced through this area. As a result of this extensive edema the glottis will be much smaller than normal; therefore, a wide selection of endotracheal tubes with a small diameter (3.0–4.5 mm) but sufficient length (28 cm) must be available.

Table 2.10
Potential Problems in a Patient with an Airway Obstruction

- Airway edema
- Secretions
- Distorted anatomy
- Hypoxia
- Decreased functional residual capacity
- Dehydration
- Fatigue
- Metabolic Acidosis
- Sepsis: increased oxygen demand, decreased level of consciousness

Intravenous Access We proceed with a slow inhalational induction of anesthesia, initially with the child in the upright position. The ideal moment to place an intravenous catheter continues to be a subject of debate. One school of thought maintains intravenous placement before induction of anesthesia in a child with a critical airway is worth the risk of upsetting the child, but that further airway compromise would be unlikely as long as the child is upright. Another school strongly argues that there is sufficient time to place an intravenous catheter when the child is sufficiently anesthetized.

Endotracheal Tube Placement When the patient is sufficiently anesthetized, a bolus of isotonic fluid is administered. If the laryngoscopist can identify the glottic structures, the endotracheal tube is placed, cultures are obtained, and antibiotics are administered. If glottic structures are not identified and the patient is well saturated, the otolaryngologist can attempt to place a ventilating bronchoscope and establish control of the airway. If this proves impossible, or if severe oxygen desaturation intervenes, the otolaryngologist proceeds with an emergency cricothyrotomy or tracheostomy.

Timing of Extubation After successful airway management, the child is admitted to the pediatric intensive care unit, where he or she is sedated with a minimum amount of benzodiazepine without neuromuscular blockade. Once the child's fever has decreased, evidence for toxicity has abated, intravascular volume has been repleted, and a leak around the endotracheal tube is present, extubation is contemplated. This process usually takes between 12 and 24 hours. Extubation should be performed only when the personnel and equipment are available should acute airway obstruction occur.

Sequelae Approximately 10% of children have some postextubation stridor attributable to the trauma of intubation, which is treated with racemic epinephrine and continued corticosteroids.

Acute pulmonary edema has been described in children with the relief of airway obstruction, such as secondary to an obstructed endotracheal tube, croup, epiglottitis, or laryngospasm. Usually, this postobstructive pulmonary edema manifests itself immediately or within a few hours of the relief of obstruction.

The Child with a Cervical Spine Injury

Conventional management practices include oral intubation after the application of cricoid pressure and manual in-line stabilization. The concern with this approach has been the potential for further exacerbation of neurologic injury during laryngoscopy.

The Child with Down Syndrome

Atlanto-occipital instability occurs in 10 to 20% of patients with Down syndrome who are at risk for atlantoaxial subluxation. To identify patients at risk for subluxation, guidelines have been adapted from the recommendations of the American Academy of Pediatrics and the Special Olympics Inc., which include preoperative neurologic assessments and cervical radiographs in the neutral, flexion, and extension positions. Children with an atlanto-dental interval of greater than 4.5 mm or with peripheral neurologic findings should be further evaluated. In the face of uncertainty and impending airway compromise, it is prudent to treat all children with Trisomy 21 as if they do in fact have atlanto-occipital instability. Our approach to these patients is identical to those with cervical spine injuries.

TRACHEOSTOMY

Indications for tracheostomy include subglottic stenosis, bilateral vocal cord paralysis, congenital airway malformations, airway tumors, and a requirement for prolonged ventilator therapy.

Morbidity and Mortality

A tracheostomy performed in a child has a complication rate ranging from 10 to 33% and a mortality rate of 1 to 3%. The mortality has been significantly reduced as a result of the advancements in the postoperative critical care management of these children. Young children have the highest complication rate.

Early complications of the procedure include subcutaneous emphysema of the neck and face, pneumothorax pneumomediastinum, poor positioning of the tube, postoperative bleeding, self extubation, and thyroid injury.

Early Postoperative Period

Immediate postoperative care of the child with a new tracheostomy involves evaluation of a chest radiograph for air accumulation and tube position. The tracheostomy tube should be tied securely around the neck and the neck protected from irritation. As the normal humidifying mechanisms of the mouth and nose are bypassed, humidified oxygen should be supplied. Airway secretions are frequently increased for 24 to 48 hours, necessitating intensive pulmonary supportive care.

Because tracheostomy tube obstruction is a life-threatening complication in the postoperative period, suction equipment, scissors, tracheal dilators, and replacement tracheostomy tubes should be available at the bedside. Multiple sizes and types of tubes should be available to ensure a tube of the appropriate diameter and length for each patient (Table 2.11).

Tube Patency

If tachypnea, respiratory distress, cyanosis, or decreased breath sounds are observed in a child with a tracheostomy, the tracheostomy tube is assumed

Table 2.11
Suggested Tracheostomy Tube Size

Age	Shiley Tube		Internal Diameter (mm)	Length (mm)
Premature	Neonatal	00	3.1	30
infant	Pediatric	00	3.1	3.9
Newborn	Neonatal	0	3.4	32
	Pediatric	0	3.4	40
Newborn–6 months		1	3.7	41
6–12 months		1–2	3.7–4.1	41–42
12 months–2 years		3	4.8	44
3–6 years		4	5.0	46
7–10 years		4	5.0	46
10–12 years		6 (single cannula tube)	7.0	67

to be obstructed until proven to be patent. This obstruction is common because of increased secretions. The child should be ventilated with 100% oxygen, the head and neck extended to expose the tracheostomy site, and the suction catheter passed. If the suction catheter will not pass, a new tracheostomy tube is inserted through the tract to allow ventilation. If the tract narrows, a smaller cannula or endotracheal tube may be necessary to allow ventilation.

Within the first week of tracheostomy creation, the tract has not had an opportunity to epithelize. As such, this tract may not be readily identifiable, making reintubation through the stoma difficult. It is for this reason that otolaryngologists place tracheal sutures to assist in reexposing the actual orifice. An assistant should firmly but gently pull these tracheostomy sutures up and away from the midline, reexposing the stoma. If neither an endotracheal tube nor a new tracheostomy tube will pass, an oxygen catheter with a high flow should be passed into the tract to allow oxygenation in the spontaneously breathing patient. If assisted ventilation is needed for a child on ventilator support, the stoma should be covered with a gauze pad and the patient ventilated by a face mask.

As the tracheostomy tract matures later in the first postoperative week, the first tracheostomy tube change is usually performed by the otolaryngologist in the intensive care unit. Other equipment necessary for tracheostomy tube change is noted in Table 2.12.

Late Complications

Tracheitis, skin ulceration, wound infection, aspiration, accidental decannulation, and tracheal granulations are common. Innominate artery

Table 2.12
Equipment Available for Tracheostomy Tube Change

- Suction—source, catheters
- Oxygen—source, bag
- Tracheostomy tubes—appropriate sizes
- Laryngoscope—blade, handle, bulb, battery
- Endotracheal tubes—appropriate sizes
- Tracheal dilator and wound retractors
- Ties—to secure tube
- Mask—for ventilation with stoma covered if unable to replace tracheostomy tube

erosion secondary to the tip of the tracheostomy tube may also occur. If sudden, rapid bleeding from the lumen of the tracheostomy tube occurs, a cuffed tube should be passed beyond the vessel erosion and the cuff inflated to prevent blood aspiration to the remainder of the tracheobronchial tree.

SUPPORT OF THE PATIENT WITH AN ARTIFICIAL AIRWAY

Endotracheal intubation bypasses several functions of the upper airway, including warming and humidification. These functions are replaced by warming and humidifying the oxygen supplied to the artificial airway. As the artificial airway also interferes with ciliary action and tracheal mucous flow, it is important to change the child's position to mobilize secretions and to suction frequently for secretions. Saline instillation may be necessary to suspend secretions.

EXTUBATION

Extubation is attempted when the indications for intubation have resolved. The criteria for extubation are outlined in Table 2.13.

Table 2.13
Criteria for Extubation

- Intact cough and gag
- Negative inspiratory force of 25 to 50 cm H_2O
- Forced vital capacity breath in excess of 15 mL/kg
- Air leak around the tube at inflating pressures <25 cm H_2O
- Maintenance of acceptable oxygenation and ventilation on minimal ventilatory support
- Adequate antagonism of neuromuscular blockade, demonstrated by sustained head lift or, in an infant, leg lift

Preparation

Feedings are withheld and sedation is weaned so that the risks of pulmonary aspiration and upper airway obstruction are minimized. During the final preparation for extubation the FiO_2 should be increased to 1.00 to minimize the risk of postextubation hypoxemia. All personnel and equipment necessary for reintubation must be immediately available at the bedside should the child's airway compromise recur.

Procedure

The oropharynx should be suctioned and cleared of secretions. If a cuffed endotracheal tube is present, the cuff is deflated as indicated by collapse of the pilot balloon. Oxygen is applied by mask or hood after extubation. Chest physical therapy is continued because ciliary function is often ineffective secondary to the mucosal changes resulting from intubation.

Immediate Complications

Pulmonary aspiration, laryngospasm, bronchospasm, and postextubation croup should be anticipated and the appropriate therapies be immediately available.

Laryngospasm

Laryngospasm results from the stimulus of extubation or residual secretions draining onto the epiglottis and vocal cords. Most commonly, laryngospasm occurs in patients who are in a "light" stage of sedation and is usually characterized by high-pitched sounds ("crowing"). The incidence of laryngospasm is reduced by ensuring the adequate recovery of upper airway reflexes and minimizing the presence of oral secretions at the moment of extubation. Under most circumstances laryngospasm can be successfully treated with gentle positive end-expiratory pressure of 5 to 10 cm H_2O delivered by bag-mask ventilation. Should precipitous desaturations occur, succinylcholine is given to facilitate effective bag-mask ventilation. Aspiration may also occur because of ineffective cough and upper airway reflexes.

Postextubation Croup

Postextubation croup occurs in 1 to 6% of pediatric patients and more commonly in children between 1 to 4 years of age. Hoarseness, stridor, and croupy cough, with or without inspiratory retraction, begin immediately to 3 hours after extubation and peak at 8 hours. These symptoms usually resolve by 24 hours, although residual hoarseness may persist for up to 72 hours.

Children are at an increased risk for the development of postextubation croup if there is an excessive air leak ($\geq$ 30 cm H_2O), excessive movement and coughing with an endotracheal tube in place, and after neck surgery. No relationship has been noted between the occurrence of postextubation croup and the use of lubricant on the tube, tracheal analgesic spray, humidification, or a history of upper respiratory infection.

Treatment of postextubation croup includes cool mist or humidified oxygen, racemic epinephrine, and corticosteroids. The action of racemic epinephrine is unclear but may be related to topical vasoconstriction. The efficacy of corticosteroids in the prevention and treatment of postextubation croup has not been resolved. Edema resulting from endotracheal intubation in animals has been reported to decrease after use of dexamethasone. It has also been suggested that clinical improvement occurs in children treated with steroids. Use of a helium-oxygen gas mixture by mask or headbox may also allow decreased respiratory work, because the low-density helium allows increased airflow through the narrowed airway. This may provide additional time for resolution of edema without requiring replacement of an artificial airway for respiratory distress.

3.

Lower Airway Disease: Bronchiolitis and Asthma

Mark A. Helfaer, David G. Nichols, and Mark C. Rogers

BRONCHIOLITIS

A number of different viral pathogens cause bronchiolitis and bronchiolitis-like illnesses. Respiratory syncytial virus (RSV) accounts for most cases of bronchiolitis in which a specific agent can be identified. It is estimated that in 40 to 75% of infants admitted to hospitals with bronchiolitis, RSV is the cause. Other viruses that cause bronchiolitis are rhinovirus; parainfluenza virus type 3; adenovirus types 3, 7, and 21 influenza virus; and, occasionally, mumps. Although *Mycoplasma pneumoniae* is usually associated with lower respiratory tract disease in older children, it rarely causes bronchiolitis in infants.

Transmission of Respiratory Syncytial Virus

RSV epidemics occur each winter and parainfluenza virus outbreaks occur in the fall. The disease is highly contagious. Once the virus is introduced in a day-care setting, virtually all exposed children (98%) become infected. Transmission of RSV within families is also significant, with 46% of the other family members becoming infected when one family member has acquired the disease.

The rate of nosocomial spread is also high. During a community outbreak of RSV infections, 45% of previously uninfected hospitalized infants became ill with RSV respiratory disease. The risk of infection increased with length of hospital stay. Hospital staff members are probably the major carrier source during nosocomial spread of RSV infection through contamination with secretions from infected infants. The hospital staff suffers approximately the same attack rate (42%) as do infants.

Clinical Manifestations

The affected infant is typically infected by exposure to an older child or an adult with an upper respiratory infection. Cough, sneeze, and rhinorrhea develop initially. Subsequent respiratory distress is characterized by tachypnea, flaring of alae nasi, chest wall retractions, wheezing, and irritability. A low-grade fever may be present, and marked dyspnea can make feeding difficult. During breathing, thoracoabdominal asynchrony correlates with the degree of airflow obstruction. The lungs are hyperinflated and the liver may be palpable several fingerbreadths below the costal margin. Auscultation of the lungs reveals diffuse wheezes, prolonged expiration, and rales.

Diagnostic Findings

Radiography

Radiologic examination of infants with acute bronchiolitis demonstrates air trapping in most patients (Fig. 3.1). About half the patients will have evidence of peribronchial thickening. Consolidation and collapse are seen less commonly on chest x-rays. Bacterial pneumonia cannot be excluded on radiologic grounds alone, however, which necessitates bacterial cultures.

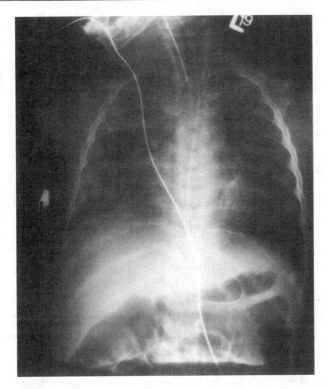

Figure 3.1. Chest x-ray of infant with bronchiolitis and respiratory failure, showing air trapping and peribronchial thickening.

Laboratory Tests

The complete blood count is generally normal. RSV may be identified by complement fixation or indirect immunofluorescent antibody testing on nasal wash specimens as well as culture of the organism.

Arterial blood gas measurements are necessary to make the diagnosis of respiratory failure in bronchiolitis. Based on a series of 32 infants with RSV bronchiolitis, Hall et al. concluded that all infants were hypoxemic, with a mean oxygen saturation of 87%. Hypoxemia was persistent, lasting 3 to 7 weeks, even after clinical improvement had occurred. Approximately one-third of patients develop "acute" or "impending" respiratory failure based on a P_aCO_2 of 65 mm Hg or higher. Acid-base analysis reveals a severe uncompensated respiratory acidosis in the group with respiratory failure.

Pulmonary Function Studies

The results of these studies follow predictably from the small airway obstruction and hyperinflation in bronchiolitis. The thoracic volume at end expiration is increased almost twofold above normal. Most studies demonstrate an increase in inspiratory and expiratory resistance, the expiratory resistance to a greater extent.

Most infants, in spite of an increased physiologic dead space:tidal volume ratio ($V_D:V_T$), are able to maintain normocarbia by increasing minute expired ventilation (V_E) significantly. Hypercarbia and respiratory failure develop when the infant becomes fatigued and minute V_E falls to predicted basal levels. The high V_E is due mainly to the increased respiratory rate, while tidal volume is unchanged or somewhat lower than normal. Respiratory muscle fatigue is not surprising, considering the infant may increase work of breathing up to sixfold during acute bronchiolitis. Apnea in RSV bronchiolitis is not because of upper airway obstruction but rather to a complete absence of respiratory effort.

Management and Treatment

The infant with acute bronchiolitis and respiratory distress should be hospitalized, particularly if the infant's age is less than 6 months, respiratory rate is elevated, or there is a history of chronic cardiorespiratory disease. Admission to the pediatric intensive care unit (PICU) is warranted for younger infants and particularly for those showing signs of impending respiratory failure. If the high risk of nosocomial spread of the disease is taken into consideration, these infants should be cohorted, and staff members involved in their care should employ strict hand-washing procedures.

Prematurely born infants less than 3 months postnatal age are at increased risk for RSV-associated apnea, particularly if they have a history of apnea of prematurity. These patients, therefore, should receive cardiorespiratory monitoring when admitted to the hospital. Agitation of the child should alert the clinician to the possibility of hypoxia; an oxygen saturation monitor or an arterial blood gas should be used. The use of sedation in these infants should be discouraged and reserved for the most difficult cases. Sedation not only will mask the signs of hypoxia, but also will depress respirations and worsen ventilation and oxygenation. Even chloral hydrate, often touted as a drug with minimal respiratory effects, will decrease the oxygen saturations of wheezy infants.

Supplemental Oxygen

Because hypoxemia is the most common abnormality detected on arterial blood gas analysis, supplemental oxygen administration is the mainstay of therapy. Oxygen may be conveniently administered in a croup tent; however, there is no evidence indicating that a mist tent is more beneficial than normally humidified supplemental oxygen alone.

Bronchodilators

Because expiratory resistance in particular is increased in bronchiolitis, aerosolized isoproterenol and salbutamol have been tried as bronchodilators. Nebulized albuterol (0.015 mg/kg) results in modest symptomatic improvement in infants with bronchiolitis, although the safety of its continuous use is controversial. In one study in a PICU, there were no electrocardiogram changes or dysrhythmias during this therapy. However, three of the 16 patients demonstrated elevation of creatinine kinase and two patients demonstrated elevated levels of creatine kinase-myoglobin.

Racemic epinephrine (0.1 mL/kg) was found to be superior to salbutamol in the treatment of infants having their first episode of acute bronchiolitis. Even intubated patients with bronchiolitis benefit from aerosolized β_2-agonists. Ipratropium bromide, an aerosolized anticholinergic agent, has not been demonstrated to be helpful in managing a wheezy infant.

Although statistics fail to demonstrate a compelling effect of bronchodilators, it seems reasonable to administer these agents on a trial basis to individual patients with bronchiolitis and gauge the clinical response.

Corticosteroids

Although statistics demonstrate steroids' lack of efficacy in bronchiolitis, careful evaluation of the response of individual patients shows that some patients do indeed respond favorably to steroids. Nebulized beclomethasone, of questionable benefit in the acute illness, may have salutary effects long after an attack of bronchiolitis.

Ribavirin

Antiviral chemotherapy with ribavirin aerosol, a nucleoside analog, has shown minimal success in clinical trials. The Centers for Disease Control and Prevention, however, recommend that health care workers who are or may be pregnant be advised of the potential risks of exposure during direct patient care. The place of ribavirin in the therapeutic approach to RSV infection, therefore, remains controversial. The American Academy of Pediatrics Committee on Infectious Diseases recommends consideration of ribavirin in RSV-infected infants (Table 3.1).

Immunoglobulin

The use of RSV immunoglobulin at high doses (500 to 750 mg/kg) has demonstrated promise. It has been used to prevent RSV in patients at risk

Table 3.1
American Academy Recommendations for Consideration
of Treatment with Ribavirin*[a]*

The intent of the new recommendations is to allow practitioners to decide whether
ribavirin therapy is appropriate by taking into account the particular clinical situation and
their own preferences.

Recommendations may be modified as new information becomes available. Ribavirin
aerosal therapy may be considered in the following list of selected infants and young
children at high risk for serious respiratory syncytial virus (RSV) disease.

- Those with complicated congenital heart disease (including pulmonary hypertension) and
  those with bronchopulmonary dysplasia, cystic fibrosis, and other chronic lung disease.
  Previously healthy premature infants ($\leq$ 37 weeks' gestational age) and those younger
  than 6 weeks of age are also at greater risk for severe RSV illness, but less so than
  patients with underlying disease.
- Those with underlying immunosuppressive diseases or undergoing therapy (e.g., those
  with acquired immunodeficiency syndrome, severe combined immunodeficiency
  disease, or organ transplantation) who have high mortality and/or prolonged RSV illness.
- Those who are severely ill with or without mechanical ventilation. Because severity of
  illness is often difficult to judge clinically in infants with RSV infection, useful guidelines
  include blood gas measurements and the infant's response to other therapies.
- Hospitalized patients who may be at increased risk of progressing from a mild to a more
  complicated course because they are younger than 6 weeks or have an underlying
  condition, such as multiple congenital anomalies or certain neurologic or metabolic
  disease (e.g., cerebral palsy or myasthenia gravis).

*[a]From Committee on Infectious Diseases. Reassessment of the indications for ribavirin therapy in respiratory syn-
cytial virus infections. Pediatrics 1996;97(1):137–140.*

for this disease, including premature infants less than 6 months of age with
bronchopulmonary dysplasia. The role in congenital heart disease remains
extremely controversial and may contribute to increased morbidity and
mortality in these patients.

Positive Pressure Ventilation

When the PCO_2 rises above the normal 40 to 45 torr in a patient with tachypnea and respiratory distress, impending respiratory failure exists. Most infants with bronchiolitis do not require intubation. If endotracheal intubation is necessary, attention should be directed to the size of the endotracheal
tube. Many premature infants are at risk for or have preexisting subglottic
narrowing that dictates the need for a smaller endotracheal tube than that
predicted solely on the child's age.

Symptoms such as lethargy, increasing respiratory distress, apneic spells,
or cyanosis all point to the need for mechanical ventilation. In general,
when the PCO_2 reaches 60 to 65 torr, frank respiratory failure has occurred
and positive pressure ventilation is instituted.

Although mechanical ventilation remains standard therapy for respiratory failure in most centers, nasal continuous positive airway pressure

may be successful in managing these patients. When the patient is mechanically ventilated, however, positive-end expiratory pressure (0, 3, 6, or 9 cm H_2O) contributes to air trapping and does not improve pulmonary mechanics.

High-Frequency Oscillatory Ventilation

When significant hypoxemia persists despite maximum conventional treatment methods, high-frequency oscillatory ventilation can be attempted. Extracorporeal membrane oxygenation also has been instituted with some success. This highly aggressive therapy should be reserved for those patients whose underlying lung disease is mild enough to allow full recovery from their acute bronchiolitic illness. Inhaled nitric oxide also has been attempted with some success.

Fluid Management

Infants with bronchiolitis are in the state of hypervolemia because of elevated antidiuretic hormone levels; yet, they also have elevated renin levels that lead to secondary hyperaldosteronism. Clinically, these infants typically display weight gain and diminished urine output, but a normal urine sodium level. Reversal of some of the hypervolemia, which decreases lung water, can be accomplished by judicious use of diuretics or careful fluid restriction after pre-existing fluid deficits have been repleted. Fluid administration must be tightly controlled to ensure euvolemia without risking overhydration, especially in patients diagnosed with impending respiratory failure.

Monitoring

Respiratory failure from bronchiolitis usually resolves within 48 to 72 hours. Nevertheless, meticulous surveillance of vital signs, sensorium, breathing pattern, skin color, fluid intake and output, heart rate, and respiratory rate—particularly in view of the high incidence of apnea in the very young or prematurely born infant—is mandatory.

Arterial blood gas value remains the standard means of measuring oxygenation and ventilation. Pulse oximetry offers a noninvasive means of measurement. In patients who have been intubated, end-tidal carbon dioxide is measured by placement of an infrared sensor directly between the endotracheal tube and gas delivery tubing or, alternatively, by inserting a catheter proximal to the endotracheal tube that conveys the sampled gas to the analyzer. Accurate measurement requires the absence of leaks from the tubing and endotracheal tube so that the exhaled CO_2 may reach a true plateau at end expiration. If this condition is met and there is normal pulmonary perfusion, the end-tidal carbon dioxide closely reflects arterial PCO_2. Central venous and pulmonary artery catheter placements are generally unnecessary in these patients with respiratory failure, because the critical phase of the disease is not associated with major hemodynamic changes.

ASTHMA

Asthma is the most common chronic disease of childhood; it is a leading cause of school absence, is a common cause for hospital and intensive care admission of older infants and children, and is associated with significant morbidity and mortality from its complications.

Disease Course and Progression

A history of recurrent attacks with a relatively symptom-free period in between is the hallmark of asthma. Pulmonary function studies during asymptomatic periods usually show signs of improvement, although some abnormalities still may persist. The asthmatic episodes may be progressive and may result in an impairment of respiratory function ranging from a moderate degree of disability to life-threatening respiratory failure. Asthma is reversible, however, and appropriate intensive management minimizes associated morbidity and mortality.

Risk Factors for Fatal Asthma

Factors that identify patients at greatest risk of fatality are young men, severe mixed acidosis with extreme hypercapnia (P_aCO_2 97 ± 31 mm Hg), and a silent chest on admission. In children, risk factors include greater frequency of respiratory failure requiring intubation, a decrease in steroid use in the month before the attack, failure to vomit with initial therapy, a history of family disturbances, and abnormal reaction to separation or losses expressed as helplessness and despair.

Characteristic Pathophysiologic Findings

The diffuse, obstructive pulmonary disease of asthma is characterized by airway inflammation and hyperreactivity manifested by difficulty in breathing resulting from generalized narrowing of the airways. The character of this airway obstruction is intermittent and reversible, either spontaneously or as a result of treatment.

Deranged Autonomic Nervous System

It is well known that airway smooth muscle tone is regulated by the autonomic nervous system (Table 3.2). The cholinergic receptor, specifically the M_3 muscarinic receptor, mediates a potent bronchoconstriction. The M_2 muscarinic receptor serves an inhibitory function and decreases the cholinergic outflow to the airway smooth muscle. The M_2 receptor provides im-

Table 3.2
Neurologic Regulation of Airway Smooth Muscle Tone[a]

System	Effect on Airway Smooth Muscle	Airway Innervation	Humoral Receptors
Sympathetic α_1 and α_2	Constrictor	First six generations not significant without β-blockade	Major resistance airways; significance in distal airway unknown; causes bronchoconstriction after β-blockade
β_2	Dilator	First six generations	All airway smooth muscle; causes substantial bronchodilatation after stimulation
Cholinergic vagus nerve	Constrictor	≤ first nine generations; peripheral airways not innervated	All airways
Histamine	H_1 Constrictor	No direct innervation	Released from mast cells; tissue concentration of histamine increases from trachea to periphery
	H_2	May partially inhibit mast cell release of histamine; may have a dilator effect on human airway smooth muscle	
Nonadrenergic (purinergic) Inhibitory	Dilator	Major resistance	Airway

[a]Adapted from Leff A. Pathophysiology of asthmatic bronchoconstriction. Chest 1982;82:13S.

portant feedback inhibition to vagally mediated bronchoconstriction. The loss of M_2 receptor function from viral pneumonia or inhalation of ozone leads to unopposed M_3 stimulation and airway hyperresponsiveness.

On the other hand, stimulation of β-adrenergic receptors on bronchial smooth muscle (β_2-subtype) causes bronchodilatation. Szentivanyi proposed a theory of reduced β-adrenergic responsiveness in asthmatic patients based on animal experiments and other supportive studies.

Airflow Obstruction

Airway Resistance Airway resistance (R_{aw}) is the important component in lung resistance that contributes to airflow obstruction. Lung resistance is composed of airway resistance and tissue resistance. A constant-volume, variable-pressure plethysmograph measures airway resistance at low flow rates (i.e., 1 to 1.5 L/sec) and represents the static or resting airway resistance.

Airway resistance varies inversely with lung volume and airway caliber. Both high lung volume and a decrease in airway diameter are found in asthmatic patients. The increase in airway resistance is related to the severity of the attack and correlates well with the decrease in large airway diameter, but is unrelated to narrowing of the small peripheral airways unless those changes are extensive.

Ventilatory Capacity During Forced Maximal Expiration Standard indices from measuring ventilatory capacity during a forced maximal expiration are forced vital capacity (FVC), forced expiratory volume in 1 second (FEV$_1$), maximum expiratory flow rate (MEFR), maximum midexpiratory flow rate (MMEFR), and the FEV$_1$/FVC ratio. The spirogram is sensitive to dynamic events and is influenced by the resistance of the airways, the elasticity of the lungs and chest wall, the absolute volume of the air in the bronchi, and the cooperation of the patient. The types of alterations seen during an acute asthmatic attack are prolonged forced expiratory time, low FVC, marked depression of the FEV$_1$, and decreased flow rate. The most important factor in determining the early part of the maximum expiratory flow volume curve is the patency of major airways at or near full lung inflation, whereas the subsequent part of the curve reflects the resistance within the peripheral airway (< 2 mm in bronchial diameter).

In acute asthma, the MMEFR demonstrates the most severe fall, followed by MEFR, FEV$_1$, and FVC (Fig. 3.2); after treatment, FEV$_1$, MEFR, and

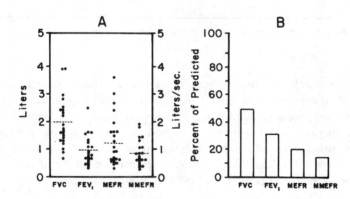

Figure 3.2. Alterations in spirometric measurements seen during acute asthma. (A) Absolute value. (B) Pattern obtained using percentages of normal FEV$_1$. (From McFadden ER Jr. Asthma: Airway dynamics, cardiac function and clinical correlates. In: Middleton E Jr, Reed CE, Ellis EF, eds. Allergy: Principles and practice. St Louis: CV Mosby, 1983:843.)

airway resistance tend to improve initially, while the MMEFR remains markedly depressed for up to 2 weeks after the onset of acute attack.

Peak Expiratory Flow Rate Portable peak flow meters can be used to follow the clinical course of a given asthmatic patient by measuring the peak expiratory flow rate (PEFR). When this value is less than 30 to 50% of predicted or the patient's personal best, a severe asthma attack is present. Extremely dyspneic patients should not be forced to carry out the PEFR maneuver because it may exacerbate bronchospasm in that setting.

Increased Lung Volume

Hyperinflation of the lung as seen on physical examination and x-ray (Fig. 3.3) is a prominent feature of an asthma attack and is responsible for the symptoms of respiratory distress.

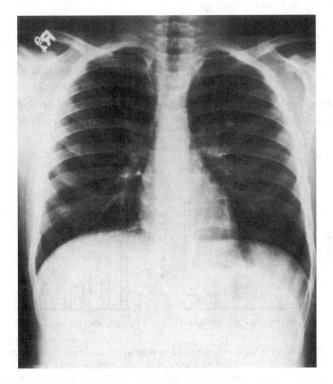

Figure 3.3. A typical chest x-ray of patient with uncomplicated asthma demonstrates hyperaeration of both lung fields.

Indices Residual volume (RV) and functional residual capacity (FRC) are increased during the acute symptoms, with the increase in RV exceeding the change in FRC. Vital capacity, inspiratory capacity, and expiratory reserve volume are all reduced to the same extent. Total lung capacity is variably increased (Fig. 3.4).

Mechanisms of Change Although the mechanisms responsible for the change in lung volume still are not known, it is postulated that the decrease in elastic recoil of the lung secondary to airflow obstruction causes more air to be trapped in the alveoli and alveolar ducts and subsequently causes increases in FRC and RV. In addition, the premature closure of the airway because of bronchial spasm, mucosal edema, and mucous plugging also results in an increase in air trapped within the lungs. In addition, lung compliance is reduced at high lung volumes. These events cause the asthmatic patient to try to overcome the airway obstruction by generating more negative pleural pressures. They also cause the symptoms of respiratory distress and the continued increase in FRC unless the airway obstruction is reversed.

Abnormality in Gas Exchange

Ventilation/Perfusion Mismatch Hypoxia, hypocapnia, and respiratory alkalosis are usually seen early in uncomplicated acute asthma attacks. Nonuniform airway obstruction during an acute asthma attack accounts for the abnormal gas exchange. Simultaneous changes in pulmonary blood flow result from the high intra-alveolar pressure causing the maldistribution in perfusion.

The degree of hypoxemia correlates well with the degree of airway obstruction, as assessed by the reduction in FEV_1. Hypocapnia is caused by alve-

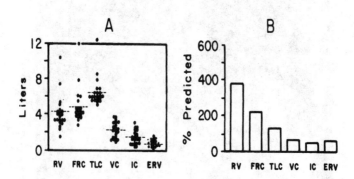

Figure 3.4. Alterations in lung volume seen during acute asthma. (A) Absolute value. (B) Pattern obtained using percentages of normal. *ERV,* expiratory reserve volume; *IC,* inspiratory capacity; *TLC,* total lung capacity; *VC,* vital capacity. (From McFadden ER Jr. Asthma: Airway dynamics, cardiac function and clinical correlates. In: Middleton E Jr, Reed CE, Ellis EF, eds. Allergy: Principles and practice. St Louis: CV Mosby, 1983:843.)

olar hyperventilation secondary to the activation of pulmonary reflexes and does not seem to be well correlated with the degree of airway obstruction. A normal level of P_aCO_2 in the presence of respiratory distress indicates severe airway obstruction, with an inability to eliminate CO_2 sufficiently. Elevated P_aCO_2 normally occurs when the FEV_1 falls below 20% of the predicted value. Some severe asthmatic patients may also exhibit a metabolic acidosis, the etiology of which is unclear.

Types of Intervention Patients with respiratory acidosis with or without metabolic acidosis should be monitored closely in an intensive care unit. Hypercapnia by itself is not necessarily an indication for intubation and mechanical ventilation if the patient is responding to therapy and remains conscious and hemodynamically stable. Conversely, normocapnic patients who are deteriorating rapidly and exhibit hypoxemia, unconsciousness, or hemodynamic instability require immediate intubation and ventilatory support.

Abnormal Cardiovascular Function

Strain placed on the right half of the heart is the product of hypoxic pulmonary vasoconstriction, acidosis, and an elevated lung volume, each of which contributes to an increased pulmonary vascular resistance. Strain placed on the left ventricle results from the increased work required to maintain an elevated cardiac output necessary to deliver oxygen and substrates to the respiratory muscles. Left ventricular strain is exaggerated by the effective increase in afterload imposed with each inspiration by the markedly negative intrathoracic pressures. The combination of an inspiratory leftward shift of the interventricular septum and an increased afterload leads to a reduced left ventricular output with each inspiration. It also produces a subsequent sharp increase during the ensuing expiration, producing the clinical sign of pulsus paradoxus in peripheral arterial blood pressure.

STATUS ASTHMATICUS

In this life-threatening form of asthma, a progressively worsening attack is unresponsive to usual appropriate therapy with β_2-adrenergic drugs and theophylline and leads to pulmonary insufficiency. The term "status asthmaticus" has been given various definitions by different authors.

Clinical Presentation

Cough, dyspnea, and wheezing are the major clinical features of asthma, but the presentation varies with age, from persistent cough at night or during exercise to shortness of breath. In infants, the first asthmatic attack is frequently associated with viral respiratory infection. In older children, attacks are usually preceded by symptoms of upper respiratory tract infection (i.e., runny nose and coughing followed by bronchospasm). Other common precipitating causes include exposure to allergens, cigarette smoke, dust, exercise, and infection.

Physical Findings

During an acute attack, the cough usually sounds tight and generally is nonproductive. The degree of wheezing does not correlate well with the severity of the attacks, but the relative absence of wheezing in the presence of respiratory distress and poor air entry on auscultation of the lungs is indicative of severe obstruction. The use of the accessory muscles of respiration, the presence of pulsus paradoxus, and evidence of cyanosis signify severe compromise of respiratory function.

Diagnosis

Laboratory Tests

The routine complete blood count usually is normal but rarely useful in the assessment of acute asthma. The differential white blood cell count usually shows eosinophilia and leukocytosis. Leukocytosis may be induced by adrenaline, corticosteroid administration, or stress; therefore, elevated white blood cell count alone does not always signify the presence of infection.

Initial urinalysis may show high specific gravity with ketonuria, which indicates dehydration and previous poor intake. These abnormalities should disappear as the treatment begins and the attack resolves.

Nasal secretions usually have a great number of eosinophils, which are sometimes confused with polymorphonuclear cells. The presence of eosinophils in the sputum of a child suggests accompanying nasal allergy, whereas the presence of polymorphonuclear cells and intracellular bacterial organisms suggests associated infection.

Arterial blood gas measurement evaluates the ability of the lung to maintain adequate blood-gas tension and helps to set important guidelines for planning the treatment of the patient. Typical blood gases during an acute uncomplicated asthmatic attack reveal low P_aO_2 and respiratory alkalosis. Hypoxemia is the result of ventilation/perfusion mismatching, whereas low P_aCO_2 is secondary to hyperventilation. A progressive increase in P_aCO_2 is an early warning sign of severe airway obstruction and fatigue of the patient. Hypercapnia and metabolic acidosis in the presence of aggressive medical treatment correlate well with severity of illness and may indicate a need for an artificial airway and mechanical ventilation.

Radiography

Chest radiographs at the time of admission to the PICU help to define the extent of the associated parenchymal disease and any complications and to differentiate other disease entities (e.g., foreign bodies). In uncomplicated asthma, only minor abnormalities are seen, including hyperinflation and peribronchial thickening. Right middle lobe atelectasis is common in young children and may cause a recurrent problem. Small segmental areas of atelectasis are frequently observed during the acute attack and may be misinterpreted as pneumonia. Radiographic examination of the paranasal sinuses is usually indicated for children in whom sinusitis is suspected.

Spirometry

This useful pulmonary function test may not be reliable in very young children and may be too difficult to perform in the older child in severe respiratory distress. PEFR measured with a small hand-held flow meter is easier to obtain and can be used to assess the severity of status asthmaticus because the clinical impression alone frequently is misleading.

When spirometry is accomplished successfully, the measurements obtained are useful in

- assessing the degree of airway obstruction and impairment of gas exchange,
- measuring airway response to allergens and other etiologic agents,
- quantifying airway hyperreactivity,
- determining the acute effect of bronchodilator treatment, and
- evaluating the treatment over the course of the disease.

Abnormal findings include a decrease in FEV_1, a decrease in FVC, and an increase in RV and total lung capacity. The fall in FEV_1 has been shown to correlate well with the degree of airway obstruction and hypoxemia.

Differential Diagnosis

Wheezing is a prominent finding in asthma, but it is not the pathognomonic sign of this disease. Various respiratory tract infections or obstructions, especially in infants and young children, can cause wheezing that may be confused with asthma. Careful history-taking, thorough physical examination, and laboratory tests can differentiate asthma from other disease entities in infants and young children (Table 3.3).

Determining Need for Urgent Care

The following features of a severe acute attack may indicate the need for hospitalization and intensive care:

- History of frequent repeated attacks, previous severe asthma that resulted in hospitalization, excessive daily use of bronchodilator and corticosteroids for control of symptoms, and failure to respond to previous effective therapy
- Use of accessory respiratory muscles

Table 3.3
Differential Diagnosis of Asthma in Infants and Young Children

Congenital malformations
  Laryngotracheomalacia
  Vocal cord paralysis
  Tracheal or bronchial stenosis
  Lobar emphysema
  Lung cysts
  Vascular ring
  Gastroesophageal reflux
Foreign bodies
Infections
  Viruses
  Bacteria
  Fungi
Croup
Acute bronchiolitis
  Respiratory syncytial virus
  Other respiratory viruses (e.g., parainfluenza, influenza)
Bronchitis and asthmatic bronchitis

- Pulsus paradoxus more than 18 mm Hg in teenagers and more than 10 mm Hg in children
- Change in consciousness and/or obvious exhaustion
- Cyanosis
- Pneumothorax and pneumomediastinum
- FEV_1 or PEFR less than 20% predicted value, with little or no response to acute therapy
- Hypoxemia, P_aO_2 less than 60 mm Hg
- Hypercapnia, P_aCO_2 more than 40 mm Hg in the presence of dyspnea and wheezing
- Metabolic acidosis
- Electrocardiographic abnormalities

Treatment Methods

Pharmacotherapy

The pharmacologic agents used to treat acute and severe asthma, as well as the route of administration and dosage, are detailed in Table 3.4.

Mechanical Ventilation

In children who develop rapidly progressive respiratory failure, which leads to coma and death, mechanical ventilation reduces the work of breathing and allows bronchodilator drugs to reverse the basic pathophysiology of status asthmaticus. Because it remains a source of iatrogenic morbidity and

Table 3.4
General Pharmacologic Agents for Treatment of Acute and Severe Asthma in Children

Agent	Parenteral	Aerosol Inhalation
Adrenergic drugs		
Epinephrine hydrochloride	Subcutaneous (1:1000) solution, 1 mg/mL, 0.01 mg/kg/dose (maximum 0.5 mL) every 15–20 min; repeat three times as necessary	Not indicated
Sus-Phrine	Subcutanous (1:200) solutions, 5 mg/mL, 0.005 mL/kg/dose (maximum 0.15 mL) every 6 h	Not indicated
Terbutaline	Subcutaneous (0.05%) solution, 0.5 mg/mL 0.01 mg/kg/dose (maximum 0.25 mg) every 20–30 min for three doses, as necessary	1% solution, 11 mg/mL, 0.03 mL/kg (maximum 1 mL); diluted with 1.5 mL saline every 4–6 h
Albuterol (salbutamol)	Intravenous (0.1%) solution, 1 mg/mL, 0.2 μg/kg/min (maximum 2 μg/kg/min or 10 μg/kg diluted and given over 10 min)	0.5% solution, 5 mg/mL, 0.01–0.03 mL/kg (maximum 1 mL); diluted with 1.5 mL saline every 4–6 hr
Isoproterenol	Intravenous (0.02%) solution, 0.2 mg/mL, 0.05–0.1 μg/kg/min, increase by 0.05–0.1 μg/kg/min every 15–20 min	0.5% solution, 5 mg/mL, 0.01–0.02 mL/kg (maximum 0.5 mL); diluted with 1.5 mL saline every 2–6 h
Isoetharine	Not available	1% solution, 10 mg/mL, 0.01 mL/kg (maximum 0.5 mL); diluted with 1.5 mL saline every 2–6 h
Metaproterenol	Subcutaneous (0.10%) solution, 1.0 mg/mL, 0.01 mL/kg every 20–30 min for three doses, as necessary	5% solution 50 mg/mL, 0.005–0.010 mL/kg (maximum 0.4 mL); diluted with 1.5 mL saline every 4–6 h
Theophylline	Intravenous (aminophylline USP 25 mg aminophylline/mL), loading dose 6–7.5 mg/kg over 20 min by constant infusion pump; modifying loading dose on basis of previous medication history or initial serum theophylline level, or 1 mg/kg for each 2 μg/mL, increased if desired in previous serum theophylline level; continuous infusion (monitor serum levels); <10 kg body weight—0.65 mg/kg/h; <10 kg body weight—0.9 mg/kg/h	No

continued

Table 3.4
General Pharmacologic Agents for Treatment of Acute and Severe Asthma in Children

Agent	Parenteral	Aerosol Inhalation
Anticholinergic drugs		
Atropine		0.03–0.05 mg/kg nebulized
Ipratropium bromide		20–40 μg metered dose every 6 h (>6 y old); 250 μg nebulized (<6 y old)
Corticosteroid drugs		
Hydrocortisone	Intravenous loading dose, 5–7 mg/kg; maintenance, 5 mg/kg every 6 h	No
Methylprednisolone	Intravenous loading dose, 1 mg/kg; maintenance, 0.8 mg/kg every 4–6 h	No
Beclomethasone dipropionate	No	50–100 μg every 6 h inhaler dose; provided 42 μg metered dose
Cromolyn sodium (useful for prevention of attacks)	No	1% solution, 10 mg/mL; 2 mL every 6 h
Leukotriene blockers	Not studied in acute asthma	

mortality, however, mechanical ventilation should be used only when bronchodilator therapy alone has failed to prevent worsening hypercapnia.

Decision to Initiate There are no absolute guidelines for initiating mechanical ventilation in status asthmaticus patients, except in cases of cardiopulmonary arrest and coma. The following criteria, however, should be considered:

- Intubation
- Decrease in respiratory effort because of progressive exhaustion
- Deterioration in mental status
- Absence of breath sounds and wheezing
- Cyanosis in 40% oxygen
- Hypoxemia with P_aO_2 less than 60 torr on 6 liters oxygen per minute
- Hypercapnia with P_aCO_2 over 65 torr and increasing by more than 5 torr/hr

Choice of Ventilator Successful mechanical ventilation for patients with status asthmaticus depends less on the type of ventilator or even on the ventilatory mode than on limiting the risk of lung hyperinflation (volutrauma) and barotrauma.

The appropriate respiratory rate depends on the patient's age and usually ranges from 10/min to 20/min with an inspiratory:expiratory ratio of 1:2 to 1:6. This longer expiratory time usually allows adequate time for expiration and reduces further air trapping in an already hyperinflated lung. An appropriate initial tidal volume is approximately 10 to 15 mL/kg. Subsequent adjustment should be performed on the basis of clinical adequacy of ventilation by chest auscultation and arterial blood gases. An indwelling arterial catheter is essential for frequent blood samples and continuous arterial pressure monitoring. Appropriate bronchodilators and steroids should be continued.

Maintaining Airway Patency Chest physical therapy and frequent suctioning are necessary to keep the patient's airway patent. This procedure can increase bronchospasm, but gentle manipulation and intratracheal administration of 1 mg/kg of lidocaine in 5 to 10 mL of normal saline 5 minutes before suctioning can diminish this bronchospastic response.

Permissive Hypercarbia This principle of ventilator management is also used in the ventilatory management of adult respiratory distress syndrome. In an effort to minimize barotrauma, the peak pressures are minimized by accepting a range of P_aCO_2 in the high 60s. In addition, the goals include maintenance of pH ≥ 7.2 and inflation pressures less than 30 cm H_2O.

Sedation/Muscle Relaxation A sedative and/or a muscle relaxant is required for the frightened and uncooperative patient to promote synchronization of breathing with the ventilator, which will ultimately result in decreased oxygen consumption and less barotrauma. Choice of sedative varies; intravenous diazepam (0.2 to 0.3 mg/kg) is preferred because of its anxiolytic, hypnotic, and amnestic properties. Even though morphine (0.1 to 0.3 mg/kg) is frequently used, it must be administered with caution because of the possibility of worsening bronchospasm from morphine-induced histamine release. The neuromuscular blocker, pancuronium bromide (0.1 mg/kg), is favored over *d*-tubocurarine because the latter also causes histamine release and may aggravate the bronchospasm.

Mode of Administration Initially, the patient should receive controlled ventilation. Subsequent changes can be made based on physiologic and clinical criteria that signify the reversal of bronchospasm. At that point, the volume-cycled respirator can be placed on the intermittent mandatory ventilation mode or pressure support, which facilitates weaning from the respirator. Most children require mechanical ventilation for approximately 24 to 48 hours.

The use of positive end-expiratory pressure (PEEP) is generally not recommended in mechanically ventilated patients with asthma. The reliability and safety of continuous positive airway pressure and PEEP in severe asthma still need further studies before they can be recommended or prohibited.

Monitoring Continuous monitoring during mechanical ventilation is required for assessment of the patient's condition and early detection of complications. Monitoring should include the following:

- Continuous arterial pressure measurement via an indwelling catheter, which permits determination of arterial blood gases and the degree of pulsus paradoxus
- Electrocardiogram, which is helpful in the early detection of cardiotoxic effects of theophylline and isoproterenol (such as ST-T-wave changes)
- Chest radiography after intubation and then daily, and as determined by the clinician when complications are suspected
- Peak inspiratory pressure, which is directly related to increased airway resistance and to the risk of pneumothorax
- Hourly intake and output to keep the patient at near-normal water balance and not overhydrated
- Serum electrolytes, especially in patients receiving steroids

Weaning and Extubation Criteria for weaning status asthmaticus patients from mechanical ventilation should be based on reliable physiologic data and evidence of clinical improvement of reversible airway obstruction. These include:

- Decreased bronchospasm
- Normal arterial blood gases in 40% oxygen
- Inspiratory pressure of less than 30 cm H_2O
- Pulsus paradoxus of less than 10 mm Hg
- Chest radiograph shows reduced hyperaeration with minimal or no atelectasis

When these conditions are present, the effects of sedatives and muscle relaxants are reversed and the patient may be weaned.

Extubation may be considered under the following conditions:

- Arterial blood gases remain stable
- Tidal volume is greater than 5 mL/kg
- Vital capacity is more than 15 mL/kg
- Negative inspiratory pressure is more than −25 cm H_2O
- Patient is alert
- Good cough and gag reflex, which is determined during endotracheal suction or stimulation

The patient should stay in the intensive care unit for at least 24 hours after extubation. If the patient's condition remains stable, he or she can be weaned gradually from the isoproterenol infusion or the nebulized bronchodilator administration and the arterial line may be withdrawn.

Complications Complications associated with positive pressure ventilators in status asthmaticus children include pneumothorax, pneumomediastinum, and subcutaneous emphysema, which is found in 10 to 15% of cases. Such barotrauma is related to the use of high peak inspiratory pressures. The incidence of subglottic stenosis or granulation is approximately 10%, compared with an incidence of postextubation subglottic stenosis in 3 to 5% in children who have been intubated because of other diseases. The mortality rate ranges from 0 to 30%, depending on the period of study.

Halothane

In pediatric and adult patients with status asthmaticus whose condition has failed to improve through other forms of aggressive medical therapy, halothane concentrations of 0.5 to 1.5% and oxygen may produce prompt bronchodilator response, with the rapid improvement in P_aCO_2 and pH within 15 to 20 minutes. After the P_aCO_2 is stabilized and clinical airway obstruction is diminished, as indicated by decreased peak inspiratory pressure or decreased wheezing, halothane inhalation can be discontinued.

Side Effects Side effects associated with use of halothane include:

- Myocardial depression
- Arrhythmia
- Hypotension (secondary to depression of myocardial function)
- Increased ventilation/perfusion mismatching (secondary to inhibition of hypoxic pulmonary vasoconstriction)
- Impaired macrophage and ciliary function in the bronchial tree (dose related and reversible after cessation of therapy)

Risks versus Benefits The adverse effects of halothane must be considered before it is used. The decision to use halothane should be based on the risks and benefits of this mode of therapy in patients with severe status asthmaticus who are not responding well despite mechanical ventilation and aggressive medical treatment.

The failure of aggressive medical treatment necessitating halothane is rare. A person experienced with halothane administration and continuous monitoring of blood pressure, electrocardiogram, and arterial blood gases is mandatory for the success and safety of this mode of treatment.

Isoflurane

Isoflurane also has been used for its bronchodilatory effects. The most serious adverse effect of isoflurane is hypotension. Unlike halothane, however, this effect is mediated by vasodilatation and is treated with intravenous fluids and phenylephrine infusions. Neither isoflurane nor phenylephrine is arrhythmogenic, however.

Ketamine

Ketamine introduced by continuous infusion (40 µg/kg/min) has been reported to sedate children in the PICU and to contribute favorably to successful treatment of bronchospasm.

Local Anesthetics

Local anesthetics largely can block the reflexes that would otherwise stimulate bronchospasm. This effect has been observed in the trachea, which has prompted many physicians to administer lidocaine before suctioning the endotracheally intubated patient to prevent bronchospasm.

Helium

Helium (60%) in 40% oxygen has been reported to decrease airway pressures and carbon dioxide retention in intubated asthmatic patients because a reduction of gas density leads to less resistance to airflow.

Magnesium

Intravenous magnesium sulfate (0.615 mmol/min for 20 min) in addition to conventional therapy (β-agonists and theophylline) has been reported to improve FEV_1 more than conventional therapy alone in adult asthmatics. The role of magnesium in the treatment of asthmatic children remains to be seen.

4.

Acute Respiratory Distress Syndrome

*James C. Fackler, John H. Arnold, David G. Nichols,
and Mark C. Rogers*

GENERAL CONSIDERATIONS

Introduction

Acute respiratory failure after injury to the alveolar capillary unit may occur after a variety of insults in patients with previously healthy lungs. The severity of the alveolar-capillary injury varies; acute respiratory distress syndrome (ARDS) is the most severe manifestation of such parenchymal injury. The radiographic and histologic pictures are nonspecific, but the pathophysiology of the alveolar-capillary injuries is similar. Given these similarities, ARDS is often a convenient heading under which a wide array of insults leading to alveolar damage and acute respiratory failure are grouped. Terms such as "shock lung," "traumatic wet lung," and "noncardiogenic pulmonary edema" describe a subset of the same pathophysiologic changes. These pathologic changes reflect the limited repertoire of the lung in responding to a variety of insults. Grouping diverse pathophysiologies within the same syndrome, however, complicates the study of underlying mechanisms and possible therapies.

Definition

An expanded definition of ARDS offers a more precise understanding of the pathogenesis and prognosis of the syndrome and includes a three-part notation of an acute or chronic course, severity of lung injury using lung injury score (Table 4.1), and cause or associated event (e.g., aspiration pneumonitis, sepsis).

At an American-European Consensus Conference on ARDS, it was recognized that any definition of ARDS was arbitrary, but ARDS represents a subset of acute lung injury (ALI). ARDS and ALI both require the following characteristics:

- Acute onset of respiratory symptoms
- Frontal chest radiograph with bilateral infiltrates
- No clinical evidence of left atrial hypertension (or pulmonary artery wedge pressure less than 18 mm Hg)

ALI further requires the following:

$$PaO_2/FIO_2 \leq 300 \text{ mm Hg}$$
(regardless of the positive end-expiratory pressure [PEEP] level)

ARDS, as a subset of ALI, requires more severe respiratory failure:

$$PaO_2/FIO_2 \leq 200 \text{ mm Hg (regardless of the PEEP level)}$$

Because ARDS is a clinical syndrome for which no specific marker exists, it is unclear whether the precipitating events are truly causative or are

Table 4.1
Components and Individual Values of the Lung Injury Score[a]

		Value
1. Chest roentgenogram score		
No alveolar consolidation		0
Alveolar consolidation confined to 1 quadrant		1
Alveolar consolidation confined to 2 quadrants		2
Alveolar consolidation confined to 3 quadrants		3
Alveolar consolidation in all 4 quadrants		4
2. Hypoxemia score		
P_aO_2/F_IO_2	>300	0
P_aO_2/F_IO_2	225–299	1
P_aO_2/F_IO_2	175–224	2
P_aO_2/F_IO_2	100–174	3
P_aO_2/F_IO_2	<100	4
3. PEEP score (when ventilated)		
PEEP	>5 cm H_2O	0
PEEP	6–8 cm H_2O	1
PEEP	9–11 cm H_2O	2
PEEP	12–14 cm H_2O	3
PEEP	>15 cm H_2O	4
4. Respiratory system compliance score (when available)		
Compliance	>80 ml/cm H_2O	0
Compliance	60–79 ml/cm H_2O	1
Compliance	40–59 ml/cm H_2O	2
Compliance	20–39 ml/cm H_2O	3
Compliance	<19 ml/cm H_2O	4

The final value is obtained by dividing the aggregate sum by the number of components that were used.

	Score
No lung injury	0
Mild-to-moderate lung injury	0.1–2.5
Severe lung injury (ARDS)	>2.5

[a]P_aO_2/F_IO_2, ratio of arterial oxygen tension to inspired oxygen concentration; PEEP, positive end-expiratory pressure; ARDS, adult respiratory distress syndrome. (From Murray JF, et al. An expanded definition of adult respiratory distress syndrome. Am Rev Respir Dis 1988;138:720–723.)

merely associated phenomena. Shock, sepsis, and drowning are the most common causes of ARDS in pediatric literature.

PATHOPHYSIOLOGY

Dysfunction of the cardiorespiratory system is the major pathophysiologic feature of ARDS and is marked by severe arterial hypoxemia. Biochemical and cellular abnormalities lead to a reduction in lung volumes and the disruption of normal gas exchange, which are factors that culminate in acute respiratory failure and associated cardiovascular disturbances.

Mechanism of Pulmonary Edema

The Starling formula characterizes movement of fluid across the alveolar capillary membrane so that the rate of flow is a function of the filtering properties of the alveolar capillary membrane and the balance of hydrostatic and oncotic forces in pulmonary capillary and interstitium:

$$\dot{Q} = K(P_C - P_{IS}) - \sigma(\pi_{PL} - \pi_{IS})$$

where $\dot{Q}$ equals filtration rate across capillary membrane, K equals filtration coefficient, P_C equals capillary hydrostatic pressure, P_{IS} equals interstitial hydrostatic pressure, σ equals reflection coefficient, π_{PL} equals plasma oncotic pressure, and π_{IS} equals interstitial oncotic pressure.

Diminished Surfactant Activity and Airway Collapse

Surfactant is a surface-active material that lines alveoli and promotes alveolar stability. Its primary chemical constituent is a phospholipid called dipalmitoyl lecithin, which is produced by type II alveolar pneumocytes. The physiologic importance of surfactant is appreciated from the Laplace equation:

$$P = 2T/r$$

In the absence of surfactant, the surface tension (T) would remain constant, despite changes in alveolar size. The result would be that alveoli of small radius (r) would require greater transpulmonary pressure (P) to stay open. Small alveoli would regularly empty into larger ones, leading to the collapse of the smaller alveoli and the overdistention of larger alveoli. This clearly does not happen under normal circumstances because of the presence of surfactant, in which surface tension is proportional to surface area. As the alveolus gets smaller, therefore, surfactant is concentrated over a smaller area, which results in a decrease in surface tension. The alveolus remains inflated at the same transpulmonary pressure.

Phospholipid composition of lung tissue in patients with ARDS is abnormal, with low lecithin:sphingomyelin ratios. Total phospholipid content of the lung in patients with ARDS may be low, remain unchanged, or even increase compared with patients with normal lungs. The phospholipid shows poor surface activity, however.

Lung Volumes and Mechanics

Patients with ARDS consistently exhibit reduced lung volumes, especially a reduction in functional residual capacity (FRC). A low FRC is associated with a large intrapulmonary shunt fraction ($\dot{Q}_S/\dot{Q}_T$) and hypoxemia. Because raising the FRC with PEEP greatly improves arterial oxygen tension, it is assumed that a low FRC reflects closure of many terminal gas-exchanging units and is a major cause of hypoxemia. Measurement of low FRC is fully consistent with the histologic appearance of fluid-filled alveoli, acinar destruction, and alveolar collapse, and with the impairment of surfactant activity.

The lowered lung volumes in ARDS imply a change in the mechanical properties of the diseased lung, which are evident in a plot of transpulmonary distending pressure ($P_{airway} - P_{pleural}$) against lung volume. Under static conditions (i.e., no airflow), a curve is produced with an inspiratory limb and an expiratory limb (Fig. 4.1). Compared with normal individuals, patients with ARDS exhibit several abnormalities:

- The slope of the curve ($\Delta V / \Delta P$) or compliance is flatter, indicating that a greater transpulmonary pressure is required to produce a given lung volume. Patients with ARDS, therefore, have relatively noncompliant, stiff lungs.
- Marked hysteresis occurs (i.e., during inflation of the lung, a much higher transpulmonary pressure is needed to reach a given lung volume than is needed during expiration).
- In normal individuals, the inspiratory and expiratory limbs of the pressure-volume (PV) curves are exponential above FRC and concave at lung volumes less than FRC, the latter due to airway closing. The point on the PV curve where shape changes from concave to exponential is the inflection point (I). Lung volume at this point virtually coincides with the closing volume as determined by xenon-133 or nitrogen washout curves. PV curves of patients with ARDS and pulmonary edema are concave above FRC and have an inflection point at lung volumes greater than FRC.

These data imply that the lung volume at which small dependent airways close (i.e., closing volume) is in the range of tidal breathing in ARDS (Fig. 4.2).

Total respiratory system resistance ($R_{rs,max}$) and elastance (E_{rs}) have

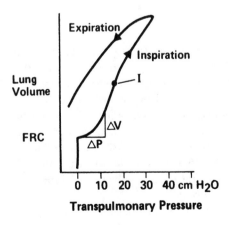

Figure 4.1. Inspiratory and expiratory static pressure (P)-volume (V) curves of the respiratory system in a patient with adult respiratory distress syndrome. Concave portion of the curve lies above the functional residual capacity (FRC); slope of curve ($\Delta V / \Delta P$) is relatively flat at lung volumes in the tidal breathing range. Inflection point (I) is where the PV curve changes from concave to exponential.

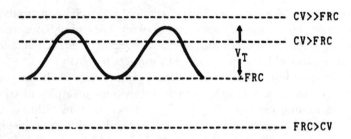

Figure 4.2. Relationship between tidal volumes (V_T), closing volume (CV), and functional residual capacity (FRC) in normal lungs and diseases characterized by low FRC, such as adult respiratory distress syndrome. In normal lungs, FRC is greater than the CV. In lungs with low FRC, the CV is greater than FRC, corresponding to complete atelectasis.

been determined with the end-inflation occlusion method, in which inflation of a relaxed respiratory system is followed by rapid airway occlusion. The postocclusion decline in tracheal pressure until a plateau value is reached allows partitioning of $R_{rs,max}$ into a component caused by airways and tissue-resistance factors ($R_{rs,min}$), and a component caused by mechanical unevenness of the system ($R_{rs,u}$). Patients with ARDS experience increased $R_{rs,max}$ primarily because of increased mechanical unevenness of the respiratory system, which reflects a reduction in distal airway caliber presumably secondary to bronchoconstriction, reduced lung volumes, or peribronchiolar edema accumulation. These data suggest that mechanical ventilation with high inspiratory flow rates may allow more uniform gas distribution and improved gas exchange, which in turn may explain the beneficial effects of such techniques as inverse ratio ventilation in patients with ARDS.

Gas Exchange Abnormalities

Venous Admixture

Arterial hypoxemia with a large venous admixture Q_S/Q_T) and a consistent finding in ARDS could be explained by either V/Q mismatching or right-to-left intrapulmonary shunting. Standard blood gas analysis is usually inadequate to define precisely the cause of arterial hypoxemia in ARDS, because venous admixture Q_S/Q_T) measured at an F_IO_2 of less than 1 may be due to either shunt units or low V/Q units, and 100% O_2 may convert low V/Q units to shunt through absorption atelectasis. More sophisticated techniques used to study gas exchange in ARDS, however, demonstrate that intrapulmonary shunt is clearly the predominant cause of venous admixture, particularly in patients with the most severe ARDS.

Venous admixture in patients with acute respiratory failure changes as a function of F_IO_2. If the inspired oxygen rises to 40%, venous admixture decreases and remains unchanged until the inspired oxygen is 60%. Thereafter, venous admixture increases again as F_IO_2 is raised to 100%. The initial decrease in venous admixture with F_IO_2 up to 40% occurs because the venous admixture contribution from some lung units with low but finite V/Q is eliminated as O_2 tension rises within these low V/Q units. Venous admixture increases again with inspired oxygen concentrations greater than 60%, presumably because denitrogenation of unstable alveoli results in complete collapse.

Inhibition of hypoxic pulmonary vasoconstriction (HPV) is another explanation for the increase in venous admixture with increasing F_IO_2. Regional HPV represents a protective mechanism that directs pulmonary blood away from collapsed or poorly ventilated lungs to well-ventilated lungs and thereby improves V/Q matching. Raising the P_AO_2 in low V/Q units inhibits vasoconstriction of arterioles supplying those segments. Therefore, a fraction of the pulmonary blood bypasses better ventilated segments and the venous admixture increases.

Dead Space

Hypercarbia is seldom found early in the course of ARDS. Hypoxemia and pulmonary reflexes stimulate the patient to hyperventilate, so that PCO_2 is normal or low. After days or weeks, fibrosis and pulmonary capillary obliteration may occur. More segments with elevated V/Q ratio appear, and the $V_D{:}V_T$ ratio increases. If the patient is unable to hyperventilate sufficiently, arterial PCO_2 will rise.

Cardiovascular Alterations

Pulmonary Hemodynamics

Although the initial derangement in ARDS involves increased permeability of the alveolar capillary membrane, increases in pulmonary artery pressure (PAP) and pulmonary vascular resistance (PVR) may occur even during the early phases of ARDS.

Consequences of Pulmonary Hypertension

An increase in PVR from active vasoconstriction or thrombosis in ARDS patients results in a rise in PAP in the face of constant pulmonary blood flow. To maintain pulmonary blood flow at constant levels, the work of the right ventricle must increase although the ability of the right ventricle to augment its stroke work is limited. Right ventricular output begins to fall with increased PVR (i.e., afterload) or with venous return (i.e., preload) limited. At this point, volume loading may fully restore cardiac output by increasing right ventricular end-diastolic volume, which in turn leads to an increase in right ventricular stroke volume, even though ejection fraction remains depressed by increased afterload.

The increase in right ventricular end-diastolic volume is not without cost, however. As the right ventricle dilates, expansion of its free wall is limited by a noncompliant pericardium. Further right ventricular dilatation requires leftward displacement of the interventricular septum. Septal displacement, in turn, decreases the compliance of the left ventricle, so that a given filling pressure corresponds to a smaller, "left ventricular" end-diastolic volume. This phenomenon has been called ventricular interdependence. Septal displacement may be exaggerated by PEEP therapy. Russell et al. suggested that survivors of ARDS have greater ventricular compliance than nonsurvivors because they exhibit greater end-diastolic volumes, stroke volumes, and cardiac indexes than nonsurvivors despite similar right atrial and pulmonary artery occlusion pressures.

CLINICAL MANIFESTATIONS
Physical Findings

The history of the patient with ARDS will vary depending on the inciting event. In some cases, the time of onset and the nature of the previous injury are unknown. Direct or indirect lung injury is usually followed by a latent period in which the patient seems to be in little respiratory distress, except for hyperventilation. Auscultation of the chest may be normal. During the next several hours to days, hypoxemia gradually progresses, and unequivocal respiratory distress becomes evident. The patient appears cyanotic, dyspneic, and tachypneic. Chest examination reveals diffuse rales. Supplemental oxygen through nasal prongs or mask fails to improve the clinical appearance.

Arterial blood gas measurements reveal profound hypoxemia refractory to the use of supplemental oxygen alone. The PO_2 is less than 50 mm Hg on an F_IO_2 of greater than 0.6. The ratio of $P_aO_2:F_IO_2$ is significantly reduced. A $P_aO_2:F_IO_2$ ratio of less than 200 correlates with a Q_S/Q_T of greater than 20%. Other physiologic measurements reveal stiff lungs with decreased total compliance.

Radiographic and Tomographic Findings

The radiographic picture of ARDS is nonspecific immediately after the inciting event. In other words, the chest radiograph may be entirely normal. Subsequently, interstitial and alveolar pulmonary edema without cardiomegaly become apparent (Fig. 4.3). Whereas the chest radiograph may show diffuse pulmonary infiltrates, computerized tomography (CT) scans of the lungs in early ARDS reveal most of the infiltrates in posterior (i.e., de-

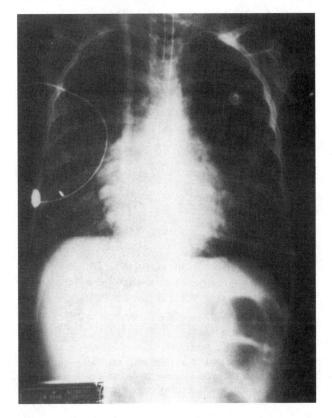

Figure 4.3. Chest radiograph of a patient with early adult respiratory distress syndrome shows mild pulmonary edema with normal heart size.

pendent) regions of the lung. A picture suggestive of diffuse interstitial fibrosis may develop after several days or weeks (Fig. 4.4).

If the patient survives, the complications of mechanical ventilation may be seen radiographically, including pulmonary hyperinflation with interstitial gas, pneumothorax, pneumomediastinum, and subcutaneous emphysema. During convalescence, the appearance of the chest radiograph may return to normal.

MANAGEMENT

Although the inciting event may specifically be treatable, ARDS itself is amenable only to supportive care. For patients with ARDS, a major goal of the physician is to deliver oxygen sufficient to satisfy metabolic demands of tissue. The P_aO_2 alone is potentially misleading in determining the adequacy of oxygen delivered to peripheral tissue.

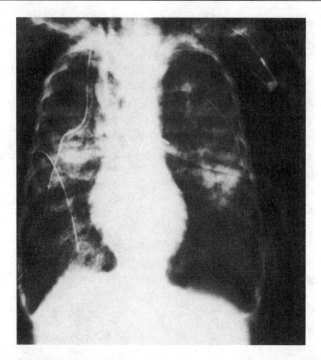

Figure 4.4. Chest radiograph of a patient with late adult respiratory distress syndrome with diffuse interstitial fibrosis and severe barotrauma consisting of pulmonary interstitial emphysema, left pneumothorax, and marked subcutaneous emphysema.

Physiologic Approach

The physician uses the concepts of oxygen delivery (DO_2), consumption, and extraction to treat the patient with ARDS. DO_2 is the product of cardiac output ($\dot{Q}$) and arterial oxygen content (C_aO_2):

$$DO_2 = \dot{Q} \times C_aO_2$$

From this formula, it is apparent that a major therapeutic goal is to optimize C_aO_2 without depressing $\dot{Q}$, so that DO_2 may supply tissue needs.

Oxygen consumption ($\dot{V}O_2$) is the product of the arterial-venous oxygen content difference ($C_{a-v}O_2$) and cardiac output ($\dot{Q}$):

$$\dot{V}O_2 = C_{a-v}O_2 \times \dot{Q}$$

Shoemaker et al. noted that both very high and very low $\dot{V}O_2$ seem to be associated with poor prognosis. These authors strongly support the position that increasing oxygen delivery (i.e., to supraphysiologic levels) decreases mortality.

The ratio of oxygen consumption to oxygen delivery, the oxygen extraction ratio (E), represents that portion of delivered oxygen that has actually been consumed:

$$E = C_{a-v}O_2/C_aO_2$$

The extraction ratio (normal is about 0.25) is a measure of circulatory efficiency, because its value increases when delivery of O_2 is inadequate to meet metabolic demand. Conversely, the extraction ratio is decreased when $\dot{V}O_2$ falls in relation to delivery, such as might be seen with a disturbed microcirculatory pattern in which arterial blood bypasses tissue capillaries while being shunted through arterial channels that are normally closed.

Oxygen Delivery-Consumption Relationship

In the normal individual, O_2 consumption ($\dot{V}O_2$) does not change over a wide range of DO_2 because tissue O_2 extraction is able to rise despite falling DO_2, thus maintaining constant $\dot{V}O_2$. If DO_2 falls to critically low values such that O_2 extraction can no longer compensate for the reduced delivery, $\dot{V}O_2$ falls even in the normal individual (Fig. 4.5). Hence, patients with ARDS may have inadequate tissue oxygenation despite apparently adequate arterial O_2 content and cardiac output.

General conclusions to draw about oxygen delivery and consumption follow:

1. Delivery-dependent oxygen consumption is probably overestimated when the Fick equation is used, but it does exist in some patients with ARDS.
2. Although no direct proof exists that raising oxygen delivery in patients with delivery-dependent oxygen consumption will improve outcome, the observation that survivors had significantly higher oxygen delivery and consumption within the first 24 hours of ARDS argues for therapeutic attempts at raising delivery.
3. No data on delivery-dependent oxygen consumption have been generated in pediatric ARDS.

Oxygen Therapy

All patients with acute respiratory failure require supplemental oxygen, the dose and duration of which must be titrated carefully. Increased inspired concentrations of oxygen denitrogenate the lungs and lead to atelectasis, which in turn worsens right-to-left shunting. This absorption atelectasis cannot be fully prevented by the application of PEEP. Furthermore, prolonged exposure to high inspired concentrations of oxygen is directly toxic to lung tissue.

In the initial stages of the disease process, oxygen may be delivered successfully with nasal prongs or a face mask. Most patients with ARDS deteriorate rapidly to a stage in which an inspired oxygen concentration of up to 50% delivered by a face mask is no longer sufficient to prevent hypoxemia. At that

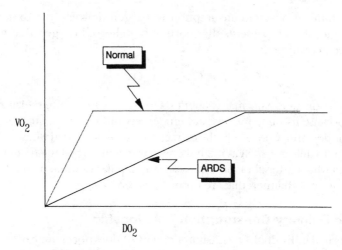

Figure 4.5. Relationship between oxygen delivery (DO$_2$) and oxygen consumption (VO$_2$) in normal individuals and patients with adult respiratory distress syndrome (ARDS). In normal individuals, VO$_2$ is constant over a wide range of delivery and is limited only at very low levels of delivery. Conversely, some ARDS patients have delivery-dependent VO$_2$, in which a linear relationship exists between delivery and consumption over a wide range of oxygen delivery. Hence, limitation of VO$_2$ by inadequate delivery may occur at relatively high levels of delivery.

point, endotracheal intubation by the addition of PEEP usually is required to improve oxygenation but without incurring the risks of oxygen toxicity.

Pulmonary oxygen toxicity can be avoided by using the following guidelines:

1. The lowest F$_I$O$_2$ consistent with adequate tissue oxygenation should be used.
2. Consider the use of PEEP to permit a lower F$_I$O$_2$.
3. Never deny a patient 100% O$_2$ if this is necessary to prevent hypoxemia.

Positive End-Expiratory Pressure

No gas exchange occurs in collapsed or fluid-filled alveoli. To achieve and maintain alveolar patency, transpulmonary distending pressure (P$_{airway}$ − P$_{intrapleural}$) must be raised, particularly at end expiration, when transpulmonary pressure is lowest and alveolar collapse is most likely to occur. The concept of PEEP was applied 60 years ago by Barach et al.

Respiratory Effects

It is rational therapy to attempt to increase the volume of ventilated lung, particularly during expiration, in an effort to improve gas exchange in patients with low FRC.

Increased FRC and Static Compliance PEEP succeeds in increasing FRC and the static compliance of the lung. That is, the end-expiratory point is on a steeper portion of the PV curve such that a given transpulmonary pressure change is associated with a larger increment in volume (Fig. 4.6). Greater increases in PEEP level produce greater increases in compliance to a limit, at which point further PEEP increases lead to a fall in compliance. Presumably, that limit represents the point at which maximal air space recruitment has been achieved and further increases in PEEP merely overdistend already open air spaces.

PEEP lowers Q_S/Q_T and increases P_aO_2 by recruiting terminal airways and alveoli, leading to an increase in FRC and compliance. The PEEP level that accomplishes this goal seems to correspond to the transpulmonary pressure that raises the patient's lung volume above closing volume.

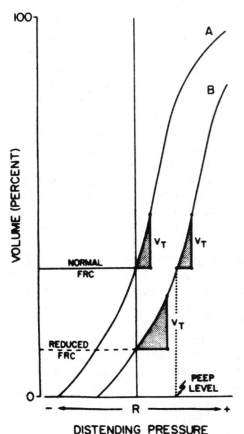

Figure 4.6. Inspiratory static lung compliance curve in normal individuals (A) and patients with adult respiratory distress syndrome (ARDS) (B). PEEP raises the end-expiratory point in ARDS patients to a more favorable position on the compliance curve. V_T, tidal volume. (From Douglas ME, Downs JB. Applied physiology and respiratory care. In: Shoemaker WC, Thompson WL, eds. Critical care state of the art. Fullerton, California: Society of Critical Care Medicine, 1982;3:E15.)

CPAP and Work of Breathing Continuous positive airway pressure (CPAP) allows an additional mechanical benefit. By increasing the CPAP level up to 10 cm and expanding lung volume, the total work of breathing decreases by about half. In contrast, a PEEP system that lacks a high-pressure reservoir bag on the inspiratory limb forces the patient to drop airway pressure below ambient pressure to inspire. Predictably, the large pressure gradient required for inspiration during spontaneous breathing with a PEEP system increases the patient's work of breathing.

Hemodynamic Effects

Improved Oxygenation Because of the pulmonary edema-associated increase in PVR in the gravity-dependent portions of the lung, ARDS causes a redistribution of pulmonary blood flow away from dependent lung regions into nondependent regions. PEEP may lower PVR in the dependent lung, therefore increasing pulmonary blood flow, because increasing lung volume in dependent areas increases the diameter of extra-alveolar vessels. Under these circumstances, PEEP improves $\dot{V}/\dot{Q}$ matching by shifting pulmonary blood flow from nondependent lung regions to dependent regions.

Increased Dead Space PEEP may also increase both anatomic dead space and alveolar dead space. Presumably, anatomic dead space enlarges as positive pressure distends the airways. Conversely, alveolar dead space expands as high PEEP levels (greater than 15 cm H_2O) produce alveolar overdistention and raise alveolar pressure to exceed pulmonary capillary pressure such that pulmonary circulation in the affected lung regions is interrupted. Nevertheless, hypercarbia is seldom seen in patients with ARDS receiving PEEP early in their course because hypoxemia and pulmonary reflexes stimulate hyperventilation such that the increase in total ventilation exceeds the rise in dead space ventilation. If ARDS progresses to a chronic fibrotic stage, dead space increases significantly because of pulmonary vascular obliteration and obstruction.

Decreased Cardiac Output The effects of PEEP on right ventricular function have been the subject of conflicting reports for many years. There is general agreement, however, that the application of PEEP may result in decreased cardiac output, principally because of decreased venous return.

In children with ARDS receiving PEEP, systemic oxygen delivery is maximized at PEEP levels ranging from 0 to 15 cm H_2O. At higher PEEP levels, systemic oxygen delivery falls because the fall in cardiac output exceeds any rise in arterial oxygen content. Volume loading restores cardiac output in patients and experimental animals who receive PEEP. Left ventricular preload is expanded, as measured by an increase in left ventricular end-diastolic area (or volume), despite the presence of PEEP.

Effect on Extravascular Lung Water

Overwhelming evidence indicates that PEEP favors the development of pulmonary edema.

Mechanical Ventilation

Clinical Application

The clinician must decide when to intubate the child with ARDS and whether spontaneous ventilation with PEEP (CPAP) or some form of mechanical ventilation with PEEP is indicated in the context of a complete therapeutic plan (Fig. 4.7). In either case, the optimal PEEP level must be determined.

It has been shown that patients at risk for ARDS do not benefit from early or prophylactic application of PEEP. Therefore, although it is valuable supportive therapy, PEEP will not alter the underlying disease process that led to the development of ARDS.

Endotracheal intubation and application of PEEP are appropriate in the patient with ARDS when the following conditions apply:

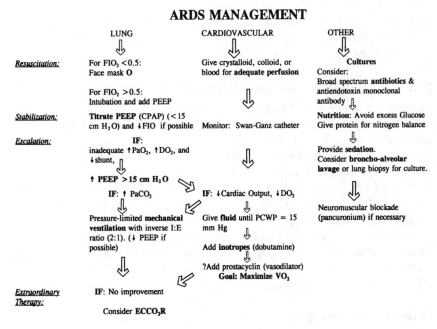

Figure 4.7. Management algorithm for adult respiratory distress syndrome. $ECCO_2R$, extracorporeal CO_2 removal; PCWP, pulmonary capillary wedge pressure; DO_2, oxygen delivery; VO_2, oxygen consumption.

- Clinical and radiographic evidence suggest worsening lung disease
- F_IO_2 of 0.5 by face mask is required to prevent hypoxemia
- Work of breathing has increased as a result of decreasing lung compliance, increasing dead space, and respiratory muscles that are no longer able to increase minute ventilations sufficiently

Inspiratory Modes

Various inspiratory modes may be combined with PEEP. One example is the combination of inspiratory positive pressure ventilation (IPPV) and PEEP, termed controlled positive pressure ventilation (CPPV). Theoretic objections have been raised regarding use of this mode of ventilation. If the patient's arterial PCO_2 is above apneic threshold, he or she will attempt to breathe spontaneously out of phase with ventilator breaths. A frequent result is hyperventilation and alkalemia. In addition, CPPV is associated with a high incidence of barotrauma.

Intermittent mandatory ventilation (IMV) and CPAP allow the patient to breathe spontaneously through the ventilator circuit. The otherwise spontaneous breathing pattern is interrupted by intermittent mechanical breaths. The use of spontaneous ventilation with this mode allows better distribution of gas, which in turn lowers physiologic dead space compared with CPPV. With IMV and CPAP, it is easier to maintain a normal alveolar ventilation ($\dot{V}_A$) and pH. Classically, the frequency of IMV is adjusted so that pH remains between 7.35 and 7.40. The initial tidal volume for IMV may be set at 15 mL/kg.

Pressure Control Inverse Ratio Ventilation (PCIRV)

Pressure-controlled ventilation using an inverse ratio of inspiratory-to-expiratory (I/E) time is instituted by setting a peak inflating pressure limit and lengthening the I/E ratio to 2:1 or 3:1. The inspiratory pattern consists of a square wave pressure pattern with decelerating inspiratory flow. Lung compliance may improve within the first several hours of applying PCIRV, which allows peak inflating pressure and PEEP to be lowered in the face of improved P_aO_2 and unchanged CO_2 elimination. The prolonged inspiratory time results in a rise in mean airway pressure that may improve the stability of alveoli in danger of collapse, which in turn results in better compliance and P_aO_2. The hemodynamic effects of inverse ratio ventilation are similar to those of conventional volume-limited IMV with PEEP.

Permissive Hypercapnea

Efforts to reduce ventilator-induced lung injury have given rise to a reexamination of the acceptable parameters of minute ventilation. Because lower-than-normal systemic oxygen saturations can be accepted if oxygen delivery is preserved, minute ventilation may be minimized as long as P_aCO_2 is balanced by serum bicarbonate levels such that pH is acceptable (the latter possibly being as low as 7.15).

High-Frequency Ventilation

The advantages of high-frequency oscillatory ventilation (HFOV) include (a) smaller phasic volume and pressure change, (b) gas exchange at significantly lower airway pressures, and (c) less depression of endogenous surfactant production.

Typically, an increase of mean airway pressure of 5 to 8 cm H_2O is required when converting from conventional mechanical ventilation to HFOV. Interestingly, despite significant increases in mean airway pressure, hemodynamic compromise as indicated by cardiac index or oxygen delivery does not appear to be an important problem using this "ideal lung volume" strategy. In certain circumstances, such as bronchopleural fistula, high-frequency jet ventilation may have distinct advantages over conventional volume-cycled ventilation or HFOV.

Weaning Process

Weaning from mechanical ventilation may be initiated when the patient is hemodynamically stable; the effects of narcotics, sedatives, and muscle relaxants have dissipated; and clinical, pulmonary function testing, radiologic, and arterial blood gas evidence demonstrates stable or improving lung disease.

The weaning process begins with a stepwise reduction in IMV rate during which normal arterial pH is maintained. F_IO_2 is decreased to nontoxic levels consistent with adequate oxygen delivery. Finally, PEEP is reduced in small increments (e.g., 2 cm) to prevent sudden decreases in FRC or compliance.

Blood and Fluid Therapy

Patients with ARDS have increased metabolic needs and fluid losses from capillary leak and decreased venous return from PEEP. Cardiac index and DO_2 must rise to meet these needs. Ideal blood and fluid therapy for patients with ARDS would allow optimal tissue perfusion without worsening pulmonary edema and intrapulmonary shunt.

Types of Fluid

Colloid

Colloid solutions provide a more sustained increase in plasma volume after administration of a smaller amount of resuscitation solution. It is believed that both colloid and crystalloid may leak into the ARDS patient's pulmonary interstitium; however, the leakage of colloid may depend on its molecular weight. Pentastarch, a hydroxyethyl starch of intermediate molecular weight, may be associated with decreased interstitial edema compared with hetastarch, a nonhomogeneous synthetic colloid with small, large, and very large molecular weight fractions.

Hypertonic Solutions

Hypertonic solutions (i.e., 7.5% saline) have not received widespread acceptance because of mixed study results: some investigators have demonstrated beneficial increases in cardiac output sustained for several hours and others report only transient improvements.

Blood

Volume expansion with blood has clear advantages in ARDS patients who have incurred blood loss or are anemic; DO_2 is improved both by the increased hemoglobin concentration and by the augmented cardiac output. DO_2 per unit of cardiac work expended is greatest when hematocrit is maintained between 40 and 49%. Hematocrit levels in this range may optimize cerebral DO_2 and improve ARDS survival rates. Some researchers have questioned whether cellular aggregates and debris in transfused blood lead to ARDS. However, 40-μm micropore filtration of blood products during massive transfusion does not decrease the incidence or severity of ARDS.

Optimal Expanded Volume

Circulating volume is expanded until cardiac output is optimized without exceeding a pulmonary capillary wedge pressure (PCWP) referenced to an atmosphere of 15 to 18 mm Hg.

It is important to avoid overhydration. Because alveolar-capillary membrane permeability is increased in ARDS, some fraction of administered fluid may leak into the pulmonary interstitium and alveoli, ultimately worsening the intrapulmonary shunt. Cardiac filling pressure is a useful indicator. Also, the risk of excess water retention is heightened because of mechanical ventilation-stimulated antidiuretic hormone secretion, which leads to reabsorption of water in the distal tubule of the kidney.

Monitoring

Hemodynamic Monitoring

Hemodynamic monitoring requires a continuous record of the electrocardiogram. Arterial lines permit beat-to-beat measurement of blood pressure, which may fluctuate widely, secondary to the underlying disease or PEEP therapy. Knowledge of oxygen delivery and consumption, in addition to Q_S/Q_T and P_aO_2, should guide therapy in ARDS and is made available through a pulmonary artery catheter.

Respiratory Monitoring

Respiratory monitoring involves the evaluation of gas exchange and lung mechanics. Arterial blood gas levels form the foundation for monitoring gas exchange. Samples are obtained via an indwelling arterial line. End-tidal CO_2 is analyzed with infrared photometry or mass spectrometry. In the normal lung, end-tidal CO_2 closely approximates arterial PCO_2. When ventilation is poorly matched to perfusion, a gradient develops between end-tidal CO_2 and arterial CO_2. End-tidal CO_2 analysis remains useful as a trend monitor and as an additional ventilator disconnect alarm, however.

Vital capacity and static lung compliance are important measures of lung mechanics in ARDS patients. Vital capacity is determined with a hand-held spirometer. A vital capacity of less than 15 mL/kg suggests inadequate strength to cough and defend the airway. A vital capacity of less than 10 mL/kg suggests incipient CO_2 retention.

Because one of the beneficial effects of PEEP is to increase compliance and decrease work of breathing, compliance is a useful measure to follow.

$$\text{Static compliance} = V_T/(\text{PIP} - \text{PEEP})$$

in which V_T is the tidal volume and PIP equals plateau pressure at end inspiration.

Radiographic Assessment

Chest radiography is indicated:

- When a sudden change occurs in the patient's clinical status
- At least once daily to confirm proper position of the endotracheal tube and pulmonary artery catheter
- To document progression of disease
- After endotracheal tube repositioning

Drug Therapy

Steroids

Steroids do not reverse the pathologic process of ARDS, improve lung function, or increase survival in ARDS. In fact, the use of high-dose steroids for sepsis led to increased mortality in patients with serum creatinine concentrations greater than 2.0 mg/dL.

Vasodilators

Patients who do not survive ARDS exhibit the characteristic hemodynamic pattern of increasing PVR, which ultimately may limit cardiac output. Successful pulmonary vasodilator therapy in ARDS would require that PVR be lowered more than systemic vascular resistance and that vasodilation of pulmonary vasculature occur in well-ventilated lung regions in order to improve $\dot{V}/\dot{Q}$ matching. Most vasodilators, including nitroprusside, hydralazine, the calcium channel blocker diltiazem, and nitroglycerin do not fulfill these requirements, because severe pulmonary hypertension has been associated with high mortality. It has not been demonstrated that treating the pulmonary hypertension effects the clinical course of ARDS.

Many reports suggest that inhaled nitric oxide, an endothelium-derived relaxant factor (EDRF), may effectively lower PAP. Simultaneously, nitric oxide may improve Q_S/Q_T, because this inhaled pulmonary vasodilator is delivered only to well-ventilated parts of the lung. Furthermore, nitric oxide is rapidly inactivated by hemoglobin and hence does not cause systemic vasodilation. Nitric oxide, in theory, may be a bronchodilator. Although blood gases improve with nitric oxide administration, mortality may remain unchanged.

Inotropic Agents

When inotropic agents are needed to augment ventricular contractility (i.e., to maintain cardiac output), dobutamine is the preferred agent because it raises cardiac output without producing significant pulmonary vasoconstriction. Amrinone, a phosphodiesterase inhibitor with cardiovascular effects similar to those of dobutamine, may also be useful in patients with ARDS, although no clinical studies of its use in ARDS have been performed.

Surfactant

A multi-institutional study of almost 500 adults with ARDS did not show diminished mortality when given aerosolized surfactant for up to 5 days. Also, a randomized trial of surfactant in adults with sepsis-associated ARDS did not affect outcome.

Other Supportive Drugs

Underlying infection warrants treatment with appropriate antibiotics. If bronchospasm is present, bronchodilators may be tried. Neuromuscular blockade is a common practice and has been used to promote patient-ventilator synchrony. Although it may seem intuitive that pulmonary compliance is enhanced with neuromuscular blockade, in the presence of sedation sufficient to suppress spontaneous ventilation, paralysis may add nothing. Complications, although rare, may be substantial.

Nutrition

Although nutritional repletion is vital in patients with ARDS just as it is with other critically ill patients, the source of nonprotein calories may have profound effects on respiration. Intake of excessive carbohydrates in the form of hypertonic dextrose may lead to a dramatic increase in CO_2 production and the total body respiratory quotient may rise to 7. Patients with respiratory failure may not be able to increase minute ventilation sufficiently to excrete this excess CO_2 load.

Extracorporeal Membrane Oxygenation

Data from a randomized trial unequivocally demonstrated no benefit from extracorporeal membrance oxygenation (ECMO). Extracorporeal carbon dioxide removal (ECCO$_2$R) showed initial promise, but its benefit could not be reconfirmed. In fact, authors of one study concluded that ECMO should not be offered (outside a clinical trial) for adult patients with ARDS.

It is important to reiterate that the aggregate overall survival of children with ARDS treated with conventional mechanical ventilation and treated with ECMO is identical. There are, however, promising data in some trials of the use of ECMO in this situation.

Liquid Ventilation

Perfluorocarbon liquids have unique features of high solubility for both oxygen and CO_2, low resistance to gas flow, and significant surface tension-reducing properties. Perfluorocarbon-associated gas exchange (PAGE) or partial liquid ventilation uses perfluorocarbon to replace the functional residual capacity of the lung. Subsequent gas exchange is provided by the delivery of gas tidal volumes using a conventional ventilator. This type of therapy remains experimental, and evaluation in controlled trials will determine its utility.

OUTCOME

Death secondary to refractory respiratory failure is relatively rare. The major cause of death among patients with ARDS is either sepsis or failure of other major organs, such as the heart, brain, and liver.

Mortality rates seem to be approximately the same for children and adults; however, the reported series are smaller. The average mortality rate of the five published pediatric series combined is 52%, with a range of 28.5 to 90%. Presumably, better intensive care techniques have led to the gradual reduction in mortality rates, from the initial high of 90% to the more recent mortality rates of 30 to 40%.

COMPLICATIONS
Oxygen Toxicity

In patients with acute respiratory failure, the histology of O_2 toxicity is difficult to distinguish from that of the underlying disease, and, in fact, release of highly toxic oxygen radicals is part of the pathogenesis of ARDS, even in the absence of a hyperoxic environment. Pulmonary oxygen toxicity is a potential complication in patients receiving respiratory support, and lung function may be affected in several ways; therefore, toxicity prevention is a major goal.

Mechanical Ventilator-Induced Lung Injury

Pulmonary barotrauma develops in patients with ARDS as a function of both the lung pathology and the therapeutic use of mechanical ventilation. Gas dissects the mediastinum, producing pneumomediastinum. If the mediastinal pressure continues to increase and decompression does not occur via another route, then the mediastinal parietal pleura is violated and a pneumothorax results.

Pneumothorax should be suspected whenever the patient with ARDS exhibits an unexplained sudden deterioration in clinical appearance, arterial oxygen tension, or hemodynamic stability. Chest radiographs confirm the diagnosis. Successful management of the pneumothorax usually requires closed-chest thoracostomy tube evacuation of air to an underwater seal system, because a continuing leak is virtually inevitable as long as the patient is breathing against positive pressure.

There is an emerging recognition that mechanical ventilation-induced lung injury is related to cyclic volume change.

Multiple Organ Failure Syndrome

Multiple organ failure syndrome (MOFS) is not strictly a complication of ARDS. Rather, ARDS occurs as part of MOFS. Lung failure generally precedes failure of other organ systems, such as the kidney, liver, gut, and brain, although subtle signs of liver and kidney injury already are present by the time ARDS develops.

The initial injury may be associated with decreased perfusion to several organs and the release of mediators known to produce capillary injury. Within 2 to 3 days, capillary leak is evident, and the patient shows signs of hypermetabolism (e.g., hyperglycemia, hyperlactatemia, increased oxygen consumption, elevated urinary urea nitrogen excretion). The clinical picture is reminiscent of that seen in patients with fulminant sepsis, although cultures are negative; hence, the term "sepsis syndrome" has been applied. Frank organ system failure may begin during the next 14 to 21 days with encephalopathy, stress ulceration in the gut, ileus, hyperbilirubinemia, reduced hepatic protein synthesis, azotemia, and oliguria. The chances for survival are remote when four or more organs have failed.

CONDITIONS ASSOCIATED WITH ARDS
Drowning

Drowning accounts for 7000 deaths per year in the United States. Toddlers are at greatest risk. Twelve percent of near-drowning victims do not aspirate water because of laryngospasm or breath-holding after submersion.

Corticosteroids and prophylactic antibiotics are not indicated in the treatment of respiratory failure after near-drowning. If the patient has aspirated stagnant and contaminated water, the risk of bacterial pneumonia is high. It is prudent to obtain daily tracheal cultures so that specific antibiotic therapy can be started at the first sign of infection.

Pulmonary Infiltrates in the Immunosuppressed Host

Impaired host defenses may disturb lung function in infectious and noninfectious ways. Drugs used in treating patients with compromised host defenses may alter pulmonary function. Corticosteroids are immunosuppressive by virtue of their ability to stabilize lysosomal membranes within phagocytes, promote fungal invasion, and retard leukocyte migration. Prolonged use of the alkylating agent busulfan may produce cough, fever, and a potentially fatal diffuse restrictive lung disease. Cyclophosphamide may be associated with a similar fibrotic reaction in the lung. The antimetabolite methotrexate has led to reversible lung disease characterized by cough, fever, and shortness of breath. Five to 10% of patients treated with bleomycin sustain acute dyspnea after several weeks of therapy and exhibit a radiologic picture reminiscent of oxygen toxicity.

Hematologic malignancy is associated with the greatest risk of respiratory failure among all forms of immunosuppression. This problem is ominous for children because acute leukemia represents the most common form of childhood cancer. The appearance of fever and pulmonary infiltrates in a patient with leukemia or lymphoma is accompanied by a high mortality rate, and aggressive management is indicated. Three categories of pulmonary syndromes in this setting, determined on the basis of radiologic appearance, are: diffuse interstitial disease, localized consolidation, and cavitary disease.

Diffuse interstitial lung disease is the most common precursor to acute respiratory failure in the immunosuppressed child. Several studies have identified *Pneumocystis carinii*, a protozoan, as the leading infectious cause.

Graft-versus-host (GVH) disease occurs when a T-cell-deficient patient receives foreign immunocompetent (killer T-cells), such as during bone marrow transplantation or blood transfusion. GVH is a significant risk factor for the development of interstitial pneumonitis and ARDS after bone marrow transplantation. A variety of infectious agents, including cytomegalovirus, *P. carinii*, herpes simplex virus, *Aspergillus*, and *Candida* have been isolated from the lungs of bone marrow transplantation patients with interstitial pneumonitis. However, most cases do not yield an infectious agent and are classified as idiopathic. The combination of cytomegalovirus infection and GVH may, through unknown mechanisms, lead to severe, diffuse interstitial pneumonitis and acute respiratory failure.

Sepsis in the Normal Host

Studies have shown that sepsis is the most frequent event precipitating the development of ARDS. The nonbacterial pathogens associated with ARDS include rickettsiae, mycoplasma, and such viruses as herpes simplex and measles.

Fat Embolism

Fat embolism is a rare cause of ARDS, occurring after long-bone fracture. The classic triad of neurologic dysfunction, respiratory insufficiency, and petechiae after skeletal trauma suggests this diagnosis. Fat embolism remains a clinical diagnosis of exclusion because no readily available laboratory test is sufficiently sensitive and specific to be of value.

In most instances, hypoxemia develops over a 12- to 48-hour period after injury to bone. Other associated laboratory abnormalities in ARDS patients with fat embolism include isolated thrombocytopenia and disseminated intravascular coagulopathy.

Chest Trauma

ARDS may occur after severe blunt chest trauma and bilateral lung contusion. The incidence of acute respiratory failure after chest trauma is 10.7%. Motor vehicle accidents account for the major cause of blunt chest trauma.

"Flail chest" is the most common associated injury in patients with severe lung contusion. This disruption in chest wall integrity occurs when there are three or more double fractures of adjacent ribs or combined sternum and rib fracture. Lung function is further compromised because the flail segment moves inward with inspiration and outward with expiration. Such ineffective, paradoxical movement leads to atelectasis and $\dot{V}/\dot{Q}$ mismatching in the lung beneath the flail segment. Respiratory failure after chest trauma is an ominous sign because it is associated with a 32% mortality rate.

Head Trauma

Permeability pulmonary edema after head trauma and increased intracranial pressure has been described in children. Most investigators of the mechanism of neurogenic pulmonary edema have focused on the massive sympathetic discharge associated with intracranial hypertension. The sympathetic discharge may be attenuated or blocked by central nervous system depressants or α-adrenergic blockers. As a result of this massive sympathetic discharge, intrathoracic vascular pressures rise. Increased pulmonary capillary pressure disrupts pulmonary capillary endothelium, leading to permeability pulmonary edema. Thus, neurogenic pulmonary edema persists, even after vascular pressures have returned to normal.

In this setting, PEEP should be applied with caution because increased intrathoracic pressures may decrease cerebral venous return and lead to increased intracranial pressure. However, if PEEP is required to improve oxygenation, it should be used, and continuous intracranial pressure monitoring should be considered.

Smoke Inhalation and Surface Burns

Smoke inhalation and burns may result in direct thermal injury, chemical pneumonitis, and carbon monoxide poisoning. Inhalation of hot gases (greater than 300°F) injures the upper respiratory tract. The lower respiratory tract is relatively uninvolved because most heat has been dissipated by the time gas reaches the lower airway. Laryngeal edema and airway obstruction may occur. Steam has a higher heat capacity than hot dry air and therefore produces a more serious burn.

Chemical pneumonitis is caused by the various noxious fumes, gases, and soot in smoke. Cilia are paralyzed and mucosal edema develops. By 24 hours after inhalation of smoke, extensive sloughing of necrotic mucosa occurs in the conducting airway. The peribronchial connective tissue space becomes distended with edema fluid. Tracheobronchitis, bronchospasm, and airway compression result.

Acute respiratory failure in the burn victim requires the same supportive respiratory care as in other causes of acute respiratory failure. Endotracheal intubation and application of PEEP may improve oxygenation. In the presence of carbon monoxide poisoning, 100% inspired oxygen concentration should be administered. Overhydration can be avoided by monitoring pulmonary artery wedge pressure with a Swan-Ganz catheter. Prophylactic antibiotics may select resistant organisms and, therefore, are not used. When bronchopneumonia is diagnosed, appropriate antibiotic therapy is begun immediately, pending bacterial culture results. Bronchodilators may be tried if the patient wheezes. Corticosteroids seem to offer no benefit and may, in fact, be detrimental.

5.

Neuromuscular Disease and Respiratory Failure

Donald H. Shaffner

INTRODUCTION

Although the term "respiratory failure" usually implies pulmonary pathology, it also applies to situations characterized by normal lung parenchyma with impaired respiratory pump function. The respiratory pump is the system that brings external gas (i.e., oxygen) into contact with the alveolar membrane for exchange with waste gas (i.e., carbon dioxide) through a common intake/exhaust channel. The gas is moved by a series of muscles that either participate in gas propulsion or maintain patency of the airway through which the gas moves. Both sets of muscles are regulated by controllers that respond to input from sensors and feedback loops and produce output to the muscles. A graphic representation of this "respiratory pump" is provided in Fig. 5.1. Input pertaining to the systemic P_aCO_2, P_aO_2, and pH from the central and peripheral chemoreceptors and regarding the presence of airway irritation and stretch applied to the intercostal muscles is supplied to the respiratory control centers. The cerebral cortex provides voluntary control and the pons and medulla maintain involuntary regulation of the respiratory rhythm. The output from the respiratory control centers is passed through the cranial and peripheral nerves to the muscles that provide airway patency or produce gas movement.

Disorders that affect the neuromuscular system have an impact on ventilatory gas exchange by impairing the central control of breathing, the pa-

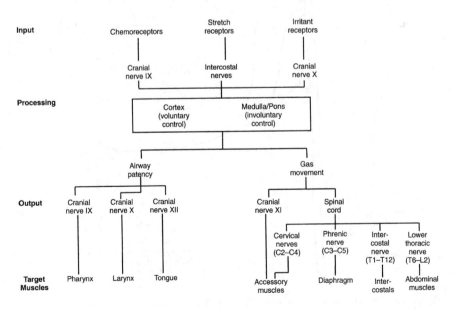

Figure 5.1. Neuromuscular framework of the respiratory system.

tency of the proximal airway, or the effectiveness of the respiratory muscles. Considering neuromuscular diseases from an anatomic perspective is useful when developing a therapeutic approach to respiratory failure associated with these disorders (Fig. 5.2). The five anatomic sites of the neuromuscular framework involved are the brain, spinal cord, peripheral nerves, neuromuscular junction, and muscles. A summary of the major features of various neuromuscular causes of respiratory failure is provided in Table 5.1.

Children with primary neuromuscular disorders frequently suffer res-

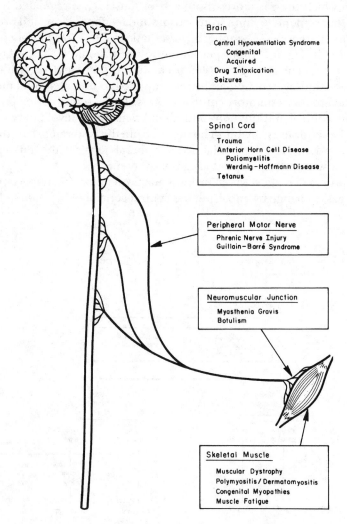

Figure 5.2. Anatomic representation of selected neuromuscular disorders associated with respiratory failure in children.

Table 5.1
Characteristics of Various Neuromuscular Causes of Respiratory Failure[a]

Disease	Prodome	Onset	Presentation	DTRs	Sensory	Autonomic	Lab	EMG/NCV
Cortical lesion (UMN)	Mental status change, headache, seizures	Varies	Contralateral hemiplegia, aphasia	↑	Maybe	Variable	CT scan, EEG	NI
Brainstem lesion (UMN)	Cranial nerve symptoms	Varies	Ipsilateral cranial nerve, contralateral hemiplegia	↑	Maybe	Variable	MR scan	NI
Spinal cord lesion (UMN)	Trauma, back pain	Varies	Quadriplegia/paraplegia	↑	Abnl	Variable	Radiographs, myelogram	NI
Tetanus (spinal cord, UMN)	Contaminated wound	3 days–3 wk	Trismus, muscle spasms	↑	Abnl	No	Culture positive in 1/3 of cases	Abnl
Poliomyelitis (anterior horn cell, LMN, bulbar, cortex)	URI or GI symptoms	1–2 wk	Asymmetric paralysis, may involve bulbar muscles	↓	Abnl	Yes	↑ Protein and cells in CSF, virus in stool and oropharynx	Abnl
Guillain-Barré (peripheral nerve, LMN)	URI or GI symptoms, surgery	1–3 wk	Symmetric ascending paralysis, usually proximal	↓	Abnl	Yes	↑ Protein in CSF, NI CSF cells	Abnl
Infant botulism (NMJ)	Honey, switch from breast-feeding	Days	Ileus, dry mouth, descending paralysis	NI	NI	Yes	Neurotoxin in stool and serum	Abnl
Myasthenia gravis (NMJ)	Exacerbations and remissions	Varies	Proximal weakness, occular findings, fatigability	NI	NI	No	Serum antibody, response to edrophonium (Tensilon)	Abnl
Myopathy (muscle)	May be hereditable	Gradual	Symmetric, proximal weakness	NI	NI	No	↑ Serum, CPK, NI CSF, abnl biopsy	Abnl

[a]DTRs, deep tendon reflexes; EMG/NCV, electromyogram/nerve conduction velocity; UMN, upper motor neuron; CT scan, computed tomography scan; EEG, electroencephalogram; NI, normal; MR scan, magnetic resonance scan; Abnl, abnormal; LMN, lower motor neuron; URI, upper respiratory infection; GI, gastrointestinal; CSF, cerebrospinal fluid; NMJ, neuromuscular junction; and CPK, creatinine phosphokinase.

piratory complications requiring intensive care. Although certain principles of respiratory therapy are applicable in all forms of neuromuscular disease, it is important to consider specific aspects of each disorder to plan individual therapy and anticipate potential complications.

CENTRAL HYPOVENTILATION SYNDROME

Central apnea is a failure of the respiratory control centers to stimulate ventilatory efforts. Obstructive apnea occurs when the airway is blocked and spontaneous respiratory efforts are made that fail to generate respiratory gas flow. Obstructive apnea may be *partial*, with some gas exchange occurring, or *complete*, with no gas exchange occurring. Mixed apnea, as the name implies, has characteristics of both central and obstructive apnea. In the case of mixed apnea, a central apneic episode is usually followed by inspiratory efforts that do not generate respiratory gas flow because of superimposed airway obstruction.

Clinical Features

Central hypoventilation syndrome is characterized by dysfunction of the respiratory centers responsible for the automatic control of breathing during sleep. This syndrome may be congenital, with onset in the perinatal period, or acquired, and associated with any of a variety of diseases.

Congenital Central Hypoventilation Syndrome

Congenital central hypoventilation syndrome usually takes the form of cyanosis at birth and responds readily to mechanical ventilatory support. Frequently, however, weaning the patient from respiratory support results in repeated failure. In less severe cases, abnormalities in the respiratory pattern during sleep are noted and lead to a presumptive diagnosis of an acute life-threatening event.

Acquired Central Hypoventilation Syndrome

In the acquired form of this syndrome, sleep-related respiratory dysrhythmias are seen in association with or following recovery from the underlying disease. Acquired central hypoventilation syndrome can be idiopathic or can occur in association with posterior fossa tumors, encephalitis, severe asphyxia, medullary infarction, the rare syndrome of idiopathic hypothalamic dysfunction, and inborn errors of metabolism (e.g., pyruvate dehydrogenase deficiency).

Structural brain pathology associated with the acquired form is usually related to the underlying central nervous system (CNS) disease. By contrast, the congenital form frequently shows variable degrees of destructive changes in the brainstem that are presumably developmental in origin.

Central hypoventilation syndrome must be differentiated from reversible disorders that can be associated with apnea or hypoventilation. Reversible systemic processes include sepsis, hypothermia, electrolyte abnormalities, hypocalcemia, hypoglycemia, and seizures.

Management
Pharmacologic Agents

Pharmacologic agents have been used to try to stimulate the respiratory control centers to prevent hypoventilation. Agents directed at stimulating medullary respiratory center (i.e., caffeine, theophylline, amphetamines, progesterone, doxapram) have mixed results, with salutary effects of theophylline and progesterone reported. Intravenous doxapram has improved respiratory drive in some cases, although severe gastrointestinal side effects also have been reported.

Phrenic Nerve Pacing

Phrenic nerve stimulation has been attempted to bypass the control centers because the distal neuromuscular framework is intact. Radiofrequency bilateral phrenic nerve pacing has been performed in children suffering from central hypoventilation, including infants with congenital forms of the disorder. In infants, pacing electrodes generally are placed on the phrenic nerve by means of a thoracotomy.

Mechanical Ventilation

Mechanical ventilation produces support without involving the control centers or the neuromuscular framework. Chronic mechanical ventilatory support with positive or negative pressure devices has been used successfully in managing central hypoventilation syndrome. The need for mechanical ventilatory assistance often is permanent in congenital forms of the disease, although recovery of adequate respiratory function has been reported in one instance. Although most patients initially require ventilatory assistance only during sleep, periods of hypoventilation often progress into wakeful states, necessitating the use of continuous ventilatory support.

Chronic positive pressure ventilation has been achieved by using a nasal mask and the more traditional tracheostomy. In older children the nasal mask is well tolerated and may obviate the need for tracheostomy.

TETANUS
Clinical Features

Tetanus is characterized by severe, painful muscle rigidity and spasms. After contamination of a wound, the vegetative form of *C. tetani* elaborates the potent neurotoxin tetanospasmin, which binds to the presynaptic terminals of inhibitory neurons at the spinal cord level. Its interference with the release of inhibitory transmitters results in the firing of opposing muscle groups simultaneously producing clinical spasms. Involvement of the laryngeal or respiratory muscles can give rise to acute respiratory insufficiency, which requires urgent intervention. Approximately half of the mortality associated with tetanus can be attributed to the respiratory complications of the disease.

Site of Entry

Tetanus has been described as occurring with virtually every type of wound. In 80% of cases, the contamination site can be identified by history or examination. In newborn infants, tetanus is most frequently linked to contamination of the severed umbilical cord after delivery in the home. Less conspicuous sites of entry for the organism include the tympanic membrane (i.e., otitis media), the uterus (i.e., septic abortion), and venipuncture sites (i.e., illicit drug use).

Symptomatology

The incubation period is variable, ranging from 3 days to 3 weeks, with an average of 8 days. In the neonate, clinical presentation of tetanus generally occurs at the end of the first week of life. A shorter incubation period may be predictive of more severe disease. Early symptoms usually are attributable to muscle rigidity and spasm. In 50 to 75% of patients, trismus (i.e, masseter spasm, lockjaw) is noted at the time of clinical presentation.

Diagnosis

The diagnosis of tetanus is usually made on clinical grounds. Other causes of muscle rigidity and trismus, such as electrolyte disorders, poisoning, and seizures, can usually be excluded on the basis of the clinical picture and appropriate laboratory studies. Wound cultures do not reliably yield the causative organism (i.e, less than one-third of cases).

Management

In severe cases of tetanus, life-threatening respiratory and cardiovascular complications can ensue with disturbing rapidity after the initial presentation. Prediction of eventual disease severity early in the course is difficult, however. For these reasons, observation in the intensive care unit (ICU) is recommended at least during the early phase of hospitalization. Passive immunization to tetanus toxin, administration of appropriate antibiotics, wound debridement, sedation, muscle relaxation, and control of sympathetic nervous system dysfunction represent critical aspects of specific therapy in tetanus.

Acute Care

The focus of intensive care in tetanus is directed at managing respiratory complications and situations associated with respiratory failure.

Spasms of the laryngeal muscles can precipitate acute airway obstruction and asphyxia. In addition, muscle spasms of the chest wall and respiratory muscles may interfere with ventilation, either primarily or secondarily, as the result of retained secretions, atelectasis, and pneumonia. Newborn infants afflicted with tetanus seem to be particularly prone to the development of aspiration pneumonitis. The use of sedation in the treatment of tetanic spasms can lead to obtundation and central respiratory depression. Finally, the use of muscle relaxants and controlled positive pressure ventilation for prolonged periods in the treatment of severe reflex spasms is associated with a particularly high incidence of atelectasis and pneumonia in infants.

Tetanic contractions of the laryngeal muscles can result in acute upper airway obstruction. These so-called respiratory convulsions often arise unexpectedly and may be associated with severe hypoxemia. Episodes of laryngeal spasm require the prompt cessation of muscle contraction. A rapidly acting muscle relaxant is recommended in this setting and should be followed by immediate endotracheal intubation. Continued muscle relaxation after intubation is advised to avoid vocal cord damage from recurrent laryngeal spasms.

Progression of respiratory muscle spasms will interfere with ventilatory gas exchange and should be managed with the administration of a nondepolarizing muscle relaxant and controlled positive pressure ventilation. Duration of mechanical ventilation varies considerably but generally ranges from 3 to 5 weeks. Because this period is complicated by a high incidence of atelectasis and pneumonia, considerable attention must be directed toward chest physical therapy, frequent postural changes, and tracheal toilet.

Chronic Care

The approach to chronic management of the airway in patients with tetanus varies. As noted previously, maintenance of an artificial airway usually is required for a minimum of several weeks. In adults, early tracheostomy has been recommended. In neonates, prolonged nasotracheal intubation compared favorably with tracheostomy in the management of tetanus. Because similar comparisons in older children are lacking, the advantages of prolonged endotracheal intubation outside the newborn period require further clarification.

Weaning from positive pressure ventilatory support is attempted when heavy sedation and muscle relaxants are no longer required to control severe spasms, usually 2 to 4 weeks after the initiation of mechanical ventilation.

POLIOMYELITIS

Clinical Features

In its most severe form, this acute viral infection of the CNS results in widespread muscle paralysis and secondary respiratory failure. As a result of modern immunization practices, poliomyelitis is a rare cause of respiratory failure in industrialized nations, although it continues to plague the childhood population of developing countries. Sporadic cases have been reported in the United States in immunocompromised patients exposed to live attenuated virus used for active immunization, in unimmunized foreign travelers, and in individuals emigrating from endemic areas.

Causes of Respiratory Failure

The clinical expression of the disease is variable. Depending on the location of nervous system involvement, respiratory failure can arise from deficiencies in airway control, clearance of secretions, central control of ventilation, and inspiratory muscle weakness. In acute paralytic poliomyelitis, muscle weakness often progresses with alarming rapidity after the onset of neurologic symptoms; therefore, patients can arrive in the ICU with acute respiratory collapse of unknown cause. In addition to the acute disease, the paralytic residua of poliomyelitis can result in chronic respiratory disability.

Abnormalities in breathing control have been well described during acute paralytic poliomyelitis and have been incriminated as a cause of sudden infant death syndrome (SIDS) in isolated instances. Bulbar palsy can result in loss of airway control as a result of pharyngeal muscle paralysis and can lead to airway obstruction or aspiration of oropharyngeal secretions.

GUILLAIN-BARRÉ SYNDROME

This acute, inflammatory peripheral neuropathy, also known as "acute postinfective neuritis" and "acute inflammatory polyradiculoneuropathy," affects both adults and children. The cause of Guillain-Barré syndrome is unknown. Autoimmune mechanisms have been postulated in the disease process, which is characterized by diffuse peripheral nerve demyelination and motor dysfunction. Although associated autonomic nervous dysfunction can produce life-threatening complications, mortality from Guillain-Barré syndrome is largely attributable to respiratory muscle weakness and secondary respiratory failure. Careful attention to the progression of respiratory muscle weakness and timely intervention at the first signs of respiratory failure, therefore, are the cornerstones of management.

Clinical Presentation

Historical features and clinical presentation of patients with Guillain-Barré syndrome follow a well-defined pattern. Onset of acute neuropathic symptoms often is preceded by a recent viral-type illness, usually an acute upper respiratory infection or gastroenteritis. Other infectious prodromal diseases include mononucleosis, scarlet fever, and a variety of exanthemas. The prodromal illness can occur several days to 4 weeks before the onset of neurologic symptoms. Clinical disorders similar to Guillain-Barré syndrome have also been described in postsurgical patients approximately 2 to 3 weeks after a variety of operative procedures and/or spinal anesthesia, and represent a subset of acute inflammatory polyneuropathy.

Classically, the earliest neurologic sign of Guillain-Barré syndrome is weakness in the lower extremities, usually symmetric, involving the distal musculature to a greater degree than the proximal musculature, followed by progressive ascending paralysis. Deviation from the classic presentation and characteristic ascending progression of weakness, however, is not uncommon. Sensory symptoms such as numbness or paresthesias frequently accompany the early onset of weakness and are distributed distally. Owing to these early symptoms, the child comes to medical attention because of nonspecific lethargy and inactivity, loss of previously achieved gross motor functions (e.g., walking, use of the distal extremities), or subjective complaints about paresthesias or diminished sensation in the distal extremities.

Physical Findings

Findings encountered at presentation include areflexia, muscle weakness in the previously described distribution, and numbness in a stocking-glove distribution pattern, as well as cranial nerve palsies, altered level of consciousness, ataxia, loss of vibratory and/or position sensation, and, less frequently, urinary retention. After the onset of motor symptoms, weakness generally progresses over a period of several days to 2 weeks. This process culminates in a period of maximal weakness, which is followed by slow remission. Severe respiratory muscle paresis develops during the progressive stage in approximately one-third of Guillain-Barré syndrome patients.

Diagnostic Studies

Laboratory and electrophysiologic studies provide supportive evidence for the diagnosis of Guillain-Barré syndrome, although these results may not be positive for several days to weeks after initial presentation. Of particular note is the finding of an elevated cerebrospinal fluid (CSF) protein level (more than 45 mg/dL) in the absence of pleocytosis (i.e., the so-called albuminocytologic dissociation). Elevated CSF protein at some point during the course of the disease is encountered in approximately 90% of patients. Although the CSF cell count is generally normal, pleocytosis is encountered in approximately 5% of patients. Abnormalities in electrophysiologic studies become particularly pronounced with progression of the disease. The majority of patients demonstrate delayed nerve conduction 2 to 3 weeks after onset of the disease, and electromyography is consistent with lower motor neuron disease.

Because no test is pathognomonic, the diagnosis of Guillain-Barré syndrome generally is established on the basis of history, clinical presentation, and characteristic disease progression.

Differential Diagnosis

Other causes of peripheral neuropathy and weakness in childhood, such as heavy-metal poisoning, thiamine deficiency, porphyria, botulism, and poliomyelitis, can usually be differentiated from Guillain-Barré syndrome on the basis of clinical and laboratory findings.

ICU Management

Any child with a clinical picture suggesting Guillain-Barré syndrome requires immediate hospitalization, but specific indications for admission to the ICU in patients without respiratory failure have not been firmly delineated. Inpatient care areas must be capable of providing frequent assessment of respiratory muscle strength, protective airway reflexes, and hemodynamic status.

Indications for admission to the ICU include rapidly progressive weakness, difficulty clearing oral or pulmonary secretions, frank respiratory failure, marginal respiratory muscle reserve, onset of atelectasis or pneumonia, loss of protective reflexes of the airway, and life-threatening signs of autonomic instability (e.g., arrhythmias, systemic hypotension).

Supportive Care

General supportive care is directed at preventing complications of immobilization and decreased motor activity; careful monitoring of the motor weakness progression, particularly as it affects respiratory muscle function (and appropriate intervention in the event of respiratory failure); observation for other complicating conditions, such as autonomic dysfunction; and consideration of specific therapeutic interventions directed at speeding the onset of recovery and reversing muscle weakness.

Acute Respiratory Failure

Care of acute respiratory failure secondary to atelectasis and/or respiratory muscle fatigue is the most important aspect of the intensive care management of patients with Guillain-Barré syndrome. Approximately 20% of children with Guillain-Barré syndrome ultimately progress to frank respiratory failure, requiring mechanical ventilatory assistance; therefore, frequent assessment of respiratory reserve is imperative.

In addition to nonspecific clinical signs of respiratory embarrassment, bedside evaluation of respiratory muscle strength can provide early warning of impending respiratory failure. Recommended techniques for such assessment in children include determination of forced or crying vital capacity and maximum negative inspiratory pressure. Although measurement of maximum expiratory pressure is a particularly sensitive index of respiratory muscle weakness and has been widely used in assessing adult patients with neuromuscular disease, abnormalities in this parameter are not necessarily specific for detecting the onset of acute respiratory failure and alveolar hypoventilation. Assessment of forced or crying vital capacity and maximum negative inspiratory pressure is recommended every 2 to 4 hours, along with generalized neurologic assessment of muscular strength.

Ventilatory Assistance

Provision of mechanical ventilatory assistance should be considered when:

- Forced vital capacity falls to less than 15 to 20 mL/kg
- Maximum negative inspiratory pressure falls to less than 20 to 30 cm H_2O
- Alveolar hypoventilation (P_aCO_2 greater than 50 torr) ensues

In addition, endotracheal intubation should be performed whenever there is evidence of retention of pulmonary secretions refractory to chest physical therapy, weakness of protective reflexes of the airway (i.e., cough and gag), or atelectasis.

Mechanical ventilatory support should be directed at providing adequate alveolar ventilation and oxygenation and at avoiding atelectasis and pneumonia. Initially, complete ventilatory support should be provided, followed by the partial withdrawal of positive pressure support by intermittent mandatory ventilation in patients who can generate effort.

With appropriate monitoring, indications for endotracheal intubation can be detected early, allowing the elective performance of the procedure. Administration of depolarizing muscle relaxants in cases of chronic or relapsing polyneuropathy has been associated with ventricular arrhythmias; therefore, succinylcholine should be avoided when endotracheal intubation is performed in patients with Guillain-Barré syndrome. Because of autonomic instability, circulatory responses to intravenous sedatives and anesthetics can be exaggerated, and the administration of these agents for obtundation during intubation should be undertaken with extreme caution.

Reports of prolonged nasotracheal intubation in children with Guillain-Barré syndrome have suggested that this technique of airway management can be used safely for several weeks. The duration of mechanical support in cases with respiratory failure varies widely, ranging from 2 weeks to 9 months. Tracheostomy can be avoided completely in selected patients who require shorter periods of mechanical ventilatory assistance. Patients with a lack of protective reflexes of the airway, poor tracheal toilet, or frank respiratory failure for prolonged periods, however, should be considered for tracheostomy. No complications were found in 15 consecutive children who underwent tracheostomy (i.e., median duration of tracheostomy 39 days, range 11 to 94 days) for Guillain-Barré syndrome.

Complications

Pneumonia is a complicating factor in two-thirds of patients admitted to an ICU and requires prompt detection and initiation of antibiotics. Chest physical therapy should be employed to help avoid atelectasis and retention of bronchial secretions.

Certain complications of Guillain-Barré syndrome are attributable to autonomic dysfunction, manifested by swings in peripheral vasomotor tone and abnormalities in cardiac rhythm, such as sinus tachycardia (50%), bradycardia (20%), S-T segment and T-wave abnormalities (64%), hypertension (61%), and postural hypotension (43%). These signs of autonomic dysfunction usually are limited to minor alterations in blood pressure and heart rate. Infrequently, hypotension and severe vasomotor collapse occur, presumably due to lack of sympathetic tone, requiring prompt expansion of intravascular volume.

Therapy

The cornerstone of Guillain-Barré syndrome treatment is supportive care, avoidance of respiratory complications, and provision of mechanical ventilation. Specific therapy for Guillain-Barré syndrome remains a topic of controversy.

Steroids

Because of the inflammatory nature of the Guillain-Barré syndrome, corticosteroids and adrenal corticotropin have been used in an attempt to improve the clinical course.

Plasmapheresis

Plasmapheresis improves the clinical course of acute Guillain-Barré syndrome as measured by time to recovery of muscle strength and independent ambulation and by outcome at 6 months. Beneficial effects of plasmapheresis were noted in patients treated within 7 days of the onset of disease and in those who subsequently required mechanical ventilation.

Immunoglobulin Therapy

In a randomized trial, gamma globulin administration was demonstrated to be more effective than plasmapheresis. The plasmapheresis group in this study did worse than groups in other studies. If immunoglobulin administration is effective, the ease of administration may make it preferable to plasma exchange.

Outcome

In spite of reports of prolonged respiratory failure, recovery of adequate respiratory function is the rule, provided life-threatening complications are avoided during the acute phase of the disease.

UNILATERAL DIAPHRAGMATIC PARALYSIS

Although bilateral weakness of the diaphragm is encountered in a wide range of systemic neuromuscular disorders, unilateral diaphragmatic paralysis in children is most often a result of direct trauma to the phrenic nerve. Although uncomplicated loss of hemidiaphragmatic function can be well tolerated in older children and adults, Guillain-Barré syndrome causes severe respiratory embarrassment in infants.

Etiology

Diaphragmatic paralysis usually occurs as a result of birth trauma or injury to the phrenic nerve sustained during cardiothoracic surgical procedures. In approximately one-third of phrenic nerve palsy cases, traction injury to the phrenic nerve is sustained during delivery. Simultaneous injury to the brachial plexus, resulting in Erb's palsy, is commonly observed. In the remainder of patients, diaphragmatic paralysis is noted after cardiothoracic surgery, usually for palliation or correction of congenital heart disease. Phrenic nerve injury in this situation can arise from traction, transection, or the application of topical cardiac hypothermia.

Clinical Presentation

The clinical manifestations of diaphragmatic paralysis in children depend on their ages and the presence of underlying lung disease. In uncomplicated cases occurring in older children, signs of diaphragmatic dysfunction often are confined to mild tachypnea and orthopnea. The newborn infant generally manifests severe respiratory distress after a difficult delivery with suspected birth trauma. When diaphragmatic paralysis results from inadvertent phrenic nerve injury during surgical manipulation, the condition often presents as inability to wean from mechanical ventilatory support in the postoperative period. Persistent unilateral pleural effusion and basilar atelectasis are common secondary findings.

Diagnostic Findings

Typically, abnormal elevation of the affected hemidiaphragm is noted on a patient's chest radiograph; however, this finding can be obscured in patients receiving positive pressure ventilatory support. For this reason, the disorder frequently is not suspected until unsuccessful attempts have been made to wean the patient from mechanical ventilation. The diagnosis usually is confirmed by fluoroscopic examination of diaphragmatic motion, which demonstrates paradoxical upward movement of the involved hemidiaphragm with inspiration. This upward movement may be accompanied by a concurrent shift of the mediastinal structures toward the contralateral hemithorax.

Certain conditions can generate misleading results from fluoroscopic examination. Continuous positive airway pressure (CPAP) may obscure paradoxical diaphragmatic motion; therefore, the examination should be performed when the patient is breathing spontaneously (i.e., without ventilatory support). Also, during the expiratory grunting maneuver, increased intra-abdominal pressure results in upward motion of the paralyzed hemidiaphragm, followed by descent of the paralyzed diaphragm and outward abdominal motion with relaxation of the abdominal musculature during inspiration. This pattern mimics normal diaphragmatic motion and could confound the interpretation.

Management

Acute management of the patient with diaphragmatic paralysis usually requires a 2-week to 4-week trial of positive pressure ventilation and positive end-expiratory pressure to establish adequate ventilation and oxygenation. Treatment of any associated pulmonary disease (e.g., pneumonia, atelectasis, pulmonary edema) is provided before making aggressive attempts at weaning from positive pressure support.

CPAP

CPAP provides a form of "internal fixation" of the flaccid diaphragm and compliant chest wall of the infant, allowing adequate ventilatory exchange with spontaneous breathing. After acute stabilization and clearing of associated lung disease, normal gas exchange usually can be sustained with CPAP at 5 to 10 cm H_2O.

Surgical Plication

Resolution of respiratory failure resulting from diaphragmatic paralysis sometimes requires surgical plication of the diaphragm to offset the paradoxical inspiratory motion. This technique usually is unnecessary after infancy. In older children, successful weaning from positive pressure ventilatory support eliminates the immediate need for plication.

MYASTHENIA GRAVIS

Clinical Features

Classical myasthenia gravis is a chronic disorder characterized by exaggerated fatigability of skeletal muscles, which, in its extreme, can lead to acute respiratory failure. The functional deficiency in muscle strength is attributed to immunologic interference with neuromuscular transmission associated with acetylcholine receptor antibodies.

In addition to classic myasthenia gravis, other myasthenic disorders unique to the pediatric age group can be associated with respiratory failure.

Management

Postoperative Intensive Care

Patients with myasthenia gravis require intensive care under two circumstances: First, myasthenia patients undergoing major surgical procedures (e.g., thymectomy) usually require intensive care in the immediate postoperative period. In addition to general supportive care, approximately one third of these patients require mechanical ventilatory support beyond the first several postoperative hours. Pediatric patients may require postoperative intensive care after thymectomy for myasthenia gravis, including mechanical ventilatory support.

Second, in particularly refractory cases or in those complicated by progression of muscle weakness or excessive treatment with anticholinesterase therapy, severe respiratory muscle weakness can be encountered, necessitating frequent monitoring of respiratory muscle strength, vigorous chest physical therapy for clearance of pulmonary secretions, or mechanical ventilatory support.

Ventilatory Support

Indications for mechanical ventilatory support in patients with myasthenia gravis include apnea, hypoventilation, or evidence of severe respiratory muscle fatigue. Predictive indices have not been identified in children; therefore, standard indices of respiratory muscle strength, such as maximum negative inspiratory pressure, forced or crying vital capacity, and arterial blood gases, are used to determine the need for mechanical ventilatory support.

Postoperative laryngeal muscle weakness and vocal cord paralysis have been described following anesthesia and can be mistaken for postextubation croup. This complicating manifestation of myasthenia gravis should be considered in any patient exhibiting stridor on extubation in the postoperative period.

Nonspecific indices of respiratory muscle weakness that can signal impending respiratory failure include decreased forced or crying vital capacity (less than 15 mL/kg) and decreased maximum negative inspiratory pressure (less than -20 to -30 cm H_2O). Muscle strength typically deteriorates with repetitive contractions in the myasthenic patient.

Endotracheal Intubation

Endotracheal intubatin usually is required in the presence of acute hypoventilation and may be necessary for clearance of pulmonary secretions in patients with impaired expiratory muscle function and cough capabilities. Performance of semielective or emergent endotracheal intubation of the myasthenic patient requires attention to several points.

First, succinylcholine is not recommended when performing endotracheal intubation because of the poorly predictable response of myasthenic patients to depolarizing muscle relaxants. The underlying abnormality of neuromuscular transmission in myasthenia gravis causes extreme sensitivity to competitive, nondepolarizing neuromuscular blockade; therefore, these agents may be required for intubation but generally are avoided.

In patients requiring endotracheal intubation and mechanical ventilatory support, extubation usually can be performed within several weeks, thereby precluding the need for tracheostomy. Nonetheless, the occasional patient requiring prolonged maintenance of an artificial airway because of inadequate muscle function or ongoing need for tracheal toilet should be considered for tracheostomy.

Therapeutic Interventions

Pharmacologic Agents

Myasthenic Crisis Myasthenic crisis generally is associated with a recent viral illness, surgery, or other systemic stress in a known or previously asymptomatic myasthenic patient. For these individuals and newly diagnosed patients, administration of anticholinesterase agents usually results in prompt improvement in muscle strength and effort-dependent respiratory function.

Use of the short-acting anticholinesterase edrophonium (i.e., Tensilon) generally is reserved for establishing the diagnosis at the time of initial presentation. Ongoing therapy with longer acting anticholinesterases (e.g., neostigmine, pyridostigmine) is necessary. Dosage of specific anticholinesterase agents is determined largely by patient response. Because anticholinesterases can be associated with bronchoconstriction, patients should be monitored carefully for this potential complication.

Cholinergic Crisis Cholinergic crisis usually can be differentiated from myasthenic crisis by signs of excessive parasympathetic activity, including lacrimation, salivation, diarrhea, and bradycardia. Symptoms attributed to excessive parasympathetic activity usually are responsive to atropine administration. Weakness associated with cholinergic crisis frequently responds to the temporary withdrawal of anticholinesterase medications.

Corticosteroids Steroid preparations have been used extensively because of the autoimmune nature of myasthenia gravis. Studies indicate that prednisone can be a valuable adjunct to anticholinesterase therapy in patients with refractory disease. Although specific indications for steroids vary, prednisone should be considered in severely affected patients with acute respiratory failure. Exacerbation of muscle weakness on initiation of steroid therapy is a risk and requires particular attention.

Drugs to Avoid A variety of drugs commonly used in the critically ill patient can impair neuromuscular transmission. The administration of these agents to myasthenic patients poses particular risks of exacerbating or precipitating respiratory failure.

In addition to the nondepolarizing muscle relaxants previously discussed, the neuromuscular blocking effects of aminoglycoside antibiotics are exaggerated in myasthenia gravis and may lead to respiratory depression; therefore, their use should be avoided.

Thymectomy

When thymectomy has been performed in patients with juvenile myasthenia gravis, patients have shown progressive improvement in muscle weakness and arrest of disease progression over several years. Development of the transcervical approach for this procedure has decreased the associated complications and simplified the postoperative course.

Plasmapheresis

Plasmapheresis has been used on a limited basis in adult patients with severe refractory respiratory failure or with advanced disease before thymectomy. Preliminary trials with plasmapheresis indicate that the technique is highly effective in improving muscle strength and decreasing the duration of postoperative mechanical ventilatory support in severely affected patients. The precise role of plasma exchange in the management of myasthenia gravis is unclear, but current applications include presurgical preparation and exacerbation of disease with respiratory failure or failure to wean from mechanical ventilation.

BOTULISM

This acute paralytic disorder involves disruption of neuromuscular transmission by the neurotoxin *Clostridium botulinum*. This bacterial toxin binds irreversibly to target sites in the peripheral nervous system, causing diffuse muscle weakness that often culminates in loss of protective airway reflexes and respiratory muscle function. Botulism can be encountered in the pediatric population in several settings defined by the specific portal of entry of the *C. botulinum* toxin. A prolonged course of respiratory failure occurs in all forms, requiring mechanical ventilatory support in addition to general supportive care.

Clinical Features

The potent *C. botulinum* toxin inhibits the release of acetylcholine. Consequently, symptoms of botulism arise from dysfunction of the autonomic nervous system and weakness of skeletal muscles. Recovery depends on the development of new synaptic connections, which at least partially explains botulism's prolonged clinical course.

Infant Botulism

This unique form of the disease accounts for the majority of cases reported in children. Infant botulism has received considerable attention both as a cause of respiratory insufficiency in infants and as a consideration in SIDS. The unique feature of infant botulism is the intestinal portal of entry of the toxin. It is formed in vivo after ingestion of organisms contained in such vehicles as contaminated honey, soil or dust, and nonhuman foods.

Diagnosis

The diagnosis of all forms of botulism is based primarily on clinical recognition of the signs and symptoms in conjunction with appropriate confirmatory testing.

Physical Signs and Symptoms Reports of infant botulism have been limited to children 9 months of age or younger. Onset of the disease usually occurs between 2 and 4 months of age. Constipation caused by the parasympatholytic effects of the toxin is the most frequent early symptom, usually occurring several days after onset. By this time, evidence of neuromuscular dysfunction has characteristically appeared, resulting in poor feeding, lethargy, and generalized hypotonia. In very severe cases, infant botulism can mimic SIDS.

Other common findings in afflicted infants include decreased lacrimation or salivation (25%) and severe muscular weakness culminating in respiratory failure (50 to 90%). In one study series, more than 90% of infants required endotracheal intubation and ventilatory assistance to maintain airway patency.

About 10% of patients with infant botulism display signs of autonomic instability: skin flushing, tachycardia or bradycardia, and fluctuations in systemic blood pressure. Aggressive treatment of these fleeting signs of dysautonomia should be tempered by the fact that they frequently resolve spontaneously.

Diagnostic Studies An acute motor disorder with early bulbar involvement, followed by descending symmetrical muscle weakness, should suggest botulism. Serum electrolytes and CSF examination typically are normal. Electrophysiologic studies can be particularly helpful in diagnosing botulism; electromyography shows the typical pattern of "brief, small-amplitude, overly abundant motor unit action potentials." Evoked muscle action potentials elicited by rapid repetitive nerve stimulation typically show an incremental response, in contrast to the pattern seen with myasthenia gravis. Normal peripheral nerve conduction velocities differs from the conduction slowing found in Guillain-Barré syndrome. Administration of anticholinesterase agents (e.g., neostigmine, edrophonium) does not consistently lead to improvement in muscle strength.

Differential Diagnosis

Appropriate screening tests and clinical observations usually allow differentiation from other disorders that can be confused with botulism initially, such as organic acidurias, heavy-metal or insecticide intoxication, sepsis, meningitis, primary myopathies, and poliomyelitis.

Management and Treatment

General Supportive ICU Care Provision of adequate nutrition during botulism treatment generally requires nasogastric or intravenous alimentation because of swallowing abnormalities frequently encountered because of involvement of the patient's pharyngeal muscles. Oral feedings should be avoided because of the high risk of aspiration pneumonia (i.e, 25% of infants). The anticholinergic effects of *C. botulinum* toxin on the urinary bladder may cause urinary retention and require bladder decompression. At the earliest sign of infectious complications, patients should receive appropriate antibiotic therapy. Use of aminoglycoside antibiotics should be avoided, however, because they are known to exacerbate the neuromuscular blocking effects of *C. botulinum* toxin and are associated with the precipitation of acute respiratory insufficiency.

Antitoxin and Other Treatment Measures Recommendations for the treatment of botulism with equine antitoxin vary. Administration of trivalent *C. botulinum* antitoxin usually is recommended in cases of wound and foodborne botulism, but is avoided in cases of infant botulism because of its lack of proven efficacy and the relatively high incidence of anaphylactic complications.

Other measures occasionally used in botulism include catharsis, enemas, and antibiotics directed at *C. botulinum,* although the benefits of these measures have not been substantiated. Guanidine has been used on a limited basis in adults because of its theoretic ability to enhance the release of acetylcholine from cholinergic nerve terminals. Improvements in strength with guanidine have been confined to nonrespiratory muscles, however, and have not altered the course of respiratory failure.

Respiratory Care

The cornerstone of management in all forms of botulism is timely and expert respiratory care.

Causes of Respiratory Failure Respiratory failure in botulism can arise from bulbar palsy, which carries a high risk of aspiration and airway obstruction, and from descending paralysis, which frequently progresses to the primary muscles of respiration, leading to hypoventilation and respiratory failure. This process also can interfere with the clearance of pulmonary secretions and result in secondary respiratory failure from atelectasis or pneumonia.

Endotracheal Intubation and Assisted Ventilation Indications for mechanical ventilatory support for patients with botulism are the same as for patients with respiratory failure associated with peripheral neuromuscular disease. Because bulbar palsy is a common finding in all forms of botulism, endotracheal intubation is recommended whenever significant depression of the gag reflex is noted.

The duration of endotracheal intubation required in patients with botulism varies. Ventilatory support may be required for 2 months or more; in one series, the average duration of assisted ventilation was 2 weeks.

MISCELLANEOUS PERIPHERAL NEUROMUSCULAR DISEASES
Treatable versus Degenerative Disorders

Numerous peripheral neuromuscular disorders are complicated by acute respiratory failure. Such diseases as tick paralysis and dyskalemic periodic paralysis can be controlled or definitively treated, and respiratory muscle failure can be limited in duration and recurrence. Other conditions, such as Duchenne's muscular dystrophy and infantile muscular atrophy (i.e., Werdnig-Hoffmann disease type 1), represent progressive degenerative processes culminating in profound, irreversible muscle weakness and chronic respiratory insufficiency.

Comparative features of some unusual neuromuscular causes of respiratory failure in children are highlighted in Table 5.2. Although each of these disorders represents a distinct pathologic entity, the pathogenesis and management of respiratory failure associated with the various neuromuscular diseases are similar in many respects.

Table 5.2
Neuromuscular Disorders Causing Respiratory Failure

Site	Course	Noted
Anterior horn cell	Spinal muscular atrophy (Werdnig-Hoffmann disease)	Acute 　Rapidly progressive, fatal 　Onset <1 year old 　Proximal muscle preference Intermediate 　Slowly progressive 　Autosomal recessive 　Survival into adulthood 　Secondary kyphoscoliosis
Peripheral motor nerve	Multiple sclerosis	Chronic relapsing 　Rare in childhood
	Intoxications	Tick paralysis 　Acute, rapidly progressive 　Neurotoxin from engorged tick 　Recovery after tick removal Heavy metal 　Acute, rapidly progressive 　Ingestion history Organophosphate 　Acute, rapidly progressive 　Salivation, lacrimation
	Uremia	Acute, rapidly progressive 　Rare
	Acute intermittent porphyria	Acute, fulminant 　Attacks precipitated by multiple drugs 　Abdominal pain 　Recovery over weeks to months
Neuromuscular junction	Antibiotic intoxication	Acute, self-limited 　Aminoglycosides, polypeptides
	Hypermagnesemia	Acute, self-limited 　Iatrogenic, cathartic/antacid abuse
Muscle cell	Duchenne muscular dystrophy	Chronic, steadily progressive 　Sex-linked recessive 　Respiratory failure 　Myocardial failure
	Myotonic dystrophy	Variable, usually gradual 　Autosomal dominant 　Different clinical forms
	Other congenital myopathies	Variable 　Multiple forms
	Inborn errors	Acid maltase deficiency 　Rapidly fatal (infant), late-onset respiratory failure (adult) 　Autosomal recessive Glycogen storage disease 　Infant, child, and adult types Carnitine deficiency 　Childhood onset, remitting fatal 　Autosomal recessive

continued

Table 5.2
Neuromuscular Disorders Causing Respiratory Failure

Site	Course	Noted
Electrolyte disorders	Hypokalemia and hyperkalemia	Acute, self-limited Diuretic use Electrocardiogram abnormalities
	Hypophosphatemia	Acute, self-limited Malnutrition Inadequate replacement
	Dermatomyositis/ polymyositis	Acute or gradual Proximal weakness Variable progression Therapy: steroids, immuno- suppression

Management

The management of the patient with neuromuscular disease should be anticipatory. Because acute respiratory failure frequently ensues with extreme rapidity, intermittent determination of arterial blood gases is usually inadequate for signaling impending respiratory failure. Early detection of marginal respiratory muscle function is achieved only by appropriate monitoring of bedside indices of respiratory muscle strength.

Inspiratory Muscle Capacity

This inspiratory muscle capacity index is evaluated by measuring maximum negative inspiratory airway pressure under static airflow conditions. When this parameter decreases to 50% of its predicted level, further decreases in negative inspiratory pressure are related linearly to arterial PCO_2. Values less negative than -20 to -30 cm H_2O are generally recognized as a sign of severe inspiratory muscle weakness and impending respiratory failure.

Expiratory Muscle Capacity

Expiratory muscle function is evaluated by measuring the maximum positive expiratory airway pressure generated at total lung capacity. A decreasing trend in this parameter signals a progressive loss of expiratory muscle strength, and a value less than 40 cm H_2O correlates with inability to generate an effective cough for the clearance of secretions.

Vital Capacity

Forced vital capacity less than three times the predicted tidal volume is associated with impaired coughing capability and retention of secretions. An inability to generate a vital capacity more than two times the predicted tidal vol-

Table 5.3
Causes of Unanticipated Prolonged Ventilator Dependence

Potentiation of residual neuromuscular junction blockade
    Acidosis, respiratory, or metabolic
    Hypothermia
    Aminoglycoside toxicity
    Calcium channel blocker toxicity
Metabolites of neuromuscular junction blockade accumulation
    Prolonged use
    Renal failure
    Liver failure
Acquired myopathies
    Steroid myopathy
    Disuse (immobilization) myopathy
    Catabolic (nutritional) myopathy
    Septic pyomyositis
    Critical illness myopathy (reversible)
      • associated with high doses of steroids and neuromuscular junction blocking agents
      • proximal generalized weakness, respiratory muscle dysfunction (rarely extraocular), attenuated reflexes
      • elevated creatine kinase level
      • normal nerve conduction; type 2 fiber atrophy, with possible muscle necrosis and vacuolization
Acquired neuropathies
    Guillain-Barré polyradiculoneuritis
    Critical illness polyneuropathy
      • manifests in adult and pediatric patients with sepsis or multiorgan failure after critical illness resolves
      • unknown etiology, but neuropathy resolves in most cases
      • distal limb weakness, hyporeflexia, areflexia, and respiratory muscle weakness; no effect in facial and extraocular muscles
      • cerebrospinal fluid is normal; motor axonal polyneuropathy, sensory potentials may vary
      • diminished sensory function
Metabolic abnormalities
    Hypermagnesemia
    Hypophosphatemia
    Pancreatic dysfunction (hypocalcemia)
Unmasking of underlying neuromuscular disease
    Porphyria
    Myasthenia gravis

ume signals severe impairment in respiratory capacity and impending acute respiratory failure. Vital capacity less than 50% of that predicted for the patient's size is associated with alveolar hypoventilation and hypercapnia.

Therapy

Intervention with mechanical ventilatory support has been associated with increases in inspiratory and expiratory muscle capacity and maximum voluntary ventilation after several weeks. Therefore, "resting" the respiratory muscles in these types of disorders seems to have a rational basis. Weaning the patient from mechanical ventilatory support should be preceded by providing adequate nutrition; correction of any metabolic or electrolyte abnormalities, particularly those associated with decreased respiratory muscle function (see Table 5.2); and adequate time to clear any acute coincidental pulmonary parenchymal disease.

NEUROMUSCULAR FAILURE IN THE ICU
Causative Factors

Critically ill patients can develop a neuromuscular disorder during treatment for respiratory failure. These individuals usually have sepsis, multisystem organ failure, or status asthmaticus and experience a generalized weakness with respiratory muscle involvement as the primary process is resolving. These patients are slow or unable to be weaned from the ventilator. Weakness and hyporeflexia not previously present are discovered as sedation and paralysis are withdrawn. A list of differential diagnoses for this condition, and details related to acquired myopathies and neuropathies and metabolic and underlying neuromuscular disorders, are provided in Table 5.3.

Principles of Prophylaxis

Prophylaxis may be easier than treatment, especially for the critical illness neuromuscular disorders. The prophylactic principles are as follows:

- Keep neuromuscular blocking agents to the lowest possible doses and the shortest possible durations, and use less than a complete blockade.
- Monitor neuromuscular transmission to keep the myotactic reflex intact.
- Avoid combining neuromuscular blocking agents and aminoglycoside.
- Employ extra vigilance when liver or renal failure occurs.
- Avoid acidosis, hypermagnesemia, and accumulation of metabolites.
- Use special caution with patients who have had a previous episode of these complications.
- Minimize exposure to and interaction with steroids.

6.

Principles and Practice of Respiratory Support and Mechanical Ventilation

Lynn D. Martin, Susan L. Bratton, and L. Kyle Walker

Behold, the child was dead . . . and he went up and lay upon the child, put his mouth upon his mouth . . . and the flesh of the child waxed warm. . . .

Kings 4:32–35

149

RESPIRATORY THERAPY

Normobaric Oxygen Therapy

Oxygen therapy is the most common intervention used in the management of respiratory disease. Despite its ubiquitous nature in pediatric intensive care, it is important to recall that the administration of an enriched concentration of oxygen has well-characterized (and potentially catastrophic) toxic effects on the lung and, in the newborn, on the retina. Consequently, oxygen therapy must be administered as conscientiously as any pharmacologic agent.

Technical Aspects of Oxygen Therapy

Medical gas sources for oxygen therapy are of two types: wall oxygen and gas cylinders. Wall oxygen sources in inpatient facilities are supplied by bulk liquid oxygen stores that gradually are warmed and evaporated. Regulations in the United States require a working pressure of 50 psi to all outlets in these facilities, which guarantees at least 35 psi driving pressure required by most commercially available mechanical ventilators.

Oxygen cylinders, which operate at internal pressures of 1800 to 2400 psi, are available in sizes providing 350 to 7000 liters of gas at room temperature and pressure. The usable duration of a given cylinder is determined by its gas capacity and the rate of gas flow. A full E cylinder contains 620 liters of oxygen and has a pressure of 2200 psi.

Medical gas sources must be interfaced with administration devices that reduce the system working pressure between the gas source and the patient. In its simplest form, this pressure-reducing function is performed by one or more *reducing valves* that drop working pressure from high-pressure gas sources (i.e., cylinder or wall oxygen outlet) to the commonly used medical gas driving pressure of 50 psi. These spring-loaded valves can be placed at single stages in the circuitry or in series with one another to provide multistage reduction in working pressure.

A further drop in system pressure is provided by a flowmeter; generally consisting of a needle valve assembly that allows regulation of flow distal to the reducing valve and visualization of the gas flow rate from the system. Manipulation of the flow control allows opening and closing of the valve orifice and adjustment of flow rate. Most commercially available flowmeters incorporate "back pressure compensation" so that introduction of flow resistance distal to the needle valve does not result in spuriously elevated flow readings. Consequently, impedance to flow in the circuitry distal to the flowmeter is detected by noting a drop in system flow, and this is accurately indicated on the flowmeter.

Devices that combine the functions of a reducing valve (i.e., reduction of system working pressure) and a flowmeter (i.e., control and measurement of delivered flow) are known as gas regulators. Gas regulators usually incorporate a pressure gauge for monitoring system working pressure and a downstream needle valve flowmeter for regulation of flow to the patient.

Oxygen Delivery Systems

Oxygen delivery systems may be thought of in two categories: (a) high-flow systems in which the gas flow from the device meets all patient inspiratory requirements; and (b) low-flow systems in which gas flow may be insufficient to meet total patient inspiratory requirements. Room air or gas in the surrounding atmosphere, therefore, is entrained and mixed with that of the delivery system to provide an inspiratory concentration of oxygen. Reference to a system as either high flow or low flow in no way reflects the fraction of inspired oxygen (FiO_2) potential of inspired gases from the delivery device. The decision to employ either a low-flow or high-flow delivery system is determined by consideration of (a) patient comfort, (b) desired FiO_2,

(c) need to control the FiO_2, and (d) need for humidification of inspired gases.

High Flow Oxygen Delivery These systems usually incorporate a Venturi-type device using the Bernoulli principle to entrain atmospheric gases. The result is augmented bulk gas flow. High-flow systems may be used with masks, tracheostomy collars, tents, and hoods. High-flow systems include such devices as oxygen nebulizers used for aerosol generation or simply "Venturi masks" themselves. Venturi masks deliver fixed concentrations at 24%, 28%, 31%, 35%, 40%, and 50% oxygen. Nebulizers using the Venturi principle are capable of delivering FiO_2 levels in the range of 30 to 100%.

Advantages of the high-flow systems follow:

- FiO_2 delivery is consistent and accurate, independent of changes in the patient's ventilatory pattern
- Temperature and humidity may be controlled as the total inspired atmosphere is being provided
- FiO_2 is measured easily and directly

Disadvantages of high-flow systems are that augmented gas flow yields are expensive and high gas flow may be uncomfortable.

Low-Flow Oxygen Delivery Low-flow oxygen delivery systems may yield concentrations of oxygen between 25 and 100%. Low-flow delivery devices are more economical and enhance patient comfort; however, in the absence of reservoir capabilities, they do not provide a consistent and accurate FiO_2 reading.

Low-flow technology includes nasal cannulae (i.e., nasal prongs), simple face masks, and nonrebreather/partial rebreather face masks.

Oxygen Delivery Equipment

Venturi Systems Operating on the Bernoulli principle, oxygen is introduced through a "jet" orifice with subsequent entrainment of atmospheric gases through side ports in the device, distal to the strictured orifice (Fig. 6.1). Dependable oxygen concentrations in the range of 24 to 50% are available by manufacturers of Venturi mask systems as long as total gas flow exceeds the patient's peak inspiratory flow. Because the FiO_2 level is dependent on a given oxygen-to-air entrainment ratio, manufacturers usually recommend operating flow rates.

Oxygen nebulizers, which generally are used to power aerosol delivery devices, also use the Venturi adaptation of the Bernoulli principle. In these systems, the FiO_2 level is independent of the patient's minute ventilation—provided the patient's inspiratory flow rate does not exceed that of the delivery device. Venturi systems are capable of providing consistent and accurate FiO_2 levels; however, any degree of distal back pressure will inhibit the

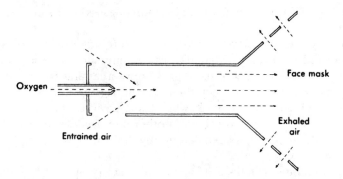

Figure 6.1. Gas delivery system of air entrainment mask. High oxygen flow velocity results in entrainment of air through the entrainment ports, thereby diluting oxygen concentration delivered to the patient. Increasing the velocity of oxygen flow, or increasing the size of the air entrainment ports, results in increased air entrainment and lower inspired oxygen concentration. (From Egan DF. Fundamentals of respiratory therapy. 3rd ed. St. Louis: CV Mosby, 1977:306.)

entrainment of atmospheric gases and thus elevate FiO_2 levels for any given flow rate.

Nasal Cannulae Nasal prongs operate at flow rates of 0.1 to 6 L/min. Most nasal prongs have a curve in the prong design that directs air posteriorly toward the turbinates, where the gas will be properly humidified.

Nasal cannulae have the advantage of being less restrictive than mask devices and, therefore, potentially are better tolerated by children. The major disadvantage of nasal cannulae is not being able to measure the FiO_2 level clinically; however, nasal cannulae generally are thought to deliver FiO_2 levels in the range of 24 to 50%. FiO_2 delivery is a function of the entrainment of atmospheric gases (i.e., those occurring with patient inspiratory flow rate and volume) mixing with source gas in the anatomic dead space.

Nasal oxygen delivery has not been proven less effective when used in patients who are "mouth breathers." The upper airway is in communication with the remainder of the airway and the delivery system is based on the entrainment of atmospheric gases.

Simple Face Masks These low-flow oxygen delivery systems operate at approximately 6 to 10 L/min. The FiO_2 level depends on the capacity of the oxygen delivery flow rate to flush dead space and the inspiratory flow rate of the patient, but it can approach 35 to 55%. Typically, the patient's inspiratory flow rate exceeds that of the delivery system with subsequent oxygen dilution by entrainment of atmospheric air through ports in the mask or around the periphery of the mask. Exhalation of gases occurs in the reverse direction.

Nonrebreathing Face Masks Incorporating a reservoir bag with a gas inflow system and a face mask, exhaled gases are eliminated and each patient's inspiratory volume consists of fresh gas. Nonrebreathing face masks typically have a one-way valve between the reservoir bag and the face mask. Gas enters the dead space of the mask, while a one-way valve prevents exhaled gas from entering the reservoir bag. Another one-way valve on the exhalation port of the mask allows exhalation of gases while preventing entrainment of atmospheric gases.

Nonrebreathing systems are capable of delivery up to 100% oxygen, provided the gas flow to the reservoir system is sufficient to maintain bag distention throughout the respiratory cycle. It is common practice to leave one port open in the event that gas flow to the system is interrupted, thereby allowing the patient access to an inspiratory gas source.

Partial Rebreathing Masks Similar in design to the nonrebreathing system in that it incorporates a reservoir bag with a gas inflow system and a face mask, partial rebreathing masks differ in the absence of one-way valve mechanisms that provide unidirectional gas flow. Part of the patient's exhaled gas or the anatomic dead space gas volume is allowed to reenter the reservoir bag. Because anatomic dead space gas does not participate in gas exchange, it is assumed to be almost entirely source gas (with the exception of a negligible quantity of CO_2). This exhaled gas, combined with the fresh gas, flows into the reservoir bag, forcing the remaining two-thirds of exhaled gas through the exhalation ports in the mask.

The danger with partial rebreathing systems is that they are often mistaken for nonrebreathing systems. This risk has led some authorities to believe the partial rebreathing system has no place in the critical care setting.

Oxygen Hoods Generally supplied with source gas from high-flow nebulizer systems incorporating the Venturi adaptation of the Bernoulli principle, oxygen hoods provide an unencumbered alternative for gas delivery to the infant (0 to 6 months). Hoods cover the patient from the neck up, are generally made of plastic, and have a removable lid that allows easy access to the patient. The patient's trunk and extremities are not involved and, therefore, remain available for access and examination. The volume contained within the hood is small enough for quick recovery time of oxygen concentration, yet large enough such that the patient's entire tidal volume may be taken from within the enclosure. Although accurate control of inspired oxygen is possible, oxygen concentration can vary as much as 20% from the top to the bottom of the hood. Also, source gas should be heated to minimize heat loss from the large surface area of the head and face of the infant.

Oxygen Tents Oxygen tents, or "croup tents," require high flows of 20 to 40 L/min to deliver 40 to 50% oxygen while maintaining CO_2 less than 1%. They are no longer used routinely because maintenance of body temperature is difficult, FiO_2 levels are variable and cannot exceed approximately 50%, access to the patient without removal from the oxygen-rich environment is limited, and observation of the child is compromised.

Hazards of Oxygen Therapy

Attendant risks include physical risks associated with enhanced support for combustion, physiologic effects of changes in PaO_2, and cellular toxicity from hyperoxia. Elevation of PaO_2 stimulates the reflexes that regulate ventilation and perfusion. Ventilatory depression can occur in patients with chronic pulmonary disease who depend on a hypoxic stimulus to breathe. Hyperoxia decreases pulmonary vascular resistance, while systemic vascular resistance increases with a resulting drop in cardiac output. Oxygen administration is also known to depress erythropoiesis and cause retinal damage in addition to the well recognized toxicity in the lungs.

Hyperbaric Oxygen Therapy (HBO)

Therapeutic Goals

This highly specialized extension of conventional oxygen therapy is used to compress gasses in isolated body cavities (the rationale for HBO therapy in decompression sickness and air embolization) and to deliver extremely high partial pressure of oxygen (greater than 760 torr) in the blood and tissues.

Limitations

The therapeutic potential of HBO is limited by the following factors:

- Severity and rapidity of oxygen toxicity
- Requires specialized equipment and personnel
- Limited number of programs offer HBO, particularly to pediatric patients
- Delivery of intensive care therapies within the chamber is technically difficult

Approved Use

Multiplace or monochambers allow delivery of 100% oxygen when increasing arterial or tissue oxygenation has theoretic therapeutic advantages. Recommendations for the use of HBO therapy are reviewed by the Undersea and Hyperbaric Medical Society. Conditions approved by the society and for payment by Blue Cross/Blue Shield funding have been defined (Table 6.1).

Table 6.1
Disorders Approved for Hyperbaric Oxygen Therapy

Decompression illness
Air embolism
Clostridial myonecrosis
Necrotizing soft-tissue infections
Osteomyelitis (refractory)
Acute traumatic ischemias (compartment syndrome)
Skin grafts and flaps (compromised)
Radiation tissue damage
Smoke inhalation
Carbon monoxide poisoning
Cyanide poisoning
Thermal burns
Anemia caused by excessive blood loss

Contraindications

Absolute contraindications for HBO therapy include:

- Untreated pneumothorax, which can progress to a tension pneumothorax while in the chamber
- Use of certain medications (disulfiran, cis-platinum or adriamycin). Hyperoxia appears to increase the toxicity of some chemotherapeutic agents (e.g., disulfiran inhibits superoxide dismutase and increases oxygen toxicity).

Relative contraindications include:

- Upper respiratory tract infection and chronic sinusitis because it impedes equalization of pressure in the middle ear. Myringotomy may be required, especially in infants or children with an endotracheal tube that may further obstruct sinus drainage.
- Seizure disorders
- Chronic lung disease because hyperoxia inhibits the hypoxic drive to breathe
- Cystic lung disease because failure to decompress slowly can cause pneumothorax
- Spherocytosis because of risk of acute hemolytic crisis

Carbon Monoxide Poisoning

Carbon monoxide (CO) is a common and potentially fatal poisoning. This colorless, odorless, tasteless, and nonirritating gas diffuses rapidly across the alveolar-capillary membrane and binds to hemoglobin (Hb), shifting the oxyhemoglobin dissociation curve to the left and exacerbating tissue hypoxia.

Carbon monoxide toxicity cannot be attributed solely to COHb-mediated hypoxia, because a poor correlation exists between CO concentration and clinical toxicity. Furthermore, delayed onset of neurologic deficits are not uncommon in CO poisonings and occurs in the absence of demonstrable COHb levels.

Clinicopathologic Evidence The pathologic hallmark of CO intoxication is bilateral necrosis of the globus pallidus. Other areas of the brain that may be affected include the cerebral cortex, hippocampus, cerebellum and substantia nigra.

Acute symptoms of carbon monoxide poisoning include:

- Headache
- Ataxia and dizziness, which can progress to seizures and coma
- Dysrhythmias
- Decreased cardiac output

HBO Therapy Although HBO therapy dramatically decreases the half life of COHb, it can also prevent granulocyte adhesion to integrins, decreasing the inflammatory response, and, at greater than 2 atm, HBO decreases lipid peroxidation and may affect CO binding to cytochromes. The exact means by which HBO therapy alleviates CO toxicity, however, remain poorly understood.

Indications for HBO therapy in CO poisoning are as follows:

- Syncope
- Myocardial ischemia
- Arrhythmias
- Severe neurologic symptoms at presentation, including coma, focal deficits or seizures, or persistent deficits several hours into 100% oxygen therapy

Usually patients with CO poisonings are treated with one session of HBO therapy. No consensus exists regarding additional treatments for persistent neurologic deficits.

Helium

Helium can be administered as a gas mixture with oxygen (heliox). The density of the gas depends on the relative percentage of helium compared to oxygen; a mixture of 80% helium and 20% oxygen will have the least density and the greatest decrease in airway resistance (oxygen/helium: 20/80 = 0.429 micropoise, 40/60 = 0.678 micropoise, and 80/20 = 1.178 micropoise). Because heliox is less dense than air, the resulting decrease in the density of the "carrier" gas and decreased resistance to gas flow may result in an increase in bulk gas flow, oxygen flow, and decreased work of breathing.

Use of heliox is limited in patients who require high inspired oxygen concentrations, because the decrease in density is generally considered clinically insignificant with less than 60% helium. In most clinical settings, heliox with a minimum concentration of oxygen of 20% is blended with pure oxygen to deliver the desired concentrations of oxygen and helium, thereby preventing the accidental delivery of hypoxic gas delivery. An additional safety is the continuous monitoring of the inspired FiO_2.

Clinical Use

Upper Airway Laboratory studies suggest that heliox would be beneficial in reducing resistance associated with turbulent gas flow, such as the upper airway of a child with croup. A 20% oxygen and 80% helium blend has proven to relieve airway obstruction. In a crossover randomized controlled study, heliox as 30% oxygen and 70% helium significantly decreased symptoms of postextubation stridor in children.

Lower Airway Studies of normal adults breathing heliox demonstrated an increase in FEV_1 and peak inspiratory flow rates. In studies of patients with severe asthma, heliox improved ventilation at lower airway pressures in both intubated and spontaneous breathing subjects.

Caution Regarding Use

The use of heliox in children requiring mechanical ventilation necessitates caution. Ventilator blenders are calibrated for air/oxygen so a separate oxygen analyzer is needed. A more notable problem is the change in density of the gas and inaccuracy in tidal volume measurement. The decrease in gas density results in a smaller pressure differential and thus leads to a falsely low flow and volume reading. Many clinicians may misinterpret the data and inappropriately increase the tidal volume, thereby defeating one of the potential therapeutic advantages of heliox. Ideally, this problem can be overcome by recalibrating the ventilator or defining conversion factors for the specific heliox blend. In the absence of this information, monitoring peak airway pressures and $PaCO_2$ offers the only alternative method of monitoring therapy.

Nitric Oxide

Nitric oxide (NO), a well-recognized industrial and cigarette pollutant, participates as a second messenger in many physiologic reactions throughout the body, including regulation of vasomotor tone, neurotransmission, immune function, and platelet aggregation. In this discussion, however, only the effects of NO in the lung are addressed.

Physiology and Toxicity

Within the lungs, the vascular endothelium as well as inflammatory cells (neutrophils, macrophages), structural cells (fibroblasts, epithelial, vascular and airway smooth muscle), anatomic nerves, and platelets produce NO. A highly lipid soluble molecule, NO diffuses through the pulmonary interstitium and vascular serosa into the vascular smooth muscle, where it binds to the heme iron of guanylate cyclase stimulating the production of cyclic 3,5'-monophosphate (cGMP). Cyclic GMP causes relaxation of vascular and airway smooth muscle through activation of cGMP- dependent protein kinase. As a result of the unstable nature of the compound, NO has a half-life ranging from 0.1 to 5.0 seconds in physiologic systems.

The activity of NO is limited by rapid and avid binding to hemoglobin. Eighty to ninety percent of inhaled NO reacts with hemoglobin to form nitrosyl-hemoglobin and methemoglobin. Further reactions with oxygen lead to formation of nitrates and nitrites. These are mostly excreted in the urine, but small amounts are excreted in saliva and stool.

Nitrogen dioxide (NO_2) and methemoglobinemia are the major known toxic byproducts of NO. The rate of conversion of NO to NO_2 is proportional to the square of the NO concentration, the O_2 concentration, and the residence time of NO and O_2. Nitrogen dioxide levels should be maintained at less than 1 part per million (ppm). Nitrogen dioxide can be removed from the breathing circuit with soda lime. Methemoglobin levels must be monitored. Populations with low methemoglobin reductase concentration (e.g., neonates, Native Americans) may develop high methemoglobin concentrations during administration of NO.

Fifty to sixty percent of inhaled NO_2 is retained in the lung, reacting with water to form nitric and nitrous acids. Although the Occupational Safety and Health Administration has recommended that work safety limits of NO_2 less than 5 ppm, inhalation of 2 ppm is associated with terminal bronchial epithelial hypertrophy and alveolar hyperplasia in rats. Animal studies also have demonstrated increased inflammatory cells and increased cytokines with exposures of 1.5 ppm.

Administration

Administration of NO should include:

- Calibrated tanks of NO that do not exceed 1,000 ppm
- Delivery systems that allow accurate NO delivery with as low as possible O_2 and NO concentrations as well as short residence time of the gases in the circuit and lungs to minimize NO_2 production
- Minimal contamination of the environment by scavenging exhaust gases
- Frequent or continuous monitoring of NO and NO_2 concentrations as can be done with chemiluminescence or electrochemical analyzers
- Periodic measurement of methemoglobin levels
- Lowest effective concentration of NO

Safe and reliable methods of delivery of NO for intubated patients breathing with various ventilators spontaneously or mechanically or in the nonintubated patient have been described.

Clinical Uses

Nitrous oxide is used both to diagnose and treat primary pulmonary hypertension and leads to clinical improvement in the majority of neonates with severe persistent pulmonary hypertension, avoiding the need for ECMO support. Unfortunately, the criteria for NO therapy are not well established. Inhaled NO also has been used in children with elevated pulmonary vascular resistance after cardiac surgery.

Inhalation of NO is particularly appealing in the setting of acute respiratory distress syndrome (ARDS) because the vasodilatory effects of NO improve perfusion only of ventilated areas of the lung, creating a diversion of blood flow from poorly ventilated areas, thereby improving matching of ventilation to perfusion. Trials in both adults and children have demonstrated increased oxygenation and decreased pulmonary artery pressure. Furthermore, vasodilatation is greatest in patients with severe pulmonary hypertension.

Humidification

Normally, inspired gases from the environment contain some degree of humidity (i.e., water vapor in ambient gas). As these gases pass through the upper respiratory system, they heat to body temperature and concomitant humidification to 100% relative humidity. Medical gases, however, are virtually dehumidified. In addition, delivery of medical gases to the critically ill patient with an artificial airway involves bypassing of upper respiratory pathways responsible for heating and humidification during spontaneous breathing.

Adequate humidification of inspired gases must be provided with all forms of respiratory therapy equipment used in the intubated patient to avoid such serious potential complications as enhanced respiratory insensible water loss and drying of respiratory secretions, which lead to airway obstruction and impaired mucociliary function. Several humidification devices have been developed that can be categorized by the presence or absence of heating elements as well as by the mechanisms of humidification.

Aerosol Therapy

Aerosols are used widely in health care, in both diagnosis and therapy, to deliver medication in large doses to their site of action with diminished systemic toxicity. Aerosols also allow delivery of active medication which may not be administered by another route.

Description of Particles

All aerosols, whether generated from solutions, suspensions, or a powdered drug, form heterodisperse, which are nonspherical water droplets or particles that are irregular in size and shape. These physical properties, as well as parameters of ventilation and airway geometry, determine the degree and site of deposition within the respiratory tree.

Aerosol particles generally are described in terms of an aerodynamic diameter, which allows description regardless of shape and density, to one of equivalent unit density sphere with the same terminal settling velocity in still air. Particles are characterized by the mass median aerodynamic diameter (MMAD) and the geometric standard deviation of their median aerodynamic diameter (GSD).

Deposition of Particles

Three physical forces determine particle deposition within the lung: impaction, sedimentation, and diffusion. Particles with MMADs greater than 10 microns have an impact on the oropharynx and proximal airways and are eliminated from aerosol. Respirable particles have MMADs less than 5 microns. Particles ranging from 0.5 to 1.0 microns are deposited by sedimentation under the influence of gravity. Deposition of still smaller particles will be determined primarily by diffusion. Approximately 80% of the extremely small particles (smaller than 1 micron) will be expired because the time required to diffuse to an airway is greater than the inspiratory phase of a breath.

Factors Affecting Deposition

Particle deposition is also affected by the following:

- Gas velocity. Higher respiratory flow rates increase turbulent gas flow, leading to increased particle deposition in the proximal airways.
- Airway geometry. Numerous bifurcations and narrowing of airways increase both turbulent flow and the likelihood of impaction in the more proximal airways.
- Inspiratory rates and airway size. Higher inspiratory rates and smaller airways of children impede deposition in the lower airways more so than in adults.

Nebulizers and Inhalers

Therapeutic aerosols are produced by nebulizers and metered-dose inhalers (MDI). Nebulizers use air or an enriched oxygen source as the vehicle with aerosolization of drug from a solution. Nebulized aerosols are produced by Venturi-type jet nebulizers or ultrasonic nebulizers. Jet nebulizers use compressed gas to create a jet of fluid carried by the airstream, whereas ultrasonic nebulizers use a piezoelectric crystal that vibrates at high frequencies, creating waves on the surface of the liquid to produce particle droplets. Although MMADs vary with equipment, jet nebulizers generally produce particles between 2 to 4 microns and the ultrasonic nebulizers generate slightly larger particles of 4 to 6 microns. Drug aerosols are generated from MDIs by an artificial surfactant such as soya lecithin, sorbiatan trioleate, or oleic acid with a fluorocarbon propellant liquid. MMADs from MDIs range from 1 to 10 microns.

Effects of Mechanical Ventilation

During mechanical ventilation, the endotracheal tube, ventilator circuit, and ventilation parameters all have an impact on aerosol deposition. Early studies demonstrated that delivery of nebulized medication through an adult endotracheal tube was decreased to approximately 3% of the original dose. Smaller pediatric endotracheal tubes further decreased drug delivery from the endotracheal tube. Studies have demonstrated that drug delivery from an MDI into a ventilator is significantly improved when a spacer is used with the MDI and when the MDI is discharged just before inspiration, with low inspiratory flow rates, low respiratory rates, and longer inspiratory times.

Nebulized therapy through a ventilator circuit requires careful adjustment of tidal volumes because of the intermittent addition of the flow from the nebulized gas into the ventilator circuit. Furthermore, filters are required to protect the expiratory valve from crystallization of medication within the ventilator. These factors and cost of administration favor MDI use over nebulized medications in ventilator circuits.

Medications Delivered

Medications administered in nebulized form include: beta adrenergic agents, anticholinergic agents, steroids, antibiotics, pentamidine, DNAse, and ribavirin.

Ribavirin, a synthetic nucleoside with antiviral properties against both RNA and DNA viruses such as respiratory syncytial virus, is typically administered with an expensive multijet small-particle aerosol generator (SPAG-2), which reliably produces a small aerosol (MMAD of 1 to 72 microns). Ribavirin may be administered safely in mechanically ventilated patients, but requires meticulous attention to prevent occlusion of the endotracheal tube or to the expiratory flow valve by crystallization of medication. Studies of ribavirin efficacy have yielded conflicting results.

Chest Physiotherapy

Chest physiotherapy refers to a constellation of maneuvers that include postural drainage, chest percussion, chest vibration, and deep breathing exercises.

Goals

The three major goals of chest physiotherapy are to clear pulmonary secretions, to avoid and reverse alveolar collapse, and to improve matching of ventilation and perfusion.

Positioning

Frequent positional changes prevent atelectasis and improve ventilation-perfusion matching. Patients receiving mechanical ventilation frequently are positioned supine, for ease of both nursing care and access to intravascular catheters and tubes. Prone positioning, however, may improve oxygenation in patients with high ventilation perfusion mismatch.

In adults with unilateral lung disease, positioning with the normal lung in the dependent position results in improved oxygenation, presumably because ventilation and perfusion is better matched. In small infants with unilateral lung disease, decreased oxygenation occurs, possibly because of decreased gravitational forces on regional blood flow relative to adults. Progressive hypoxia can occur in unilateral lung disease that impedes pulmonary perfusion from overdistention of the better functioning lung.

MECHANICAL VENTILATOR THERAPY

Physiologic Effects

Weighing the risks and benefits of mechanical ventilation helps the clinician establish a set of goals for mechanical ventilation (Table 6.2) and forms

Table 6.2
Goals and Complications of Assisted Mechanical Ventilation[a]

Goals to Achieve
  Complications to avoid
Improve alveolar ventilation and avoid significant hypercapnia and respiratory acidosis
  Hyperventilation and decreased cerebral blood flow
Reduce $\dot{V}/\dot{Q}$ mismatch and maintenance of normal hemoglobin saturation
  Hypoxemic tissue injury
  Oxygen toxicity to the lungs or other organs
Reexpand atelectatic or collapsed lung segments
  Alevolar overdistention
    Pulmonary hypoperfusion
    Reduced venous return/cardiac output
    Volutrauma to alveolar structures
Reduced work of breathing and eliminate respiratory muscle fatigue
  Suppressed ventilatory drive
  Respiratory muscle disuse atrophy
  Increased upper airway resistance (i.e., subglottic edema/stenosis)

[a]Modified with permission from Chatburn RL. Principles and practice of neonatal and pediatric mechanical ventilation. Respir Care 1991;36:569.

the framework for a complete description of the physiologic effects of mechanical ventilation on the growing and developing child.

Maintenance of Oxygenation Adjusting the inspired oxygen concentration is the most straightforward means to control oxygenation. Despite the simplicity of this system, there is rarely a direct relationship between FiO_2 and PaO_2. To start, consider the calculation of the partial pressure of inspired oxygen (PiO_2):

$$PiO_2 = FiO_2(P_b - P_H2_O),$$

where P_b is barometric pressure and P_H2_O is water vapor pressure. The P_H2_O is 47 torr at 37°C. This equation shows that some of the inspired oxygen is displaced by water vapor as the gas traverses the upper airways. Thus, solving the equation for room air at sea level (0.21×760 torr $- 47$ torr) results in a PiO_2 of approximately 150 torr. As the gas continues into the alveolar region of the lungs, more of the oxygen is displaced by carbon dioxide. The P_AO_2 in the alveolus is determined by the equation:

$$P_AO_2 = PiO_2 - P_ACO_2,$$

where P_ACO_2 is the alveolar partial pressure of carbon dioxide. For clinical purposes, this equation is simplified by the substitution of P_ACO_2 with the arterial partial pressure of carbon dioxide, which can be directly measured and dividing by the respiratory quotient (RQ):

$$P_AO_2 = PiO_2 - PaO_2/RQ.$$

The RQ is determined by the mix of substrates for metabolism (i.e., carbohydrates, proteins, fats) and generally is estimated to be approximately 0.8 in most clinical situations. Thus, using the estimated RQ, 40 torr for the PaO_2 and the 150 torr previously calculated for PiO_2 yields a value of approximately 100 torr for P_AO_2.

Maintenance of Alveolar Ventilation

A principal goal of mechanical ventilation is to augment or control alveolar ventilation. In fact, respiratory failure is frequently defined in terms of $PaCO_2$, which is inversely related to alveolar ventilation (V_A):

$$PaCO_2 \text{ proportional to } V_{CO2}/V_A,$$

where V_{CO2} is carbon dioxide production. Alveolar ventilation can be defined (in normal ventilatory frequencies) as:

$$V_A = (V_T - V_D)f,$$

where V_T is tidal volume, V_D is dead-space volume, and f is respiratory frequency. Therefore, it is clear that $PaCO_2$ can be altered by regulating V_T and f, which are the components of minute ventilation (V_E).

Simplified equations can be used to predict changes in $PaCO_2$ with changes in frequency and constant tidal volume: $nPaCO_2 = oPaCO_2 \times of/nf$ where n is the new or desired value, o is the old or measured value, $PaCO_2$ is the arterial partial pressure of carbon dioxide, and f is the respiratory frequency.

Dead-space volume is not routinely measured. In normal individuals, most V_D is a result of the volume of the conducting airways (anatomic V_D). This volume is relatively constant with increasing V_T, however, V_D/V_T tends to decrease and rarely exceeds 0.3. In ventilated patients, the configuration of the ventilator circuit (i.e., apparatus dead space) can affect V_D, although this is usually a minor consideration. In mechanically ventilated patients with intrinsic lung disease, V_D/V_T has been found to exceed 0.6 and principally is related to ventilated but poorly perfused lung regions (i.e., alveolar V_D).

Work of Breathing

The pressure-volume characteristics (i.e., compliance and resistance) of the respiratory system determine the work of breathing, which in reality represents afterload on the respiratory muscles. The work of breathing overcomes two major sources of impedance:

1. elastic recoil of the lungs and chest wall (Fig. 6.2, *area ADC*), and
2. the frictional resistance to gas flow in the airways (Fig. 6.2, *area ABC*).

Total work of breathing (Fig. 6.2, *area ABCD*) is increased either by an increase in resistance properties or by a decrease in respiratory compliance.

If minute volume is constant, the work done against compliance is increased when breathing is deep and slow. Conversely, the work done against airflow resistance is increased when breathing is rapid and shallow. In patients with restrictive lung diseases (i.e., low compliance) such as pulmonary edema or ARDS, the optimal respiratory frequency is increased, often leading to rapid, shallow breaths. With obstructive lung diseases (i.e., high resistance) such as asthma or bronchiolitis, the optimal strategy is decreased respiratory rate with slow, deep breaths.

Classification

The classification system of Chatburn is based on the physiologic principles of the equation of motion (i.e., pressure = volume/compliance + resistance × flow) and includes five broad categories to provide a thorough discussion (Table 6.3).

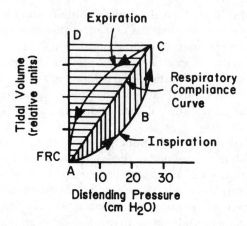

Figure 6.2. Inspiratory/expiratory pressure-volume loop recorded during respiratory cycle. The normal respiratory cycle entails the expenditure of work during inspiration to overcome resistive and elastic impedance to inflation of the lungs. Total work of breathing (pressure × volume) is defined by the sum of resistive work (*area* defined by *ABC*) plus elastic work (*area* defined by *ACD*). Total work of breathing (*area* defined by *ABCD*) is increased either by an increase in resistive properties of the respiratory system or by a decrease in respiratory compliance (*slope of line* between *A* and *C*). (Modified from Goldsmith JP, Karotkin EH. Assisted ventilation of the neonate. Philadelphia: WB Saunders, 1981:29.)

Table 6.3
Classification Scheme for Mechanical Ventilators

Power input
Power transmission
Control scheme
  Control variable
  Phase variable
  Conditional variable
Output waveform
Alarms
  Input power alarms
  Control circuit alarms
  Output alarms

Control Variables

These variables are those set or controlled by the ventilator to deliver the predetermined energy to the respiratory system. Four possible options for the control variable are available:

- Pressure-controllers control either the airway pressure (i.e., increasing it above the ambient pressure for inspiration) or the pressure surrounding the body surface (i.e., decreasing it below airway opening pressure for inspiration). These ventilators are classified as either positive or negative pressure type ventilators.

- Volume-controllers maintain a relatively constant tidal volume regardless of the varying workload (i.e., change in compliance and/or resistance) and measure volume to control the waveform.
- Flow controllers have a constant volume waveform, even with alterations in compliance and/or resistance, but volume is not measured or used as a feedback signal to alter flow.
- Time controllers time inspiration and expiration and are used when both pressure and volume are affected by changes in lung mechanics.

Phase Variables

Four phase-variable categories can be defined:

1. the trigger variable,
2. the limit variable,
3. the cycle variable, and
4. the baseline variable.

Trigger Variable The selected variable (i.e., pressure, volume, flow, time) that initiates or triggers inspiration is the trigger variable. Time was the first trigger variable used (i.e., the ventilator initiates a breath according to a set frequency independent of the patient's inspiratory efforts). To allow mechanical ventilation synchronized to the patient's inspiratory efforts, pressure became a trigger variable (i.e., a preset drop in the baseline circuit pressure secondary to the patient's inspiratory effort starts inspiration independent of the set frequency). Improved ventilator capabilities have led to the development of flow as a trigger variable. Flow triggering is more sensitive and associated with less imposed work for the patient with a standard ventilator circuit than pressure triggering. The sensitivity of the ventilator to the trigger variable and the amount of imposed work for the patient is adjustable by changing the ventilator's sensitivity.

Limit Variable During inspiration, pressure, volume, and flow all increase above their baseline end-expiratory values. One or more of these variables may rise up to a preset limit, which is the limit variable. To meet the criteria of a true limit variable, however, inspiration must not be terminated because this variable has achieved its preset limit value as seen with a cycle variable. For consistency, pressure, volume, and flow limits must be specified relative to their end-expiratory values. To maintain consistency and avoid any potential confusion, pressure limits must always be measured relative to the end-expiratory pressure (i.e., above positive end-expiratory pressure [PEEP]).

Cycle Variable The cycle variable is the specified variable used to terminate inspiration when a preset value is reached, in contrast to the limit variable, which attains its peak value before end-inspiration. Determining which variable terminates inspiration in a given ventilator can be confusing. Most microprocessor ventilators allow the clinician to set a tidal volume and inspiratory flow rate, leading one to believe that the ventilator is volume-cycled. In fact, these ventilators do not measure volume, but set the inspiratory time necessary to achieve the set tidal volume using the set inspiratory flowrate. Thus, the cycle variable actually is time.

Baseline Variable During expiration, the ventilator may alter the way the control variables return to their respective baseline values. The baseline variable is that controlled during the expiratory time. Pressure is the typical baseline variable in the vast majority of clinical situations. Control of the baseline variable allows the ventilator to control end-expiratory transrespiratory pressure and thus end-expiratory volume. The term transrespiratory is used to accommodate the situation in which a negative pressure ventilator is used to maintain a negative body-surface pressure during expiration or when negative pressure is applied to the airway to facilitate expiration.

Breath Types Depending on whether the ventilator or the patient controls the triggering, limiting, and cycling variables, four different breath types have been described (Table 6.4).

Conditional Variables Modern microprocessor ventilators combine the control and phase variables to deliver the predetermined waveform for each breath. The ventilator may keep this pattern constant for each breath or it may introduce other patterns (i.e., mandatory and spontaneous breaths, assisted and supported breaths). The ventilator must determine which pattern of control and phase variable to use before each breath, depending on the value of some preset conditional variables. A common example is in the synchronized intermittent mandatory ventilation (SIMV) mode of ventilation. If the ventilator fails to detect a patient's inspiratory effort during a predetermined time (i.e., the SIMV window), a mandatory breath is delivered. If the patient's inspiratory efforts are sensed while the SIMV window is open, an assisted breath is provided; however, if the patient's inspiratory effort oc-

Table 6.4
Classification of the Available Mechanical Ventilator Breaths[a]

Breath Type	Trigger	Phase Variable Limit	Cycle
Mandatory	Machine	Machine	Machine
Assisted	Patient	Machine	Machine
Supported	Patient	Machine	Patient
Spontaneous	Patient	Patient	Patient

[a]Modified with permission from Branson RD & Chatburn, RL. Technical description and classification of modes of ventilator operation. Respir Care 1992;37:1029.

curs after the SIMV window is closed, then a spontaneous breath is allowed. Under these circumstances, the conditional variables are pressure (or flow) and time.

Output Waveform

Output waveform analysis (Fig. 6.3) is a useful tool to examine the characteristics of ventilator operation and provides a graphic display of the various modes of ventilation. It can be used to optimize mechanical ventilatory support and analyze ventilator incidents and alarm conditions. Simultaneous display of pressure, volume, and time waveforms may signal the need to alter the form of ventilatory support to improve patient-ventilator synchrony,

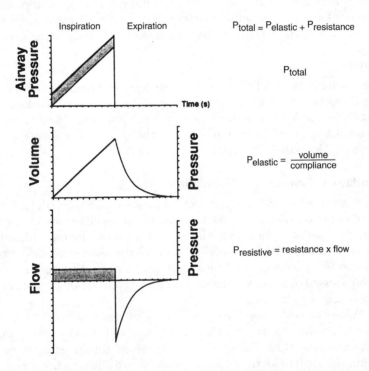

Figure 6.3. The theoretical output waveforms for flow-controlled inspiration presented as specified by equation of motion (i.e., pressure-top, volume-middle, flow-bottom). Note that the volume waveform is the same shape as the transthoracic or lung pressure waveform (i.e., pressure is due to elastic recoil) and the flow waveform is the same shape as the trans-airway pressure waveform (i.e., pressure due to airway resistance). If all the pressure scales are equal, then the height of the airway pressure waveform at any instant in time is the sum of the heights of the two waveforms as indicated by the shaded and unshaded portions of the figure. (From Chatburn RL. Classification of mechanical ventilation. Respir Care 1992;37:1022.)

reduce work-of-breathing, and calculate an assortment of physiologic parameters associated with respiratory mechanics.

Optimal measurement of these data is obtained when the pressure and
flow measuring device is positioned between the patient and the ventilator.
Measurement of esophageal pressure and integration of the intrapleural
pressure enhances output data analysis and enables measurement of the patient's work-of-breathing.

Alarms

Nearly every aspect of a patient's ventilatory pattern can be assessed, monitored, displayed, and alarmed. These alarms may be audible, visual, or both,
depending on the seriousness of the alarm condition. The alarm event may
be technical (i.e., inadvertent change in the ventilator's performance) or
patient related (i.e., denoting a change in the patient's status as detected by
the ventilator). Alarm types include input, control, and output alarms.

Modes

The ventilator may deliver four different types of breaths—mandatory, assisted, supported, or spontaneous. Most of the commonly used modes are
actually a combination of these four types of breaths (Table 6.5). This classification system will be used to describe the modes of mechanical ventilation available to the clinician.

Mandatory (Controlled) Ventilation

In this mode of ventilator operation, all breaths are triggered, limited, and
cycled by the ventilator (i.e., the machine performs all the work). Any of the
control modes of ventilation are intended for use in patients with limited or
absent ventilatory drives. In reality, many of the assisted modes of ventilation also become controlled modes when the patient's inspiratory efforts
are suppressed by sedatives, analgesics, or hyperventilation or otherwise prevented (e.g., by paralysis).

Volume Control Ventilation Volume control ventilation (VCV) delivers a
preset tidal volume during a set inspiratory time with a set frequency and constant inspiratory flow. The ventilator controls all timing parameters of the
breath, although modern ventilators respond to a patient's inspiratory effort
(see discussion of assisted ventilation). VCV is typically used only for patients
who are apneic from sedation or anesthesia; have nervous system injury, drug
overdose, or neuromuscular blockade; or have had deliberate mechanical hyperventilation so that the patient's spontaneous ventilator drive is suppressed.

Pressure Control Ventilation Pressure control ventilation (PCV) is designed
for patients with suppressed ventilatory drive although patient inspiratory efforts will trigger the ventilator to deliver the same pressure-limited breath. In
this mode the ventilator delivers positive pressure up to a predetermined pres-

Table 6.5
Classification System for Common Modes of Mechanical Ventilation[a]

Modes	Mandatory			Assisted			Supported			Spontaneous			Conditional Variable
	trigger	limit	cycle	trigger	limit	cycle	trigger	limit	cycle	trigger	limit[b]	cycle[b]	
VCV	time	flow	volume[c]	—	—	—	—	—	—	—	—	—	—
PCV	time	pressure	time	—	—	—	—	—	—	—	—	—	—
PRVC	time	pressure	volume[c]	—	—	—	—	—	—	—	—	—	minute volume
ACV (volume)	time	flow	volume[c]	patient[d]	flow	volume[c]	—	—	—	—	—	—	patient effort or time
ACV (pressure)	time	pressure	time	patient[d]	pressure	time	—	—	—	—	—	—	patient effort or time
IMV (volume)	time	flow	volume[c]	—	—	—	—	—	—	patient[d]	pressure	pressure	—
SIMV (volume)	time	flow	volume[c]	patient[d]	flow	volume[c]	—	—	—	patient[d]	pressure	pressure	patient effort or time
IMV (pressure)	time	pressure	time	—	—	—	—	—	—	patient[d]	pressure	pressure	—
SIMV (pressure)	time	pressure	time	patient[d]	pressure	time	—	—	—	patient[d]	pressure	pressure	patient effort or time
APRV	time	pressure	time	—	—	—	—	—	—	patient[d,e]	pressure	pressure	—
APRV (synch.)	time	pressure	time	patient[d]	pressure	time	—	—	—	patient[d,e]	pressure	pressure	patient effort or time

continued

Table 6.5
Classification System for Common Modes of Mechanical Ventilation[a]

Modes	Mandatory			Assisted			Supported			Spontaneous			Conditional Variable
	trigger	limit	cycle	trigger	limit	cycle	trigger	limit	cycle	trigger	limit[b]	cycle[b]	
MMV	time	flow	volume[c]	patient[d]	flow	volume[c]	—	—	—	patient[d]	—	—	minute volume
PSV	—	—	—	—	—	—	patient[d]	press.	flow[f]	—	—	—	—
VSV	—	—	—	—	—	—	patient[d]	press.	flow[f]	—	—	—	minute volume
VAPS	—	—	—	—	—	—	patient[d]	press.	flow[f]	—	—	—	tidal volume
CPAP	—	—	—	—	—	—	—	—	—	patient	pressure	pressure	patient effort

[a]Modified with permission from Branson RD, Chatburn RL. Technical description and classification of modes of ventilator operation. Respir Care 1992;37:1029.

[b]Pressure-limited only on demand-valve systems in which the ventilator limits and cycles to maintain constant airway pressures (applies to all modes in this column).

[c]Cycling can also be caused by set inspiratory time in the setting of a fixed flow.

[d]May be either patient-generated pressure or flow in the ventilator circuit.

[e]Allows spontaneous breaths during mandatory inspiratory and expiratory time.

[f]Flow reflects the interaction of the patient's effort with the respiratory system impedance and ventilator flow rate.

VCV, volume-controlled ventilation; PCV, pressure-controlled ventilation; PRVC, pressure-regulated volume control; ACV, assist-control ventilation; IMV, intermittent mandatory ventilation; SIMV, synchronized IMV; APRV, airway pressure release ventilation; MMV, mandatory minute ventilation; PSV, pressure support ventilation; VSV, volume support ventilation; VAPS, volume-assisted pressure support; CPAP, continuous positive airway pressure.

sure limit above PEEP during a selected inspiratory time and at a set frequency. The inspiratory flow depends on airway pressure and lung compliance, normally achieving high levels from the beginning of the breath and then decelerating toward zero at the end of inspiration. Because inspiratory pressure is the limiting variable, changes in respiratory system mechanics (i.e., compliance and/or resistance) will result in alteration in the delivered tidal volume and thus minute ventilation.

Pressure Regulated Volume Control Ventilation Pressure regulated volume control (PRVC) combines the characteristics of both volume- and pressure-limited ventilation. This mode uses a decelerating inspiratory flow waveform to deliver a set tidal volume during the selected inspiratory time and at a set frequency. The ventilator monitors airway resistance and compliance and uses a predetermined algorithm to deliver the preset tidal volume. Airway pressure is limited below a selected high pressure threshold and may vary by as much as 3 cm H_2O from the previous breath. Thus, the ventilator is continuously adapting the inspiratory pressure to changes in the volume/pressure relationship of the patient's respiratory system.

Assisted Ventilation

Assisted ventilation is essentially identical to the respective controlled modes of ventilation except that patient inspiratory efforts trigger the ventilator to deliver assisted breaths using the preselected limit and cycle variables (i.e., the patient performs only the triggering work while the ventilator completes the remaining work). Assisted ventilation can be provided with either pressure or flow as the limit variable.

One potential drawback with this class of ventilation is that the inspiratory time is fixed. Rapid respiratory rates with the fixed inspiratory times lead to shorter expiratory times and may result in the delivery of mechanical tidal volumes with inspiratory times in excess of expiratory times (i.e., inverse inspiratory/expiratory [I/E] ratios).

Assist Control Ventilation In this form of mechanical ventilation, the ventilator provides a preset tidal volume or pressure in response to every patient-initiated breath. Should the patient fail to initiate a breath within a preselected time, the ventilator delivers the mechanical tidal volume at a predetermined frequency (i.e., controlled ventilation). In essence, the controlled mode of ventilation on the recent generation of ventilators is assist control ventilation (ACV) when the patient is breathing spontaneously. Because every spontaneous respiratory effort by the patient triggers a mechanical tidal volume, minute ventilation essentially is determined by the patient regardless of the selected ventilator rate—as long as the ventilator rate is lower than the patient's spontaneous rate.

When compared to synchronized intermittent mandatory ventilation (SIMV), ACV has been associated with a respiratory alkalosis with equal minute ventilation (presumably secondary to a lower deadspace to tidal volume ventilation ratio) and a higher mean airway pressure and resultant lower cardiac output. A perceived problem with a mode of ventilation is the inability to "wean" the mechanical portion of the minute ventilation. Thus, patients typically are extubated from ACV following either a continuous positive airway pressure (CPAP)/t-piece trial or "when they are judged to be ready."

Intermittent Mandatory Ventilation Intermittent mandatory ventilation (IMV) allows spontaneous breathing between positive pressure breaths with a preset inspiratory time and frequency. The positive pressure breaths may be either pressure or volume limited. Delivery of the mechanical breaths can be triggered at a predetermined time interval (i.e., asynchronous IMV) or in response to the patient's spontaneous inspiratory efforts (i.e., synchronous IMV). Between mechanical breaths, the patient may breathe spontaneously from either a continuous-gas flow or a demand-flow system.

The gradual decrease in positive pressure ventilatory support and concomitant increase in spontaneous breathing allows smooth, continuous progression from assisted to independent ventilation and circumvents problems with asynchrony between the patient and ventilator, decreasing the necessity for sedatives and muscle relaxants in the management of mechanical ventilatory support. In addition, IMV offers the advantage of diminishing the level of positive intrathoracic pressure associated with positive pressure ventilatory support; consequently, it has been suggested that circulatory impairment resulting from impedance to venous return during positive pressure ventilation might be diminished with IMV. Finally, spontaneous breathing is associated with improved distribution of ventilation to dependent lung regions where greater perfusion occurs, while controlled positive pressure ventilation has been found to favor ventilation of nondependent regions (e.g., dead space). The fact that SIMV allows a certain degree of spontaneous breathing offers the theoretical attraction of improving V/Q matching in the lungs. For all practical purposes, SIMV has become the standard mode of mechanical ventilation in most neonatal and pediatric centers worldwide.

Airway Pressure Release Ventilation Airway pressure release ventilation (APRV), as originally described, provides a continuous gas flow circuit to vary the airway pressure between two different CPAP levels (known as CPAP and release pressure) for set periods of time while allowing spontaneous ventilation for the patient at both levels. Airway pressures are decreased or "released" intermittently from the preset CPAP to a lower (release) or ambient pressure. Lung volume transiently decreases, allowing gas to exit the lungs passively, thereby augmenting alveolar ventilation.

Airway pressure release ventilation was designed to open and stabilize the collapsed alveoli associated with acute lung injury without excessive peak airway pressures and to augment spontaneous minute ventilation with the brief, intermittent releases of airway pressure. One benefit of the continuous gas flow circuit is that the patient may breathe spontaneously throughout the ventilatory cycle with minimal imposed work of breathing, and therefore, minimal or no sedation or paralysis is required.

Airway pressure release ventilation has been incorporated into several ventilators with demand circuits with synchronized patient triggering capabilities. Preset variables that physicians control include the CPAP level, the frequency of the airway pressure releases, the level to which airway pressure is reduced during release, and the duration of airway pressure release. The limit variable is pressure, thus the degree of augmented ventilation depends on these variables plus the patient's respiratory system compliance and resistance. Timing (i.e., synchronized with the patient's inspiratory efforts) and duration of the release time (i.e., as a function of the time constant of the respiratory system) may affect the efficiency of this mode of ventilation significantly.

Mandatory Minute Ventilation   This mode allows the mandatory delivery of a predetermined minute volume that is distributed variably between spontaneous and mechanical breaths and depends on the patient's spontaneous ventilation. With mandatory minute ventilation (MMV), the machine measures the volume of gas breathed spontaneously by the patient over a predetermined time period. If this timed spontaneous volume falls below a preset volume, the machine delivers breaths of either fixed volume or pressure until the preset minute volume is achieved. Mandatory minute ventilation "guarantees" that a predetermined minute ventilation will be delivered to the patient by either spontaneous or mechanical positive pressure means. Used primarily for the purpose of weaning, MMV has been used infrequently in the United States but has received some attention in Europe.

Supported Ventilation

Supported ventilation is defined as a breath triggered by the patient, limited by the ventilator, and cycled by the patient (i.e., the patient provides the triggering work and interacts with the ventilator to perform a variable amount of the remaining work). Ventilation is spontaneous in that the patient initiates and terminates each breath and is only used in patients with adequate ventilatory drives.

Continuous Positive Airway Pressure   During CPAP, the clinician selects a level of pressure that is maintained constant in the ventilator circuit while the patient breathes spontaneously. To avoid confusing CPAP with PEEP, which is defined as the elevation in baseline pressure during mechanical ventilation, consider that CPAP represents a mode of ventilation, whereas PEEP is simply the control of the baseline pressure during mechanical ventilation. Although defined as separate entities, both CPAP and PEEP are used for the same purpose, to increase end-expiratory lung volume.

Technically, CPAP or PEEP is provided by mechanical ventilatory devices using a modification of standard expiratory valve mechanisms in conjunction with either continuous-flow or inspiratory demand-valve circuitry. Expiratory valves can function either as threshold resistors, which allow unimpeded expiration prior to achieving the preset end-expiratory circuit pressure, or as expiratory flow resistors, which act to impede flow during expiration such that inspiration begins before expiratory airway pressure reaches atmospheric levels (Fig. 6.4). The latter expiratory valve system is undesirable in most clinical settings because it is associated with higher mean intrathoracic pressures, greater circulatory embarrassment, and increased physiologic dead space.

Pressure Support Ventilation In this mode of positive pressure ventilation, the patient triggers the ventilator to deliver a flow of gas sufficient to

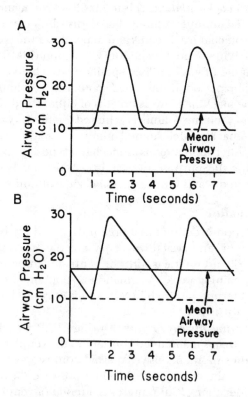

Figure 6.4. Airway pressure pattern during mechanical ventilation with PEEP generated by expiratory threshold valve (A) and expiratory flow resistor (B). Both systems generate 10 cm H_2O PEEP. However, the ventilatory pattern generated with the expiratory flow resistor results in increased mean airway pressure.

meet inspiratory demands while the exhalation valve closes, thus pressurizing the circuit to a preset pressure limit. Each cycle is terminated when inspiratory flow decreases to a percentage of its initial peak value rather than by volume, pressure, or time. Therefore, the patient retains control of the cycle length as well as its depth and flow characteristics. The patient's effort, the preset positive pressure limit, and the respiratory system impedance determine the delivered tidal volume.

The degree of machine support depends on the level of preset pressure, which can range from partial support with low-pressure limits to nearly complete mechanical support with high-pressure limits. Pressure support ventilation (PSV) can decrease inspiratory work and abolish diaphragmatic muscle fatigue, which may be related to the ability to change the pressure-volume characteristics during PSV and enhance the endurance conditioning of the diaphragm. Pressure support ventilation also has been used to compensate for inspiratory work because of endotracheal tube impedance and inspiratory demand valves.

Pressure support ventilation may be of help in patients who have been difficult to wean from mechanical ventilation. Two methods of weaning from ventilation with PSV have been advocated.

1. Patients initially are ventilated at PS_{MAX} (defined as the pressure support level required to produce a tidal volume of 10–12 mL/kg). As clinical status dictates, the pressure support level gradually is decreased to a minimal value determined by the diameter of the endotracheal tube, at which time extubation can be performed.
2. SIMV plus PSV is used when complete machine support is required. "Trials" with PSV can be provided periodically in between periods of SIMV until the patient no longer requires SIMV and the pressure support level is minimal.

Volume Support Ventilation   Several "new" modes of volume support ventilation have been introduced in which the patient spontaneously triggers the ventilator to provide a pressure-limited and flow-cycled breath with a conditional "if, then" variable. These modes have all the theoretically beneficial characteristics of PSV (i.e., the patient controls the inspiratory flow, time, and frequency) with the unique asset of providing a guaranteed minimal minute ventilation. They also provide backup mandatory breaths should the patient become apneic. No clinical experience with these theoretically attractive modes of ventilation have been published.

Indications

The most common and obvious indication for mechanical ventilatory support is respiratory failure. This condition can be defined qualitatively as any respiratory condition associated with inadequate alveolar ventilation, failure of arterial oxygenation, or both (Table 6.6).

Table 6.6
Indications for Initiating Positive Pressure Ventilation, Continuous Distending Pressure, or Both

Absolute
Inadequate alveolar ventilation
   Apnea
   $PaCO_2 > 50–55$ torr (in the absence of chronic hypercapnia)
   Impending hypoventilation
      Increasing $PaCO_2$
      Vital capacity < 15 mL/kg
      Dead space/tidal volume ratio > 0.6
Failure of arterial oxygenation
   Cyanosis with $FiO_2 \geq 0.6$
   $PaO_2 < 70$ torr with $FiO_2 > 0.6$
   Other indices of severely impaired oxygenation
      $AaDO_2 > 300$ torr with $FiO_2 = 1.0$
      $\dot{Q}_s/\dot{Q}_T > 15$–20%
Relative
Secure control of ventilatory pattern and function
   Intracranial hypertension
   Circulatory insufficiency
Decrease metabolic cost of breathing
   Chronic respiratory failure
   Circulatory insufficiency

Application

After the decision to initiate ventilatory support has been made, preset mechanical ventilatory parameters should be determined in a systematic fashion (Table 6.7).

As a general rule, deviations from physiologic respiratory patterns with regard to rate and inspiration time are avoided. Excessive prolongation of inspiratory time can result in significant elevations in mean airway pressure, decreased venous return and depressed cardiac output. Short inspiratory times and prolonged expiratory times (i.e., low I/E ratio) may be associated with an increased ratio of physiologic dead space and thus hypercapnia. The relationship between the inspiratory and expiratory times employed during positive pressure ventilation must be tailored to the patient's underlying physiologic abnormality.

Normal Respiratory Mechanics

Postoperative Setting Most patients do not require mechanical ventilation after surgery. In a few patients, residual anesthetic effects, usually a result of narcotics and suppression of respiratory drive or neuromuscular blocking agents with respiratory pump failure, may result in the need for mechanical ventilation for a variable period of time. Although anesthetic-induced

Table 6.7
Guidelines for Initiating Positive Pressure Support

Provision of adequate alveolar ventilation
Select rate—physiologic norm for age
Select tidal volume—10–15 mL/kg
Select inspiratory time (I/E ratio)—age-specific norm generally resulting in I/E ratio = 1:2
Obstructive diseases—prolong expiratory time, avoid prolonged inspiratory time
Immediately assess for signs of adequate ventilation (e.g., chest excursion, breath sounds)
Measure $PaCO_2$; adjust SIMV rate and/or tidal volume as needed to maintain level
  between 35 and 45 torr
Decrease SIMV rate to level tolerated as determined by $PaCO_2$
Maintenance of adequate oxygenation
FiO_2—1.0
PEEP—3 cm H_2O, or higher level if needed, and ability to tolerate hemodynamic effects
  are anticipated
Immediately assess for signs of adequate oxygenation (e.g., color, pulse oximetry) and
  circulatory depression (e.g., hypotension, diminished peripheral pulses)
Measure PaO_2
  Decrease FiO_2 maintaining $PaO_2 > 70$ torr
  Restrictive disease (low FRC, low compliance)—increase PEEP as needed to achieve
    $PaO_2 > 70$ torr at $FiO_2 = 0.4$–0.5
  Consider direct monitoring of cardiac output if $\bar{P}_{aw} > 25$ cm H_2O; adjust PEEP further to
    maintain $\dot{Q}_S/\dot{Q}_T < 20\%$
Decrease PEEP while maintaining $PaO_2 > 70$ torr

SIMV, synchronized intermittent mandatory ventilation; PEEP, positive end-expiratory pressure; FRC, functional
residual capacity.

changes in respiratory mechanics have been reported, in many cases these are
of little or no consequence and easily managed. Examples include surgeries
involving the face or airway (e.g., craniofacial and tracheal reconstruction,
cricoid split, tumors) in which the patency of the airway is of paramount importance or when deliberate hyperventilation is required for specific therapeutic purposes (i.e., intracranial and pulmonary hypertension). Patients
more commonly remain intubated receiving mechanical ventilation postoperatively because of actual or suspected alterations in respiratory mechanics.

Respiratory Pump Failure Patients with respiratory pump failure generally fall into one of the categories of acute (e.g., spinal cord trauma, Guil-
lain-Barre syndrome, botulism) or chronic (e.g., the various muscular dys-
trophies, myasthenia gravis, polio) neuromuscular disease. These patients
usually have normal ventilatory drives and lung function, but respiratory
muscle weakness making atelectasis and pneumonia common. Maintenance of a patent airway and provision of adequate lung volume are of primary importance for these patients. No evidence exists to suggest that either
positive or negative pressure ventilation is superior in this situation.

Circulatory Pump Failure The provision of a patent airway and mechanical ventilation is one of the primary therapeutic interventions for shock.

Children with circulatory failure frequently have impaired oxygen delivery from hemodynamic impairment, but also from respiratory muscle dysfunction secondary to hypoxia and acidosis-both metabolic and respiratory in etiology). Respiratory failure in shock may also be a result of the development of noncardiogenic pulmonary edema as seen in ARDS with its resultant intrapulmonary shunting. Although the increase in intrathoracic pressure during mechanical ventilation commonly is associated with a decrease in venous return and cardiac output, the large negative intrathoracic pressures seen in patients with increased respiratory work leads to increased left ventricular transmural pressure, increased wall stress and afterload with subsequent deleterious effects on myocardial function. In fact, this phenomenon has been documented in critically ill adults. Finally, the reduction in metabolic expenditures and blood flow to the respiratory muscles following initiation of mechanical ventilation in patients with cardiogenic shock may serve to abate further ischemic or anoxic injury to other vital organs.

The decision to institute mechanical ventilation for these patients must be tempered by the potential hemodynamic consequences associated with many of the medications used to facilitate airway management and the physiologic changes seen when converting from a largely negative to positive intrathoracic pressure.

Neurologic Injury Hypercapnia is the most potent stimulus for cerebral vasodilatation; consequently, one of the most effective means of acutely decreasing intracranial pressure (ICP) is to lower the arterial carbon dioxide tension artificially via hyperventilation. Decreases in ICP do not necessarily reflect increases in cerebral perfusion pressure. Although it is reasonable to introduce hyperventilation to decrease ICP until other therapies (e.g., diuretics, sedatives) administered for the same purpose have time to take effect in the acute situation, the *chronic* application of prophylactic hyperventilation in patients with head injury without raised ICP is detrimental. If the head-injured patient has been hyperventilated prophylactically to a $PaCO_2$ of 25 to 30 mm Hg, a dramatic increase in minute ventilation may be required to further decrease $PaCO_2$. The increase in mean airway pressure and intrathoracic pressure associated with this increase in minute ventilation may provoke a paradoxical increase in ICP. Thus, stable head-injured patients without elevations in ICP should receive mechanical ventilation sufficient to produce normocapnia while preventing hypoxemia. Care must be exercised when $PaCO_2$ has been lowered for acute ICP management, the return to normocapnia should be gradual so that the ensuing cerebral vasodilation will not increase ICP.

Abnormal Respiratory Mechanics

Most children who require mechanical ventilation do so because of alterations in their respiratory mechanics that result in hypoxemia or hypercapnia. Mechanical ventilation for these children should be tailored to compensate or correct the underlying pulmonary pathophysiology.

Restrictive Lung Disease Restrictive lung diseases are characterized by a decrease in lung volume with a proportionate reduction in airflow, often resulting from abnormalities in either thoracic (e.g., obesity, abdominal distention) or lung (e.g., alveolar filling, fibrosis) mechanics. Reduction in compliance usually results in a decrease in the time constant of the respiratory system, lower functional residual capacity in conjunction with increased closing volume (defined as the volume at which conducting airways in the dependent regions of the lung begin to collapse), increased V/Q mismatch and intrapulmonary shunting, and increased work of breathing.

For discussion purposes, the provision of mechanical ventilation for patients with ARDS is used as the model for this category of disease.

Clinical Picture Patients with ARDS exhibit reduced lung volumes associated with atelectasis and an elevation in closing volume. These changes lead to a generalized decrease in the lungs V/Q ratio, increased intrapulmonary shunting, and hypoxemia. The reduction in lung volumes causes:

1. decreased lung compliance,
2. alterations in regional resistances secondary to reduction in distal airway caliber by bronchoconstriction, peribronchial edema, and reduced lung volume, and
3. marked hysteresis (i.e., higher transpulmonary pressures are required during inspiration compared to expiration).
4. The net result of these alterations in respiratory mechanics is the development of a heterogenous decrease in respiratory system time constant and a significant increase in the transpulmonary pressure (i.e., work of breathing).

Alveolar Recruitment The primary goal of alveolar recruitment is achieved via increases in mean airway pressure ($\bar{P}_{aw}$). Under passive conditions, $\bar{P}_{aw}$ correlates closely to the forces holding the lung distended and is associated with the level of oxygenation. In clinical practice, $\bar{P}_{aw}$ is manipulated through changes in inspiratory and expiratory pressure and times as well as alteration in inspiratory waveform. While the benefits of alterations in inspiratory waveform (i.e., volume- versus pressure-limited ventilation) and/or inspiratory/expiratory ratio (i.e., inverse I/E ratio ventilation) remain controversial (see below), the regulation of expiratory and more recently inspiratory pressures appears well established by clinical and experimental evidence.

Use of PEEP

BENEFITS Positive end-expiratory pressure prevents airway pressure from falling below the alveolar closing pressure, thus maintaining airway patency and alveolar volume throughout the ventilatory cycle. Positive endexpiratory pressure not only redistributes pulmonary edema fluid from the alveoli to the interstitium, but also may help to maintain surfactant activity by limiting alveolar collapse and concurrent surfactant film collapse. The result is improved distribution of ventilation to low V/Q compartments of the lung and better overall V/Q matching in the lung. Positive end-expiratory pressure is of primary importance in improving oxygenation, diminishing the necessity for high concentrations of oxygen, increasing EEV, and improving total respiratory compliance in respiratory diseases with decreased resting lung volume and compliance.

HAZARDS Selection of the proper level of PEEP is important in achieving optimal results. High levels of PEEP, even when indicated, can depress cardiac output and oxygen delivery to peripheral organs. Application of continuous distending pressure beyond its optimal level can lead to increased physiologic dead space and decreased lung compliance as the result of alveolar overdistention. Worsening of oxygenation has also been reported with excessive PEEP, presumably because blood flow is shunted to poorly ventilated alveolar units from overdistended regions of the lung.

Optimal PEEP Physiologically defined first in terms of total oxygen delivery (i.e., arterial O_2 content times cardiac output), in association with maximal oxygen delivery—which coincided with the achievement of maximum total respiratory compliance, and then as the level that allows support of oxygenation with nontoxic levels of inspired oxygen without inducing refractory circulatory depression, optimal PEEP has been defined most recently in terms of respiratory mechanics (i.e., static pressure-volume curves of the respiratory system). Because the routine measurement of the static pressure-volume curve in most clinical settings is difficult, clinicians continue to use the lowest amount of PEEP necessary to achieve an easily monitored clinical goal (arterial oxygenation or saturation) with "non-toxic" inspired oxygen concentrations.

When increases are indicated, PEEP should be elevated in 2 to 3 cm H_2O increments with the goal of achieving adequate oxygenation (i.e., arterial hemoglobin saturation >90%) on nontoxic levels of supplemental oxygen (i.e. FiO_2 < 0.6); this usually corresponds roughly to an intrapulmonary shunt < 20% and an alveolar to arterial partial pressure of oxygen difference of <250 torr. Because of the risk of circulatory depression, it is recommended that cardiac output monitoring be performed by using a flow-directed, thermodilution pulmonary artery catheter when $\bar{P}_{aw}$ exceeds 25 cm H_2O or when clinical evidence of circulatory compromise is present. Decreased cardiac output in association with the application of PEEP usually responds to intravascular volume expansion with crystalloid or colloid solution, or to low-dose inotropic support (i.e., dopamine).

Limiting End-Inspiratory Alveolar Volume An airway plateau pressure of > 35 cm H_2O may be deleterious to the lung. In clinical conditions associated with decreased chest wall compliance, a plateau pressure threshold somewhat greater than 35 cm H_2O may be acceptable. The clinician may achieve this goal by using either smaller tidal volumes in volume-limited ventilation or lower peak airway pressures (in pressure-limited ventilation). This scheme of limiting plateau pressures frequently is responsible for the use of small tidal volumes, thus lowering minute and alveolar ventilation and allowing elevations in $PaCO_2$.

The term "permissive hypercapnia" has been used to describe the overall strategy of small tidal ventilation with adequate $\bar{P}_{aw}$ to achieve satisfactory oxygenation without toxic inspired oxygen concentrations while allowing $PaCO_2$ to increase if necessary.

Adverse side-effects or potential complications of hypercapnia include:

- Intracellular acidosis with potential to alter cellular oxidative metabolism, ionic conductances, excitation-contraction coupling, and cell division
- Increased sympathoadrenergic tone with elevations in heart rate and stroke volume while systemic vascular resistance decreases, which lead to an overall increase in cardiac output
- Cerebral vasodilatation, which allows cerebral blood flow to increase
- Increased arrhythmias

Many of these adverse effects are minimized by the body's ability to retain bicarbonate and compensate metabolically for a consistent respiratory acidosis. The only apparent absolute contraindication to permissive hypercapnia appears to be cerebral disorders in which increases in blood flow may lead to intracranial hypertension.

Obstructive Lung Disease Obstructive lung disease is identified by a reduction in airflow that is greater than any accompanying reduction in forced vital capacity (FVC); FEV_1 is reduced more than the FVC and the FEV_1/FVC ratio is low. As the disease progresses, increased airway resistance causes air trapping and an increase in residual volume (RV) (dynamic hyperinflation), until the elevation in RV begins to encroach on the vital capacity. Thus, the predominant change in respiratory mechanics is the increase in airway resistance and prolongation of the time constant. The dynamic hyperinflation and increase in RV also causes tidal ventilation to occur on the upper flat portion of the pressure-volume curve of the respiratory system, resulting in decreased compliance.

Acute respiratory failure in patients with asthma is associated with significant expiratory obstruction and dynamic hyperinflation. Resistance to inspiration and expiration are not only increased by bronchoconstriction but also as a consequence of airway edema and mucous. Patients benefit from mechanical ventilation strategies designed to maximize expiratory time, thereby decreasing end-expiratory lung volume (V_{EE}), intrinsic PEEP, and the risk of cardiovascular compromise. A higher V_{EE}, when using the same tidal volume, will invariably produce a higher end-inspiratory lung volume and a greater risk of volume-related lung injury (volutrauma). Principles on which we ventilate the asthmatic patient are discussed in Chapter 3.

Many of the same issues regarding deliberate hypoventilation, hypercapnia, and volutrauma discussed with respect to restrictive lung diseases also apply in this category. Thus, attempts to maintain airway plateau pressures under 35 cm H_2O theoretically should be allied with a decreased risk of volutrauma to the lung.

The consequences of dynamic hyperinflation include:

- Cycling of tidal volume closer to total lung capacity (where compliance is diminished) making higher airway pressures necessary to deliver the selected tidal volume
- Interfering with patient efforts to trigger the ventilator in assisted or supported modes of ventilation (i.e., the patient must generate enough pressure to overcome the intrinsic PEEP plus the trigger sensitivity)
- Increasing the work of breathing secondary to both preceding consequences
- Altering cardiovascular function similar to extrinsic PEEP through increases in intrathoracic pressure
- Causing overestimation of the pressure difference required for tidal ventilation and underestimation of the true compliance of the respiratory system

When assisted ventilation is used, the application of small amounts of extrinsic PEEP may be advantageous to decrease the work of breathing by improving the patient's ability to trigger the ventilator. Caution must be exercised to limit the application of extrinsic PEEP to a level less than intrinsic PEEP or dramatic increases in FRC and dynamic hyperinflation can occur. Regardless of the specific mode of ventilation, careful application with low frequency normal tidal volume ventilation with long expiratory times and the tolerance of hypercapnia has been associated with decreased morbidity and mortality in adults and children.

Focal Lung Disease In patients with unilateral lung disease developing respiratory failure, the physiologic change responsible for the initiation of mechanical ventilation is in almost every situation a result of hypoxemia and not hypercapnia. Therapeutic efforts typically are directed toward positional changes of the patient and alterations in inspiratory flow rates in order to improve overall lung function. Simultaneous independent lung ventilation via double-lumen tracheal tubes and differential application of positive airway pressure has been described in both adults and children, but is technically difficult and has not been shown to improve outcome. Therefore, most clinicians continue to use conventional ventilatory techniques. When difficulties in oxygenation are encountered, options include:

- A trial of ventilation with the least involved lung in the dependent position is appropriate in larger patients and the diseased lung in the dependent position in infants
- Reinflating the diseased lung (i.e., flexible fiberoptic bronchoscopy for clearing of involved airways)

- Other experimental methods of cardiorespiratory support (i.e., independent lung ventilation, high frequency ventilation, extracorporeal life support)

Weaning

The successful weaning of positive pressure support depends on the careful consideration of general patient status, the presence of adequate ventilatory reserve, and the attainment of favorable pulmonary mechanics. Greater understanding of respiratory muscle performance in infants and children may improve the decision making during the process of withdrawal (i.e., weaning) from mechanical ventilation. The determinants of the ability to resume and sustain spontaneous ventilation are the converse of the indications for mechanical ventilation; therefore, the pathophysiologic factors that determine ventilator dependence can be divided into hypoxemic failure and hypoventilation.

Physiology

Hypoxemia during a weaning trial may be the result of three separate processes:

1. hypoventilation,
2. impaired pulmonary gas exchange (typically lung volume loss), or
3. decreased mixed venous O_2 content.

Hypoventilation because of respiratory muscle pump failure is the most common cause of failure to wean from mechanical ventilation. The etiology of respiratory muscle pump failure can be divided into decreased ventilatory capacity or increased respiratory muscle load (Table 6.8).

Predictive Indices

The indices directed at ensuring adequate gas exchange (i.e., oxygenation) and the presence of adequate respiratory reserve (i.e., ventilatory pump function) are summarized in Table 6.9.

Techniques

Techniques used to wean patients from mechanical ventilation include T-tube weaning, intermittent mandatory ventilation, and pressure support ventilation. Despite conflicting data, SIMV has emerged as the standard mode of ventilatory support used for weaning mechanical ventilation in infants and children (Table 6.9).

Synchronized Intermittent Mandatory Ventilation Synchronized intermittent mandatory ventilation mode allows the withdrawal of a portion of the positive pressure breaths shortly after initiation, and further withdrawal can progress

Table 6.8
Etiologies of Respiratory Pump Failure

Decreased ventilatory capacity
Neurologic
   Decreased respiratory center output
     Narcotics
   Cervical spinal cord surgery
   Phrenic nerve dysfunction
     Diaphragmatic paralysis
Respiratory muscle
   Hyperinflation
   Malnutrition
   Metabolic derangements
     Hypomagnesemia
     Hypophosphatemia
     Hypocalcemia
     Hypokalemia
   Decreased oxygen supply
     Shock
     Hypoxemia via decreased energy supply
     Hypercapnia
   Disuse atrophy
   Respiratory muscle fatigue
   Abdominal wall defects
Increased respiratory muscle load
Increased ventilatory requirements
   Increased CO_2 production
     Malnutrition
     Fever
     Excessive muscle activity
   Increased dead space ventilation
     Asthma
     Bronchiolitis
     Bronchopulmonary dysplasia
   Inappropriately elevated ventilatory drive
     Psychologic stress
     Neurologic lesions
     Pulmonary irritant receptor stimulation
Increased work of breathing
Decreased efficiency of breathing
   Increased chest wall compliance
   Respiratory pattern

at a pace tailored to the capabilities of the patient. In general, the frequency of positive pressure breaths is decreased in increments of 2 to 5 breaths/min following the assessment of the patient by using clinical signs and blood gas determination. The appearance of signs of respiratory distress or carbon dioxide retention at any point should temporarily halt attempts to withdraw support. In the older child, the ultimate goal is to withdraw positive pressure ven-

Table 6.9
Guidelines for Discontinuing Positive Pressure Support

Weaning
Decrease SIMV rate
  Infants: wean to 2–4 breaths/min
  Older child: wean to CPAP mode
Decrease continuous distending pressure (CPAP or PEEP)
  Infants: wean to 2–3 cm H_2O
  Older child: wean to 5 cm H_2O or less
Discontinuing support
Evidence of adequate ventilatory reserve
  Infants:
    Normal $PaCO_2$
    Crying vital capacity > 15 mL/kg
    Maximum negative inspiratory pressure against occluded airway > 45 cm H_2O
  Older child:
    Normal $PaCO_2$
    Vital capacity > 10–15 mL/kg
    Maximum negative inspiratory pressure against occluded airway > 20 cm H_2O
  Minute ventilation < 10 L/min
  Ability to double resting minute ventilation
  Thoracic compliance > 25 mL/cm H_2O
  Airway occlusion pressure < 6 cm H_2O
  Tidal volume > 300 mL
  Respiratory frequency < 25 breaths/min
Evidence of adequate oxygenation capability
  $PaO_2 \geq 60$ torr at $FiO_2 \leq 0.35$
  Ancillary tests
  $AaDO_2 < 350$ torr at $FiO_2 = 1.0$
  PaO_2/FiO_2 ratio > 200
  $Q_S/Q_T < 10$–20%
  Dead space/tidal volume ratio < 0.6

SIMV, synchronized intermittent mandatory ventilation; CPAP, continuous positive airway pressure; PEEP, positive end-expiratory pressure.

tilation fully, leaving the patient to breathe spontaneously with CPAP. In infants, the presence of an endotracheal tube is associated with increased airways resistance and work of breathing, which may cause diaphragmatic fatigue with spontaneous breathing alone. It is recommended, therefore, that several mandatory positive pressure breaths (i.e., low IMV or PEEP mode) be maintained during the weaning of positive pressure ventilation in younger children to help offset this mechanical disadvantage.

PSV with or without SIMV PSV alone or in conjunction with SIMV allows gradual withdrawal of mechanical ventilation. PSV is particularly appealing because the patient maintains control of the ventilatory frequency and pattern while the degree of machine support depends on the preset pressure. PSV decreases the ventilator imposed work of breathing and relieves diaphragmatic muscle fatigue in patients who fail conventional weaning attempts. These facts may be because of the improved pressure-volume load characteristics and enhanced endurance conditioning of the diaphragm seen with PSV. Others use PSV simply to overcome the work imposed by endotracheal tube resistance and gradually decrease the SIMV rate as the means of weaning support. Regardless of the method selected, the clinician must monitor continuously for signs of increased work and halt weaning to avoid respiratory muscle fatigue.

Complications

Mechanical ventilation, while frequently lifesaving, is also associated with numerous real and potential complications, some of which are themselves life-threatening. Although complications are well recognized in adults, little work is available in the pediatric literature.

Complications range from patient discomfort to unnecessary prolongation of mechanical ventilation with excessive use of limited health resources. This discussion is limited to complications related to positive intrathoracic pressure and required adjunctive therapies.

Positive Intrathoracic Pressure

The side effects of mechanical ventilation related to continuous positive intrathoracic pressure are presented in Tables 6.10 and 6.11.

Cardiovascular Function

Cardiovascular and peripheral circulatory complications associated with the use of CPAP or PEEP (i.e., elevated mean airway pressure) are well described. Decreased cardiac output accompanies the administration of continuous distending pressure with regularity. A variety of mechanisms have been evoked to explain the effects of $\bar{P}_{aw}$ on cardiac output. Decreased cardiac filling associated with increased intrathoracic pressure during positive pressure assistance has been documented and increased intrapleural pressure associated with CPAP or PEEP has been shown to decrease systemic venous return and ventricular preload. Increased pulmonary vascular resistance and right ventricular afterload have also been implicated in the depression of cardiac output accompanying PEEP.

Required Adjunctive Therapies

The single most important intervention associated with delivery of mechanical ventilation is airway intubation to assure patency and allow application of positive pressure. Patients with severe alteration in respiratory function may require imposition of an abnormal frequency or pattern of breathing. Most children who receive mechanical ventilatory assistance require sedation, and

Table 6.10
Adverse Effects that May be Encountered During the Application of Continuous Distending Pressure (CPAP or PEEP)

Decreased cardiac output
Decreased systemic venous return
Increased pulmonary vascular resistance
Interventricular septal displacement impeding left ventricular filling
Neural and/or humoral depression of left ventricular function
Decreased myocardial blood flow
Decreased cerebral perfusion pressure
Increased intracranial pressure
Systemic hypotension
Altered renal blood flow and/or function
Decreased renal blood flow
Redistribution of renal blood flow
Decreased free water clearance
Decreased creatinine clearance
Decreased sodium excretion
Decreased splanchnic blood flow
Decreased hepatic arterial flow
Decreased intestinal blood flow
Alveolar overdistention
Pneumothorax
Pneumomediastinum
Pneumopericardium
Subcutaneous emphysema
Increased physiologic dead space

Table 6.11
Conditions Associated with Pulmonary Barotrauma

Impedance to exhalation
Small artificial airway
Ball-valve obstruction of endotracheal tube
Failure to clear tracheobronchial mucus
Intrathoracic obstructive airway diseases
Positive pressure ventilation
    Inadequate expiratory time (prolongation of inspiratory time or high ventilatory rate)
    Mechanical expiratory retardation
Excessive alveolar volume or pressure
Positive pressure support
    High inflating pressure
    Prolonged inspiration
    Inspiratory pressure hold
    High CPAP or PEEP
    Patient-ventilatory respiratory phase asynchrony
Decreased respiratory compliance
Regional disparities in pulmonary volume distribution
Marked inhomogeneity in regional compliance (focal lung diseases)
Marked inhomogeneity in regional resistance (focal lung diseases)
Mainstem bronchus intubation

in some cases neuromuscular blockade is needed to achieve the desired therapeutic goals. Unfortunately, these interventions and therapies are accompanied with their own set of side-effects and complications.

Perhaps the most widely reported complication of the use of neuromuscular blocking drugs (NMBDs) in the intensive care unit is prolonged muscle weakness. This clinical entity also has been commonly associated with the co-administration of aminosteroid NMBDs (e.g., pancuronium, vercuronium) and corticosteroids. Many have suggested that this combination of medications should not be used in critically ill patients.

High-Frequency Ventilation

Low tidal volume HFV involves the delivery of low tidal volume breaths at frequencies far in excess of physiologic respiratory rates. Conventional positive pressure ventilation stands in marked contrast to high-frequency ventilation in which the usual tidal volume approaches or is less than the dead space volume.

Classification

Many high-frequency ventilators—each with unique and overlapping characteristics—have been developed for clinical use. These characteristics can be used to classify different high-frequency ventilators into broad categories to help clarify and define principal techniques used to deliver high-frequency ventilation (Table 6.12). Practitioners also must remember that circuit and delivery system designs may have a major impact on the functioning of high-frequency ventilators.

High-Frequency Positive Pressure Ventilation Originally developed to minimize arterial blood pressure fluctuations with positive pressure ventilation, high-frequency positive pressure ventilation (HFPPV) is effective in achieving normal blood gas values with reduced airway pressures. High-frequency positive pressure ventilation typically uses a standard conventional ventilator with low-compliance tubing, so that adequate tidal volumes can be delivered with very short inspiratory times. High-frequency positive pressure ventilation has been developed for use intraoperatively and in the intensive care unit.

A pneumatic valve system delivers compressed gas during inspiration while allowing passive expiration (Fig. 6.5). With HFPPV, the ventilatory frequency is 60 to 150 breaths/min with tidal volumes of 3 to 4 mL/kg; I/E ratios are usually 0.3. Most conventional neonatal ventilators have been modified to include the capacity to deliver rates up to 150/min.

Limitations with HFPPV have been recognized. For example, with increasing frequency, tidal volume delivery may be compromised so that actual alveolar ventilation decreases despite an increase in minute ventilation.

Table 6.12
Technical Features of HFV

Feature	HFPPV	HFJV	HFFI	HFO
Flow generator	High-pressure gas source	High-pressure gas source	High-pressure gas source	Piston pump acoustic speaker
Fresh gas delivery system	Continuous or valved fresh gas flow	Jet catheter with continuous fresh gas bias flow	Valved flow interruptor	Continuous fresh gas flow
Tidal valve	> dead space	> or < dead space	> or < dead space	< dead space
Expiratory phase	Passive	Passive	Passive	Active
Airway pressure waveform	Variable	Triangular	Triangular	Sine wave
Entrainment	None	Possible	None	None
Frequency (cycles/min)	60–150	60–600	300–1200	60–3600

HFPPV, high-frequency positive pressure ventilation; HFJV, high-frequency jet ventilation; HFFI, high-frequency flow interruption; HFO, high-frequency oscillator.

High Frequency Jet Ventilation

Widely used high-frequency jet ventilation (HFJV) system generates flow by using a high-pressure, air-oxygen gas source. A reducing valve allows the adjustment of inspiratory driving pressure from 0 to 50 psi, and a rapidly responding solenoid valve provides timed flow interruption. The flow interrupter can be adjusted to vary the frequency between 60 and 600 insufflations/min (the usual frequency is 100 to 150/min) with a relatively short inspiratory time (10 to 50% of the respiratory cycle). Manipulation of the inspiratory driving pressure provides the primary means for regulating tidal volume delivery. Insufflated gases are delivered through a low-volume, noncompliant tubing system connected to a small-diameter (i.e., 1.0 to 1.7 mm internal diameter) jet catheter housed within the airway adapter and extending into the endotracheal airway. Alternatively, specially designed endotracheal tubes incorporating a side lumen within the wall of the tube allow the delivery of jet gases into the distal portion of the endotracheal tube.

Manipulation of various ventilatory parameters in HFJV has consequences. Elevation of inspiratory driving pressure increases the volume of insufflated gases and enhances carbon dioxide elimination. Carbon dioxide elimination as a function of ventilatory frequency is less predictable. A linear rise in carbon dioxide tension, with increasing frequency beyond 100 breaths/min, has been attributed to expiratory gas trapping, increased physiologic dead space, and a relative decrease in insufflated gas volume with increasing frequency. Positioning the jet cannula orifice distally in the airway

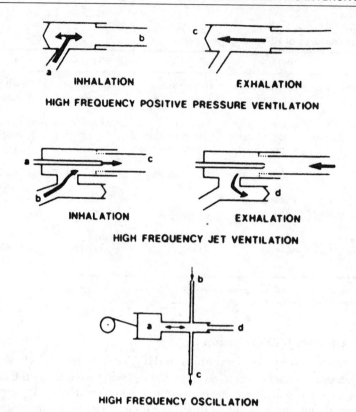

INHALATION   EXHALATION

HIGH FREQUENCY POSITIVE PRESSURE VENTILATION

INHALATION   EXHALATION

HIGH FREQUENCY JET VENTILATION

HIGH FREQUENCY OSCILLATION

Figure 6.5. Schematic diagrams of HFV circuits. *Top panel:* With HFPPV, gas is delivered during inhalation from a low compliance ventilator. Exhalation is passive; (a) low compliance circuit; (b) endotracheal tube; (c) one-way valve. *Middle panel:* During HFJV, high-pressure gas enters from a cannula (a) along the endotracheal tube or trachea (c). Additional gas (b) is entrained. Exhalation is passive. *Bottom panel:* During HFO, the piston (a) oscillates while fresh gas (termed the bias flow) enters (b) and exhaust gas exits (c). The bias flow can be positioned anywhere along the airway (d), but gas transport is enhanced as the bias flow is positioned further into the lung. (From Villar J, Winston B, Slutsky AS. Non-conventional techniques of ventilatory support. Crit Care Clin 1990;6:579.)

or increasing the internal diameter of the jet cannula has resulted in decreased $PaCO_2$. The response of $PaCO_2$ in different studies to changes in relative inspiratory time (i.e., percent inspiration), however, has been erratic. Under pathologic conditions, changes in jet ventilation parameters that result in increased mean airway pressure and mean lung volume tend to diminish intrapulmonary shunting and improve oxygenation much like CPAP or PEEP in conventional modes of mechanical ventilation.

High-Frequency Flow Interrupters High-frequency flow interrupters (HFFIs) are similar to jet ventilators in that they provide small tidal volumes (2 to 5 mL/kg) delivered at high frequency by interrupting a flow or high-pressure source. In contrast to HFJV, no injector jet cannula or gas entrainment is present. Expiration is passive and frequencies vary from 300 to 1200/min.

High-Frequency Oscillation High-frequency oscillation (HFO) is unique in that both inspiration and expiration are active; gas is forced into the lungs during inspiration and sucked out of the lungs during expiration. High-frequency oscillation uses a reciprocating device (i.e., piston pumps, acoustic speaker cones) to produce sinusoidal pressure waves at the airway opening at frequencies of 60 to 3600 cycles/min. A continuous fresh gas (i.e., bias flow) is delivered to the proximal airway to supply O_2 and remove CO_2 while tidal volumes are less than dead space volume (1 to 3 mL/kg).

Two different types of bias flow—low and high impedance—have a profound impact on the performance of the HFO ventilator. The low-impedance flow is used more widely because of safety and simplicity, although less of the tidal volume is delivered to the patient because some volume is "lost" to the low-impedance bias flow. Because of its greater complexity, high-impedance flow is used predominantly to investigate gas transport mechanisms during HFO. The high-impedance circuit has negligible loss of tidal volume to the bias flow; therefore, it is easier to measure tidal volume.

High-Frequency Ventilation Devices

Most data regarding the use of HFV in the United States have involved one of five high-frequency devices (Table 6.13). The principal differences between the various devices are related to the control of mean airway pressure

Table 6.13
Clinical Characteristics of Available High-Frequency Ventilatory Devices[a]

Ventilator	Type[b]	Mean Airway Pressure Control	Expiratory Phase	Frequency (Hz)	Variable Inspiratory Time
Sensor Medics 3100A	HFO	direct	active	3–15	yes
Senko Med. Instr. Humming II	HFO	direct	active	—	no
Bunnell Life pulse	HFJV	indirect	passive	4–11	yes
Infrasonics Infant Star HFV	HFFI	indirect	active (venturi)	2–22	no
Bird Space Tech. PVDR-4	HFFI	indirect	passive	2–22	yes

[a]Data with permission from Clarke RH. High-frequency ventilation. J Pediatr 1994;124–661.

HFO, high frequency oscillator; HFJV, high frequency jet ventilator; HFFI, high frequency flow interrupter.

and expiration. Both variables are associated directly with lung volume and the risk of overdistention. Passive exhalation and indirect control of mean airway pressure potentially complicate the clinician's ability to control intrinsic PEEP and mean lung volume, thereby theoretically increasing the risk of volutrauma.

Clinical Applications

Although HFV has been used extensively for intraoperative management during laryngoscopy and bronchoscopy and with complicated tracheal and bronchial surgery, application of the technique in the management of acute respiratory failure is still in the evaluative stage, and most of the theoretic benefits have yet to be demonstrated in clinical settings.

Liquid (Perfluorocarbon) Ventilation

In an attempt to eliminate air-fluid interfaces and decrease surface tension, thereby enhancing lung compliance, liquid ventilation with oxygenated perfluorocarbon has been investigated in the laboratory and in the clinical arena. Initial attempts were geared toward complete replacement of the gas FRC and tidal ventilation with the oxygenated perfluorocarbon (i.e., total liquid ventilation). Subsequent investigations have been directed toward a liquid FRC while using a conventional mechanical ventilator for gas tidal ventilation (i.e., partial liquid ventilation).

Total Liquid Ventilation

Pulmonary gas exchange using perfluorocarbon liquid ventilation has been investigated for more than 25 years. Various studies in premature newborn animals have demonstrated improvements in compliance, gas exchange, and a reduction in airway pressures with total liquid ventilation (TLV) when compared to gas ventilation. Controlled clinical trials demonstrating clear advantages over conventional therapy are needed before this technique assumes a role in clinical practice.

Partial Liquid Ventilation

This method was developed to apply mechanical gas tidal ventilation with liquid perfluorocarbon filled lungs via conventional instruments (i.e., partial liquid ventilation [PLV]). In contrast to total liquid ventilation, PLV has few adverse cardiovascular side effects.

Extracorporeal Life Support

This relatively simple concept has required multiple technical advancements to make this idea a clinical reality. The term initially used to describe long-term extracorporeal support (ECMO) focused on the function of oxygenation and the type of oxygenator used. In some patients, the emphasis shifted to CO_2 removal, and extracorporeal CO_2 removal ($ECCO_2R$) was coined to describe the use of extracorporeal circulation and a membrane oxygenator to function primarily for CO_2 removal instead of oxygenation. Extracorporeal support also began to be used for cardiac assist in postoperative cardiac surgical patients. With these different methods of cardiopulmonary support offered by the use of extracorporeal circuitry, a new term, extracorporeal life support (ECLS) has become the standard term to describe this technology.

Classification

The basic classifications of ECLS, venoarterial (VA), veno-venous (VV), and arteriovenous (AV) are based on the site of blood withdrawal and return, each with distinct advantages and disadvantages (Table 6.14).

Venoarterial Techniques This technique of ECLS has been the most common form of support and is the most common in neonatal ECLS. Blood is routed from the right atrium through the oxygenator and returned to the arterial circulation, usually into the right common carotid artery (Fig. 6.6). The cannulation is extrathoracic, usually resulting in permanent ligation of the vessels used. This form of ECLS can provide a significant amount of cardiac support as well as pulmonary support and has been used in postoperative cardiac surgery patients with myocardial failure. The benefits of this therapy (cardiac support, excellent oxygenation, relatively low ECLS flows) are associated with significant risks (i.e., ligation or the need for repair of a large artery, the risks of arterial embolization, questions concerning the risks/benefits of decreasing pulmonary blood flow). Pulsatility often is decreased for significant periods during the procedure, raising questions about the effects on vascular beds that may depend on pulsatility for autoregulation.

Venovenous Techniques During this form of ECLS, venous blood is withdrawn from and returned to the venous circulation after oxygenation, and depends on the patient's native cardiac output for oxygen delivery to the periphery. Because of a varying rate of "recirculation" of previously oxygenated blood, VV-ECLS requires higher extracorporeal flows—if the pulmonary bed

Table 6.14
Comparison of Technical and Physiologic Aspects of Venoarterial and Venovenous ECMO Techniques

Venoarterial Technique	Venovenous Technique
Bypasses pulmonary circulation	Maintains pulmonary blood flow
Decreases pulmonary artery pressure	Elevates mixed venous PO_2
Assists systemic circulation	Lacks circulatory assist capability
Requires arterial cannulation	Requires only venous cannulation
Decreases pulmonary blood flow (?)	Presents total venous return to lungs

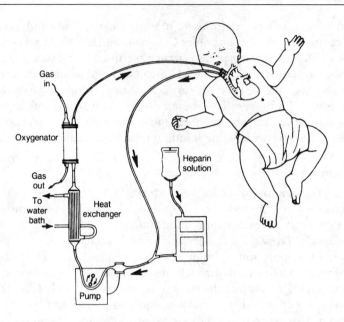

Figure 6.6. Extracorporeal membrane oxygenation perfusion circuit for infant. (From Krummel TM, Greenfield LJ, Kirkpatrick BV, Mueller DG, Ormazabal M, Salzberg AM. Clinical use of an extracorporeal oxygenator in neonatal pulmonary failure. J Pediatr Surg 1982;17:525.)

is totally nonfunctional—to maintain adequate oxygenation. The use of VV support does reduce the risk of embolization except in the presence of large right to left shunts and does not require sacrifice/repair of a large artery. It maintains well oxygenated pulmonary blood flow that may be of benefit but requires the right ventricle to function in the face of pulmonary hypertension.

Arteriovenous Techniques Arteriovenous ECLS is currently not a clinical entity, but it has been explored in the laboratory setting. It would require an intact cardiovascular system to tolerate the large arteriovenous fistula that would be necessary to achieve gas exchange. Because of the large blood flow requirements for support of gas exchange, its use may be restricted to partial CO_2 removal.

Clinical Applications

ECMO

Infants versus Children The dichotomous picture of more than 9,000 reported cases of neonatal ECLS and almost 900 pediatric ECLS cases relates to several factors:

- Higher success rates in neonatal ECMO than in pediatric ECMO (80% versus 50%)
- Greater frequency of neonates with conditions severe enough to warrant support
- Treatment of PPHN is more successful than the treatment of multifactorial diseases leading to pediatric respiratory failure and the pathophysiology of the disease
- Introduction of a continuous flow, double lumen catheter that provides venovenous support has increased the number of cases in which ECLS is applied

Principle Uses The primary pathophysiologic condition being treated by ECMO is reversible pulmonary hypertension. Other primary diagnoses include meconium aspiration syndrome (MAS), congenital diaphragmatic hernia (CDH), respiratory distress syndrome (RDS), persistent pulmonary hypertension of the neonate (PPHN), and sepsis.

Complications The most common complication remains a neurologic abnormality on imaging (i.e., cranial ultrasound, computed tomographic scan), with 24% of patients showing this finding. Other common complications include hemorrhage, chronic lung disease, and renal insufficiency. Except for hemorrhage, many of these complications can be related to injury suffered secondary to the severity of the illness which necessitated ECLS support. The heparinization, as well as platelet dysfunction seen with ECLS, contributes to the bleeding that continues inexorably, thus intracranial hemorrhage early in the course of therapy leads to severe morbidity or mortality.

Extracorporeal CO_2 Removal The major focus in $ECCO_2R$ is the use of the circuit and membrane lung to ventilate or remove CO_2 instead of oxygenating the patient. There is some oxygen delivery with this technique, but the primary source of oxygenation is the inflated but apneic lung. Humidified oxygen is insufflated near the carina at a rate equal to the amount of oxygen consumed. The ventilator is set to deliver a low number of pressure limited breaths per minute to avoid atelectasis. Because there is little alveolar ventilation, the alveolar gas composition is determined by the composition and flow of gas ventilating the oxygenator.

7.

Unusual Causes of Myocardial Ischemia, Pulmonary Edema, and Cyanosis

Jayant K. Deshpande, Mark A. Helfaer, Randall C. Wetzel, and Mark C. Rogers

Intensivists often are confronted with three categories of cardiovascular disease that mimic the symptoms of congenital heart disease and/or respiratory disease but may not be caused by congenital heart disease: myocardial ischemia, pulmonary edema, and cyanosis. This chapter reviews the unusual causes of myocardial ischemia, pulmonary edema, and cyanosis likely to confront the intensivist. Although this discussion includes a review of some traditional congenital heart disease syndromes, such as cyanotic spells in the tetralogy of Fallot and myocardial infarction in anomalous left coronary artery, the focus is on more unusual causes of these conditions.

MYOCARDIAL ISCHEMIA IN CHILDREN

Myocardial ischemia, angina, myocardial infarction, and ischemic coronary artery disease occur in children of all ages. Although the leading causes of ischemic heart disease (IHD) in children (Table 7.1) differ from that in adults (i.e., atherosclerotic coronary artery disease), the physiologic factors underlying myocardial oxygen consumption and oxygen delivery are the same.

Diseases in children that clearly cause myocardial ischemia include:

- Anomalous coronary arteries
- Kawasaki disease
- Congenital heart disease
- Asphyxia

Table 7.1
Causes of Myocardial Ischemia in Childhood

Neonatal ischemic heart disease
Asphyxia neonatorum
Increased demand
   Persistent transitional circulation
   Pulmonary hypertension, i.e., respiratory distress syndrome, meconium aspiration
Congenital heart disease
Cyanotic heart disease
   Total anomalous pulmonary veins
   Transposition of great vessels
Obstructive disease
   Aortic or pulmonary stenosis
Anomalous coronary arteries
Increased demand
Catecholamine-induced ischemia, i.e., isoproterenol treatment of asthma
Head injury
Vascular disease
Kawasaki disease
Infantile periarteritis nodosa
Embolism
Atheroma (rare)
Trauma
Trauma and head injury

- Trauma
- Asthma
- Cardiac tachydysrhythmias
- Shock

Physicians dealing with critically ill children must understand the factors that govern myocardial oxygen consumption (MVO_2) and myocardial oxygen delivery (MDO_2):

- Wall tension
- Contractility
- Heart rate
- External workload

Neonatal Ischemic Heart Disease

Even with normal coronary arteries and in the absence of congenital anomalies, myocardial ischemia and necrosis do occur, are not uncommon, and may even be a significant factor in the mortality of acutely ill infants. The unusual stresses imposed on the transitional circulation perinatally can lead to both increased myocardial oxygen demand and impaired oxygen delivery. Superimposition of hypoxia, hypovolemia, sepsis, and respiratory distress during this period can severely impair myocardial perfusion.

Clinical Presentation

The clinical picture of IHD in neonates, which is not remarkably different from other causes of neonatal respiratory distress, is as follows:

- Tachypnea
- Hypoxemia
- Heart failure, characterized by cardiomegaly, tricuspid, or mitral insufficiency, and cardiogenic shock
- Electrocardiographic evidence, including right ventricular hypertrophy (RVH), S-T segment depression, T-wave inversion, and even frank myocardial infarction (Fig. 7.1)
- Elevated creatine phosphokinase (CPK) (CK-MB) level, although this indicator is less reliable in children than in adults

Differential Diagnosis

The differential diagnosis includes structural heart diseases such as total anomalous pulmonary venous drainage (TAPVD), hypoplastic left heart syndromes, and anomalous origin of the coronary arteries. Angiography and radionuclide imaging may be of help in diagnosis.

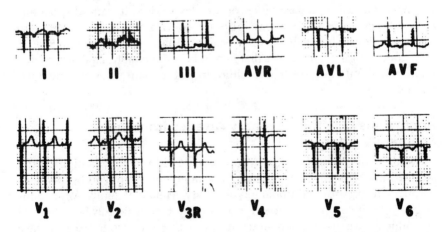

Figure 7.1. ECG of a 13-day-old neonate. Note Qs in I, V5, V6, and inverted T waves in I, II, aVL, aVF, V5, and V6, which are consistent with inferolateral myocardial infarction. (From Kilbridge H. Myocardial infarction in the neonate with normal heart and coronary arteries. Am J Dis Child 1980;134:759, © 1980, American Medical Association. With permission.)

Therapy

Therapy is primarily supportive, with increased FIO_2, ventilatory support, and fluid restriction. Digoxin, diuretics, and inotropic agents have been beneficial. Application of therapies that are traditionally used in adults, such as nitroglycerin, β-blockade, and calcium channel blockers have not been reported. The outlook is generally good, and supportive therapy is usually associated with resolution of symptoms in 48 to 72 hours and radiographic and electrocardiographic resolution within 2 weeks.

Prognosis

The high incidence of myocardial necrosis at postmortem indicates that IHD may be an underdiagnosed condition. The long-term prognosis is unknown. It is tempting to speculate, however, that several conditions of unknown etiology, such as mitral valve prolapse, idiopathic cardiac dysrhythmias, and cardiomyopathies in older children, may be related to neonatal IHD and unsuspected myocardial infarction.

Myocardial Ischemia Associated with Congenital Heart Disease

It is unusual to consider myocardial ischemia when caring for children with congenital heart disease, although hypertrophy, cyanosis, increased hematocrit (Hct), and the frequency of the postoperative state would suggest that ischemia may occur frequently. Children with congenital heart disease have an increased incidence of abnormal coronary artery changes; therefore, coronary occlusive disease does occur. Hyperviscosity and hypoxemia caused by cyanotic heart disease also are contributing factors. Although electrocardiographic evidence of myocardial infarction is present in 50% of the patients, significant myocardial ischemia and, possibly, fatal myocardial infarction should be expected in children with certain types of congenital heart disease.

Anomalous Origin of Coronary Arteries from the Pulmonary Artery

Anomalous origin of the right coronary artery is generally benign, as the low-pressure right ventricle appears to be adequately supplied by this right coronary artery with additional left coronary artery collaterals. Anomalous origin of both coronary arteries is rare and uniformly rapidly fatal. Several anatomical variants of anomalous origin of the left coronary artery have been described, including left anterior artery descending from the pulmonary artery and left coronary artery originating from the right main pulmonary artery.

The natural history of this disease is determined by cardiovascular developmental changes. By 4 months of age, most infants have developed an abnormal flow pattern that leads to a large left-to-right shunt, which simultaneously increases myocardial workload and impairs left ventricular perfusion. Myocardial damage is inevitable, and at least 80% of these children do not survive the first year of life.

Clinical Presentation

In the first few months of life, the infants seem normal. They subsequently manifest symptoms, however, that fall into three categories: recurrent respiratory infections, discomfort, and heart failure. Clinical findings include:

- Irritability
- Screaming (especially with feeding)
- Drawing up of the legs
- Apparent anxiety
- Pain
- Pallor
- Sweating
- Dyspnea
- Tachycardia
- Wheezing
- Coughing
- Poor perfusion
- Shock
- Edema
- Hepatomegaly
- Grunting respirations
- Rales

Diagnostic Methods

Chest radiography may reveal cardiomegaly and pulmonary edema with possibly concurrent respiratory tract infection. Electrocardiography (ECG) usually reveals a pattern that is consistent with an anterior myocardial infarction pattern, characterized by a Q-R pattern and inverted T-waves in leads I and aVL. Frequently, a left ventricular hypertrophy (LVH) pattern is seen with deep Qs in V5 and V6 and S-T changes in the precordial leads. Radionuclide imaging reveals myocardial hypoperfusion, and angiography defines the anatomy.

Differential Diagnosis

The differential diagnosis includes defects associated with LVH, such as aortic stenosis, tricuspid atresia, coarctation of the aorta—especially associated with a patent ductus arteriosus-and ventricular septal defects, although these are readily differentiated. More difficult and frequently clinically undiscernible are endomyocardial fibroelastosis and myocarditis, which can often only be differentiated angiographically, although the presence of Q-waves strongly suggests anomalous coronary arteries.

Therapy

Medical management directed at initial resuscitation and stabilization traditionally includes oxygen, digoxin, fluids, and diuretics. Logical extension of the therapy for IHD in adults would indicate that optimizing fluid balance, afterload reduction, and antidysrhythmia therapy could be useful. Definitive therapy requires surgical intervention, preferably before massive infarction and aneurysm formation. Early recognition and correction remains the basis of managing this form of childhood IHD.

Catecholamine-Induced Ischemia

In addition to defects in substrate delivery, increased myocardial oxygen demand also could lead to ischemia. The underlying cause of catecholamine-induced injury is multifactorial. For example, in untreated status asthmaticus, desaturation and acidosis may adversely affect myocardial oxygen balance. In addition, negative intrapleural pressures are associated with profound cardiorespiratory interactions; the overall effect of which is to increase left ventricular afterload and, thus, oxygen consumption.

Adding isoproterenol to this scenario has several effects. Increased heart rate and enhanced myocardial contractility may dramatically increase MVO_2 while compromising delivery by a direct $\beta2$-vascular effect lowering diastolic pressure. In addition, isoproterenol inhibition of hypoxic pulmonary vasomotor responses increases intrapulmonary shunting and regularly decreases PaO_2. In children with a chronically stressed heart (e.g., from asthma), isoproterenol clearly can present a risk.

The use of epinephrine and norepinephrine also poses a threat to myocardial oxygen balance. Isoproterenol-marked salutary effects in status asthmaticus must be balanced against the possibility of induced myocardial ischemia. Theophylline also increases MVO_2 and, in animals, has led to myocardial necrosis. It is conceivable that theophylline and isoproterenol present an additional challenge to the myocardium in these patients.

Kawasaki Disease

The leading cause of IHD in children, Kawasaki disease was first described by Tomisaku Kawasaki in 1967 as an acute, febrile, mucocutaneous lymph node syndrome predominantly affecting infants and small children. Although it is a multisystem disease, its predominant morbidity and mortality rates are related to its catastrophic coronary vascular involvement.

Epidemiology

Eight percent of all cases of Kawasaki disease occur in children 4 years of age and younger, and 75% of all deaths occur in children younger than 2 years of age. Its increased frequency in warm weather, its occurrence in clusters, and its clinical symptoms (e.g., fever, leukocytosis, erythematous rash) indicate an infectious process, although extensive effort has been unable to demonstrate either a viral, rickettsial, mycoplasmal, bacterial, protozoal, or chlamydial infectious agent.

Clinical Course

The clinical picture of Kawasaki disease consists of three well-defined phases: the acute febrile stage, which usually lasts from 1 to 2 weeks; a subacute phase; and a convalescent phase, occurring usually after 6 weeks.

Pathology

The main pathologic feature of Kawasaki disease is a nonspecific panvasculitis. Endarteritis of major arteries, especially in the coronary arteries, occurs during the subacute phase and may lead to aneurysms, central destruction, thrombosis, and embolization.

The pathologic evolution of Kawasaki disease appears to undergo four distinct postmortem stages. Stage 1 (lasting fewer than 10 days) shows a panvasculitis of the microcirculation and includes the coronary arteries. Acute myocarditis, pericarditis, and endocarditis with valvulitis are evident. In stage 2 (11 to 28 days), aneurysm formation and coronary artery stenosis with persistence of pancarditis is found. In stage 3 (28 to 45 days), global evidence of myocardial ischemia with thrombosis and intimal proliferation is obvious. The pancarditis is resolving, and the vasculitis is absent during stage 3. During stage 4 (more than 50 days), resolution of the ravages of the first three stages in the coronary circulation is seen with calcifications, stenosis, scarring, recanalization, and chronic aneurysm formation. Endocardial fibroelastosis and ischemic myocardial changes are prominent. Capillary muscle dysfunction with mitral and tricuspid regurgitation can occur. Although seen throughout all three stages, ischemia and inflammatory changes in the conducting tissue generally are in the process of resolving by the fourth stage.

During the first stage, conduction abnormalities in arrhythmias are a common cause of death; myocardial infarction and aneurysm rupture are the predominant causes during stage 2. Ischemic heart disease caused by coronary artery occlusion is the cause of death in stages 3 and 4. Although the natural history of the aneurysms formed during Kawasaki disease is resolution, rupture and sudden death can occur many years later. Aneurysms also occur throughout the circulation and have been found in hepatic, peripheral circulatory, cerebral, iliofemoral, renal, testicular, and splenic vessels. Clinically evident peripheral aneurysms of the brachial, cervical, and femoral arteries should prompt a search for associated central and coronary aneurysms.

Diagnostic Criteria

At least five of the following six criteria are required for diagnosis of Kawasaki disease:

1. A spiking remittent fever of 101 to 104°F, lasting from 5 days to 2 weeks
2. Mucosal changes in the oropharynx, often with bleeding, cracked lips, fissuring, pharyngeal hyperemia, and a strawberry tongue
3. Cervical lymphadenopathy, with a hard tender lymph node mass greater than 1.5 cm that is frequently unilateral
4. Conjunctival involvement with edema and injection of both the bulbar and palpebral conjunctiva
5. Deep red erythema of the palms and soles, accompanied by induration and edema of the hands and feet, which often limit the ability to walk and are frequently followed by periungual desquamation approximately 2 weeks after the onset of the illness
6. An erythematous rash that is polymorphous, nonvesiculated, generally pruritic, migratory, occasionally urticarial, and usually truncal

Other manifestations of Kawasaki disease include:

- Aseptic meningitis (25%)
- Diarrhea (40%)
- Meatal ulceration (20%)
- Urethritis (25%)
- Arthralgia (30%)
- Sporadic central nervous system (CNS) involvement with symptoms of lethargy and emotional irritability
- Hydrops of the gallbladder
- Jaundice
- Uveitis
- Hepatitis
- Pleural and pericardial effusions
- Pneumonia

In infants (i.e., children younger than 6 months of age), the clinical features of the disease may be atypical, making diagnosis difficult in this high-risk population. Also, a syndrome of atypical Kawasaki disease may not have all of the above diagnostic criteria but may have cardiac involvement alone.

Cardiac Complications

Fatal cardiac complications can arise in patients initially free of clinical cardiac symptomatology. These considerations mandate careful observation and electrocardiographic monitoring, best performed in a PICU.

Myocardial Involvement

Myocardial involvement may be obvious clinically as patients develop tachycardia and a gallop rhythm. More serious arrhythmias and myocardial involvement usually after the ninth day may occur with pericardial effusion, mitral regurgitation, and heart failure. Electrocardiographic abnormalities found in 30 to 50% of patients are atrioventricular block, arrhythmias, P-R prolongation, prolonged Q-T interval, and voltage changes compatible with left ventricular strain. Pericardial effusions, pericarditis, and nonaneurysmal cardiac dilatation also have been reported.

Coronary Artery Involvement

Coronary artery aneurysms, with or without thrombosis, and myocardial infarction usually develop in the convalescent period. Aneurysmal coronary artery dilation has been seen in up to 26% of Kawasaki disease patients, accompanied by biopsy evidence of myocarditis, cellular infiltration, and fibrosis.

Coronary artery involvement and cardiac abnormalities are more common in children with Kawasaki disease when they have the following profile:

- Males
- Younger than 1 year of age
- Have had a fever for more than 2 weeks or have had a recurrent fever
- Have prolonged elevation in the erythrocyte sedimentation rate (ESR) or an ESR greater than 100 mm/hour
- Show significant cardiac involvement in the early stages

Follow-up studies in large numbers of children with Kawasaki disease revealed that cardiovascular complications are found in more than 50% of patients, and coronary artery aneurysms are more frequent than thought previously. In addition, aortic regurgitation caused by myocarditis seems to be a frequent follow-up finding. Remember, children can suffer severe and occasionally fatal complications many years after initial involvement with Kawasaki disease.

Laboratory Findings

Although there are no specific diagnostic tests for Kawasaki disease, several abnormalities have been reported:

- Leukocytosis with a white count higher than 15,000 cells/mL
- Leftward shift that may persist for several weeks
- Elevation of all acute-phase reactants, such as C-reactive protein, α2-globulin, and ESR
- Thrombocytosis during the second and third weeks
- Platelet abnormalities detected for months after the acute phase associated with higher risk of coronary artery aneurysms

- Normocytic, normochromic anemia
- Hyperbilirubinemia
- Increased hepatic enzyme levels
- Proteinuria and sterile pyuria, although marked renal involvement with abnormalities in serum electrolytes is abnormal
- Cerebrospinal fluid (CSF) pleocytosis

Noninvasive Test Results

The chest radiograph of a child with Kawasaki disease is frequently normal, although pneumonitis has been reported in a few patients. Cardiomegaly, caused by either left ventricular failure or hypertrophy, and pericardial effusions occasionally are seen during the second or third week. Other noninvasive diagnostic tests specifically designed to detect underlying cardiac abnormalities and an ECG are essential and may show the abnormalities mentioned previously.

Echocardiography can help to identify children who develop coronary aneurysms and should be performed serially in children with Kawasaki disease. In addition, echocardiographic abnormalities of ventricular wall motion appear to be a sensitive method of detecting cardiac involvement in Kawasaki disease. Two-dimensional echocardiography demonstrates coronary aneurysms, follows patients during the recovery phase, and provides follow-up.

Follow-up

More than half of these demonstrable coronary aneurysms can be expected to resolve within the first year. Echocardiographic anomalies alone do not necessarily indicate the need for angiography, and serial follow-up seems the wisest course in the absence of clinical findings. More ominous is the development of irritability, pallor, and hypotension during the subacute phase of Kawasaki disease, which may herald myocardial infarction. Electrocardiographic monitoring should probably be continued throughout the first 10 days of the illness. The development of Q-waves during electrocardiographic monitoring is an ominous sign, associated with full-thickness myocardial infarction in more than 30% of the cases in which it is seen.

Treatment

Therapy for Kawasaki disease necessitates prompt treatment with 100 mg/kg/day of aspirin, followed by prolonged treatment with 30 mg/kg/day during the convalescent stage. This program apparently inhibits inflammatory reaction and platelet aggregation. Also, therapy appears to be able to prevent the associated coronary artery disease, coronary thrombosis, and thromboembolism.

Although the use of steroids has been recommended in the past, coronary angiography performed in children 2 months after the onset of fever has demonstrated a 65% incidence of aneurysms in those treated with prednisolone, compared with 20% in those treated with antibiotics and only 11% in those treated with aspirin.

Aspirin should be continued beyond the convalescence stage. Malabsorption of salicylates seems to be a common problem in these children; therefore, serum levels should be followed in the initial period. In addition, high-dose intravenous γ-globulin is safe and effective in reducing the prevalence of coronary artery abnormalities when given early in the course of this syndrome. A single large dose (2 g/kg) of intravenous γ-globulin is even more effective in the treatment of Kawasaki disease than the standard four daily doses.

Prognosis

The prognosis for children with Kawasaki disease seems to be excellent, with about a 1% mortality (down from 3 to 4% in 1975). The long-term implication of coronary artery disease in children who have suffered from Kawasaki disease, however, is unknown. There has been some early enthusiasm for the correction of coronary artery lesions, and coronary artery bypass grafting has been undertaken, especially in those patients with severe ischemic evidence, such as S-T wave changes, myocardial infarction, myocardial failure secondary to ischemia, aneurysm rupture, and angina. The fact, however, that many aneurysms apparently resolve and can be followed accurately with two-dimensional echocardiography, coupled with the overall favorable prognosis of the disease, indicates that conservative management is appropriate, although long-term follow-up is necessary.

Trauma

Head injury, subarachnoid hemorrhage, and elevated intracranial pressure cause ST-T wave changes on the ECG that are consistent with myocardial ischemia. Myocardial CPK levels are elevated in children after head injury and cerebral vascular injury, indicating myocardial damage in this setting.

Head Injury

Head injury causes a rather accentuated autonomic response with direct sympathetic cardiac stimulation and enhanced levels of circulating catecholamines. MVO_2 levels increase because of elevated heart rate, increased contractility, and increased afterload. This increased demand could lead to relatively insufficient perfusion.

Chest Trauma

Myocardial injury occurs in this setting, although the incidence is lower than that in adults. Radionuclide angiography has revealed myocardial dysfunction in 74% of chest trauma victims. This is frequently not accompanied by abnormalities on the ECG (28% abnormal) or an increase in the CK-MB enzyme (i.e., 8% abnormal).

Several forms of injury can accompany chest injuries, including myocardial contusions, myocardial concussion (commotio cordis), valvular damage, rupture, and coronary vascular occlusion; frequently, the diagnosis is missed. The long-term results include myocardial scarring, arrhythmias, and ventricular aneurysms.

Although direct myocardial injury occurs, some have speculated that coronary vascular lesions result in trauma-associated damage. Certainly, traumatic coronary artery aneurysm occur (Fig. 7.2). In the setting of trauma, unexplained hemodynamic compromise should suggest possible myocardial damage or ischemia. Radionuclide angiography is the most sensitive test available to discover traumatic myocardial dysfunction.

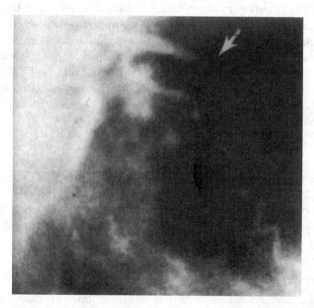

Figure 7.2. Coronary angiogram in a child admitted to the PICU with hypotension, ECG S-T wave depression, and chest pain. Note the abrupt occlusion of the left anterior descending coronary artery, which is the branch most commonly occluded. (From Sutherland GR, Calvin JE, Driedger AA, Holliday RL, Sibbald WJ. Anatomic and cardiopulmonary responses to trauma with associated blunt chest injury. J Trauma 1981;21:1. With permission.)

Other Causes

Hyperlipidemia

Children with familial hyperlipidemia, especially type II, are at great risk for the early involvement of the coronary arteries by disease. Unusual causes of myocardial ischemia include coronary sinus thrombosis caused by a central hyperalimentation, a complication that leads to myocardial infarction by elevating coronary venous pressures and reducing coronary perfusion.

Cocaine Use

Cocaine abuse prenatally produces cardiovascular problems for the infant. Ventricular hypertrophy (RVH and LVH) occurs in a significant number of these children, who also are at higher risk for having atrial septal defect, patent ductus arteriosus, or ventricular septal defect. Some infants also have conduction or rate disturbances (e.g., sinus tachycardia, ventricular ectopy, ventricular tachycardia, prolonged QTc interval).

In older patients, the persistent sympathomimetic and vasoconstrictive effects of chronic cocaine abuse may induce hypertension or coronary artery spasm, leading to cardiac arrhythmias, myocardial infarction, or sudden death.

The pathogenesis of ischemic heart disease may include one or a combination of the following:

- Nonatherosclerotic intimal proliferation of smooth muscle
- Obstructive platelet thrombosis
- Microfocal fibrosis of the myocardium observed at necropsy

Chest pain associated with cocaine abuse may be chest wall and not myocardial in origin.

Therapy for Ischemic Heart Disease

There is no reason to suspect that the recommended therapy for IHD in children would differ from that of adults, which is outlined as follows:

- Assure A, B, Cs
- Optimize hematocrit and volume status (possible transfusion)
- Control dysrhythmias
- Consider β-blockade
- Afterload reduction (intubation or pharmacologic)
- Consider anticoagulation
- Surgical correction for amenable lesions

PULMONARY EDEMA

Pulmonary edema may be defined as the accumulation of abnormal amounts of fluid and solute in the extravascular spaces of the lung.

The sequence of formation of pulmonary edema conceptualized as the progress from interstitial edema to alveolar flooding is shown in Figure 7.3. A more comprehensive approach is shown in Table 7.2.

Important Causes of Heart Failure and/or Pulmonary Edema in the Pediatric Intensive Care Unit

Anthracycline Cardiotoxicity

Anthracycline antimetabolites doxorubicin (adriamycin) and daunomycin, commonly used antitumor agents, can cause bone marrow suppression and cardiotoxicity.

Clinical Signs Early signs of anthracycline cardiotoxicity are generally changes on the ECG, which can be transient. Cardiomyopathy is a serious, dose-dependent, life-threatening complication, particularly in a patient who has received more than 500 mg/m^2 of doxorubicin.

Therapy Monitoring to prevent anthracycline toxicity is preferable to therapy for heart failure and pulmonary edema. Once present, however, fluid and salt restriction, diuretics, and judicious use of digitalis may be all that is required after anthracycline therapy is discontinued. When admission to the PICU is required, intensive inotropic support with dopamine or dobuta-

Figure 7.3. Sequence of fluid accumulation in pulmonary edema. (A). Normal lung. (B) Interstitial edema with fluid accumulation in the perivascular, peribronchial interstitial space. (C) Early alveolar edema, which begins in alveolar "corners" and follows filling of the interstitial space. (D) Alveolar flooding with a critical change in the pressure-volume relationship of some alveoli and a loss of alveolar volume. (From Staub NC, Nagano H, Pearce ML. Pulmonary edema in dogs, especially the sequence of fluid accumulation in the lungs. J Appl Physiol 1967;22:227. With permission.)

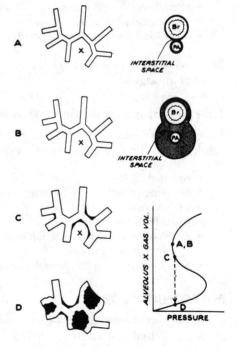

Table 7.2
Causes of Pulmonary Edema Based on Mechanism[a]

Increased pulmonary capillary pressure
Systemic hypertension, aortic coarctation
Left ventricular outflow obstruction
Myocardial failure secondary to ischemia, myocarditis, high output, shunt, valvular
  regurgitation or obstruction, toxic antimetabolites (anthracycline)
Cortriatriatum, obstruction to or high resistance in pulmonary veins
Noncardiogenic pulmonary venous disease, such as secondary to mediastinal tumors
Altered permeability
Infectious bacterial and viral pneumonia
Inhaled toxic agents, such as phosgene, ozone, and oxides of nitrogen, and prolonged
  high-concentration oxygen administration
Circulating toxins, such as alloxan, snake venom, and α-naphthylthiourea
Vasoactive substances, such as histamine, kinins, and arachidonic acid metabolites, such
  as leukotrienes
Diffuse capillary leak syndrome, such as endotoxemia
Immunologic reactions, drug reactions, including salicylate pulmonary edema, allergic
  alveolitis, leukocyte sensitivity states, and blood transfusion reactions
Smoke inhalation and associated thermal injury
Disseminated intravascular coagulation
Near-drowning
Aspiration, including acid pneumonitis
Radiation pneumonia
Adult respiratory distress syndrome
Uremia
Decreased oncotic pressure
Hypoalbuminemia secondary to renal or hepatic disease, protein-losing enteropathy, or
  malnutrition
Lymphatic insufficiency
Congenital or acquired
Increased negative interstitial pressure
High negative pressure—croup or epiglottitis, reexpansion pulmonary edema
Mixed or unknown mechanisms
Neurogenic pulmonary edema
Heroin (narcotic) pulmonary edema
High-altitude pulmonary edema
Pulmonary embolism
Eclampsia
Hypoglycemia
Pancreatitis

[a]Modified from Robin ED, Cross CE, Zelis R. Pulmonary edema. N Engl J Med 1973;288:239, 292 (2 parts). With permission.

mine and forced diuresis can be used. Both acute and chronic afterload reduction can be particularly beneficial. Because anthracycline cardiomyopathy may be reversible in children, intensive cardiac support including intubation and mechanical ventilation may be warranted to treat an acute episode of pulmonary edema.

Oxygen Toxicity

Although the systemic effects of oxygen toxicity can include a variety of physiologic alterations (i.e., ranging from paresthesias and seizures to retrolental fibroplasia), in the PICU setting, the most important toxic effects of oxygen involve the lung. In this section, we review generalized lung toxicity to oxygen and oxygen-induced pulmonary edema. A pattern of lung response to oxygen exposure is shown in Figure 7.4.

An early clinical sign of oxygen toxicity is pulmonary capillary leakage with pulmonary edema. The toxicity of oxygen is probably related to free radical-generated lipid membrane injury.

Immune Responses, Hypersensitivity, and Pulmonary Edema

Many allergic reactions that involve the lung include a series of cellular and biochemical events such as vasodilation, increased vasopermeability, and edema formation. Regardless of the initiating event, many allergic reactions can lead to pulmonary edema formation by this mechanism. The interaction of immunoglobulin E (IgE) antibody and an antigen on the surface of a mast cell results in primary mediator release, release of prostaglandin D_2, and the activation of other cell types, and the secondary release of leukotriene and other oxidative arachidonate metabolites from pulmonary interstitial mononuclear cells.

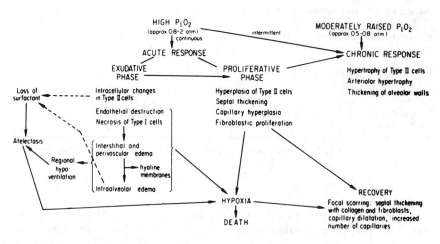

Figure 7.4. Lung response to increased oxygen exposure. Note that the response to diffuse injury is limited and not specific to the injurious agent. (From Winter PM, Miller JD. Oxygen toxicity. In: Shoemaker WC, Thompson WL, Holbrook PR, eds. Textbook of critical care medicine. Philadelphia: WB Saunders, 1984:218. With permission.)

Salicylate-Induced Pulmonary Edema

A review of clinical studies indicates that in adult patients with salicylate pulmonary edema, distinguishing characteristics included an acute intoxication on top of chronic administration, a history of smoking, an increased incidence of neurologic abnormalities, and proteinuria. Higher salicylate levels (more than 40 mg/dL) were also associated with a higher incidence of pulmonary edema. In a group of 36 consecutive adult patients with serum salicylate levels more than 30 mg/dL, eight patients developed pulmonary edema. Four of these patients had Swan-Ganz catheters placed, and none had elevated wedge pressures. The authors of this series concluded that pulmonary edema clears in response to measures designed to lower the salicylate level.

Croup, Epiglottitis, and Pulmonary Reexpansion

In 1977, Travis et al. described pulmonary edema associated with croup and epiglottitis in two patients (Fig. 7.5). These changes increase the volume of

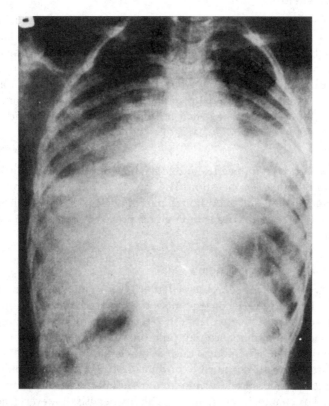

Figure 7.5. Radiograph of chest showing bilateral pulmonary edema in a patient with upper airway obstruction. (From Travis KW, Todres ID, Shannon DC. Pulmonary edema associated with croup and epiglottitis. Pediatrics 1977;59:695. With permission.)

blood in the pulmonary capillaries, increase the pore size in the pulmonary capillaries, and increase the hydrostatic driving pressure of fluid into the lungs. The authors postulated that it was likely that the same physiology could be responsible for pulmonary edema associated with other forms of upper airway obstruction, such as chronic enlargement of the adenoids and tonsils. This same explanation has been applied to the observation that sudden reexpansion of a collapsed lung (such as in application of suction to a chest tube for a pneumothorax) may result in pulmonary edema.

Heroin- and Narcotic-Induced Pulmonary Edema

The edema fluid in heroin overdose is virtually identical with serum proteins. In fact, although heroin overdose can cause renal failure, myocardial infarction, brain infarction, and rhabdomyolysis, the lungs are the organ most frequently affected.

Causative Factors

Several mechanisms are postulated for the production of lung fluid, but most involve the cerebral edema documented in these patients and the lack of elevated wedge pressure in this syndrome. Most data suggest that the cause is not primary myocardial failure. The consensus is that narcotic-depressed respiration, caused by CNS hypoxia, produces a variety of neurogenic pulmonary responses. Additionally, CNS depression can cause loss of airway control and aspiration. Both of these factors may be implicated in the syndrome.

Therapy

Patients with heroin-induced somnolence may develop pulmonary edema up to several hours after ingestion. The treatment requires intubation, ventilation, and airway control. Although narcotic reversal can help arouse the patient, naloxone can cause vomiting and provoke aspiration in nonintubated comatose patients.

Neurogenic Pulmonary Edema

Pulmonary edema has been observed after head trauma in adults and children. The hemodynamic consequences of increased intracranial pressure and massive sympathetic discharge involve marked increases in aortic, systemic arterial, pulmonary arterial, pulmonary venous, and superior vena cava pressures. These hemodynamic effects last only 5 to 15 minutes, after which vascular pressures return to normal. Central venous and pulmonary wedge pressures measured during ongoing neurogenic pulmonary edema are normal. A change in vascular permeability persists, however, leading to ongoing pulmonary edema in spite of these normal vascular pressures.

The mechanism of neurogenic pulmonary edema is a process in which trauma, hypoxia, or increased intracranial pressure initiates a hypothalamic reflex, which results in massive sympathetic discharge. The resulting increase in systemic and pulmonary vascular pressures leads to capillary wall damage and increased permeability, which persists and causes ongoing pulmonary edema. As vascular pressures return to normal values, heart failure is averted. Unfortunately, the pulmonary edema persists and can be life threatening in itself.

High-Altitude Pulmonary Edema

High-altitude pulmonary edema can be reversed on return to a lower altitude or by administration of oxygen. Pulmonary artery wedge pressure is normal, suggesting lack of left ventricular failure despite documented pulmonary vascular hypertension. The many pathophysiologic theories include hypoxia-induced disruption of arteries and arterioles and hypoxia-induced increase in capillary permeability. Sympathetic nervous system discharge causing central hypervolemia is also said to be a contributing cause.

Treatment

Patients with unexplained or unusual causes of respiratory distress thought to be pulmonary edema require admission to the PICU earlier than do patients with more usual forms of cardiac failure because of the rapidity with which altered permeability pulmonary edema can develop. Early observation of these patients and assessment of the rate of change in the pulmonary edema are critical to their treatment plan.

Evaluation and Management

All patients admitted to the PICU require frequent assessment of vital signs and a chest radiograph to document baseline radiographic signs of pulmonary edema and associated cardiomegaly, if applicable. In addition, the patient should have a baseline arterial blood gas determination. It is useful to have samples obtained on room air, if possible, to evaluate the degree of intrapulmonary shunting. Samples obtained with nasal oxygen or on oxygen masks are frequently assumed to represent preset inspired oxygen concentrations, but this is unreliable in anxious children who may have one sample with the mask on and another with the mask over the side of the face. The authors have avoided placing indwelling arterial lines in patients for longer periods because of noninvasive oximetry, but they still believe that an indwelling arterial line for arterial blood gas monitoring is indicated if blood gas analyses are required more frequently than every 2 or 3 hours.

Catheter Techniques of Measurement

In seriously ill or rapidly changing patients, particularly those who will need or already need respiratory support with positive end-expiratory pressure (PEEP) or continuous positive airway pressure (CPAP), the authors frequently use a balloon-tipped thermodilution cardiac output catheter. The ability to measure left atrial "wedge" pressure for diagnosis and therapy and the ability to measure intrapulmonary shunt, systemic vascular resistance, and other hemodynamic variables often are invaluable. The various catheter techniques used to measure lung water in patients with pulmonary edema have proven useful in the treatment of infants and children with pulmonary edema.

Supplemental Oxygen

The primary therapy for pulmonary edema is supplemental oxygen. Oxygen masks with reservoir bags allow high levels of supplemental oxygen to be delivered. Face mask CPAP circuits may be effective.

Intubation Indications

Indications for intubation include:

- Progressive hypoxemia despite supplemental oxygen
- Increasing $PaCO_2$
- Respiratory rate and pattern indicating the likelihood of impending respiratory fatigue
- Young children out of the neonatal period in distress who will not tolerate their face mask

Rapid Sequence Techniques

Intubation of patients in cardiorespiratory distress requires a knowledge of the rapid-sequence intubation techniques. After the patient is intubated, CPAP may be successful in older children who will breathe spontaneously and cooperate with medical direction. Infants and small children often require positive pressure ventilation and have a higher incidence of need for paralysis to avoid inefficient ventilatory patterns. PEEP does not improve hypoxemia and decrease right-to-left shunting by pushing fluid out of the alveoli as originally postulated. PEEP increases functional residual capacity (FRC), expands fluid-filled alveoli, and improves compliance. The net effect is improved arterial oxygen tension.

Other Measures

Specific measures beyond this depend on the cause of the pulmonary edema. Cardiac failure may require digitalis, catecholamine, diuretics, and even afterload-reducing agents, depending on the specific nature of the cardiac failure. Morphine, which is used commonly in adults, is not generally used in small children because of concern about respiratory depression, although other supportive measures, such as head elevation, can be useful. Steroids directed at capillary permeability injury generally has not proved useful in any specific pulmonary edema syndrome, and because they may impair responses to infection, they are not widely used. For similar reasons, the indiscriminate use of wide-spectrum antibiotics is rarely indicated because of the possibility of subsequent nosocomial infections.

Pulmonary Edema During Weaning from PEEP or CPAP

The increased venous return, which develops as PEEP or CPAP, is decreased, often requires a decrease of fluid administration, diuresis, or both. Similar concerns are present in critically ill patients with pulmonary edema, hypoxia, and hypercarbia who receive high levels of PEEP and CPAP. The harmful CNS effects of hypoxia or hypercarbia, when combined with the potential for elevated airway pressure to decrease blood pressure and increase intracranial pressure, must be considered when neurologic symptoms develop that are not explainable by the degree of hypoxia or hypercarbia.

CYANOSIS

Cyanosis is "a bluish purple discoloration of the mucous membranes and skin, due to excess amounts of reduced hemoglobin in capillaries, or less frequently to the presence of methemoglobin." The presence of 4 to 5 g reduced hemoglobin/dL blood is necessary to produce the cyanosis. Cyanosis is clinically significant because it implies severely decreased oxygen content of blood (i.e., hypoxemia), an important consequence of which is inadequate oxygen delivery to tissues for metabolic needs (i.e., hypoxia). A review of the physiologic causes of cyanosis is presented in Table 7.3.

Factors Altering Normal Oxygen Delivery

Decreased Availability of Oxygen in Inspired Air

Oxygen in adequate concentrations and partial pressures in the inspired gases is essential for adequate oxygen delivery to tissues. A decrease in the partial pressure of inspired oxygen may cause a significant decrease in arterial oxygen content. With increasing altitude, the partial pressure of oxygen decreases while its concentration (%) remains unchanged. Therefore, arterial PO_2, which depends on the PO_2 of ambient air, will decrease as the altitude increases. Similarly, inhalation of nonphysiologic gas mixtures, such as automobile exhaust, will decrease the PO_2.

Table 7.3
Physiologic Causes of Cyanosis

Environmental decreased availability of oxygen
Altitude
Inhalation of nonphysiologic gas mixtures
Alveolar hypoventilation
Central nervous system (CNS) depression (e.g., trauma, drugs, infection)
Upper airway obstruction (e.g., tracheal rings, epiglottitis, etc.)
Hypotonia (e.g., CNS insults, spinal cord insults, drugs)
Restricted lung movement (e.g., diaphragmatic hernia, tension pneumothorax)
Major diffusion abnormalities
Interstitial fibrosis
Oxygen toxicity
Adult respiratory distress syndrome
Pulmonary edema
Abnormalities of hemoglobin and oxygen-carrying capacity
Abnormal hemoglobin (e.g., methemoglobin, carboxyhemoglobin, sulfhemoglobin)
Alterations in oxyhemoglobin affinity (e.g., changes in 2,3-diphosphoglycerate content, pH, temperature)
Too much reduced hemoglobin (e.g., hyperviscosity)
Abnormalities of pulmonary blood flow
Congenital obstruction to heart disease with pulmonary blood flow (and/or right-to-left shunting, e.g., tetralogy of Fallot, pulmonary atresia)
Primary pulmonary hypertension
Persistent fetal circulation
Intracardiac chronic heart disease with right-to-left shunts
Hypotension
Abnormalities of $\dot{V}/\dot{Q}$ matching
Pharmacologic effects, e.g., sodium nitroprusside
Poor tissue perfusion
Shock with inadequate compensation for tissue perfusion (e.g., septic, hemorrhagic, cardiac etiology)
Impaired rheology (hyperviscosity)

Hypoventilation

Hypoventilation may cause a reduction in PAO_2 by delivering less oxygen to the alveolus than is needed to meet metabolic demands. Clinical situations associated with hypoventilation include:

1. Upper airway obstruction from choanal atresia, meconium aspiration, laryngeal or tracheal web, vascular rings, and tumors and masses of the neck
2. CNS depression from sedative medications (e.g., phenobarbital), perinatal hypoxia (with or without intracranial hemorrhage), and infection (e.g., meningitis or cerebral abscess)
3. Hypotonia of central or neuromuscular origin
4. Disorders that restrict normal lung movement (e.g., diaphragmatic hernia or eventration, pneumothorax, lobar emphysema, hypoplastic lung, and intrathoracic tumors)

If the hypoventilation caused by any one of these conditions leads to systemic desaturation, cyanosis occurs.

Major Diffusion Abnormalities

Primary abnormalities of diffusion are extremely rare in children. Interstitial fibrosis (Hamman-Rich syndrome) usually is seen in adult patients. Other clinical entities commonly included under this heading are really abnormalities in the V/Q relationship, in that alveolar hypoventilation is associated with a decreased alveolar surface area. Congenital lobar emphysema, hypoplasia of a lung, diaphragmatic hernia and atelectasis in hyaline membrane disease, ARDS, and aspiration pneumonia result in reduced alveolar surface area and hamper normal oxygenation of blood because of decreased V/Q ratio.

Hemoglobin and Oxygen-Carrying Capacity

The effect of Hb concentration on oxygen content (CaO_2) is shown in Table 7.4.

Anemia

A consequence of this relationship is that an anemic patient may manifest inadequate CaO_2 and tissue oxygen delivery in the presence of an adequate arterial O_2 and saturation. Tissue hypoxia will occur in the absence of cyanosis. An anemic patient is also susceptible to tissue hypoxia caused by significant Hb desaturation associated with low PaO_2. Cyanotic discoloration will not occur because the patient does not have the necessary 4 to 5g desaturated Hb.

Table 7.4
Oxygen Content of Blood at Various Hemoglobin Concentrations

Hb (g/dL)	C_aO_2(mL/dL)[a]
30	40.5
25	33.8
20	27.1
18	24.4
16	21.7
14	19.1
12	16.4
10	13.4
8	10.8
6	8.1

[a]Assuming an oxygen-carrying capacity of 1.34 and 100% saturation.

Polycythemia

Conversely, polycythemia can produce cyanosis even in the absence of profound hypoxia. Polycythemia involves an increased number of circulating erythrocytes and an associated elevated blood volume. In an adult, an Hct of 60% or above strongly suggests this condition. In neonates who normally have high erythrocyte counts, an Hct of 65% or above supports a diagnosis of polycythemia.

Erythrocytosis can be divided into primary and secondary causes. Primary polycythemia, or polycythemia vera, is a myeloproliferative disorder that commonly begins in middle life and is rare in the pediatric population. In the neonate with Down's syndrome or trisomy D, a transient marrow dysfunction may produce primary polycythemia. Secondary polycythemia results from an increased production of erythropoietin or from transfusion of red cells. The stimuli for erythropoietin formation include hypoxia and various endocrine abnormalities. Congenital heart defects with significant right-to-left shunts produce a chronic hypoxic state and polycythemia in the neonate and child. Endocrine abnormalities such as congenital adrenal hyperplasia, neonatal thyrotoxicosis, and maternal diabetes are associated with an increased metabolic demand for oxygen and increased erythropoiesis and polycythemia.

Under normal conditions, the PO_2 in the venous circulation is approximately 40 to 50 mm Hg, and Hb saturation is reduced to 70 to 80%. In the polycythemic patient, even this normal 30% desaturation provides the minimum 4 to 5 g total desaturated Hb/dL needed to produce cyanosis. In the neonate with a normal Hct of approximately 60%, this is responsible for the commonly observed discoloration in the hands, feet, and skin (acrocyanosis or peripheral cyanosis).

2,3-DPG

Within the erythrocyte, the influence of organic phosphates, particularly 2,3-diphosphoglycerate (2,3-DPG), alters these affinities. The interaction of 2,3-DPG with Hb produces a decrease in oxygen affinity. The higher the concentration of 2,3-DPG in the erythrocyte, the greater the rightward shift of the O_2-Hb dissociation curve (lower P50), indicating more O_2 is released per unit change of PO_2. However, HbF is less affected by 2,3-DPG, and the resultant decrease in oxygen affinity is much less, producing the functional differences. Elevation of 2,3-DPG levels in response to tissue hypoxia is discussed later.

Temperature and pH

An increased body temperature will facilitate oxygen release and may be beneficial in cases of hyperthermia, with its accompanying increased metabolic demand for O_2. Lower temperatures have the reverse—and potentially adverse—effect. The P50 is reduced because of a greater affinity for oxygen, which reduces the amount of O_2 released for a given change in PO_2.

Hypothermia

During states of reduced oxygen consumption, such as hypothermia, dissolved O_2 may contribute more significantly to the total oxygen content. Basal oxygen consumption is approximately 3 to 4 mL/kg body weight/min in adults. The requirement is decreased by 50% at 31°C (approximately 2 mL/kg/min) and by an additional 25% at 20°C (to 1 mL/kg/min). Thus, during hypothermia, the oxygen requirements may be satisfied in large part or solely by the dissolved O2 (assuming a cardiac output of 100 mL/kg/min).

Redox of Heme Iron

A change in the redox state of the heme iron will alter O_2 delivery by affecting oxygen content. Methemoglobin (MetHb) contains oxidized iron (Fe3+), which cannot reversibly bind oxygen. It is constantly formed under normal circumstances but comprises less than 1 to 2% of total Hb. The concentration is maintained at low levels by active enzymes, NADH- and NADPH-dependent methemoglobin reductase, which reduce Fe3+ to Fe2+, a form that can transport oxygen. If MetHb levels rise (methemoglobinemia), cyanosis occurs. The discoloration is evident with as little as 1.5 g MetHb/dL, compared with the 4 to 5 g desaturated normal Hb. Methemoglobinemia may be produced by a variety of causes including a congenital defect in Hb formation (M-hemoglobinopathy), a defect in the reducing enzyme, nitrite toxicity, or exposure to other toxins (Table 7.5). Cyanide toxicity also results in the accumulation of MetHb.

Table 7.5
Amino and Nitro Compounds Producing Methemoglobinemia[a]

Aromatic Drugs	Aliphatic and Inorganic Drugs
Aniline	Sodium nitrite
Phenacetin	Hydroxylamine
Sulfanilamide	Dimethylamine
Sulfapyridine	Nitroglycerin
Sulfathiazole	Sodium nitroprusside
Phenylenediamine	Amyl nitrite
Phenylhydroxylamine	Ethyl nitrite
Nitrobenzene	Bismuth subnitrate
Dinitrobenzene	Ammonium nitrate
Trinitrotoluene	

[a]Adapted from Finch CA. Methemoglobinemia and sulfhemoglobinemia. N Engl J Med 1972;239:470. With permission.

Abnormalities of Pulmonary Blood Flow

A shunt that produces cyanosis permits mixing of blood from the venous and systemic (arterial) circulations. Therefore, venous blood must bypass normal flow pathways to cause cyanosis. Mixing desaturated blood with systemic blood produces variable degrees of systemic desaturation, depending on the fraction of desaturated blood. If significant portions of cardiac output are diverted through a shunt, cyanosis occurs. Shunts that produce cyanosis may be divided into those of intrapulmonary origin and those of intracardiac origin.

Intrapulmonary Shunts Intrapulmonary shunts include anatomic and physiologic pulmonary arteriovenous connections. There are normally left-to-right shunts in the lung. Potential right-to-left anatomic shunts that are normally closed are also present in the lung. These shunts can open and may accommodate up to 20% cardiac output during conditions of elevated pulmonary pressure and produce cyanosis. Abnormal ventilation/perfusion relationships also produce intrapulmonary shunts.

Prominent factors determining appropriate pulmonary perfusion include:

- Matching perfusion to ventilation in the alveolar-capillary unit
- Transit time of blood in the pulmonary capillary
- Pulmonary vascular resistance

Vasodilator drugs (e.g., sodium nitroprusside, nitroglycerin, dobutamine) attenuate pulmonary vasoconstrictor response to alveolar hypoxia, leading to perfusion of poorly ventilated lung regions and hindering oxygenation of blood. If the fraction of blood thus diverted is significant, systemic desaturation and cyanosis result.

The final saturation of systemic blood depends on

1. The fraction of shunted blood (e.g., the amount of blood not exposed to ventilated lungs)
2. The oxygen content of the venous ("shunted") blood
3. The oxygen content of the pulmonary venous blood

If there is either low cardiac output or increased oxygen consumption, mixed venous oxygen content may be very low, and thus the impact of any given shunt will be greater.

Pulmonary perfusion may be compromised by inappropriate hypoxic pulmonary vasoconstriction, which usually is localized and reversible in children and adults. In neonates and infants exposed to alveolar hypoxia, however, severe, diffuse vasoconstriction can occur in response to hypoxia. Even after the hypoxia has been corrected, pulmonary vasoconstriction and its associated reduction in total pulmonary flow may persist, producing elevated pressures in the pulmonary artery, right ventricle, and right atrium. In the neonate, if right-sided pressures become greater than left-sided, the foramen ovale and ductus arteriosus may open to produce a right-to-left shunt. This can perpetuate a pathophysiologic state termed persistent fetal circulation (PFC). Diminished total effective pulmonary flow lowers oxygen saturation of blood and subsequently produces cyanosis.

Intracardiac Shunts Anatomic shunts of cardiac origin also divert blood away from the regular flow pathway. Right-to-left shunts that divert venous blood to the systemic circulation are common causes of cyanosis. These cyanotic congenital heart defects include tetralogy of Fallot, truncus arteriosus, TGA, tricuspid atresia, total anomalous pulmonary venous return, and single ventricle. Admixture also can occur in the absence of pathologic intracardiac shunts, because obstruction to right ventricular outflow resulting from pulmonic stenosis or pulmonic atresia increases right ventricular and right atrial pressures and cause the foramen ovale to open.

The presence and extent of admixture and cyanosis in many conditions with communications between the right and left heart may be understood by examining the ratio of pulmonary vascular resistance (PVR) to systemic vascular resistance (SVR). Normally, the SVR is several times greater than the PVR. When pulmonary resistance increases or systemic resistance decreases, blood flow may be shunted into the systemic circulation if a communication exists. These "dependent" or "dynamic" shunts can determine the level of arterial desaturation and cyanosis in conditions such as persistent fetal circulation or tetralogy of Fallot.

Poor Tissue Perfusion Secondary to Inadequate Perfusion Pressure

Inadequate tissue perfusion secondary to inadequate perfusion pressure results in insufficient flow to meet metabolic needs, a condition that occurs during congestive heart failure and in classic shock conditions. Congestive heart failure with low cardiac output, poor perfusion, and cyanosis may result from a primary myopathy, such as endocardial fibroelastosis, or from numerous other causes. A set of events common to the various causes may be observed. Peripheral perfusion is decreased. Increased sympathetic activity causes tachycardia and vasoconstriction of various arteriolar beds, further compromising peripheral blood flow. The net result may be a child with cool extremities, decreased blood pressure, and diminished peripheral pulses; secondary cardiomegaly may occur. If congestive heart failure is prolonged, growth delay can also ensue. Because of the reduced perfusion, oxygen delivery is significantly impeded. When congestive heart failure is of moderate severity, cyanotic discoloration may be seen peripherally (acrocyanosis). More severe failure may result in systemic desaturation and "central cyanosis."

Poor Tissue Perfusion Secondary to Altered Rheology

The rheologic properties of blood normally determine the flow characteristics through microcirculation. Blood viscosity depends on red cell deformability, the dynamics of viscoelastic fluid flow through vessels, and the influence of the individual blood components. Tissue flow (and thus cardiac output) is inversely affected by viscosity. In particular, increased blood viscosity may impede flow through small vessels, which will decrease oxygen transport to the tissue. A primary determinant of blood viscosity is the erythrocyte concentration (Hct). In the neonate, a significant rise in viscosity is observed above an Hct of 63%, and adverse effects may be observed at an Hct of 65% or greater.

Adaptive Changes to Hypoxia

Optimizing Oxygen Delivery

Initial Changes When PaO_2 falls below 60 mm Hg and arterial saturation to 93%, carotid, aortic, and central chemoreceptors are activated. This triggers an increase in minute ventilation, which causes both the PaO_2 and PaO_2 to rise. Sympathetic activity is also stimulated, elevating both heart rate and systemic arterial blood pressure. In addition, tissue hypoxia causes a decrease in local tissue vascular resistance. Thus, tissue flow increases because of the increased tissue perfusion pressure and lower tissue vascular resistance. This results in a higher cardiac output if hypoxia is not profound and prolonged. In turn, pulmonary perfusion also increases, producing greater pulmonary capillary blood flow and increasing flow through the lungs, both of which promote oxygen uptake. In addition, distribution of systemic blood flow is affected by the sympathetic activity. Blood flow is preferentially shunted away from the muscular bed, while renal, hepatic, and cerebral flows increase.

Sustained Hypoxia Sustained systemic hypoxia engenders further adaptive changes designed to improve tissue oxygen availability. Minute ventilation and heart rate remain elevated and may rise further. Levels of 2,3-DPG can increase as soon as 24 hours after sustained hypoxia. The interaction of 2,3-DPG with Hb shifts the oxygen-Hb dissociation curve to the right, which facilitates release of oxygen, making more O_2 available to the tissues, and resulting in a change in PO_2. A similar effect on oxygen dissociation is seen with a decreased pH, which is normally found in tissue capillaries. Further decreases in tissue pH may result from hypoxia-associated anaerobic metabolism and lactic acid formation, effecting a greater shift to the right.

Continued Hypoxia Continued hypoxia stimulates production of erythropoietin, resulting in increased circulating Hb and red blood cell levels after 2 to 3 weeks. The elevated concentrations of Hb allow more oxygen to be transported by increasing levels of CaO_2. The polycythemia may also make the appearance of cyanosis more likely. Finally, a prolonged hypoxic challenge can also induce a greater efficiency of mitochondrial oxidative systems, which optimizes cellular use of delivered oxygen. Long-standing cyanosis, however, may produce myocardial dysfunction and be reflected in diminished left ventricular reserve.

Severe Hypoxia In the adult, acute, severe hypoxia will also result in the respiratory and cardiovascular changes mentioned previously. A rapid deterioration of clinical status occurs because of depression of the myocardium and central respiratory centers, followed closely by death. In the neonate, the cardiovascular responses to acute, moderate, or severe hypoxia are quite different. Instead of tachycardia or increased blood pressure, significant bradycardia and hypotension may occur, placing the neonate at added risk.

Physiologic Changes and Clinical Status Physiologic adaptations to hypoxia are an attempt to improve oxygen delivery and use. Failure of these changes to provide sufficient oxygen for normal function is followed by malfunction of various organ systems. In this setting, bradycardia, hypoventilation, and shock result. To care for the critically ill patient, it is of particular importance, therefore, to understand the disturbances of the CNS, pulmonary vasculature, kidney, and liver that are produced by hypoxia.

CNS Response The cerebral oxygen uptake ($CMRO_2$) is approximately 3 mL O_2/100 g/min (or 45 mL O_2/min for an adult brain). The brain has no anaerobic metabolism and requires a continuous supply of oxygen to sustain normal function. Depletion of oxygen for any reason produces abnormal cerebral function. Figure 7.6 is a graphic representation of the cerebral responses to hypoxia.

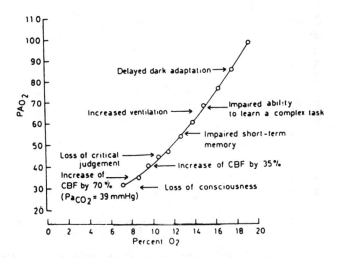

Figure 7.6. CNS responses to hypoxia. CBF, cerebral blood flow. (Adapted from Siesjo BK, Johannsson H, Ljunggren B, Norberg K. Brain dysfunction in cerebral hypoxia and ischemia. In: Plum F, ed. Brain dysfunction in metabolic disorders. New York: Raven Press, 1974:75.)

Kidney Function Renal blood flow is normally high, approximately 420 mL/kg/min. This perfusion is required to supply oxygen for the high renal O_2 consumption necessary for tubular reabsorption. The relationship of tubular reabsorption (e.g., of Na+) to oxygen consumption is correlated over a wide range of values (Fig. 7.7). From this figure, it can be seen that a reduced availability of oxygen reduces the reabsorptive work of the kidney.

Liver Function Liver blood supply is composed of flow from the portal vein and from the hepatic artery. The portal vein contributes blood with low PO_2 and comprises the larger portion (70%) of total flow. This blood perfuses first the peripheral and then the centrilobular cells, which are exposed, therefore, to an even lower PO_2 level. During hypoxic conditions, hepatic arterial flow is significantly decreased, placing centrilobular cells at increased risk of damage and possibly producing centrilobular necrosis, hepatic dysfunction, and clotting abnormalities.

Evaluation of the Cyanotic Patient

History A history of cyanotic congenital heart disease does not ensure that the current episode of cyanosis is due solely to that heart disease and not to an

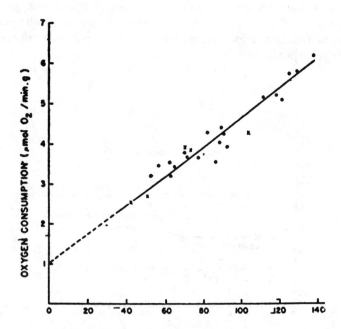

Figure 7.7. Relationship of renal oxygen consumption and tubular reabsorption of sodium. (From Thurau K. Renal Na-reabsorption and O_2-uptake in dogs during hypoxia and hydrochlorothiazide infusion. Proc Soc Exp Biol Med 1961;106:714. © Society for Experimental Biology and Medicine. With permission.)

episode of aspiration. Even cyanotic children ingest poisons, for example. The history of a patient with obvious cyanosis from pulmonary disease may seem irrelevant if the patient appears to have pneumonia, but a history may reveal an underlying immune deficiency or other additional cause of the cyanosis.

Physical Examination Physical examination can often clarify the reason for the cyanosis.

Diagnostic Physical Signs The presence of gastric contents in the nostrils or pharynx suggests aspiration. This may be the primary cause of the cyanosis or may be secondary to it. Cyanosis with hypotonia, apnea, or bradypnea is commonly associated with CNS disorders caused by asphyxia or infection, neuromuscular disease, or pharmacologic agents. Clubbing of the digits indicates hypoxia of several months' duration. Signs of progressive hyperviscosity include plethora, lethargy, tachycardia, tachypnea, grunting, and retractions. More dramatic evidence of the polycythemia-hyperviscosity syndrome is the presence of nonspecific neurologic abnormalities and arterial or venous thromboses, including those in intracranial sites.

Respiration The respiratory pattern may be of help in diagnosing the cause of cyanosis. Tachypnea, use of accessory muscles, retractions, stridor, and grunting are usually manifestations of pulmonary pathology. Nasal obstruction can produce a snorting respiratory sound; laryngeal obstruction is frequently associated with inspiratory stridor; and bronchial and lower airway obstruction can produce expiratory wheezing. However, localization of the obstruction is sometimes difficult in the neonate, who may show similar signs in the presence of many causes of airway obstruction. Asymmetrical chest movements may occur because of bronchial obstruction, pneumothorax, diaphragmatic injury, or mass lesions. Inadequate muscular effort and air movement suggest a neuromuscular disorder or drug effect as the cause of the cyanosis. No monitoring equipment in the PICU can serve as a substitute for a physical examination in detecting findings of this type.

The Abdomen Examination of the abdomen may be diagnostic. A scaphoid contour indicates that abdominal contents have possibly been displaced into the thorax because of diaphragmatic herniation. Bowel sounds heard on auscultation of the chest add further support to this diagnosis. Hepatomegaly suggests congestive heart failure as the cause of the cyanosis.

Musculoskeletal System Although not commonly remembered, examination of the musculoskeletal system may be vital in the evaluation of a patient with cyanosis. Fractured bones, particularly long bones, can produce fat emboli, which occur in children. Thromboembolism is generally more frequent in adults than in children, but pulmonary emboli also occur in children and have resulted in patients with cyanosis.

Cardiac Evaluation Rate, location, and characteristics of precordial impulses, intensity of pulses, and blood pressure levels in both the upper and lower extremities should be noted. Although tachycardia is common in patients with cyanosis of any cause, the development of bradycardia is a prognostic sign suggesting profound cyanosis. A shift of the maximal impulse may result from ventricular hypoplasia or hypertrophy related to valvular or septal abnormalities or from cardiac malposition (i.e., dextrocardia). The presence of a murmur may also indicate congenital heart disease. It is important to remember, however, that right-to-left shunts by themselves do not produce murmurs, because the flow required would be incompatible with life. This fact is important in certain disease states, such as profound respiratory failure in the neonatal period when an enormous ductal flow producing a massive right-to-left shunt is inaudible. The specifics of cyanotic spells are covered at the end of this section.

Central Nervous System CNS causes of cyanosis are well known but are not always considered. Isolated head trauma can produce both CNS-induced pulmonary edema and intrapulmonary shunting from alterations in neural control of the matching pulmonary ventilation and flow.

Cyanotic Spells Children with cyanotic congenital heart defects, particularly tetralogy of Fallot, may develop an alarming complication known by various names such as "cyanotic spells," "paroxysmal hyperpnea," "tet spells," "hypoxic spells," "anoxic spells," "blue spells," or "syncopal episodes." These episodes are characterized by paroxysmal hyperpnea and increased cyanosis. Patients often proceed to exhibit limpness, generalized stiffness, and rolling back of the eyes. Systemic acidosis accompanies these attacks. Occasionally, convulsions, cerebral vascular accidents, and/or death may occur. In the early stages, a patient may spontaneously assume the squatting (or knee-chest) position to alleviate the symptoms. Patients range in age from 1 month to 12 years, with the peak incidence occurring in patients between 1 and 3 months of age. Although the paroxysms may occur at any time, most occur in the morning, usually on awakening. The duration of an episode ranges from minutes to several hours, with most lasting 15 to 60 min. Several factors precipitating the attacks have been identified—most commonly, crying, defecation, and feeding. There seems to be no correlation between the resting arterial PO_2 and the incidence of the attacks.

Several causes have been suggested for the episodes, including spasm of the pulmonary infundibulum, acute rises of PVR, and sudden decreases in SVR. Regardless, the result is an increased ratio of PVR:SVR, with a decrease in pulmonary blood flow relative to systemic flow.

Laboratory Tests Elevated Hb and/or Hct levels suggest the possibility of polycythemia. In infants and children, polycythemia may be secondary to hypoxia of cardiac, pulmonary, or another etiology. An elevated or depressed white cell count, with or without an increase in immature forms, implicates infections. A sample of blood drawn from a patient with suspected MetHb can be placed on filter paper and exposed to air. The blood will appear chocolate brown after a few minutes.

Serum or blood glucose and calcium levels should be determined. Hypoglycemia is defined as blood glucose lower than 40 mg/dL in infants older than 4 days. However, between birth and 3 days of age, levels lower than 20 mg/dL on two determinations in premature infants and below 30 mg/dL in term infants are considered to indicate hypoglycemia. Calcium levels are normally in the range of 10 mg/dL; the ionized calcium is approximately 5 mg/dL. At levels below 3 to 4 mg ionized calcium, the patient may display symptoms of hypocalcemia, including cyanosis.

Arterial blood gas determinations provide important information concerning the etiology of cyanosis. The $PaCO_2$ usually is decreased in cyanosis of cardiac origin because of hypoxia-triggered tachypnea in the presence of normal gas exchange. Pulmonary disease associated with cyanosis indicates respiratory failure, which results in a normal or elevated $PaCO_2$ despite the associated tachypnea. Most often, cyanosis is associated with hypoxic conditions and low PaO_2. Commonly, in hypoxia resulting from hypoventilation or pulmonary disease, inspiration of 100% oxygen elevates the PaO_2 significantly (i.e., more than 100 to 150 mm Hg). In the case of congenital cardiac defects, the response to 100% inspired O_2 may be minimal because of the effects of right-to-left shunts. Cyanosis may also occur with a normal PaO_2. This apparent paradox occurs in patients with polycythemia because of the desaturated blood normally present in the venous circulation and in patients who have suffered smoke inhalation with carboxyhemoglobin elevation. Of particular concern is the effect of carboxyhemoglobin and MetHb on the oxygen saturation of Hb (SaO_2), which is determined by pulse oximetry. Pulse oximetry has become a routine tool used for monitoring arterial oxygen saturation and, in most circumstances, accurately correlates with hemoglobin saturation as measured by cooximetry. However, in the presence of carboxyhemoglobin and MetHb, the SaO_2 may be falsely and significantly elevated, thus masking the presence of hypoxemia.

Diagnostic Imaging

Radiography Anterior/posterior and lateral chest radiographs provide extremely valuable information, including the following:

- Symmetry of lung fields
- Classic signs of pneumothorax, pulmonary parenchymal disease, lobar emphysema, or hyaline membrane disease
- Bowel gas pattern in the chest and a "gasless" abdomen, which point to diaphragmatic hernia
- An elevated diaphragm is seen with eventration
- Evidence of elevated or decreased pulmonary blood flow differentiates certain cardiac lesions
- Cardiac silhouette showing a normal-sized heart with a cocked-up apex (couer-sabot or boot shape) caused by right ventricular dominance is the pathognomonic sign of tetralogy of Fallot

- Narrow mediastinal shadow
- Decreased pulmonary vascular markings
- Right aortic arch in 25% of cases

Electrocardiography Most patients with cyanosis of noncardiac etiology are expected to have a normal ECG. However, a child with upper airway obstruction or chronic hypoxia from other causes may develop cor pulmonale, which manifests as right-axis deviation and right ventricular strain and hypertrophy. A prolonged Q-T interval is observed in hypocalcemia. A decrease in body temperature below 30°C induces lengthening of all time intervals: R-R, P-R, QRS, Q-T, and "J-point deflections" may be obvious in the midprecordial leads.

Echocardiography The echocardiogram is essential in diagnosing anatomic causes of heart disease. It is also used, with increasing sophistication, to localize and quantitate shunts.

Therapeutic Considerations

Cyanosis in the neonate or in a child of any age is an emergency. Although a search for the cause is being conducted, supplemental oxygen should be administered to all patients. Respiratory failure, confirmed by low PaO_2 and elevated $PaCO_2$, requires instituting ventilatory support, usually in the form of endotracheal intubation and mechanical ventilation.

Congestive Heart Failure

Successful management of congestive heart failure requires prompt identification of the underlying cause. In the interim:

- Place the patient in a semisitting position
- Administer supplemental oxygen
- Institute ventilatory support as dictated by the clinical evaluation
- Restrict total fluid intake
- Begin digoxin therapy (guidelines and dosage schedules are presented in Table 7.6)
- Monitor the ECG, serum levels of digoxin and electrolytes, and renal function to prevent digoxin toxicity
- In severe congestive heart failure, use diuretic agents and monitor serum levels of sodium, potassium, chloride, and bicarbonate to prevent electrolyte disturbances

Additional therapeutic measures may be necessary if initial therapy of congestive heart failure proves insufficient. Intravenous sympathomimetics (e.g., dopamine, isoproterenol) can improve cardiac output. Sedation with morphine (0.05 mg/kg) or diazepam (0.1 mg/kg) may decrease metabolic demands but also must raise concerns about respiratory depression. In ad-

Table 7.6
Digoxin Therapy[a]

Preparation	Route of Administration	Effect (Onset/Maximum)	Effect (Duration)	Total Excretion	Oral Absorption	Dose (Digitalizing)	Dose (Daily Maintenance)
Digoxin (lanoxin) Available in Tablets: 0.125, 0.25, 0.5 mg Elixir: 0.05 mg/mL Ampules: 0.1, 0.25 mg/mL	IV, IM, PO	5–30 min/2–5 h 15–60 min/2–5 h 1–2 h/4–8 h	24 h	48–72 h	40–90%	PO (µg/kg) Preterm: 20–30 Full term: 25–35 1–24 mos: 35–60 2–5 yr: 30–40 5–10 yr: 20–35 10 yr–adult: 10–15 IM or IV (µg/kg) Preterm: 15–25 Full term: 20–30 1–24 mos: 30–50 2–5 yr: 25–35 5–10 yr: 15–20 10 yr to adult: 8–12 *Parenteral digitalizing doses are 80% of oral digitalizing doses; ½ TDD[b] is administered stat, then ¼ TDD is administered q 6–8 h × 2	PO (µg/kg) Preterm: 20–30% of oral loading dose Full term to adult: 25–35% of oral loading dose Maintenance dose is administered q 12 h IV (µg/kg) Preterm: 20–30% of IV loading dose Full term to adult: 25–35% of IV loading dose

[a]Adapted from Cole CH, ed. The Harriet Lane handbook. 10th ed. Chicago: Year Book Medical Publishers, 1984:132.

[b]TDD, total digitalizing dose.

dition to its sedative effect, morphine produces systemic vasodilation and increases cardiac output. Many pediatric intensivists are using afterload in this setting with good results. If the congestive failure is still inadequately controlled with medical therapy, corrective or palliative surgery of the underlying cardiac defect, which may have been scheduled for a later date, must be performed at this time.

Cyanotic Spells

Treatment of cyanotic spells is designed to improve arterial PO_2 and acidosis by decreasing obstruction to right ventricular outflow, improving pulmonary blood flow, and reducing the PVR/SVR ratio.

Improved Oxygenation

Supplemental oxygen is administered by face mask or oxygen hood. The patient is placed in a knee-chest position, which is physiologically similar to squatting. Squatting increases effective pulmonary blood flow and redistributes systemic flow to the upper body by increasing the SVR. During this maneuver, the arterial oxygen saturation remains unchanged, but the venous saturation increases, implying improved capillary and tissue oxygenation.

Intravenous Fluid Administration

Acidosis is corrected administering $NaHCO_3$ after a sample for blood gas and pH analyses has been obtained. Initially, the patient may be given 2 mEq $NaHCO_3$/kg (0.5 mEq/mL) over 5 minutes. Subsequent doses may be administered as needed according to the following formula:

$$NaHCO_3 \text{ dose (mEq)} = 0.3 \times \text{body weight (kg)} \times \text{base deficit}$$

Half the dose is administered over 30 minutes, and the remainder over 4 hours.

Pharmacologic Agents

Morphine administration (0.1 to 0.2 mg/kg subcutaneously or intravenously) is often effective in relieving a spell. The probable mechanism of action is a reduction of infundibular spasm and improved pulmonary blood flow. β-Adrenergic antagonists given intravenously may also reverse a spasm. Propranolol (0.2 mg/kg intravenously) has been shown to terminate a spell, probably by relaxing the right ventricular outlet. In addition, chronic oral therapy with propranolol (1 to 2 mg/kg four times daily) has been shown to decrease the frequency of the paroxysms. However, the use of propranolol in the newborn is discouraged because it may cause severe cardiac depression. Conversely, inotropic agents may exacerbate the obstruction to right ventricular outflow and cause further deterioration. Therefore, their use in the treatment of cyanotic spells is best avoided. Calcium blockers can alleviate pulmonary hypertension and are potentially useful in the treatment of cyanotic spells. However, hypoxia may actually be exacerbated if cardiac performance is significantly depressed by the effects of calcium blockers on the myocardium. Caution is advised, therefore, until more experience has been gained with these agents in the treatment of paroxysms. After the child with hypoxic spells has been stabilized, prompt surgical correction must be considered.

Pulmonary Causes

Cyanosis may be the result of a pulmonary parenchymal disease such as acute respiratory distress syndrome, hyaline membrane disease, pneumonia, or aspiration. Cyanosis caused by pulmonary parenchymal disease requires supplemental oxygen and may necessitate ventilatory support. Such support may take the form of CPAP or mechanical ventilation.

Surgical Approach

Surgical intervention is necessary to treat certain pulmonary causes of cyanosis:

- Intrinsic lesions such as choanal atresia or congenital webs that obstruct the airway
- Extrinsic lesions that restrict lung movement, which include lobar emphysema and diaphragmatic herniation
- A pneumothorax may be relieved by needle aspiration of the free air and/or placement of a thoracostomy tube

Pharmacologic Approach

Pharmacologic depression of ventilation sufficient to produce cyanosis requires mechanical ventilatory support until the effects of the agent have subsided. Antagonists are available for some pharmacologic agents—such as narcotics—and may be administered to reverse respiratory depression. Morphine, meperidine (i.e., Demerol), fentanyl, and other opioids may be reversed by naloxone (i.e, Narcan) at a dose of 0.01 mg/kg intramuscularly or intravenously and should be repeated as needed.

Metabolic Abnormalities

Hypothermia and Hypoglycemia Hypothermia can be reversed by the use of warming lights, warm coverings, and adjustment of the ambient temperature. Patients with symptomatic hypoglycemia should receive intravenous glucose. The usual dose is 1 to 2 mL/kg of 25% dextrose (i.e., 50%

dextrose diluted 1:1 in sterile water). We avoid direct administration of 50% glucose to minimize adverse effects of hyperosmolality. For infants of diabetic mothers, the dose is adjusted to deliver 150 mg/kg or 1 mL 15% dextrose/kg. The initial dose is followed by an infusion of dextrose delivering 4 to 8 mg/kg/min to maintain a normal serum level of glucose. The blood glucose level should be determined periodically to ascertain that the patient is normoglycemic. Further therapy with hydrocortisone may be needed to maintain normal glucose levels if dextrose therapy alone is insufficient.

Hypocalcemia Hypocalcemia severe enough to cause cyanosis is usually associated with other symptoms, including extreme irritability and convulsions. Symptoms may be reversed by a slow intravenous push of calcium gluconate (i.e., 10% in water) at 1 mL/min to a maximum of 3 mg/kg, until a clinical response is obtained. Calcium levels may then be maintained in the normal range with an infusion of calcium. Either calcium gluceptate or calcium gluconate can be used, and the infusion can be adjusted to deliver 24 to 35 mg calcium/kg/day.

Methemoglobinemia Therapy for methemoglobinemia (MetHb) starts with general supportive care and removal of any possible toxin. The latter may entail removal of contaminated clothes, washing the skin, and emptying gastric contents with induced emesis or lavage. Because normal mechanisms convert MetHb to Hb over 15 to 20 hours, no other treatment for toxin-induced methemoglobinemia is needed in the absence of hypoxic symptoms. However, if signs of hypoxia are present or the MetHb level exceeds 30%, drug therapy should be considered. Pharmacologic treatment is designed to convert the ferric iron (Fe^{3+}) in heme to the ferrous state. The preferred agent is methylene blue (tetramethylthionine chloride), which forms an NADPH-dependent oxidation reduction system for heme. This is accomplished through activation of NADPH-MetHb reductase, with methylene blue as a cofactor.

The usual dosage of methylene blue is 1 to 2 mg/kg (in a 1% solution) administered intravenously during a 5 minute period. Most MetHb should be converted within 30 to 60 minutes. If needed, the dose may be repeated after 1 hour (maximum dose 7 mg/kg). Side effects are seen with higher doses and include precordial pain, dyspnea, restlessness, tremors, and apprehension. Dysuria and urinary frequency may also be present. High concentrations of methylene blue can occasionally cause mild hemolysis and may actually produce methemoglobinemia by reversing the reaction.

Failure of methylene blue treatment may require blood transfusion or exchange transfusion therapy. Treatment failure suggests the possibility of glucose 6-phosphate dehydrogenase deficiency or sulfhemoglobinemia, for which no specific therapy exists. Therapy with transfusions, exchange transfusions, or hyperbaric oxygen may alleviate the acute symptoms. This intervention can be followed by treatment with ascorbic acid, which reduces MetHb slowly.

Polylycythemia or Hyperviscosity Treatment of polycythemia and/or hyperviscosity is directed at achieving an isovolemic reduction in the erythrocyte count. This is accomplished by performing a partial or "reduction" exchange transfusion. Catheters are placed for the withdrawal and infusion of blood. In the neonate, an umbilical venous or arterial catheter may be used. The total amount of blood to be exchanged is calculated as follows:

$$V = \text{weight} \times (80 \text{ mL/kg}) \times$$
$$[(\text{observed Hct} - \text{desired Hct})/\text{observed Hct}]$$

where V equals total volume to be exchanged.

The desired Hct level is lower than 55%. Blood is withdrawn in 5 to 10 mL aliquots and discarded. The removed blood is replaced by an equal volume of plasma solution. The process is repeated until the calculated volume has been removed and an equal amount has been reinfused. The patient's temperature should be monitored closely to maintain normothermia. Resuscitation drugs and equipment should be readily accessible in case severe hypotension, seizure, or cardiac arrest occur.

8.

Postoperative Management of the Cardiac Surgical Patient

Charles L. Schleien, Nancy A. Setzer, Gwenn E. McLaughlin, and Mark C. Rogers

The immediate postoperative intensive care of the infant or child who has undergone surgery for the palliation or correction of congenital heart disease is an important part of the overall sequence of surgical management of congenital heart disease. This care requires a multidisciplinary approach with coordination of multiple services.

The infant being readied for cardiac surgery may already have a vast array of problems (Table 8.1).

Table 8.1
Preoperative Problems in Neonates

Metabolic	↓ Glucose; poor glycogen stores
	↓ Calcium; ↓ PTH activity
	Acidosis
	Electrolyte disturbance
Temperature	Increased heat loss
	↓ Ability to generate heat
Pulmonary	Difficult airway
	Premature infant—hyaline membrane disease, BPD
	↓ PVR
	Persistent fetal circulation
	Reactive pulmonary vascular bed
	Vasoconstriction to ↑ PCO_2 ↓ PO_2
	Pneumothorax
Liver	↑ Bilirubin
	↓ Metabolism of many drugs
CNS	Intraventricular hemorrhage

PTH, parathyroid hormone; BPD, bronchopulmonary dysplasia; PVR, pulmonary vascular resistance; CNS central nervous system.

OPEN HEART SURGERY: INTRAOPERATIVE CONCERNS

The surgical procedure for the patient with congenital heart disease is divided into several distinct periods: anesthetic induction, prebypass surgery, the actual procedure during cardiopulmonary bypass (CPB), and the postbypass period. Each of these periods should be reviewed when the report is given in the pediatric intensive care unit (PICU) postoperatively.

Presurgical and Anesthetic Management

Choice of Induction Agents

Anesthesia for congenital heart repair may be induced safely by a variety of methods, including intravenous agents such as ketamine or thiopental, intramuscular injections such as ketamine, or inhalation agents, depending on the child's disease and underlying physical condition. The common goal that can be achieved with each of these anesthetics is avoiding increases in inotropy or decreased systemic vascular resistance (SVR), either of which might exaggerate right-to-left intracardiac shunting.

Anesthesia is induced in infants with poor ventricular function by using agents that are more hemodynamically "neutral," such as fentanyl or sufentanil (Table 8.2).

Table 8.2
Comparative Hemodynamic Effects of Induction Doses of Anesthetic Agents

	Heart Rate	SVR	CO
Halothane (1 MAC[a])	↓	↓⇆	↓
Isoflurane (1 MAC[a])	↑	↓	↑
Ketamine	↑	↑	↑
Thiopental	↑	↓	↓
Fentanyl	↓	↓⇆	⇆
Midazolam	⇆	↓⇆	⇆
Sufentanil	↓	↓⇆	⇆
Propofol	⇆	↓	↓
Etomidate	⇆	⇆	⇆

[a] MAC is minimum alveolar concentration, a description of the amount of anesthetic necessary to prevent movement to a given stimulus in an unparalyzed patient. It is a method of comparing equivalent "doses" of inhalation agents when serum level measurements cannot be done or are inappropriate.

Maintaining Anesthesia

Anesthesia maintenance for the open heart procedure may be performed with a variety of agents. Intravenous narcotics, such as fentanyl and sufentanil in anesthetic rather than analgesic doses, are used most frequently because of their hemodynamic stability. In contrast to the potent inhalational anesthetics (e.g., isoflurane, halothane), these drugs have minimal effect on SVR or cardiac output and they lower elevated pulmonary vascular resistance (PVR). Because of the long half-life of narcotics, however, respirations may be blunted and awakening may be delayed for several hours postoperatively. Adjunctive agents such as midazolam, given to ensure amnesia, compound these effects on the respiratory and central nervous system (CNS) (Table 8.3).

Surgery

Knowledge of the actual surgical procedure is essential in formulating a plan for care in the postoperative period. Surgery may be palliative or curative. Surgical access may be through a thoracotomy or via median sternotomy. Repair may be done with or without CPB support.

Thoracotomy entails collapse of one lung during the operation. This approach—used for PDA ligation, placement of a Blalock-Taussig shunt, coarctation of the aorta repair, and pulmonary artery banding in some instances—may result in pulmonary problems caused by atelectasis postoperatively. Additionally, intrathoracic structures, such as the thoracic duct or phrenic nerve, may be injured. These injuries may manifest as management problems in the PICU with chylothorax or diaphragmatic paralysis several days postoperatively.

Table 8.3
Physiologic Factors that May Be Altered by Anesthetic Agents

Respiratory	Airway reactivity; bronchomotor tone
	Chemoreceptor response to PCO_2
	Hypoxic pulmonary vasoconstriction
	Ciliary function
Central nervous system	Intracranial pressure
	Cerebral blood flow
	Cerebral oxygen consumption
	Seizure threshold
	Cognitive function
Cardiovascular	Heart rate
	Cardiac output
	Systemic vascular resistance
	Pulmonary vascular resistance
	Baroreceptor response
	Coronary blood flow
	Arrhythmia threshold
Endocrine	Catecholamine release
	Growth hormone, insulin, steroid release
Immunologic	Immune response
Miscellaneous	Renal blood flow
	Hepatic blood flow
	Gastric motility

Cardiopulmonary Bypass

The Bypass Circuit

CPB has several essential components (Fig. 8.1). Conceptually, anticoagulated blood is allowed to drain passively from the systemic veins or right atrium via a large cannula into a reservoir. Following its "ventilation" in a mechanical oxygenator and CO_2 removal, the blood is filtered and actively pumped back into the systemic circulation via a cannula in the aorta. During bypass, while the heart is inactive, nutrients are supplied by either continuous perfusion from bypass through the coronary arteries or by a cardioplegia solution that relaxes the heart and decreases its metabolism. During bypass, venous return to the heart from the periphery is diverted by cannulae placed in the inferior and superior venae cavae or by a single cannula in the right atrium that is drained by gravity to the venous reservoir on the circuit. Blood is not actively pumped out of the body, and any impediment to venous return may lead to venous engorgement. This may result in inadvertent cerebral venous hypertension and cerebral edema if the superior vena cava (SVC) cannula is obstructed or passive hepatic congestion if the inferior vena cava (IVC) cannula is obstructed. In addition to the venous

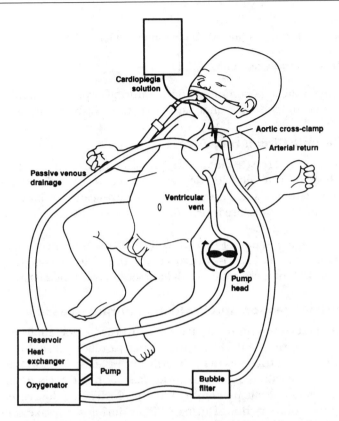

Figure 8.1. Cardiopulmonary bypass circuit schematic. Note positions of venous and arterial cannulae, aortic cross-clamp, and cardioplegia infusion site.

cannulae, blood return to the bypass machine also is delivered from a separate suction apparatus that scavenges blood from the operative field and a myocardial vent that empties the heart continuously.

Pump flow rates are generally adjusted to approximate normal cardiac output (e.g., 2 to 3 L/m^2/min) during normothermia. These can be reduced safely during hypothermia when metabolic requirements are decreased.

Monitoring

On-line continuous mixed venous saturation and periodic arterial blood gas determinations detect decreases in mixed venous saturation or development of metabolic acidosis, which may indicate inadequate perfusion and tissue oxygen delivery. Other parameters monitored episodically include:

- Hematocrit
- Serum electrolytes (including potassium and ionized calcium)
- Glucose
- Activated coagulation time (ACT)

Ionized hypocalcemia commonly occurs during bypass and may adversely affect cardiac function and alter cardiac rhythm postbypass if uncorrected.

Hypothermic Circulatory Arrest

Total circulatory arrest facilitates repair of complex lesions in the small heart. This field is totally bloodless and the venous cannulae that may obscure visualization of small intracardiac structures can be removed. Following repair, the cannulae are replaced, circulation on bypass is resumed, and the patient is warmed.

At a core temperature of 18 to 20°C, 50 to 60 minutes of circulatory arrest are tolerated with minimal risk of gross motor or intellectual defects. Approximately 5 to 10% of these patients will have seizures postoperatively, however.

Myocardial Function and Protection during Bypass

It is important to minimize the patient's myocardial metabolism and myocardial work during CPB. During the normal cardiac cycle, coronary blood flow to the left ventricle occurs primarily during diastole. Coronary perfusion pressure typically is defined as aortic diastolic blood pressure minus left ventricular end-diastolic pressure (LVEDP), which is the downstream pressure limiting coronary flow. During CPB, as during the awake state, coronary perfusion can be maximized by minimizing LVEDP.

A still, nonbeating heart is required for intracardiac repair and can be achieved by hypothermia, electrically induced ventricular fibrillation, or instillation of a cardioplegia solution into the coronary arteries to arrest the heart. All of these methods decrease myocardial oxygen consumption, particularly if the heart is empty. A left ventricular vent that ensures an empty heart is inserted to return venous blood from the heart back into the bypass circuit.

Cardioplegia Solution

The most essential components of cardioplegia solution are a high concentration of potassium and cold temperature, which will arrest the heart in diastole. Other components are lactated Ringer's solution, glucose, lidocaine, and mannitol. Steriods and β-blockers are sometimes added.

Systemic Effects

Aside from the damage caused by ongoing myocardial metabolism, additional myocardial injury can occur during bypass by several other mechanisms (Table 8.4). Although these effects generally are self-limited, subtle myocardial dysfunction requiring vasopressor support after bypass may occur, particularly with longer aortic cross-clamp times (Table 8.5).

INTENSIVE CARE UNIT COURSE AFTER BYPASS

Many of the physiologic derangements that begin during CPB continue to manifest during the initial period in the PICU.

Table 8.4
Systemic Effects of Cardiopulmonary Bypass

	Clinical Effect	Management Options
Neurologic	Cerebral and spinal cord infarcts	
	Hemorrhage	
	Choreoathetosis	
	Neuropsychiatric syndromes	
	Emboli (both air and debris)	Add CO_2 to oxygenator to maintain pH and correct blood gas temperatures
	Lower cerebral blood flow from hypothermia and mechanical obstruction	
	Lower $CMRO_2$	
	Intact autoregulation	
	Basal ganglia abnormalities	
Cardiac	Ischemia—coronary occlusion	
	Emboli	
	Direct coronary injury	
Pulmonary	Vascular exclusion during bypass	
	Complement-induced endothelial damage	
	Hemorrhage	
	Atelectasis	
	Decreased lung compliance	
Renal	Nonpulsatile perfusion	Osmotic (Mannitol) and loop (furosemide diuretics offset oliguria
	Elevated ADH levels	
	Increased renin production	
	Hematuria	
	Decreased urine production	
Gastrointestinal	Emboli	
Coagulation	Complement activation	
	Platelet consumption	
	Altered platelet aggregability	
	Coagulation factor dilution	
Endocrine	Elevated growth hormone, insulin	Increased anesthesia and profound analgesia improve outcome
	Elevated glucose	

$CMRO_2$, cerebral metabolic rate for oxygen; ADH, antidiuretic hormone.

Table 8.5
Frequently Used Cardiovascular Medications

Agent	Dosage Range (μg/kg/min)	Effects
Dopamine	1–3	Renal vasodilator
	5–10	Inotrope
	>10	$\alpha >> \beta$, ↑ PVR, ↑ SVR
		β_1-Agonist; mild β_2-agonist
Dobutamine	1–20	Inotrope, chronotrope
		Vasodilator, ↓ PVR, ↓ SVR
		Arrhythmogenic
		Weak α-effect
Isoproterenol	0.05–1	β-Agonist (nonselective)
		Inotrope, chronotrope
		Vasodilator, ↓ PVR, ↓ SVR
		Arrhythmogenic
Epinephrine	0.05–0.3	Potent β-agonist, inotrope, chronotrope
	0.3–2	$\alpha > \beta$ effect, ↑ SVR
Norepinephrine	0.05–1.0	α-Agonist, some β-effect at low doses
		Vasoconstriction
Amrinone	5–10	Loading dose: 0.75–4 mg/kg administered slowly, $t_{1/2}$ 4 h
		Vasodilator, ↓ PVR, ↓ SVR
		Inotrope (not chronotrope)
		Thrombocytopenia
Sodium nitroprusside	0.05–10	Arterial > venous vasodilator
		↑ ICP, may ↑ hypoxia by blunting HPV response, cyanide toxicity, tachyphylaxis
Nitroglycerin	1–20	Venous > arterial vasodilator ↓ preload, ↑ ICP
Esmolol	50–300	β_1-Antagonist—short $t_{1/2}$ 8 min—may load with 500 μg/kg
		Negative inotrope and chronotrope potentially useful for tachycardia, tachyarrhythmias, and infundibular spasm; causes bronchospasm
Labetalol	100–1000	β- > α-antagonist, vasodilator, negative inotrope, $t_{1/2}$ 5 h

PVR, pulmonary vascular resistance; SVR, systemic vascular resistance; ICP, intracranial pressure; HPV, hypoxic pulmonary vasoconstriction.

Hypothermia

Despite warming on bypass and subsequent passive warming measures, the child typically will display some degree of hypothermia on admission to the PICU. As warming progresses in the unit, the child's peripheral capillary beds continue to dilate, necessitating volume infusion to maintain cardiac filling pressures and volume. This can be partially offset by the use of systemic vasodilators such as nitroprusside during rewarming on bypass and while in the operating room.

Bleeding

Although the effects of heparin are reversed by protamine at the end of the bypass procedure, clinical bleeding may continue. Platelets are destroyed or rendered dysfunctional by CPB and sequestered in the oxygenator. Plasma coagulation factors may be diluted in the bypass prime or during blood loss after bypass and may require replacement. Despite initial neutralization, residual rebound heparin effect may be seen several minutes to hours after bypass, as measured by an elevated ACT. Additional protamine may be needed in this case. Samples for coagulation studies should be drawn immediately on admission and replacement given if clinically indicated.

INITIAL ASSESSMENT IN THE PICU

Immediately after surgery, a system to transfer the patient smoothly from the surgery-anesthesia team to the critical care team in the PICU should be in place (Table 8.6). Fundamental to this transfer of care is the maintenance

Table 8.6
Information Required on Transfer to PICU Team

Surgery	Type of lesion
	Procedure—correction, palliation, shunts, (takedowns?)
	Postrepair anatomy
	Cardiopulmonary bypass time
	Aortic cross-clamp time
History	Previous medical illnesses
	Medications
	Allergies
	Previous cardiac surgery
Anesthesia	Intraoperative problems—surgical, anesthetic, bypass
	Respiratory parameters
	Airway (easy?, ETT size, taped, leak?)
	Ventilator settings
	Anesthetic agents—reversal, dosage, last medications administered
	Cardiac rate and rhythm
	Intravascular lines
	Filling pressures (optimal)
	Transport problems—bleeding
	Any vasoactive agents
	Most recent monitoring of vital signs—HR, BP, temperature, urine output
	Most recent laboratory data
	Hematocrit
	K^+
	Arterial blood gases
	Temperature

PICU, pediatric intensive care unit; ETT, endotracheal tube; HR, heart rate; BP, blood pressure.

and continued monitoring of vital signs, including the electrocardiogram, blood pressure, ventilation, and oxygenation.

Particular attention should be paid to CPB time, aortic cross-clamp time, and surgical and anesthetic complications.

Clinical Evaluation

A rapid assessment of the child is made at the time of admission to PICU after CPB. In addition to the physical examination (Table 8.7) and laboratory studies (Table 8.8), chest radiography is performed to determine:

- Position of the tip of the endotracheal tube
- Location of central vascular catheters
- Position of mediastinal and chest tubes
- Heart size
- Condition of the lung fields, including the presence of atelectasis, pneumothorax, or hemothorax
- Status of pulmonary vascular markings

Table 8.7
Initial Assessment—Physical Examination

Respiratory	Breath sounds
	ETT size, taped? if no cuff, leak?
	Chest excursion
Cardiovascular	Heart rate
	Blood pressure—waveform
	Correlate with noninvasive BP
	If there is coarctation, residual upper/lower extremity gradient
	Heart sounds, murmurs, shunt flow
	Cardiac output
	Capillary refill
	Temperature of distal extremities
	Peripheral perfusion (color)
	Precordial activity
	Pulse volume
	Waveform (dicrotic notch)
	Filling pressure—RA, LA
	Rhythm—electrocardiogram
	Paced?
	Pacemaker settings
Skin	Turgor, cyanosis
CNS	Level of wakefulness
	Pupils (atropine/scopolamine given?)
	Motor, sensory (postoperative palsies), DTRs, bulbar reflexes
General	Vascular line position
Abdomen	Distended or flat
	Liver, spleen size

ETT, endotracheal tube; BP, blood pressure; RA, right atrial; LA, left atrial; CRS, central nervous system; DTRs, deep tendon reflexes.

Table 8.8
Initial Laboratory Studies

CBC	Platelets
	Hematocrit
Electrolytes	Na$^+$ ↑↓
	K$^+$ ↓ (↑)
	Ca$^+$
	Acidosis
Arterial blood gas	PO$_2$, PCO$_2$, pH
Coagulation	PT, PTT, platelets
Liver function tests	SGOT, SGPT, bilirubin
Chest radiograph	Position of ETT, chest tubes, vascular lines
	Heart size
	Lung parenchyma, congestion, atelectasis
	Pulmonary vascular markings
	Pneumothorax or hemothorax
	Pericardial effusion

CBC, complete blood count; ETT, endotracheal tube; PT, prothrombin time; PTT, partial thromboplastin time; SGOT, serum glutamic oxaloacetic transaminase; SGPT, serum glutamic pyruvic transaminase.

Postoperative Monitoring

Thorough attention to and continuous surveillance of the monitoring data is necessary to direct further therapies for the postoperative cardiac patient (Table 8.9).

PRINCIPLES OF POSTOPERATIVE MANAGEMENT
Hemodynamic Management

If cardiac output is adequate, blood pressure will be in the normal range, although normal blood pressure does not preclude decreased cardiac output. Urine output should equal or exceed 0.5 mL/kg/hr. Warm peripheral extremities and brisk capillary refill are good indicators of adequate cardiac output; however, disorientation or agitation may indicate hypoxia, hypercarbia, or inadequate perfusion.

Cardiac output depends on heart rate and stroke volume. Stroke volume, in turn, depends on adequate preload, minimizing afterload, contractility, adequate heart rate, and an optimal rhythm.

Heart Rate and Rhythm

Bradycardia in infants and children can severely compromise cardiac output. Tachycardia, although generally better tolerated in children than in adults, limits ventricular filling time, thereby decreasing stroke volume. Arrhythmias may disrupt appropriate coordination of atrial and ventricular

Table 8.9
Postoperative Monitoring after Cardiac Surgery

Noninvasive	Method	Information Gained
Electrocardiogram (12 leads)	Leads II and V_5	Ischemia
		Arrhythmias (VT, asystole)
	Atrial pacing wire	Differentiate VT and SVT
Temperature	Core: rectal PA catheter, esophageal, tympanic membrane	Cardiac output (secondary difference between core and peripheral denotes severe compromise)
	Peripheral: skin, great toe	
		Hyperthermia and hypothermia (O_2 consumption, SVR); hypothermia also heralds infection or malignant hyperthermia
BP	Manual, automated systems	Hypotension or hypertension measurement in all extremities estimates postrepair residual pressure gradient
O_2	Pulse oximeter	O_2 saturation (cardiac output, intracardiac, or intrapulmonary shunting)
		Perfusion of limb
Urine[a]	Foley, diaper weighing	Renal perfusion
		Cardiac output
End-tidal CO_2	Mainstream or sidestream	PCO_2 correlates with respiratory dead space
Invasive		
Arterial line	BP, blood sampling	
CVP (RA line)	Right atrial pressure	Elevations in patients with pulmonary BP may indicate PA pressure or RV function
	Fluid infusion	
	Monitor tracing (a and v waves)	
PA line	Pulmonary pressure	
	Cardiac output	
	Derived SVR, PVR	
	Mixed venous blood gas O_2 consumption, O_2 extraction	
	Core temperature	
LA line	Left atrial filling pressure	
	LA/RA pressure difference (differentiate pulmonary hypertension)	
Chest tubes	Blood drainage—mediastinum, pleural space	
	Blood loss > 20 mL/kg warrants return to OR; remove mediastinal tubes after transthoracic intracardiac catheters	
	15–20 cm H_2O suction pressure	

continued

Table 8.9
Postoperative Monitoring after Cardiac Surgery

	Method	Information Gained
Pacing wires	Atrial or skin ground wire connected to positive pole; ventricular wire to negative pole. Sensitivity is adjusted to ventricular demand pacing output to minimum setting. Capture rate is 20–30 bpm above intrinsic rate.	Diagnosis of atrial arrhythmias Ability to pace atria, ventricles

[a]Diuretics used at end of CPB may invalidate measurements during first few postoperative hours.

VT, ventricular tachycardia; SVT, supraventricular tachycardia; PA, pulmonary artery; SVR, systemic vascular resistance; BP, blood pressure; CVP, superior vena caval central line; PVR, pulmonary vascular resistance; LA/RA, left atrial to right atrial.

contraction. Lack of atrial-ventricular coordination decreases ventricular filling and thus cardiac output. Initial management of any arrhythmia begins with optimization of arterial blood gases, pH, and serum electrolytes. Ventricular tachycardia in the postoperative period must be treated immediately with lidocaine (1 mg/kg). If this is not successful, cardioversion should be attempted. Ventricular fibrillation should be treated with immediate cardiopulmonary resuscitation and electrocardioversion. Specific arrhythmias encountered most commonly in postoperative cardiac patients are discussed below (Table 8.10).

Bradycardia

In patients undergoing hypothermic arrest, the degree of bradycardia is proportional to the degree of hypothermia. Bradycardia occurs frequently following extensive atrial surgery, the atrial switch procedure, and repair of total anomalous pulmonary venous return. Injury to the sinus node may result from incision of the node, placement of suture through the node, or interruption of the blood supply to the sinoatrial (SA) node by surgical trauma.

If the cardiac rate is slow enough to compromise cardiac output, atropine or isoproterenol may increase the conduction rate of sinus or junctional rhythms. If medical therapy fails, then temporary or permanent pacing may be necessary. As edema around the conduction system resolves three to four days after surgery, normal sinus rhythm generally returns.

Tachycardia

Postoperative tachycardia may be due to pain, agitation, or hypovolemia and will respond to specific treatment. Tachycardia caused by conduction disturbances is usually a consequence of junctional tachycardia.

Table 8.10
Common Postoperative Arrhythmias

Anatomy	Arrhythmia	Lesion
SA node	Bradycardia	Senning or Mustard procedure (TGV)
	Sick sinus syndrome	Tetralogy of Fallot
	Sinus asystole	ASD
	Paroxysmal atrial tachycardia	AV canal
Intranodal pathway	Atrial flutter	Mustard procedure (TVG)
	SVT	TAPVR
	Junctional bradycardia	
Junctional injury	Junctional tachycardia	Mustard procedure (TGV)
AV node		Endocardial cushion defect
Bundle of His	AV block (1°, 2°, 3°)	Membranous VSD
Intraventricular conduction	RBBB	Tetralogy of Fallot
pathways	RBBB with LAH	AV canal
	Trifascicular block	Ostium primum ASD
		VSD
		Membranous VSD, associated with complex CHD
		Resection of pulmonary infundibulum
Ventricle	PVCs	Tetralogy of Fallot
	Ventricular tachycardia	Right ventriculotomy, especially with ventricular dilation or hypertension

ASD, atrial septal defect; SVT, supraventricular tachycardia; TGV, transposition of the great vessels; TAPVR, total anomalous pulmonary venous return; RBBB, right bundle branch block; LAH, left anterior hemiblock; CHD, congenital heart disease; PVC, premature ventricular contraction.

Junctional Tachycardia The electrocardiogram (ECG) shows narrow QRS complexes and the absence of P waves. The heart rate is usually 120 to 280 beats/minute. The loss of atrial contractility and rapid ventricular response rate impair ventricular filling. If hemodynamic instability exists, cardioversion should be attempted. If atrial pacing wires are present, atrial contraction can be induced or overdrive pacing can be performed. Junctional tachycardia does not respond to vagal maneuvers. Digitalization or β-blockade may reduce excessive conduction rate or induce aterio-venous (A-V) block, thereby slowing the ventricular rate.

Junctional Ectopic Tachycardia (JET) This life-threatening arrhythmia is defined as a heart rate above 200 and a narrow QRS complex with or without P waves. If P waves are present, there is invariably A-V dissociation. Treatment of this rhythm must be instituted early and includes conservative management, such as avoiding vagolytic compounds, aggressive sedation, avoiding sympathomimetics, and digitalization. Recent clinical reports suggest that propafenone, a type 1C antiarrhythmic with β-antagonist properties, can significantly lower heart rate in patients with JET. JET itself subsides spontaneously 48 to 72 hours after surgery. Occasionally, inducing hypothermia in the patient is required to resolve the arrhythmia.

Cardiac Pacing

Atrial wires may be used for either atrial pacing with an intact conduction system with a slow rate or for A-V sequential pacing when the conduction system is disrupted to augment ventricular filling. Ventricular wires can be used for A-V sequential pacing or ventricular pacing alone. Should the epicardial pacing system malfunction, transesophageal pacing may be useful. A pacing catheter is passed through the esophagus to the atrial level, which is detected by the appearance of P waves. Ventricular contraction requires an intact intracardiac conduction system. Transesophageal pacing is particularly useful for application of overdrive pacing to supraventricular tachycardia.

Stroke Volume

Preload With the decrease in the peripheral vascular resistance associated with rewarming, the right atrial pressure decreases. This initial fall in cardiac output may be compensated by an increased heart rate, but as preload falls further, peripheral perfusion eventually will be limited. Procedures involving a ventriculotomy, prolonged cardioplegia, CPB, and those with residual outflow tract obstruction require higher right atrial filling pressures.

Contractility Myocardial contractility is impaired after open-heart surgery because of ischemia, hypoxia, inflammation, and ventriculotomy. The following agents may prove beneficial:

- Dopamine at low doses, although its α-agonist effects may be detrimental
- Dobutamine improves contractility
- Isoproterenol, in addition to its inotropic effect, provides chronotropy, which is particularly useful following repair of total anomalous pulmonary venous return and in the denervated heart posttransplant.
- Epinephrine, with its α- and β-adrenergic effects, may be needed when diastolic blood pressure is so low that coronary perfusion is impaired
- Amrinone, a phosphodiesterase III inhibitor, is a potent inotropic agent as well as a peripheral vasodilator without a chronotropic effect

Afterload Elimination of physiologic factors that increase SVR, such as acidosis, hypoxia, pain, and hypothermia, should be the first step in lowering afterload.

Pharmacologic afterload can also be instituted with:

- Smooth muscle relaxants such as nitroprusside, nitroglycerin, hydralazine, and diazoxide

- α-blockers such as phentolamine, prazosin, and chlorpromazine
- The ganglionic-blocking agent trimethaphan

Aortic balloon counterpulsation, which increases coronary artery perfusion pressure and decreases afterload, has been used in older patients who have a failing circulatory system.

Cardiac Tamponade

Cardiac tamponade should always be suspected when a patient's initially benign postoperative course deteriorates, especially in the setting of diminished chest tube drainage. Clinical signs include:

- Narrowed pulse pressure or pulsus paradoxus on the arterial pressure tracing
- Rising right atrial pressure with jugular venous distention
- Decreased blood pressure
- Tachycardia
- Poor peripheral perfusion

Treatment The treatment for cardiac tamponade is prompt volume infusion to maintain cardiac output. The operating room and cardiac surgeon should be immediately notified of an impending return to the operating room for thoracotomy. Needle aspiration of the pericardial cavity is dangerous, often ineffective, and time-consuming when the chest can be readily opened.

Atypical Tamponade A clinical syndrome of poor cardiac function without evidence of tamponade has been described in infants and children. The pathophysiology of this syndrome appears to be an alteration in compliance of the left ventricle as a result of edema of the myocardium and surrounding structures. Hemodynamic improvement is observed when the sternum is opened. The sternum can be closed electively 24 to 72 hours later when hemodynamics has improved.

Postpericardiotomy Syndrome (PPS)

Late cardiac tamponade occurring more than seven days postoperatively is a recognized complication and may occur as a result of PPS (Table 8.11).

Chylothorax

Chylothorax most frequently follows corrective or palliative extrapericardial procedures, including repair of coarctation of the aorta, the Blalock-Taussig or Waterston shunts, Potts' anastomosis, the Glenn procedure, and ligation of a PDA. Postoperative chylothorax results from injury to the thoracic duct or its intrathoracic tributaries.

Table 8.11
Clinical Features of Postpericardiotomy Syndrome

Symptoms
    Persistent fever, spiking to 40°C
    Precordial chest pain
    Irritability
    Decreased appetite
    Left shoulder pain
Physical Examination Findings
    Pericardial friction rub
    Pleural friction rub
    Fever
Imaging and Laboratory Test Results
    Enlarged heart
    Electrocardiogram changes
    Elevation of ST segments
    Nonspecific T wave changes
    Low amplitude (with large effusions)
    Echocardiography—pericardial effusion
    Antiheart antibody present in high titer (confirmatory test)
Treatment
    Steroids
    Aspirin

Diagnosis Symptoms and signs include:

- Pleural effusions
- Dyspnea
- Pleural friction rub
- Shoulder pain
- Fever

Effusions usually develop in the first few days postoperatively but may develop as late as 1 month after surgery. The pleural fluid appears milky and does not clot after feedings have been instituted.

Complications Complications secondary to chylothorax include respiratory compromise and malnutrition, the latter caused by the loss of chyle, which is rich in proteins, lipids, and lymphocytes. Lymphocytes, present in the thoracic lymph in large numbers, may be severely depleted with chylothorax.

Therapy Medical management of chylothorax includes prolonged hospitalization with strict monitoring and control of nutritional intake. Pleural drainage prevents atelectasis and ventilatory insufficiency. A high-protein, high-carbohydrate, medium-chain triglyceride diet with reduced fat content decreases lymph flow. Indications for surgery include an average daily chyle loss exceeding 1500 mL in adults or 100 mL/year of age in children after a

5-day period of medical management, a flow of chyle that is not diminished after 2 weeks of medical management, or severe nutritional complications.

Chylopericardium

This condition usually is associated with intrapericardial surgery after coronary bypass surgery, aortic or pulmonary valvular surgery, or ventricular septal defect (VSD) repair. Symptoms may be associated with those of coincident chylothorax or with cardiac tamponade. A single percutaneous pericardial aspiration may be sufficient treatment. If the pericardial effusion recurs, however, partial pericardiotomy with or without ligation of the thoracic duct may be warranted.

Oxygen Consumption after Cardiac Surgery

The oxygen consumption of children after cardiac surgery may be increased by shivering secondary to hypothermia, increased respiratory and circulatory system activity, muscle activity, and endogenous secretion of catecholamines. To increase the oxygen supply:demand ratio, every effort should be made to decrease oxygen consumption while improving the level of oxygen delivery.

- Muscle relaxants may decrease oxygen consumption in some patients by abolishing voluntary and involuntary muscle activity. In infants, however, because shivering does not usually occur, muscle relaxation would not be expected to decrease oxygen consumption.
- Sedatives or analgesics may be used to decrease oxygen consumption by decreasing endogenous catecholamine secretion.

Respiratory Support

Respiratory Function

The lungs may be traumatized intraoperatively, and prolonged atelectasis may result in some postoperative improvement. In addition, the thoracic incision and accompanying chest tubes cause postoperative pain and splinting of the chest wall in spontaneously breathing patients, with a resultant decrease in deep breathing, coughing, and chest wall compliance. Anesthetic agents and muscle relaxants also depress cough reflexes, interfere with mucociliary action, and lead to diminished clearance of secretions.

Complications

Postoperatively, complications children may demonstrate:

- Upper airway complications, such as stridor (subglottic tracheal mucosal swelling, vocal cord paralysis)
- Problems with the endotracheal tube (mucus plugging, kinking of the tube)

- Diaphragmatic paralysis, which can be diagnosed by observation of paradoxical motion of a hemidiaphragm under fluoroscopy when positive pressure is not being applied during spontaneous breathing
- Increased atrial pressure or ventricular failure affects lung compliance, resulting in increased intravascular hydrostatic pressure
- Pulmonary capillary endothelial damage, leading to pulmonary edema and increased lung water, may result from prolonged CPB and subsequent low cardiac output

This syndrome, termed "pump lung," may be caused by blood transfusion, direct trauma, endotoxin injury, complement activation, or foreign protein from the oxygenator.

Care and Management

When uncuffed endotracheal tubes are used, a leak between 15 and 30 cm H_2O is recommended. When a cuffed tube is used, the cuff is inflated until the leak just disappears.

Warming and humidification of inspired gases will avoid heat loss and thickening of secretions. The temperature of these gases should be kept below 40°C.

For the most part, in the absence of pulmonary hypertension, maintenance of normal pH, PCO_2, and PO_2 is the goal of respiratory support. In patients with pulmonary hypertension or in those in whom it may be expected (e.g., preoperative VSD with a large left-to-right shunt), respiratory support is altered so that PO_2 is weaned in small increments and the patient is hyperventilated (Table 8.12).

Table 8.12
Managing Increased Pulmonary Vascular Resistance

Sedation and Analgesia
    Fentanyl: begin 1–2 μmg/kg/h infusion
    Midazolam: begin 0.05 mg/kg/h infusion
Muscle relaxation
    Pancuronium: 0.1 mg/kg bolus every 60–90 min
    Vecuronium: 0.1 mg/kg/h infusion
Hyperventilation (torr)
    PCO_2 25–30, alkalotic pH
Oxygenation
    Small increments in weaning FiO_2
    Maintain PaO_2 > 100 torr
Drugs
    β-Agonists: dobutamine, isoproterenol, low-dose epinephrine
    Direct vasodilators: PGE_1, nitroglycerin, tolazoline, nifedipine, nitric oxide gas
    Phosphodiesterase inhibitors: amrinone

The use of continuous positive airway pressure (CPAP) or positive end-expiratory pressure (PEEP) improves oxygenation by increasing functional residual capacity and decreasing atelectasis and small airway closure (see Chapter 4). Weaning the patient from mechanical support is described in Chapter 2.

Postextubation stridor occurs in about 25% of PICU patients and usually responds well to racemic epinephrine by nebulization. Supplemental oxygen is gradually withdrawn by findings of physical examination, pulse oximetry, and arterial blood gas determinations.

Prolonged endotracheal or nasotracheal intubation is a relatively safe alternative to tracheostomy in infants and children. Tracheostomy is now performed in most institutions when respiratory support is anticipated for more than 30 days or when a congenital or acquired airway lesion is documented.

Fluids, Electrolytes, and Renal Function

Fluids

Optimal intracardiac pressures are determined by clinical observation of heart rate, blood pressure, perfusion, and urine output as fluid boluses are being administered. The optimal filling pressure will vary over time and depends on myocardial function.

Patients who have undergone CPB are total body fluid overloaded, although commonly depleted intravascularly. Although acute volume expansion is often required, open-heart surgery patients should have their continuous infusion rates adjusted to provide only one-half to two-thirds of normal maintenance. In contrast, patients who have not undergone CPB (e.g., following shunting procedures or repair of moderate coarctation of the aorta) can receive maintenance fluid or have their fluids adjusted according to their volume status. Many patients have increased volume requirement as they warm and their vascular space expands with dilation. In addition, postoperative fever will increase insensible losses by 10% for each 1°C increase in body temperature.

Electrolytes

Because the CPB circuit is primed with normal saline or lactated Ringer's solution, most patients are sodium and water overloaded. During the first 24 to 48 hours postoperatively, hyponatremia reflects excess free water.

If the patient demonstrates adequate urine output, maintenance potassium is initiated on admission to the PICU to avoid hypokalemia. A decrease in total body potassium with a negative potassium balance after cardiac or other types of surgical procedures is common. Striking increases in potassium excretion or an intracellular shift of potassium during the first 2 days after major vascular procedures is common.

Hyperkalemia usually occurs as a consequence of decreased cardiac output, poor perfusion, and altered renal function. The treatment for severe, acute hyperkalemia or when life-threatening arrhythmias coexist is infusion of a 10% calcium chloride solution (0.2 to 0.5 mL/kg over 2 to 5 minutes), sodium bicarbonate (2 mEq/kg), and glucose (0.5 g/kg) and insulin (0.3 units/g glucose) administered over 2 hours.

Ionized calcium levels and total protein are diluted by pump-priming solutions. Citrate, as an anticoagulant in transfused blood, binds some available calcium. Calcium is also excreted in urine in response to diuretic therapy. The use of albumin to expand intravascular volume decreases the proportion of ionized calcium available for cellular interaction by binding calcium. Hypomagnesemia, which has been reported after cardiac surgery, can contribute to both hypocalcemia and hypokalemia and may lead to ventricular arrhythmias, especially torsade de pointes.

Regardless of the serum level of calcium, rapid infusion of calcium increases blood pressure. Rapid boluses can induce bradycardia and hypotension. For symptomatic patients with tetany, seizures, or ECG changes, a 10% calcium chloride solution of 0.1 to 0.2 mL/kg is administered, preferably via a central catheter to avoid the potential for tissue necrosis from inadvertent extravasation. Maintenance calcium requirements can be met by parenteral administration of calcium gluconate at 100 mg/kg/day or by enteral administration of calcium-containing compounds.

Hypophosphatemia has been observed in 50% of patients after surgery. Clinically, hypophosphatemia can lead to impaired oxygen delivery, myocardial depression, and respiratory insufficiency. Phosphate can be replaced by using sodium phosphate (5 to 10 mg/kg/dose over 6 hours) or by substituting potassium phosphate for potassium chloride.

Glucose Hyperglycemia and hypoinsulinemia during cardiac surgery are associated with hypothermia. High levels of hyperglycemia may result in an osmotic diuresis, increased free water loss, and intravascular dehydration. If severe hyperglycemia results in a large amount of glucose in the urine, regular insulin should be administered by intravenous infusion. Hypoglycemic coma has also been observed after cardiac surgery. Monitoring of blood glucose is part of routine postoperative care.

Renal Function

Factors that Affect Function Various anomalies of the genitourinary tract associated with congenital heart disease affect renal function. Congestive heart failure leads to decreased renal blood flow. The kidneys may be affected by chronic hypoxia, with malnutrition and growth retardation. Patients with cyanotic lesions may be polycythemic, affecting renal function by the presence of vascular thromboses and parenchymal infarcts.

Renal Failure The incidence of renal failure after cardiac surgery in adults is reportedly 1 to 30%, with an incidence of 8% in one study of infants and children. The causes, diagnosis, and treatment of postoperative acute renal failure are discussed in Chapter 24.

Hematologic Management

Hemolysis

Hemolysis most commonly manifests during bypass and immediately afterward as hematuria. Hemolytic transfusion or drug reactions are distinctly uncommon but need to be considered if hemolysis persists or there are other clinical suspicions. Ensuring adequate urine output by the use of loop or osmotic diuretics is generally the only therapy needed. Most frequently, hematuria has cleared by the time the child is admitted to the PICU.

Hematocrit levels do not signify blood volume but aid in deciding on the type of fluid replacement. The hematocrit is maintained at 35% in children and above 40% in infants. Patients who are cyanotic after a palliative procedure may remain polycythemic. In addition, following simple procedures, the hematocrit may be maintained at lower levels to avoid transfusion.

Platelet Abnormalities

Children have a high incidence of intraoperative and postoperative bleeding as the result of qualitative and quantitative platelet abnormalities. Qualitative disorders include impaired platelet adhesion and abnormalities of platelet release.

Other patients with cyanotic congenital heart disease have prolonged prothrombin time (PT0 and partial thromboplastin time (PTT), elevated fibrin degradation products, decreased fibrinogen, decreased clotting factors V, VII, VIII, and IX, and evidence of fibrinolysis. Low-grade disseminated intravascular coagulopathy (DIC) has been observed in cyanotic patients preoperatively, leading to bleeding complications in the postoperative period.

Factors Affecting Hemostasis

Aspirin and other nonsteroidal antiinflammatory agents that inhibit prostaglandin synthesis can dramatically alter perioperative hemostasis. Platelets are irreversibly deactivated for their life, lasting 10 to 14 days.

During cardiac surgery with bypass, heparin in a dose of 300 units/kg is given to prevent clotting in the bypass circuit and in the patient. Heparin prevents clotting by accelerating the formation of antithrombin III, which blocks the conversion of fibrinogen to fibrin and the conversion of prothrombin to thrombin by inhibiting thrombin and activated factor X activity. Coagulation cascade factors inhibited by heparin are factors XI, IXa, Xa, IIa, and thrombin.

Protamine binds with heparin to reverse its antithrombin III anticoagulant activity but not the effect on platelet aggregability. Side effects following protamine administration are common and include hypotension and complement activation. "Heparin rebound" has been described from several minutes to hours later, characterized by an increased ACT and clinical bleeding resulting from heparin release from body tissue.

Evaluation Before Transfusion

In the patient with postoperative bleeding, platelet count, PT, and PTT should be obtained on admission to the PICU. The ACT should be checked after protamine administration and additional protamine should be given if necessary.

Administration of platelets and fresh frozen plasma or cryoprecipitate should not be deferred until laboratory results are available in the patient with rapid diffuse oozing and no discernible bleeding site in the operating room. Component transfusion is reserved for the patient who is stable with continued oozing and laboratory evidence of coagulopathy. Platelet deficiency is probably the most common cause of continued oozing after surgery with major blood loss in children.

Neurologic Complications

Muscle Weakness

In the patient who remains flaccid or weak, the prolonged effects from muscle relaxants should be considered. Serial examinations can be performed for rapidly assessing gross abnormalities such as hemiparesis, cranial nerve abnormalities, peripheral neuropathy, or the presence of seizures.

Metabolic Derangements

All intravenous lines should be meticulously cleared of air bubbles to avoid air embolism across a right-to-left intracardiac shunt. Acid-base imbalance, electrolyte disorders, and other conditions that cause neurologic sequelae should be avoided by closely monitoring blood gases and serum electrolytes. Glucose determinations should also be monitored frequently, especially when acute hepatic failure ensues after cardiac surgery. Episodes of hypoxia and hypotension that affect all organ systems will, of course, also have a detrimental effect on the CNS.

Seizures

Anticonvulsant therapy for seizures or treatment of any metabolic derangement that causes seizures should be administered rapidly. Airway and ventilatory support with continued intubation may be necessary because of the seizures themselves or obtundation of the patient from anticonvulsant medications.

Peripheral Neuropathies

Postoperative peripheral neuropathies include:

- Diaphragmatic paralysis secondary to phrenic nerve laceration or trauma (see Chapter 5)
- Paraplegia secondary to spinal cord ischemia during coarctation repair
- Vocal cord paralysis secondary to recurrent laryngeal nerve trauma after ligation of a PDA or shunting procedure
- Brachial plexus injury, usually involving the medial cord of the plexus, is related to traction of the plexus by adverse positioning of the patient in the operating room during median sternotomy
- Ulnar nerve palsy

Gastrointestinal Complications

Initial Assessment

This evaluation includes the presence or absence of bowel sounds and measurement of abdominal girth. The liver and spleen should be percussed for position and span, specifically to assess the degree of right ventricular failure.

Postcoarctectomy Syndrome

This condition usually presents as abdominal pain, vomiting, and ileus 1 to 5 days postoperatively. Prolonged restriction of oral feedings and treatment of hypertension with antihypertensive medications is the treatment of choice.

Necrotizing Enterocolitis (NEC)

NEC caused by a local ischemic phenomenon may manifest with:

- Abdominal distention in the first 24 hours after surgery
- Peritoneal signs
- Ileus
- Bloody or guaiac-positive stools
- Radiographic evidence of bowel distention, pneumatosis intestinalis, and air in the hepatic portal system

Management includes:

- Discontinuing oral feedings
- Implementing nasogastric drainage
- Administering systemic antibiotics
- Monitoring for signs of infarction or perforation
- Delivering large-volume infusions as large amounts of fluid extravasate into the peritoneal cavity

Jaundice

Manifestations of jaundice in the early postoperative period (2 to 9% of patients with congenital heart disease) include:

- Increased bilirubin level peaking between the second and the 10th postoperative day
- Elevated alkaline phosphatase level, peaking after the seventh postoperative day
- Normal or slightly raised serum glutamic pyruvate transaminase level

Hepatic Failure

Children at particular risk for hepatic failure include those in whom a modified Fontan procedure was performed or those in whom elevated right atrial pressure was required to maintain pulmonary blood flow when high PVR coexisted (see Chapter 22). Care for these patients involves:

- Regular surveillance of bilirubin, serum transaminase levels, PT, and glucose levels
- Appropriate and timely treatment to correct a coagulopathy, hypoglycemia, or hyperammonemia
- Fluid restriction, with early institution of dialysis
- Maintain right atrial pressure at the lowest possible level to maintain cardiac output

Protein-Losing Enteropathy

This condition can occur secondary to obstruction of the superior or inferior vena caval conduit of the intraatrial baffle after the Mustard procedure.

Nutrition

After simple procedures such as a PDA ligation or simple atrial septal defect (ASD) or VSD closure, enteral feeding can begin as early as the first postoperative day. In more complicated operations, typically, mechanical ventilation is stopped and the patient's trachea is extubated before feeding is instituted around the third postoperative day. In the unstable patient or if enteral feeding cannot be started because of a primary gastrointestinal problem, parenteral feeding should be instituted as early as possible via a central venous line by the third postoperative day.

Infection

Fever

Low-grade fever in the first 48 hours postoperatively is common. Fever persisting after this time, however, should be worked up with appropriate cultures:

- Blood (multiple to rule out bacterial endocarditis)
- Urine
- Sputum
- From surgical wounds
- From intravenous catheters
- Cerebrospinal fluid, in the presence of signs and symptoms of a CNS disorder

Low-grade fever occurring 5 to 7 days after surgery may be due to PPS.

Infectious Processes

In children, most cases of mediastinitis are caused by staphylococci, but Gram-negative organisms and fungi have also been implicated. The incidence of mediastinitis after repair of congenital heart disease is 0.4 to 1%. The overall incidence of sternal infections may be increased when postoperative hemorrhage or the need for thoracic reexploration coexists. Other infectious diseases, such as hepatitis and cytomegalovirus (CMV) infection, are common following blood transfusions and should be investigated when fever presents in the postoperative period.

SPECIFIC SURGICAL PROCEDURES

Table 8.13 summarizes the types of corrective surgical interventions.

Palliative Shunt Operations

Palliative procedures correct the physiologic defects arising from cardiac anomalies without addressing the anatomic defects. These procedures are commonly used to maintain the infant until the child is large enough to un-

---

Table 8.13
Types of Surgical Corrections

Total correction—no residual abnormality
  VSD repair
  PDA repair
Total correction—mild residual abnormality
  Repair tetralogy of Fallot
Mild to moderate residual abnormality
  Mustard or Senning repair for TGA
  Aortic stenosis repair
Palliative procedures (final treatment) with persistent abnormalities
  Fontan procedure
Palliative procedure (staged treatment)
  Shunt placement
  Pulmonary artery banding

VSD, ventricular septal defect

dergo corrective surgery with greater success. Systemic-to-pulmonary artery shunts are used as palliative procedures when there is inadequate or ductal-dependent pulmonary blood flow. Critical pulmonic stenosis or pulmonary atresia and tricuspid atresia are the most common indications for shunting in the newborn period. The modified Blalock-Taussig shunt is the most common systemic-to-pulmonary artery shunt (Fig 8.2). Advances in corrective surgery have made shunt procedures beyond the newborn period uncommon (Table 8.14).

Balloon Atrial Septostomy

To lessen hypoxemia in transposition of the great vessels (TGV), an intra-atrial communication is created. In the cardiac catheterization laboratory by the Rashkind procedure, a balloon septostomy catheter is used to tear the atrial septum.

Complications are rare but include perforation of a heart chamber or A-V valve and damage to the pulmonic valve or inferior vena cava. Embolization of air or balloon fragments as a result of balloon rupture has also been reported. Balloon atrial septostomy is successful in 80 to 90% of children with TGA.

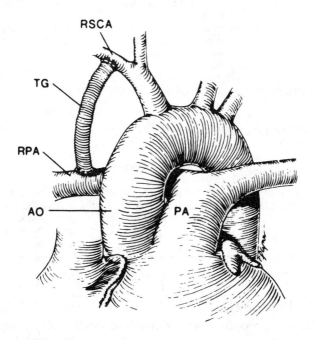

Figure 8.2. Modified Blalock-Taussig Shunt. RSCA, right subclavian artery; RPA, right pulmonary artery; AO, aorta; PA, pulmonary artery; and TG, tube graft. (From Ariniegas E, ed. Pediatric cardiac surgery. Chicago: Year Book Medical Publishers, 1985.)

Table 8.14
Shunts Procedures

Types of Shunt	Adverse Effects	Precautions/Therapy
Blalock-Taussig (subclavian artery to pulmonary artery)	Arm initially cold and pulseless, but flow improved over ensuing 48–72 h. Gangrene is rare. Ischemic changes may be reversible with reconstructive arterial surgery. Decreased muscle blood flow and arm development initially	Avoid taking blood pressure in arm on side of shunt. Monitor color and warmth of arm.
Modified Blalock-Taussig (synthetic shunt from subclavian artery to pulmonary artery	Early shunt thrombosis in neonates	Maintain adequate cardiac output and blood pressure postoperatively (dopamine)
	Leaking GORE-TEX shunts cause increased chest tube drainage and localized seroma formation around graft	Partial exchange transfusion or phlebotomy decreases hematocrit. Also use systemic anticoagulation.
	Transient unilateral increase in pulmonary blood flow and pulmonary edema in first 48 h	Maintain fluids and hydration
Waterston (ascending aorta to pulmonary artery)	Distortion/kinking of left pulmonary artery causes shift of flow to right pulmonary artery	
Potts (descending aorta to left pulmonary artery)	Inability to control size of communication orifice (tendency to grow) Distortion and aneurysm of pulmonary artery	
Glenn (superior vena cava to right pulmonary artery)	Decreased pulmonary artery pressure increases perfusion pressure	Avoid hypercarbia and hypoxia (pulmonary vasoconstrictors) as well as premature tracheal extubation

Blalock-Hanlon Operation

A Blalock-Hanlon procedure may be required should balloon septostomy fail to create an adequate communication. An interatrial septal defect is created by excising the posterior portion of the atrial septum in a closed-heart procedure.

Transient atrial arrhythmias have been described following this procedure, which are usually of no clinical significance. Children who do not have adequate mixing despite the creation of a large ASD require early corrective surgery.

Pulmonary Artery Banding

This procedure offers improved survival in the management of patients with various anatomic causes of increased pulmonary blood flow. Pulmonary artery banding is reserved for lesions deemed noncorrectable by other measures and in neonates with single ventricle or its variant to preserve low PVR and the feasibility of a future Fontan procedure.

Because of the acute increase in cardiac afterload induced by pulmonary artery banding, inotropes may be required postoperatively. This increased afterload may not be well tolerated by patients who have preexisting tricuspid or mitral insufficiency. In the PICU, because of congestive heart failure, fluids should initially be restricted to two-thirds of maintenance. However, aggressive use of diuretics may be required to control heart failure while providing adequate fluid to meet caloric requirements.

Initially, pulmonary artery banding does not usually restrict pulmonary blood flow enough to avoid pulmonary edema. As a result, weaning from mechanical ventilation may be difficult. Therefore, it is important to avoid maneuvers that lower PVR and maintain oxygen saturation in the mid-to-low 80% range. In contrast, patients who are banded too tightly are cyanotic postoperatively. Chest radiographs typically reveal a paucity of pulmonary blood flow. Reoperation may be necessary in this situation.

Atrial Septal Defect (Secundum)

Early repair of the secundum-type ASD is indicated in infants with significant left-to-right shunts (greater than 1.5:1). Primary closure by approximation and suture of the edges of the defect is sufficient for small defects. Larger defects are repaired with a pericardial or Teflon patch.

Preliminary efforts at transcatheter closure of ASDs using an umbrella device are promising. This nonsurgical approach would avoid the inherent risks of CPB and related postoperative morbidities.

Perioperative mortality for ASD repair approaches zero, and postoperative complications are uncommon. Postoperative arrhythmias include:

- Atrial flutter
- Atrial fibrillation
- Sinus tachycardia
- Paroxysmal atrial tachycardia
- Nodal rhythms

Arrhythmias that persist (i.e., 2%) are most likely due to surgical trauma to the sinus node or its arterial supply.

Simple ASD

Postoperative care following repair of a simple ASD with a short CPB period is relatively routine. Most patients can be extubated in the operating room or on arrival in the PICU. Extubation should be delayed, however, until patient rewarming is completed, the distal extremities are well perfused, and any metabolic acidosis has been corrected.

Large ASD

A large ASD with long-standing increased pulmonary blood flow can lead to pulmonary hypertension and ventricular dysfunction preoperatively that may persist in the postoperative period. In most young patients, however, right ventricular hypertrophy and dilation resolve 6 months to 1 year after operation.

Endocardial Cushion Defect

Successful repair of complete AV canal (Fig. 8.3) depends on the presence of a low PVR. Surgical repair is usually attempted at 1 year of age but has been performed earlier with low postoperative mortality and excellent long-term results.

Care after A-V Canal Repair

The postoperative course is typically uncomplicated when repair is timed appropriately. Postoperative hemodynamic insufficiency is related to the duration of CPB and the degree of mitral insufficiency postoperatively. If inotropic support is required, dobutamine and amrinone, agents that decrease afterload and do not aggravate mitral regurgitation, are preferable to dopamine.

Persistent Mitral Regurgitation

Mitral regurgitation can be detected by inspection of the left atrial tracing for the presence of v waves. Left atrial end-diastolic pressure is used as the indicator of left ventricular filling pressure, as mean pressure is elevated because of the presence of v waves. Mitral regurgitation can be managed medically by:

- Minimizing afterload
- Avoiding agitation and its increase in intrathoracic pressure
- Minimizing the use of α-adrenergic agonists
- Maximizing vasodilation

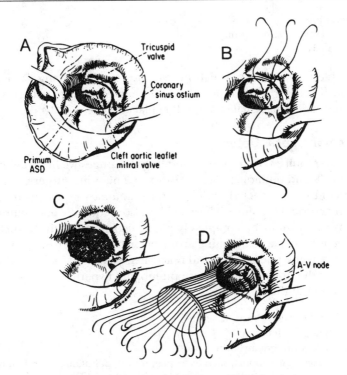

Figure 8.3. Repair of partial atrioventricular (A-V) canal. (A) Surgical exposure. (B) Closure of mitral valve cleft. (C) Prosthetic patch closure of ostium primum defect. (D) Repair completed. (From Danielson GK. Endocardial cushion defects. In: Ravitch MM, Welch KJ, Benson CD, Aberdeen E, Randolph JG, eds. Pediatric surgery. 3rd ed. Chicago: Year Book Medical Publishers, 1979;1:720.)

Pulmonary Edema

When significant mitral regurgitation occurs, prolonged mechanical ventilation can be anticipated. To avoid pulmonary edema that complicates ventilator weaning, the intravascular volume should be reduced as much as possible. Along with aggressive diuretic therapy and fluid restriction, continuous arterial venous hemofiltration may be used to reduce intravascular volume, thereby permitting adequate caloric intake.

Other Complications

Pulmonary hypertension, which can be minimized by early repair before hypertension develops, is managed with:

- Oxygen
- Hyperventilation to a $PaCO_2$ of 25 to 30

- Sedation
- Avoidance of stimulation
- Paralysis

Complete heart block, which necessitates cardiac pacing, is generally transient. If this arrhythmia persists more than 3 weeks postsurgery, however, a permanent pacemaker should be placed.

Ventricular Septal Defect

Infants who require VSD surgery generally have congestive heart failure and elevated PVR and pulmonary artery pressure. Following surgery, persistent elevation of PVR is expected, with episodic pulmonary hypertensive "crises" and right ventricular failure. These babies also frequently have pulmonary problems that cannot be completely controlled preoperatively, including left lower lobe collapse resulting from bronchial compression by an enlarged left atrium, pneumonia, and reactive airways.

Specific therapies to blunt these pulmonary hypertensive crises and to lower PVR in the PICU include:

- Mild deliberate hyperventilation
- Adequate oxygenation
- Sedation with fentanyl infusion
- Pharmacologic support, such as isoproterenol, dobutamine, and amrinone, prostaglandin E1, and nitroprusside

Tetralogy of Fallot

Through a right ventriculotomy at the level of the outflow tract, the VSD is closed with a patch, avoiding damage to the annulus or leaflets of the overriding aorta and applying techniques to relieve obstruction of the right ventricular outflow tract. At the time of repair of tetralogy of Fallot, previous palliative shunts (e.g., Blalock-Taussig) are taken down (Fig. 8.4). In addition, because ECG abnormalities are common after repair of tetralogy of Fallot, temporary pacing wires are placed in all patients.

Complications after repair of tetralogy of Fallot include:

- Diminished cardiac output from poor right ventricular function caused by ventriculotomy and CPB and residual right ventricular outflow tract obstruction or pulmonary insufficiency. Maintenance of a high postoperative CVP is important both to improve contractility and to overcome right-sided obstruction.
- Tachycardia and an increase in the dynamic component of outflow tract obstruction from the use of inotropic agents
- Right bundle branch block (RBBB), associated with right ventriculotomy with or without trauma to the right main bundle branch or proximal conducting system

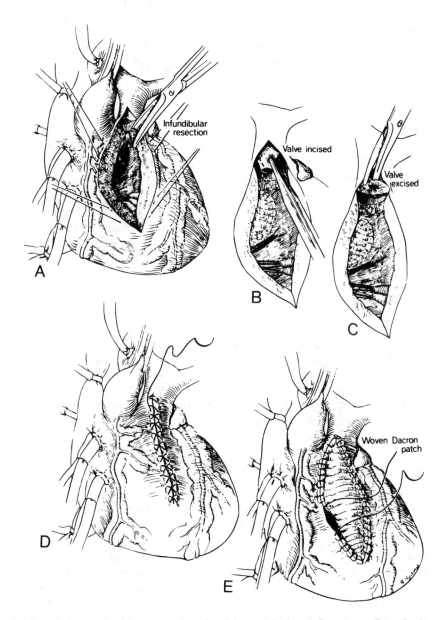

Figure 8.4. Methods of reconstructing the right ventricular outflow tract. (From Cooley DA. Total correction of tetralogy of Fallot. In: Techniques in cardiac surgery. 2nd ed. Houston: WB Saunders, 1984:135.)

- RBBB associated with left anterior hemiblock (LAH) due to peripheral injury to the A-V conduction system or secondary to a lesion of the bundle of His
- Complete heart block associated with RBBB-LAH. If complete heart block persists after 2 to 3 weeks resulting from an injury to the bundle of His, or if it recurs, a permanent pacemaker should be inserted.
- Ventricular arrhythmias, associated with a high incidence of sudden death, consequent to volume overload as seen with pulmonary regurgitation.

Truncus Arteriosus

Children with truncus arteriosus and unobstructed pulmonary blood flow do not require surgical intervention until their PVR falls at approximately 3 months of age. At that time, significant pulmonary edema may develop.

Immediate postoperative complications of truncus arteriosus repair include a diminished cardiac output caused by ventriculotomy and labile pulmonary hypertension. Postoperative management of children undergoing truncus repair is facilitated by right atrial and pulmonary artery pressure determinations. Management of pulmonary hypertension may be required for 24 to 48 hours, including:

- Hyperventilation
- Aggressive sedation
- Muscle paralysis
- Increase CVP to augment cardiac output
- Maintain PCO_2 between 30 and 35 torr and PO_2 above 90 torr

Infants who do poorly after truncus repair generally have significant truncal valve regurgitation and may benefit from truncal valve replacement. Cardiac catheterization or echocardiography can rule out a residual VSD and pulmonary conduit obstruction.

Double-Outlet Right Ventricle

Double-outlet right ventricle (DORV) occurs when all of one great artery and more than 50% of the other great artery originate from the right ventricle. DORV with a subpulmonic VSD is referred to as a Taussig-Bing malformation.

The most common type of DORV has concordant A-V relation with the d-position of the aorta, and repair depends on the orientation of the VSD with respect to the semilunar and tricuspid valves. Other variations of DORV are corrected with modifications of Rastelli, Fontan, and Mustard procedures.

The Lecompte maneuver, in which the posteriorly positioned pulmonary artery is brought anteriorly underneath the transected aorta, approximates normal arterial configuration with low postoperative mortality.

Early postoperative mortality following DORV repair is approximately 20%. Early complications include low cardiac output caused by ventriculotomy and tachyarrhythmias. As with other lesions where ventriculotomy is necessary, the CVP should be kept high postoperatively and other fluids should be restricted. Pulmonary hypertension occurs in DORV when there is no coexisting pulmonic stenosis. Management of pulmonary hypertension with oxygen, hyperventilation, and sedation is indicated; however, the presence of pulmonary hypertension greatly increases postoperative mortality.

The incidence of sudden death following repair of DORV is 18%. Sudden death generally occurs within the first postoperative year. Risk factors for sudden death include older age at time of repair, history of perioperative tachyarrhythmias, and third-degree A-V block.

Coarctation of the Aorta

Aortic coarctation generally occurs in the descending thoracic aorta opposite the insertion of the ductus arteriosus and adjacent to the origin of the left subclavian artery. Symptomatology correlates with the amount of narrowing and the presence or absence of collateral circulation. There is a bimodal age distribution at presentation.

Newborns

Coarctation in the newborn usually manifests as acute onset of congestive heart failure at the closure of the ductus arteriosus, with decreased femoral pulses. Before these patients are brought to the operating room, they should be stabilized with an infusion of prostaglandin E1 to reopen the ductus arteriosus and reduce left ventricular afterload. Severe congestive failure may require endotracheal intubation with positive pressure ventilation, inotropic support with a β-adrenergic agonist, and concomitant correction of metabolic acidosis.

Older Children

In older children with well-developed collateral circulation, coarctation is usually found initially on careful physical examination, with decreased femoral pulses and cardiac murmur. Hypertension may or may not be present with coarctation.

Subclavian Aortoplasty

This type of correction uses the proximal left subclavian artery as a patch across the narrowed segment of the aorta (Fig. 8.5). Late-onset complications from this procedure include recurrence of the coarctation in 10% of patients as a result of formation of an intraaortic shelf. Interestingly, although there is no subclavian flow to the left arm, perfusion to the arm remains adequate.

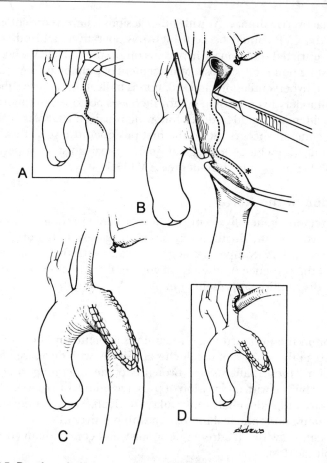

Figure 8.5. Repair technique proposed by Waldhausen. (A) and (B) The left subclavian artery is ligated distally at the level of the first branches and is then opened longitudinally. (C) The open subclavian artery is then used as a pedicle flap or patch to enlarge the stenotic isthmus. (D) A disadvantage of this method is the need to sacrifice arterial flow through a major aortic arch tributary supplying the left shoulder and vertebral artery. An end-to-side anastomosis between the divided subclavian artery and the adjacent left common carotid artery can be used to solve this problem. (From Cooley DA. Repair of coarctation of the thoracic aorta. In: Techniques in cardiac surgery. 2nd ed. Houston: WB Saunders, 1984:40.)

End-to-End Aortic Anastomosis

End-to-end aortic anastomosis, with or without a Dacron graft, is usual in the older infant and child. There is a 20% incidence of recoarctation in these children, which requirs reoperation or balloon angioplasty. Postoperative aneurysm formation seen in 5 to 16% of children has been associated with the use of a Dacron patch for repair.

Intraoperative and Postoperative PICU Considerations

Paralysis Ischemia of the spinal cord, kidneys, and gastrointestinal tract may result from hypoperfusion during aortic cross-clamp, the most severe complication of which is paraplegia (0.14% of patients postoperatively). Paralysis, with preserved proprioception and temperature sensation following coarctation repair, is termed anterior spinal artery syndrome.

Intraoperatively, several factors have been linked to the development of paralysis, including the duration of aortic cross-clamping, temperature, and the use of deliberate hypotension to limit left ventricular afterload. Measurement of distal aortic blood pressure during cross-clamp—which presumably reflects blood flow from collateral circulation—and use of a temporary shunt around the cross-clamped area has been advocated when the distal pressure is less than 40 mm Hg.

Proximal Aortic Blood Pressure

Management of proximal aortic blood pressure during aortic cross-clamping can be difficult; sudden increases in left ventricular afterload may be poorly tolerated by the patient with preexisting congestive heart failure, especially when there is poorly developed collateral circulation. Afterload reduction with vasodilators such as nitroprusside is potentially hazardous, because distal perfusion pressure below the cross-clamp may be inadequate.

Atelectasis

The left lung must collapse for the surgeon to gain access to the aorta through a left thoracotomy incision. Postoperatively, although the lung is reexpanded with manual ventilation, areas of atelectasis remain. Occlusion of the endotracheal tube with high peak inspiratory pressures should be excluded rapidly by inserting a relatively large suction catheter to a level below the end of the endotracheal tube. Endotracheal tube occlusion necessitates rapid reintubation before clinical deterioration can occur. When end-tidal CO_2 is monitored by capnography, tube occlusion should be suspected when there is a progressive decrease in end-tidal CO_2.

Other causes of decreased end-tidal CO_2 include:

- Esophageal intubation
- Endobronchial intubation
- Low cardiac output
- Pulmonary embolism
- Any cause of increased respiratory dead space

Metabolic Acidosis

Intraoperatively, metabolic acidosis may develop related to aortic cross-clamping and distal ischemia.

Persistent Hypertension

Initially, hypertension is attributed to both elevated plasma catecholamines during the surgery and elevated plasma renin levels, with abnormal barore-ceptor autoregulatory responses. If allowed to continue untreated, uncon-trolled hypertension can lead to reflex mesenteric vasoconstriction and splanchnic hypoperfusion (postcoarctectomy syndrome). Intestinal is-chemia, leading in some cases to frank bowel infarction, is a leading cause of early postoperative morbidity and mortality in this group of patients. Early preventive treatment includes leaving the child on continuous naso-gastric suction, with no feedings for 2 or more days postoperatively. Addi-tionally, early aggressive management of postoperative hypertension has been stressed.

A wide variety of agents have been used to control blood pressure post-operatively, including β-blockers, α-blockers, and direct vasodilators. Direct vasodilators such as nitroprusside offer the advantage of being simple to titrate in the operating room and in the PICU, particularly during rapidly changing physiologic circumstances such as emergence from anesthesia.

Perioperative blood pressure should be monitored in the right arm (i.e, proximal to the coarctation) and checked in the legs for presence of a resid-ual gradient. The left arm should not be used for blood pressure checks, in-travenous access, or arterial puncture when the surgical procedure was a left subclavian aortoplasty.

Interrupted Aortic Arch

Interruption of the aortic arch may occur anywhere along the transverse arch but is seen most frequently near the origin of the left subclavian artery, as is coarctation of the aorta. Distal perfusion is provided by the ductus ar-teriosus. These infants generally show sudden onset of hypoperfusion and shock at the time of duct closure.

Preoperative Stabilization

Steps are similar to those for neonatal coarctation, including:

- Use of prostaglandin E1 to maintain ductal patency
- Support of the circulation with vasopressors if necessary
- Correction of metabolic abnormalities, including acidosis, if feasible, before the patient is brought to the operating room

Intraoperative and PICU Considerations

In the postbypass period, myocardial failure may occur because of preexist-ing myocardial failure or lack of complete recovery of the myocardium fol-lowing cardioplegia intraoperatively. Hemodynamic support of the circulation with vasopressors such as dobutamine or epinephrine is similar to that used for any other newborn with congestive heart failure. The potential for elevated PVR perioperatively, as for any neonate, is present. Similarly, the baby should be screened for neurologic deficits after awakening from anesthesia, particularly if the aortic interruption was contiguous with the origin of any of the carotid vessels.

Aortic Stenosis

Preoperative Care

Because these patients with aortic stenosis usually have severe left ventricular hypertrophy and elevated left ventricular intracavity pressures, maintenance of systemic perfusion pressure and avoiding tachycardia, which decreases diastolic perfusion time, are important preoperatively. Because of limited coronary reserve, angina and myocardial ischemia can be seen—even in the absence of coronary stenosis—in young adults with this disease. Preoperative, prebypass care is directed toward maintaining coronary perfusion by maintaining systemic diastolic blood pressure and controlling heart rate to maintain diastolic perfusion time.

The ability to protect the myocardium intraoperatively with cardioplegia may be somewhat limited by severe left ventricular hypertrophy.

After Valvuloplasty

Aortic stenosis may be corrected surgically by either aortic valvuloplasty or aortic valve replacement, depending on the clinical circumstances. Valvuloplasty is used in the infant to dilate the valve orifice. A small degree of aortic regurgitation afterward is common.

Pulmonary Valvular Stenosis

Neonates with critical pulmonary valvular stenosis usually begin to deteriorate when the ductus arteriosus closes, generally on the second or third day of life.

Preoperative Stabilization

Steps include:

- Prostaglandin E1 infusion to maintain ductal patency and provide pulmonary blood flow
- Correction of electrolyte disorders, particularly systemic acidosis
- Ventilatory support if needed

A common coexisting cardiac defect is right ventricular hypertrophy with a relatively small hypoplastic ventricular cavity.

Intraoperative and PICU Considerations

Pulmonary stenosis and relative hypoplasia of the distal pulmonary arteries and arterioles requires staged repairs with systemic to pulmonary artery shunts designed to enhance pulmonary blood flow and arteriolar growth. Single-stage repair, in the face of distal pulmonary vascular hypoplasia, frequently leads to acute right-sided heart failure.

Right ventricular ischemia may occur with inadequate intraoperative myocardial preservation. Pulmonary insufficiency normally occurs after pericardial outflow patch reconstruction, although this is usually of minor clinical consequence. The need for an extensive incision in the ventricle intraoperatively will also contribute to ventricular dysfunction.

With relief of outflow obstruction, the right ventricle usually shows improved overall function, and there is little or no need for inotropic support. Factors that cause elevation of the PVR, such as hypercarbia or hypoxemia, may cause the ventricle to fail and obviously should be avoided. Otherwise, postoperative care is directed toward rewarming, volume repletion, and correction of electrolyte abnormalities, as for any open-heart procedure. For the uncomplicated procedure in a hemodynamically stable child, early extubation is anticipated.

Patent Ductus Arteriosus

The ductus arteriosus may be either ligated with suture and divided or occluded with a hemoclip.

Ventilation and Oxygen Saturation

Intraoperatively, collapse of the left lung alters ventilatory compliance, particularly in the sick premature infant with hyaline membrane disease who requires a high inspired concentration of oxygen.

Hemorrhage

Although extremely rare, tearing of the duct can occur, with exsanguinating, difficult-to-control hemorrhage. This devastating complication occurs more frequently in the older child when ductal tissue has become more friable.

Other Complications

Ligation of the ductus may cause injuries to the following structures:

- Phrenic nerve, resulting in diaphragmatic paralysis
- Thoracic duct, resulting in chylothorax
- Recurrent laryngeal nerve, resulting in vocal cord paralysis, more commonly in premature infants

Transposition of the Great Vessels

As with other cyanotic congenital heart disease, TGV generally presents with cyanosis in the neonatal period. Prostaglandin E1 infusion at this juncture frequently is given to maintain ductal patency until atrial septectomy via either balloon or Blalock-Hanlon or definitive repair (i.e., Jatene procedure) can be performed.

Surgical Correction

Jatene Procedure This procedure, which involves reimplanting both the aorta and the pulmonary artery onto their "normal" ventricle (Fig. 8.6), can only be performed when the left ventricle is able to withstand pumping against SVR rather than the lower PVR. Physiologically, this occurs under three different sets of circumstances:

1. During the weeks immediately following birth, the child's PVR is sufficiently high to maintain left ventricular muscle tone.
2. Left ventricular pressure and, consequently, muscle mass remain high in the older child with TGV and nonrestrictive VSD.
3. In older children with TGV and without a VSD in whom a Jatene-type repair is contemplated, temporary banding of the pulmonary artery allows the left ventricle to hypertrophy, and then the arterial switch is an option.

Mustard and Senning Procedures The atrial switch operation is usually performed in the older child with TGV. Generally, these children have undergone a balloon atrial septectomy as a newborn. An intraatrial baffle directs systemic venous return to the left ventricle and out the pulmonary artery to the lungs and pulmonary venous return to the right ventricle and out the aorta. The Senning and Mustard procedures differ in the choice of material used to construct the atrial baffle-pericardium or Dacron patch material in the Mustard procedure, native atrial tissue in the Senning. Although the circulation is physiologically corrected with these procedures, the child is left with an anatomic right ventricle providing systemic perfusion for life (Fig. 8.7).

Intraoperative and Intensive Care Unit Considerations

Arterial Switch (Jatene) Procedure The Jatene procedure is most commonly carried out in newborn infants, frequently with circulatory arrest. Perioperative complications include:

- Extensive hemorrhage
- Elevated PVR
- Myocardial ischemia related to coronary artery reimplantation

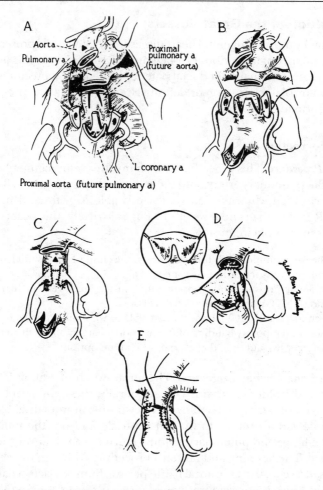

Figure 8.6. Arterial switch operative technique. Preliminary steps before the transfer of the coronary artery-aortic cuffs include transection of the main pulmonary artery distal to valve commissures with inspection of pulmonary (neoaortic) valve and subvalvar region and transection of the aorta about 2 mm (in neonate) distal to the coronary ostia. (A) The left and right coronary arteries are removed from their corresponding aortic sinus locations with a cuff of aortic wall. (B) Incisions are made into the left and right anterior sinuses of the pulmonary artery (neoaortic) stump, and the coronary cuffs are positioned for suturing in place. (C) The distal aortic segment (solid triangle), previously anterior in (A) and (B), is passed posterior to the bifurcation of the pulmonary artery. This distal aortic segment is sutured to the reconstructed (coronary ostia bearing) pulmonary artery stump of the left ventricular outflow tract. (D) A pantaloon-shaped patch of autologous pericardium is used to fill the defects in the aortic (neopulmonary) stump that were created by removal of the coronary cuffs, and the patch also forms the free edge of the stump reconstruction. (E) The distal pulmonary artery is approximated and anastomosed to the right ventricular outflow stump. (From Idriss FS, Ilbawi MN, DeLeon SY, et al. Arterial switch in simple and complex transposition of the great arteries. J Thorac Cardiovasc Surg 1988;95:29.)

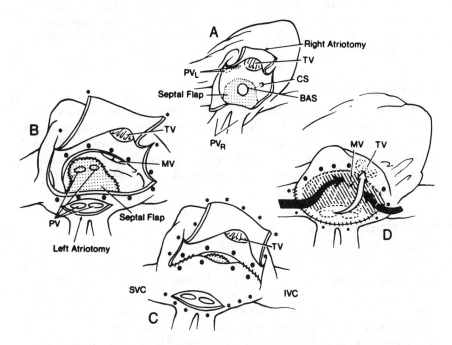

Figure 8.7. Atrial switch operation (Senning Technique) performed using cardiopul-monary bypass with cold cardioplegic myocardial protection or during profound hy-pothermia with total circulatory arrest. (A) A right atriotomy is made in front of and paral-lel to the caval veins and is extended into the atrial appendage. This exposes the atrial septum with its balloon septostomy defect. The atrial septum is now incised anteriorly, superiorly, and inferiorly to form a septal flap (dotted area) as large as possible that remains fixed pos-teriorly between the caval entrances. The wall between the coronary sinus (CS) and left atrium may be incised to provide a large posterior lip for the inferior septal flap suture line (B), and direct coronary sinus return to the newly formed systemic venous chamber and conduit to the mitral valve is formed posteriorly by the repositioned septal flap (dotted area); the con-duit is then completed anteriorly by suturing the posterior right atrial free wall flap (●●●) an-teriorly to the anterior septal limbus (●●●) as in (C) A left atriotomy is made as long as possi-ble in the internal atrial groove (exposing the orifices of the right pulmonary veins). (C) and (D) The pulmonary venous chamber and pathway to the tricuspid valve are completed with the suturing of the anterior right free wall atrial flap (***) over the right pulmonary veins to the anterior lip of the left atriotomy (***). (D) Black arrows indicate systemic venous caval flow through the newly created atrial tissue conduit and systemic venous chamber (\\\\\\\\\\\\) toward the mitral valve. White arrow indicates pulmonary venous flow path in pulmonary ve-nous atrium passing behind, rightward, and anterior to the systemic venous chamber toward the tricuspid valve (TV). BAS, balloon atrial septostomy; IVC and SVC, the inferior and the su-perior vena cava, respectively; MV, mitral valve; PV, PVL, and PVR, pulmonary veins, left and right. (From Paul MH. Complete transposition of the great arteries. In: Adams FH, Em-manouilides GC, Riemenschneider TA, eds. Moss' heart disease in infants, children, and ado-lescents. 4th ed. Baltimore: Williams & Wilkins, 1989:403. With permission.)

Atrial Switch (Mustard and Senning) Procedure Potential complications, both early and long-term, ascribed to these atrial switch operations include obstruction to venous return, systemic ventricular failure, and conduction system abnormalities.

Fontan Procedure

The Fontan procedure entails connection of all systemic venous drainage to the pulmonary arteries, either directly or through the right atrium. Pulmonary blood flow in this procedure is not provided by "pumping" of blood but instead relies on systemic venous pressure for its upstream pressure gradient (Fig. 8.8). The Glenn shunt (see below), may be considered simply the first stage of a Fontan repair.

Preoperative Findings

Normal or low PVR (less than 4 Woods units [mm Hg/L. min-1pdm-2]) and the absence of left heart obstructive lesions are considered critical requirements for this operation. As such, the Fontan procedure is not done in the neonatal period or first few months of life because of the normal neonatal elevation of PVR. Generally, infants with cyanotic obstructive lesions and inadequate pulmonary blood flow, such as tricuspid atresia, undergo palliative procedures, such as a modified Blalock-Taussig shunt.

Children and adults presenting for the Fontan procedure usually have:

- Long-standing cyanosis and all its attendant problems
- Polycythemia
- Inadequate perfusion
- Chronic metabolic acidosis
- Elevated PT and PTT
- Hypoglycemia

Intraoperative and Intensive Care Unit Considerations

Glucose Levels As with any polycythemic child, prolonged fasting preoperatively should be avoided because of the risks of hypoglycemia and dehydration that may further increase hematocrit. Similarly, because of the potential impact of severe hyperglycemia on neurologic sequelae, glucose levels should be monitored intraoperatively and glucose administered judiciously.

Superior Vena Caval Central Line (CVP) The CVP not only monitors venous pressure in the SVC (and presumably the brain) but also represents the filling pressure for the pulmonary arteries. Care must be taken in placing the CVP to position the catheter above the anticipated suture line between the SVC and pulmonary artery. Failure to recognize placement may result in the catheter being incorporated into the suture line.

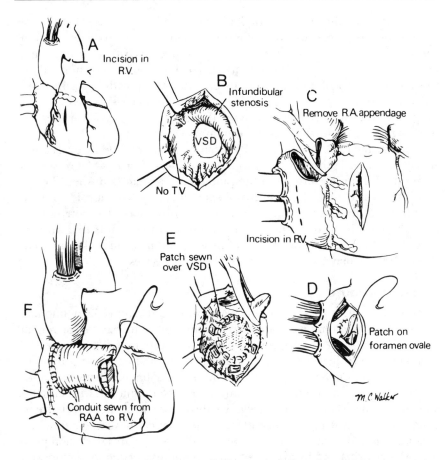

Figure 8.8. Fontan Procedure for correcting congenital tricuspid atresia. In the case depicted, the patient has a ventricular septal defect, patent foramen ovale, and normal pulmonary valve, making him an ideal patient for this technique. RV, right ventricle; RA, right atrium; RAA, right atrial auricle. (From Cooley DA. Lesion of the tricuspid valve. In: Techniques in cardiac surgery. 2nd ed. Houston: WB Saunders, 1984:218.)

Augmenting Pulmonary Blood Flow and Optimizing Myocardial Function
Right heart return and pulmonary blood flow are maintained through adequate intravascular volume repletion and patient positioning. SVC return of blood to the pulmonary vascular bed is aided by gravity, and so simply elevating the head of the bed or sitting the patient up is important. Drainage from the IVC can be promoted by the use of military antishock trousers (MAST) that are cyclically inflated or by leg elevation.

SVC pressure and cerebral venous pressure are elevated postoperatively, with pressures of 12 to 15 mm Hg being common. Although elevated

SVC pressure has the potential for decreasing cerebral perfusion because of elevated downstream pressure, this is problematic only when cardiac output and mean arterial pressure are depressed. In patients with a right atrium, normal sinus rhythm may be necessary for adequate pulmonary blood flow. Chronic elevation of systemic venous pressure often leads to ascites and pleural effusions, usually right-sided, often several days or weeks after surgery. Chest tube drainage of these effusions may be needed if they become significant enough to cause respiratory compromise.

Minimizing PVR Minimizing PVR can be accomplished by decreasing airway pressure, optimizing oxygenation, and lowering PCO_2. Pressure is transmitted from the airways to the pulmonary vascular bed when the patient's chest is closed. Early return of spontaneous ventilation is optimal. Negative intrathoracic intrapleural pressure will augment venous return from the periphery to the pulmonary arteries. Other agents that directly lower PVR, such as nitroprusside and prostaglandin E1, may also be used, although these may also lower systemic blood pressure.

Glenn Procedure

The Glenn shunt is an anastomosis between the SVC and right pulmonary artery to increase pulmonary blood flow in children with cyanotic congenital disease (Fig. 8.9). CPB support is not required except in the "bidirectional" Glenn procedure, in which the SVC is attached to both pulmonary arteries to enhance blood flow and promote "growth" of the pulmonary arteries.

SVC pressure above the suture line should be monitored with either a jugular or subclavian CVP line. Negative intrathoracic pressure (relative to atmospheric pressure) is transmitted to the pulmonary vascular tree, decreasing pulmonary artery pressure and thus increasing this perfusion pressure. Hypercarbia and hypoxia are potent pulmonary vasoconstrictors and should be avoided. Premature tracheal extubation can be deleterious if these result.

Total Anomalous Pulmonary Venous Return

Total anomalous pulmonary venous return (TAPVR) usually presents in the first days of life and requires emergency surgical correction.

Preoperative Anatomy

The three anatomic types of TAPVR are classified by the site of anomalous drainage of the pulmonary veins: supracardiac, cardiac, and infracardiac (Fig. 8.10). Infracardiac TAPVR, with pulmonary venous return to the liver, carries the highest mortality. In all instances, pulmonary venous drainage is to the right atrium, with systemic oxygenation occurring only with atrial mixing through an obligatory patent foramen ovale or ASD.

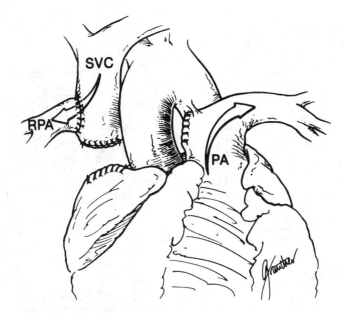

Figure 8.9. Glenn Shunt, an end-to-end anastomosis of the superior vena cava (SVC) to the distal end of the divided right pulmonary artery (RPA). The superior vena cava to right atrial junction and the proximal right pulmonary artery (PA) are ligated. (From Lowe DA. Abnormalities of the atrioventricular valves. In: Lake CL, ed. Pediatric cardiac anesthesia. 2nd ed. Norwalk, Conn: Appleton & Lange, 1993.)

Intraoperative and PICU Considerations

The surgical correction of TAPVR involves reimplanting the confluence, where all of the pulmonary veins join, into the posterior wall of the left atrium and closing the ASD. After the bypass is complete, medical therapy is directed toward augmenting cardiac output and minimizing PVR using β-adrenergic agonists and direct pulmonary vasodilators, such as dobutamine, isoproterenol, epinephrine, amrinone, and prostaglandin E1.

In the PICU, problems that can be expected are related to:

- Maintaining adequate cardiac output
- Controlling pulmonary hypertension
- Correction of a coagulopathy
- Monitoring for other organ damage that may have occurred intraoperatively
- Cardiac tamponade, demonstrated by an abrupt elevation in filling pressures and deterioration in systemic perfusion
- Elevation in PVR with episodic pulmonary hypertensive crises

Factors that contribute to pulmonary hypertension include:

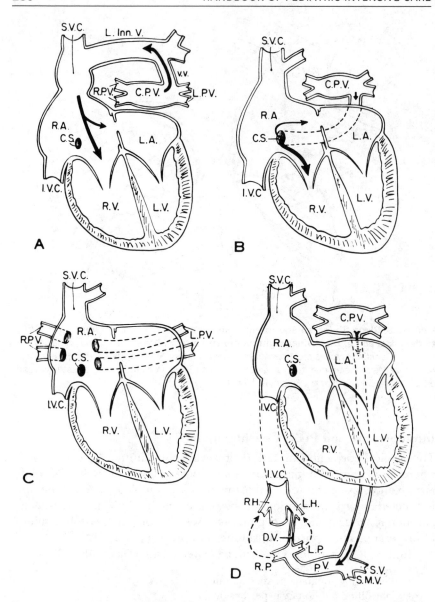

Figure 8.10. Common forms of total anomalous pulmonary venous return (TAPVR). (A)
TAPVR to the left innominate vein (L Inn V) by way of a vertical vein (VV). (B) TAPVR to coronary sinus (CS). The pulmonary veins join to form a confluence designated common pulmonary
vein (CPV), which connects to the coronary sinus. (C) TAPVR to right atrium. The right and left
pulmonary veins (LPV and RPV) usually enter the right atrium separately. (D) TAPVR to the portal vein (PV). The pulmonary veins form a confluence, from which an anomalous channel
arises. This connects to the portal vein, which communicates with the inferior vena cava (IVC)
by way of the ductus venosus (DV) or the hepatic sinusoids. SV, splenic vein; SMV, superior

- Normal neonatal PVR
- Elevated left atrial pressure
- Obstruction to pulmonary venous drainage at the anastomotic site
- Congenital pulmonary vascular hypoplasia

HEART TRANSPLANTATION
Selection of Donors

Cardiac function of the donor is considered adequate for transplantation if:

- ECG is normal, without evidence for ischemia
- Normal left ventricular shortening fraction by echocardiography
- Normal cardiac structure

The donor must be free of infection, although the recipient may be on antibiotics.

Selection of Recipients
Indications

Current indications for heart transplant are:

- Dilated cardiomyopathy
- Palliated congenital heart disease with irreversible myocardial dysfunction
- Life-threatening arrhythmias resistant to conventional medical therapy
- Lethal neonatal heart disease including hypoplastic left heart syndrome or variants of this complex

Medical Considerations

The major cause of early postoperative failure is right ventricular failure of the graft, which is associated with recipient pulmonary hypertension. Sudden exposure of the transplanted right ventricle to a very high PVR will cause it to dilate or fail.

Other contraindications to transplantation are relative. Renal and hepatic dysfunction, if secondary to myocardial dysfunction, may be reversible after transplantation. Pulmonary infarction that may increase the risk of lung abscess with immunosuppression has not precluded successful transplantation.

Figure 8.10. (continued) mesenteric vein; RP and LP, right and left portal veins; RH and LH, right and left hepatic veins; SVC, superior vena cava; RA and LA, right and left atrium; RV and LV, right and left ventricle. (From Lucas RV Jr, Krabill KA. Anomalous venous connections, pulmonary and systemic. In: Adams FH, Emmanouilides GC, Riemenschneider TA, eds. Moss' heart disease in infants, children, and adolescents. 4th ed. Baltimore: Williams & Wilkins, 1989:588. With permission.)

Donor and recipient matching is based on ABO compatibility and CMV infection status. If the recipient is serologically negative for CMV, every effort is made to obtain a CMV-negative heart.

Surgery

Excision of the Diseased Recipient Heart

After the pericardium has been appropriately dissected and secured, the aorta and right atrium are mobilized. The ascending aorta and cavae are cannulated, allowing preservation of a generous cuff of posterior right atrium for anastomosis to the donor heart. The patient is placed on CPB, the body temperature is lowered to 28°C, and the aorta is cross-clamped (Figs. 8.11 and 8.12). The recipient's diseased heart is then excised, leaving posterior cuffs of left and right atrium, aorta, and pulmonary artery. Coordination of donor and recipient operations is critical in expediting reperfusion to optimize early postimplant function.

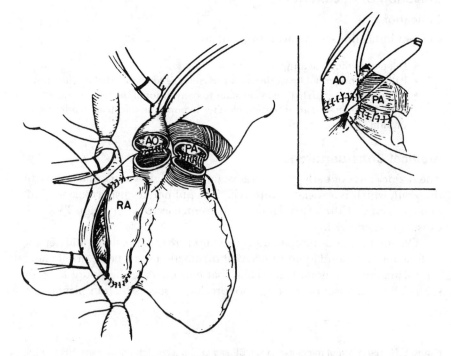

Figure 8.11. Medial aspect of the right atrial (RA) anastomosis has been completed, and the methods of the anastomosis of the aorta (AO) and pulmonary artery (PA) are shown. Insert demonstrates the technique of venting air from the ascending aorta as the aortic cross-clamp is released, restoring perfusion to the donor heart. (From Bolman RM III. Cardiac transplantation: the operative technique. Cardiovasc Clin 1990;20:140. With permission.)

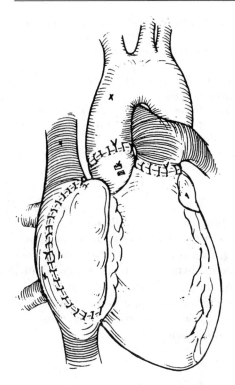

Figure 8.12. Completed right atrial anastomosis. Right atrial, aortic, and pulmonary suture lines are visible, and the cardiopulmonary bypass cannulae have been extracted. (From Bolman RM III. Cardiac transplantation: the operative technique. Cardiovasc Clin 1990;20:141. With permission.)

Implantation of the Donor Heart

The donor heart is prepared for placement into the recipient. The aorta and pulmonary arteries are separated. The superior vena caval orifice is oversewn. The cuffs of the left and right atrium are created—matching those in the recipient—by excising the posterior wall of the left atrium and making an incision in the right atrium from the inferior vena caval orifice to the right atrial appendage.

In situations in which the donor heart ischemic time is excessive, the aortic anastomosis is performed after the left atrial anastomosis, at which point the aortic cross-clamp is removed and perfusion is restored to the donor heart.

Postoperative Care

Full Reverse Isolation Precautions

Many centers adhere to a protocol as follows:

- Mechanical ventilation overnight maintains normal oxygenation and ventilation
- Patients with a reactive pulmonary vascular bed are maintained on the

pulmonary hypertension protocol, including sedation, paralysis, and limited stimulation
- Isoproterenol is infused at a rate that results in a slight tachycardia relative to age
- Low-dose dopamine is administered to maintain renal blood flow
- Atrial or sequential A-V pacing is used as needed
- Cephalosporin is delivered when invasive vascular lines are still in place
- Sulfamethoxazole and trimethoprim are administered chronically to minimize the risk of *Pneumocystis carinii* infection (see below)
- H_2-receptor blockers provide prophylaxis for stress ulcers, especially when high doses of corticosteroids are used

Characteristic Clinical Findings

Elevations in right- and left-sided filling pressures gradually recede. Reduction in right-sided pressures may be attributable to the decrease in pulmonary pressure, improvement of right ventricular contractility, and a decrease in tricuspid regurgitation. Systemic hypertension is seen frequently, mainly as a side effect of cyclosporine therapy. Cardiac denervation theoretically protects against arrhythmias. Primary malignant arrhythmias after transplantation are likely related to acute rejection, coronary artery disease, or ventricular dysfunction from some other cause.

Immunosuppression Therapy

Many institutions currently use a triple-drug therapy in children that includes cyclosporine, steroids, and azathioprine. Clinical signs of acute rejection that warrant emergency endomyocardial biopsy include:

- Fever
- Tachycardia
- Arrhythmias
- Hypotension
- Weakness
- Lethargy
- Fluid retention

Systolic function may not be affected in the early stages of rejection. Diastolic dysfunction is more typically seen as a decreased stroke volume, decrease in end-diastolic volume, and a reduction in peak filling rate. These changes follow the pattern seen with restrictive cardiomyopathy.

Rejection

The rate of rejection is probably close to 100% in children following transplantation. Clinical or histologic rejection events are treated with high-dose intravenous methylprednisolone. With persistent or progressive change, polyclonal antibody, antithymocyte globulin, or monoclonal antibody (OKT3) is used.

Denervation

Duration of Denervation

Studies measuring myocardial catecholamines and nerve density and displaying denervation physiology and pharmacology in the transplanted heart have been unable to show reinnervation at any point up to 5 years after surgery. These results refute findings in anecdotal reports of early reestablishment of sensory innervation.

Physiology of the Denervated Heart

Electrical Activity

The SA node, previously under the continual influence of the vagus nerves, is altered in the transplanted heart. The rate of the donor heart;q2s atria is generally higher than that of the recipient's. The electrical activity of the native atria does not cross the suture line. The native atria continue to respond to reflex stimuli and medications, although they play no role in the regulation of the donor ventricle. The rise in heart rate in response to exercise or stress is delayed, as is the time to return to baseline.

Denervation does not, however, alter conduction time through the AV node, nor does it affect ventricular conduction. Denervation may protect the heart from arrhythmias, although arrhythmias are reported in the transplanted heart, associated with tissue rejection, coronary artery disease, or ventricular dysfunction from other causes. Because the heart is also afferently denervated, it cannot sense pain, and so ischemia is always silent.

Effects of Drugs on the Denervated Heart

Drugs that act primarily through the autonomic nervous system are ineffective on the denervated heart. Drugs that act both directly on the heart and via the autonomic nervous system have only direct effects expressed.

Catecholamines

Optimal inotropic support following transplantation is critical, because there is both primary ventricular dysfunction in the immediate postoperative period and ventricular dysfunction secondary to tissue rejection later on. Because of loss of the presynaptic neuronal catecholamine uptake system following transplantation, nonselective agents such as epinephrine, dobutamine, or isoproterenol are more effective for inotropic support. The transplanted heart also appears to be supersensitive to norepinephrine and epinephrine, mediated by the presynaptic loss of uptake of these drugs.

Other Agents

The A-V nodal blocking property of digitalis is reduced because of the interruption of preganglionic parasympathetic efferent nerves, although its inotropic effect remains intact. The anticholinergic properties of atropine and quinidine are virtually absent. Atrial flutter could be treated, therefore, with quinidine without fear of accelerating A-V conduction. Digoxin is ineffective in treating atrial flutter. Atropine cannot be used to accelerate SA or A-V node conduction. Calcium channel blockers do not induce any major electrophysiologic effects in the denervated heart.

Coronary Artery Dynamics

Denervation does not appear to alter coronary blood flow changes associated with metabolic need. The local influences modulating autoregulation of coronary blood flow most likely play a more important role in this setting.

Endocrine Function

Studies suggest that heart transplant recipients have mechanisms by which blood volume can be regulated by altering plasma antidiuretic hormone levels independent of cardiac volume receptors.

9.

Dysrhythmias and Their Management

Randall C. Wetzel, Mark A. Helfaer, and Mark C. Rogers

Cardiac output is the product of stroke volume and heart rate. Factors that combine to determine stroke volume include:

- Inotropic state of the heart
- End-diastolic volume of the heart (preload)
- Myocardial afterload

Just as these three factors are interdependent, they also are affected by the timing and sequencing of electrical depolarization of the myocardium, and, in several instances, alterations in electrical depolarization affect preload and contractility.

In children, normal heart rates vary over a wide range in the first year of life. With age, heart rate tends to decrease, as does the range that is considered normal. Concurrently, stroke volume increases. As expected, the maximally achievable cardiac index occurs at higher heart rates in younger children than in adults (Fig. 9.1). Myocardial ischemia during rapid heart rates is occasionally noted in children, and it is important to consider myocardial oxygen supply-demand relationships when dealing with tachydysrhythmias in children.

ETIOLOGY

Many congenital heart diseases show a predilection toward cardiac dysrhythmias. These conditions and other etiologic factors are described in Table 9.1.

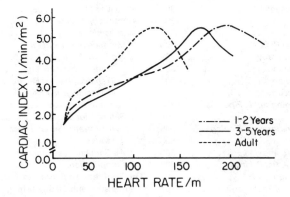

Figure 9.1. Changes in cardiac index with heart rate for three different age groups. This graph is derived from normative data and illustrates the increased dependence of cardiac output on heart rate in young children. (From Wetzel RC, Rogers MC. Pediatric hemodynamic monitoring. In: Shoemaker WC, Thompson WL, eds. Critical care—state of the art. Fullerton, California: Society of Critical Care Medicine, 1981;2:II(L)9. With permission.)

Table 9.1
Etiologic Factors in Cardiac Dysrhythmias

Etiologic Factor	Associated Cardiac Dysrhythmia
Wolf-Parkinson-White Ebstein's anomaly TGA Mitral stenosis Systemic lupus erythematosus Cardiac surgery for congenital cardiac disease	Congenital complete heart block
Ventricular repolarization disorders (associated with deafness and Romano-Ward autosomal dominant syndrome)	Sudden ventricular fibrillation; prolonged Q-T interval; prominent U waves in association with short P-R interval
Hyperkalemia	Fatal ventricular dysrhythmias; reentry dysrhythmias
Hypokalemia	Ectopic activity; prolonged repolarization; U waves and prolonged T waves; reentry VT (Fig. 9.2)
Hypercalcemia	Increase in phase 2, prolonging Q-T wave and leading VT
Low magnesium and phosphorus levels	Drug-resistant tachycardias, torsade de pointes
Pharmacologic agents (digitalis, β-blockers, sympathomimetics, aminophylline, barbiturates, tricyclic antidepressants)	Profound and fatal rate and rhythm disturbances
Thoracic trauma and myocardial contusion	Conduction abnormalities; ventricular dysrhythmias; sinus tachycardia

DIAGNOSIS

Electrocardiography (ECG) is the cornerstone of both evaluation and diagnosis of abnormalities in cardiac rate and rhythm. Frequently, the first indication of an underlying cardiac dysrhythmia is the routine ECG monitoring performed in the pediatric intensive care unit (ICU). In all critically ill children and in those who present with abnormal mental status or sudden loss of consciousness, ECG monitoring is mandatory. Rarely, for the diagnosis of difficult dysrhythmias, unorthodox positions such as the intracardiac or the transesophageal position for ECG recording may be necessary in the pediatric ICU. Postoperatively, pacing wires can also be used to record ECG patterns to aid in diagnosis.

BRADYDYSRHYTHMIAS

Asystole

The total absence of ventricular electrical activity may result from either sinoatrial node arrest or complete sinoatrial ventricular conduction blockade caused by hypoxia, ischemia, direct myocardial injury, severe electrolyte abnormalities, or severe multiple system injury.

Sinus Bradycardia

Sinus bradydysrhythmias may occur from either abnormally slow generator potential from the sinus node, the total absence of sinoatrial generator potential, or conduction failure of this potential.

A guide to the normal lower limit of heart rate in children is provided in Table 9.2.

Sick Sinus Syndrome

Either a congenital abnormality or direct injury to the sinus node results in decreased sinus impulse formation or the inability of the generator potential to exit the sinus node (so-called sinus exit block). In children, this situation most frequently occurs in association with:

- Surgery, especially after the Mustard procedure for correction of TGA
- Cardiomyopathies
- Ischemia
- Myocarditis

The ECG manifestations of sick sinus syndrome are varied and may include escape rhythms that are nodal or ventricular in origin, giving rise to tachydysrhythmias (hence the name bradycardia-tachycardia syndrome). Clinically, patients may present with either Stokes-Adams attacks or profound bradycardia and hypoperfusion. Those patients who become symptomatic almost always require permanent intracardiac pacemaking.

Conduction Abnormalities

First-degree atrioventricular (AV) block occurs when all sinus impulses are conducted but with delay, as indicated by a prolonged P-R interval. The

Table 9.2
Normal Lower Heart Rate Limit

Awake state:	
5 y of age and older	60
5 y of age and younger	80
First year of life	100
First week of life	95
Sleep state:	
5 y of age and older	< 50
Infants	< 60

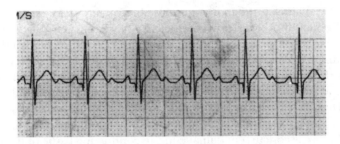

Figure 9.2. Normal sinus rhythm in a 2-year-old with a serum potassium of 2.0 mEq/mL. Note prominent U wave after each T wave and the potential for confusing U waves with P waves. U waves resolved with potassium replacement.

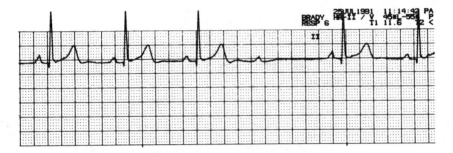

Figure 9.3. Mobitz Type II second-degree heart block. Note the sinus rhythm with a regularly timed P wave and no QRS.

rhythm is regular with normal QRS morphology. Conduction times greater than 0.20 seconds in children should always raise suspicion. A P-R interval greater than 0.14 seconds in infants, more than 0.16 second in children, and more than 0.18 seconds in adolescents is abnormally prolonged.

Second-degree AV block is associated with failure of conduction of some, but not all, atrial beats to the ventricles and is divided into Mobitz type I and Mobitz type II blocks.

- Mobitz type I block (i.e., Wenckebach phenomenon). The P-R interval becomes progressively longer until eventually the atrial impulse is not conducted and a dropped beat occurs. Mobitz type I heart block is invariably associated with conduction delay within the AV node.
- Mobitz type II block. Irregular and intermittent sudden dropping of beats follows P waves (Fig. 9.3). These are not preceded by progressive P-R prolongation. The QRS morphology may alter.

Mobitz type II block is the more ominous abnormality of AV conduction because it frequently progresses to complete AV block. It is generally thought to occur via conduction blockade in the bundle of His or the bundle branches.

Complete AV block, either congenital or acquired, is the most common bradydysrhythmia in childhood. Complete AV block (i.e., third degree) means that there is total lack of conduction between the atria and the ventricles. Diagnosis depends on the recognition of an abnormally slow QRS rate for a particular age and a regular atrial rhythm but an irregular P-R interval. If there is concurrent damage to the conducting tissue of the bundle of His, which may occur during surgery, then the QRS pattern either may be consistent with bundle branch blockade or may resemble a ventricular extrasystole.

Therapy

Indications

Hemodynamic compromise manifested by hypotension and hypoperfusion warrants treatment. In addition, certain dysrhythmias, such as Mobitz type II block, are so highly associated with catastrophic deterioration that therapy may also be indicated.

Initial Measures

All dysrhythmias require:

- Correction of hypoxia, acidosis, hyperkalemia or hypokalemia (Table 9.3), hypovolemia, hypotension, and hypothermia
- Removal of drugs where appropriate
- Treatment of elevated intracranial pressure where indicated

With these steps, oxygenation and ventilation should be assured, and intravascular volume is restored.

Table 9.3
Treatment of Hyperkalemia

Remove all potassium from all IV solutions
Calcium chloride 10 mg/kg IV
    or
Calcium gluconate 30 mg/kg slowly
Induce alkalosis (sodium bicarbonate 1 mEq/kg IV and/or hyperventilation)
Clear calcium from the line first
5% dextrose > 2 mL/kg/h IV
Insulin 0.1 U/kg/h, check glucose
Kayexalate 1–2 g/kg PO or PR

Vagolytic medications (e.g., atropine) frequently increase heart rate and are the first line of therapy. This treatment is useful in overriding lower escape rhythms of either junctional or ventricular origin. If atropine is unsuccessful in increasing heart rate, intravenous isoproterenol is often efficacious.

Severe Sinus Node Dysfunction

Frequently, severely compromised sinus node function, such as occurs in sick sinus syndrome, is refractory to such therapy. If sinus bradycardia persists and is associated with hemodynamic compromise, cardiac pacing is indicated.

Conduction Delay and Blockade

Treatment of these bradycardias follows approximately the same schema. Although atropine is frequently used initially, it is often unsuccessful. Isoproterenol or even epinephrine may be required for conduction delay and may provide sufficient time to institute either transvenous or transthoracic pacemaking. In the presence of hemodynamic compromise associated with conduction delay, the possibility of providing temporary or permanent electrical cardiac pacemaking should be strongly considered (see subsequent description of pacing options). Clearly, cardiac pacemaking must be at the ventricular level in AV conduction defects.

The duration of pacemaking after the acute onset of AV conduction delay is a matter of concern. Frequently, normal conduction may be expected to return in 1 to 2 weeks. After 2 weeks, if AV conduction has not returned to normal, permanent cardiac pacemaking will probably be required.

TACHYDYSRHYTHMIAS
Atrial Dysrhythmias
Atrial Extrasystoles

Atrial extrasystoles frequently occur in healthy individuals and children admitted to the pediatric ICU.

Identification Atrial extrasystole is recognized by the early, premature occurrence of a P wave followed by a QRS complex (Table 9.4). The premature QRS complex may have the same morphology as the preceding QRS complexes, or it may be aberrantly conducted and thus be dissimilar from preceding QRS complexes. Because of the extremely rapid rate of repolarization of the conducting tissue in the infant's myocardium, aberrant conduction rarely occurs in children under 18 months of age.

Differentiation from Ventricular Extrasystoles Differentiating atrial extrasystoles from ventricular extrasystoles may be difficult, especially in children (Table 9.5). Useful points include the following:

Table 9.4

Electrocardiogram Forms of Premature Atrial Contractions

Early P wave, normal QRS
Early P wave blocked in AV node
Early P wave, blocked in bundle branches, wide QRS with high likelihood of right bundle
  branch block (RBBB)

Table 9.5

Comparison of Premature Atrial Contraction (PAC) and Premature Ventricular Contraction (PVC)

PAC—resets sinus node, no compensatory pause
PVC—does not reset sinus node, compensatory pause
PAC—most have normal QRS; some have no QRS (blocked); some have RBBB pattern
PVC—wide and bizarre in any shape

RBBB, right bundle branch block.

- Aberrancy does not occur in children younger than 18 months of age
- Right bundle branch block (RBBB) pattern occurs more frequently in aberrantly conducted premature atrial contractions (PACs)
- Recognition of the RSR′ pattern in V1 is suggestive of an aberrantly conducted PAC (Fig. 9.4)
- Occurrence of a compensatory pause suggests that the premature beat is a ventricular ectopic beat
- PVCs generally demonstrate a different initial vector from the preceding sinus beats, whereas PACs do not

Despite these differences, it may be impossible to differentiate a given PAC with aberrancy from a PVC.

Sinus Tachycardia

Sinus tachycardia (ST), although defined in adults as heart rate greater than 100 beats/minute, cannot be so readily defined in children.

Identification ST is identified by recognizing:

- One-to-one AV conduction
- Regular R-R intervals
- Regular QRS morphology
- Abnormally fast rate

Occurrence ST frequently occurs in response to stress and is often not associated with any hemodynamic impairment. ST occurs:

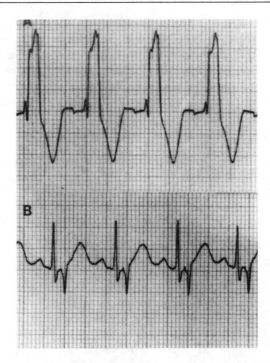

Figure 9.4. Tachycardia in a child after an AV canal repair with right bundle branch block. (A) In lead V_1, note the rsr' pattern, as would be seen in an aberrantly conducted PAC. (B) In lead 2, the PQRS relationship is obvious.

- After exercise, surgery, and ingestion of certain drugs
- With fever
- In the postanesthetic state
- During anemia, hypothyroidism, pain, and anxiety

Because ST is a normal physiologic compensation for a pathologic state, treatment is not indicated and can be disastrous.

Supraventricular Tachydysrhythmia

The most frequently observed pathologic dysrhythmia in pediatric practice is paroxysmal supraventricular tachycardia (SVT), which includes paroxysmal atrial tachycardia (PAT).SVT with aberrant AV conduction is extremely uncommon in children. SVT is caused by the "reentry" phenomenon, which occurs when the atria are excited through the aberrant, retrograde entry of an electrical impulse along a conducting pathway back into the atria, causing a circular movement of depolarization.

Clinical Presentation In general, children with SVT present with congestive cardiac failure. SVT may occur in utero and lead to the birth of a hydropic newborn infant. In older children, SVT may be confused with any of several other causes of low output, including cardiac failure, fever, sepsis, septic shock, and volume contraction. Chest pain may also be the presenting symptom in children with SVT, and screaming and irritability may be the only symptoms in infants.

Diagnosis In paroxysmal supraventricular tachycardia:

- ECG demonstrates regular R-R intervals and narrow QRS complexes (Fig. 9.5A); however, abnormal P wave morphology and a deranged P- R relationship with prolonged P-R intervals and absent or difficult- to-define P waves usually occur (Fig. 9.5B)

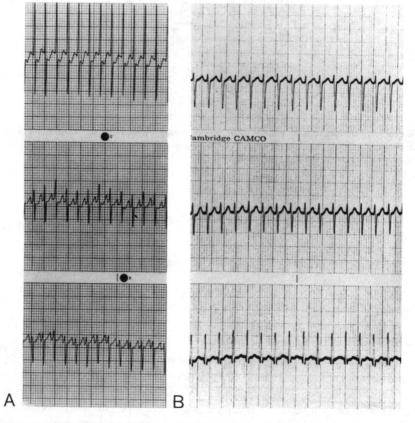

Figure 9.5. Two examples of neonatal SVT. Note narrow, regular QRS complexes, regular P-R intervals, and a heart rate of 300 beats/minute. The regular P waves that are evident in (A) are not as clearly defined in (B).

- Heart rates in infants and neonates may be 200 to 300 beats/minute; in older children, 150 to 250 beats/minute is more common.
- Normal P-R interval and a normal QRS complex, except in the Lown-Ganong-Levine syndrome, with a short P-R interval and a normal QRS complex
- P-R interval exceeds 100 ms in children between the ages of 3 and 16 years, 120 ms in adults, and 80 ms in children under 3 years

Treatment After adequate oxygenation has been assured, the first priority is to abort the SVT. Chronic SVT may cause an underlying cardiomyopathy.

In older children and in adults, these maneuvers include carotid sinus massage and the Valsalva maneuver. In younger children, firm abdominal pressure often leads to a bearing-down response in children. Ocular pressure, which carries a high risk of retinal detachment, is no longer recommended.

Elicit Diving Reflex This complex neurologic reflex is elicited by providing an iced water (0° C) stimulus to the head and/or face of the child. The physician should be prepared to treat profound bradycardias and even asystole rapidly, which may result from vagotonic methods of aborting supraventricular dysrhythmias.

Pharmacotherapy

- Edrophonium bromide (Tensilon) can be given intravenously (0.1 mg/kg). This short-acting cholinesterase inhibitor increases concentrations of endogenous acetylcholine and thus vagal tone.
- α-Adrenergic sympathomimetic agents lead to an elevation in systemic vascular resistance and reflex vagal stimulation of the myocardium. Both methoxamine and phenylephrine have been reported to be useful for this purpose.
- Digitalization was once, but is no longer, standard first-line therapy for conversion of SVT in infants and older children. Rapid digitalization intravenously, if necessary over 4 to 6 hours, frequently converts supraventricular tachydysrhythmias. The use of digoxin for initially converting SVT, atrial fibrillation, and atrial flutter in children may be contraindicated.
- Adenosine has become the drug of first choice for the reentry SVT.
- Propranolol and other β-blocking agents, such as esmolol, have proven useful in converting supraventricular tachydysrhythmias
- Propranolol is particularly effective in treating SVT resulting from Wolff-Parkinson-White syndrome.
- Quinidine and procainamide, other agents that block intraventricular conduction, may be useful in severe cases of refractory SVT.
- Verapamil, a calcium channel blocker, has been reported to be useful, although hypotension may be a complication. Because of its myocardial depressant and peripheral vasodilator effects, Verapamil must be used with great care in combination with β-blockade.

Cardioversion Synchronized direct-current cardioversion (0.5–2 J/kg) is usually effective in the child who presents with hypoperfusion or becomes acutely hypoperfused, hypotensive, or acidotic or in whom pharmacologic therapy has been ineffective. Repeated attempts are indicated, and the dose may be increased to 5 J/kg. Previous digitalization is not a contraindication to cardioversion in the face of life-threatening SVT with hemodynamic collapse.

Remember that cardioversion can result in asystole or severe bradycardia. If all of the above methods have failed, intra-atrial cardiac pacing may be required. The atrial rate is increased above the supraventricular rate and then suddenly withdrawn. A recent report of esophageal overdrive pacing for SVT provides promise.

After conversion, those children without Wolff-Parkinson-White syndrome are best treated by digitalization. Those with Wolff-Parkinson-White syndrome are best maintained on propranolol, preferably orally.

Atrial Fibrillation

Rapid chaotic depolarization of multiple atrial foci results in disorganized, ineffective, atrial contraction accompanied by a variable response from the ventricles.

Clinical Occurrence Atrial fibrillation may occur in rheumatic heart disease, mitral valve disease, hyperthyroidism, pulmonary embolus, pericarditis, atrial septal defects, Ebstein's anomaly, and cardiomyopathies. The loss of atrial filling during atrial fibrillation is usually better tolerated in children than in adults.

Electrocardiographic Findings Electrocardiography reveals the following:

- Rapid, irregular, ventricular response
- Irregular R-R intervals
- Absent P waves (Fig. 9.6)

The atrial rate may vary between 350 and 600 times/minute, with prominent (coarse), small (fine), or inapparent P waves.

Atrial Flutter

Atrial flutter is characterized by a rapid, uniform, sawtooth flutter wave that occurs between 250 and 500 times/minute. Causes include:

- Various types of congenital heart disease
- Cardiomyopathies
- Rheumatic disease
- Mitral valve prolapse
- Pericarditis

Atrial flutter appears less frequently than atrial fibrillation in children, and occasionally occurs in an anatomically normal heart. When atrial flutter occurs in a child younger than 1 year of age, it is likely to be associated with the Wolff-Parkinson-White syndrome.

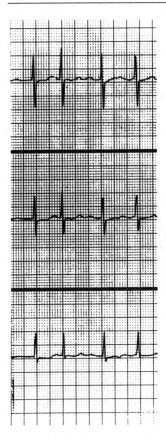

Figure 9.6. Atrial fibrillation. Note the absence of P waves and the irregular P-R interval with normal QRS morphology (V_4, V_5, V_6).

Electrocardiographic Findings Flutter waves are atrial depolarizations that last up to 180 ms (Fig. 9.7A). Leads II, III, aVF, and V_1 are the leads that most frequently show flutter waves. AV conduction is almost always blocked to some degree, resulting in an irregular ventricular response (Fig. 9.7B). QRS morphology is the same as that for normal sinus beats, though aberrant conduction may also occur.

Treatment As in other dysrhythmias, the underlying hemodynamic status and diagnosis dictate the therapy.

Pharmacotherapy In hemodynamically stable patients, atrial flutter and fibrillation may best be treated with intravenous digitalization. If the underlying diagnosis includes the Wolff-Parkinson-White syndrome, intravenous propranolol or a short-acting β-blocker is preferable. Disopyramide and verapamil have been used to treat flutter and fibrillation. Procainamide and quinidine have also been useful in treating refractory flutter and fibrillation.

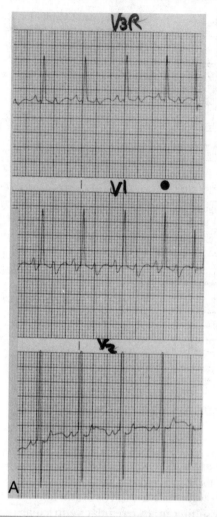

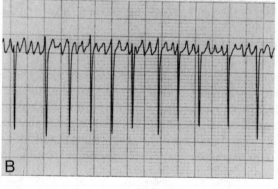

Overdrive Atrial Pacing When pharmacologic maneuvers have been unsuccessful, the safest method of converting atrial flutter is overdrive atrial pacing, which can be performed with an indwelling intracardiac catheter or via an esophageal pacing electrode. Atrial pacing should be at a rate approximately 20 to 30 beats greater than the intrinsic atrial rhythm and continued for at least 60 seconds. The pacing voltage should be three or four times greater than the atrial capture threshold. It should then be rapidly terminated.

Cardioversion The most efficacious way of converting atrial fibrillation and flutter is by synchronized direct-current cardioversion. Standby pacing should be available and appropriate anesthesia should be provided. If cardioversion is followed by rapid relapse, intravenous digitalization may be indicated as might the addition of procainamide. An alternative to this tactic is the use of propranolol, which, through slowing AV conduction, may maintain the conversion to sinus rhythm.

Multifocal Atrial Tachycardia

This condition has been reported in children as young as 1 week of age. The ECG shows more than 100 atrial beats/minute and discrete nonsinus P waves with at least three morphologies. The P-P, P-R, and R-R intervals are irregular with an isoelectric baseline. The rhythm occurs postoperatively in myocarditis and mitral valve disease.

Treatment requires correction of the underlying abnormalities. β-blockers (i.e., metoprolol, esmolol) and calcium channel blockers are the major therapeutic choices. Magnesium and amiodarone have proven to work. Electrical cardioversion and digoxin are not recommended.

Junctional Ectopic Tachycardia

This arrhythmia may be a manifestation of AV block and is most commonly seen in the postoperative period (ventricular septal defect, Mustard, and tetralogy of Fallot), but it can occur with myocarditis. It also occurs in infants younger than 6 months of age.

Electrocardiographic Findings

- QRS rate is abnormal for age, usually between 130 and 200 beats/minute and occasionally as high as 300 beats/minute
- R-R interval is regular
- QRS morphology is similar to that of normal sinus beats
- Retrograde conducted P waves follow each QRS; occasionally, P waves cannot be seen

Figure 9.7A–B. Two Examples of atrial flutter. (A) shows flutter with a regular 2:1 AV conduction block and regular P-R intervals with a rate of 104 (leads I–III). This example of flutter is more subtle than that for another patient (B) (lead V_1), showing the characteristic sawtooth pattern with variable R-R intervals.

Therapy Therapy for this dysrhythmia is generally unsatisfactory but includes:

- Correction of metabolic abnormalities that may exacerbate the dysrhythmia
- Administration of digitalis, which may lower the rate but often is unsuccessful in converting this dysrhythmia to sinus rhythm.
- Paired ventricular pacing, in which ventricular pacing is adjusted to such a rapid rate that although every beat causes an electrical QRS complex, effective ventricular contraction only occurs with every other beat. Close monitoring of cardiac output and perfusion is necessary.
- Intravenous propranolol, if pacing is unsuccessful
- Amiodarone
- Propafenone
- Intravenous magnesium
- Induced hypothermia
- Ablation of the ectopic site by surgical manipulation, in severe cases, especially postoperatively, after medical failure before the patient is moribund

Ventricular Dysrhythmias

Premature Ventricular Contraction (PVC)

A PVC is characterized by a wide, abnormal, slurred QRS complex, usually followed by a T wave with an inverted axis without a preceding P wave (Fig. 9.8). Points by which to differentiate PVC from aberrantly conducted PAC are outlined in Table 9.5.

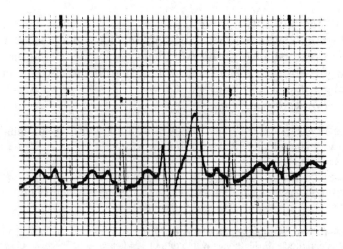

Figure 9.8. A single ventricular extrasystole. Note wide QRS with opposite vector from sinus QRS, abnormal T morphology, and fully compensatory pause.

PVCs can be described morphologically as uniform or multiform (old terms: unifocal or multifocal). Their ECG appearance results from the fusion of an ectopic ventricular beat with a supraventricular beat, and thus their morphology lies between that of a sinus beat and a PVC (Fig. 9.9). Because a fusion beat requires ventricular ectopic focus, the significance of a fusion beat is the same as that of any other PVC. These damaged foci constantly pose the risk of deterioration to a sustained ventricular tachycardia (VT) or ventricular fibrillation with hemodynamic collapse (Figs. 9.10 and 9.11).

Ventricular Tachycardia

VT can arise from an electrolyte or metabolic imbalance, cardiac tumor, cardiac damage after surgery, myocarditis, or a cardiomyopathy, or it may be idiopathic. It can also occur in the prolonged Q-T syndromes (Jervell, Lange-Nielsen, or Romano-Ward). Frequently in prolonged Q-T syndromes, torsade de pointes is seen (Fig. 9.12).

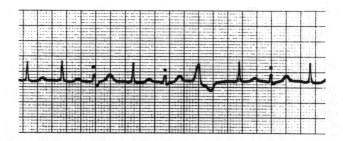

Figure 9.9. This rhythm strip shows an example of fusion beats marked with a solid dot. There is also a ventricular ectopic beat. A fusion beat represents a combination of a ventricular ectopic beat with a supraventricular beat and is intermediate in form between the two. Their significance is the same as for ventricular ectopic beats.

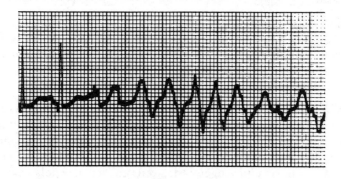

Figure 9.10. Sinus rhythm degenerating into ventricular tachycardia.

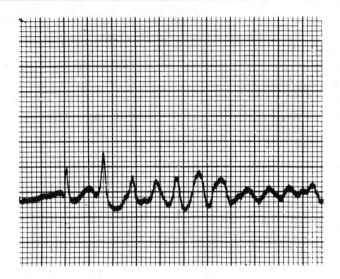

Figure 9.11. Bradycardia with a ventricular ectopic (R-on-T) initiating coarse ventricular fibrillation. Note disorganized, rapid chaotic electrical activity.

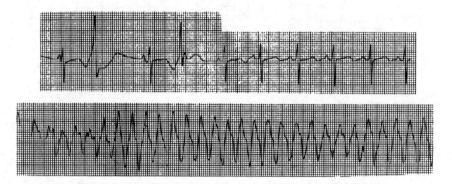

Figure 9.12. A 6-year-old who presented with syncope and an ECG suggesting bigeminy. The sinus Q-Tc is 0.52 seconds. Moments later torsade de pointes developed. This was successfully treated by intravenous magnesium, suggesting acquired Q-T syndrome. The child was receiving amiodarone.

Torsade Torsade de pointes is a variant of VT and frequently is difficult to treat. It is characterized by variation in the QRS height, so that the complexes (i.e., pointes) appear to twist (i.e., torsade) around the baseline. The mechanism is poorly understood, but the presence of prominent U waves and T-U wave abnormalities suggests delayed ventricular repolarization and a reentry mechanism. On the other hand, after-depolarizations may be occurring. This rhythm occurs in antidysrhythmic drug toxicity, especially from type I (e.g., quinidine) and II drugs, tricyclic overdose, hypovolemia, and prolonged Q-T syndromes.

Ventricular Fibrillation

Ventricular fibrillation (VF) is manifest by chaotic, irregular ventricular depolarization and is characterized by the absence of regular recognizable QRS complexes.

Differential Diagnosis Characteristic findings of both VF and torsade include:

- Rates greater than 150 beats/minute
- Wide QRS complexes
- Inadequate circulation

VT is associated with:

- Preexisting AV dissociation
- Preexisting fusion beats

SVT is characterized by:

- RSR' pattern in V1
- Preexcitation phenomenon

Vagomimetic maneuvers rarely affect VT and frequently slow or abort SVTs. Adenosine may be of particular help in diagnosing the tachycardia.

Therapy Treatment of rhythms that predispose to VT and VF is indicated when there is either hemodynamic compromise or a rhythm that may rapidly deteriorate, including:

- PVCs in couplets or triplets
- Multiform ventricular premature beats
- PVCs occurring on or near the T wave (Fig. 9.10)
- More than 6 PVCs/minute.

Although ventricular bigeminy is a stable dysrhythmia, hemodynamic compromise caused by the inadequate ventricular contractions during the ectopic beat may require therapy directed at preventing the PVCs (Table 9.6).

Premature Ventricular Contractions

After metabolic stabilization and correction of hypoxia and hypercarbia, the acute therapy for PVCs is intravenous lidocaine. If this is unsuccessful in altering the pattern of PVCs, it may be repeated, and a continuous intravenous lidocaine infusion with serum levels to guide therapy is indicated.

Table 9.6
When to Treat a Premature Ventricular Contraction

High frequency (> 6/min)
Three or more in a row (VT)
Multifocal (different QRS forms)
Vulnerable period (PVC on T wave)

Intravenous procainamide is the next therapeutic step and may be continued either orally or intravenously. Disopyramide, a quinidine-like drug, is an oral agent that prevents and suppresses PVCs and may eventually be available for intravenous use in the United States. Oral quinidine is also effective in the long-term suppression of PVCs.

Ventricular Tachycardia

Pharmacologic Treatment The treatment of VT is again guided by the hemodynamic status of the patient. If cardiac output is maintained, the first drug of choice is intravenous lidocaine repeated twice and followed by a continuous infusion. If VT persists, intravenous procainamide or phenytoin is frequently successful. Bretylium tosylate, an adrenergic nerve-blocking drug given intravenously, is effective in terminating VF and VT in children and should be considered in children with resistant VT. Although it works within several minutes in VF, it may take up to 2 hours to be effective in VT. Intravenous amiodarone has also been used occasionally to treat resistant VT in children. A short-acting blocker such as esmolol may be useful in suppressing recurrent VT. Treatment with magnesium (1 to 2 g in adults) intravenously often will treat ventricular dysrhythmias.

Cardioversion If pharmacologic treatment has been unsuccessful and hemodynamic compromise is present, electrocardioversion is the therapy of choice. VT with hypotension requires cardioversion (Fig. 9.13). Again, anesthetic and airway management aspects of the child should be ensured before defibrillation. Doses of 1 to 4 J/kg are necessary and may be repeated until sinus rhythm occurs. For ventricular fibrillation or VT refractory to defibrillation, overdrive ventricular pacing may suppress an ectopic focus, and paired ventricular pacing may also be efficacious.

Ventricular Fibrillation

The therapy for VF is the same as that for cardiac arrest (see Chapter 1):
- Correction of underlying acidosis and metabolic abnormalities
- Airway maintenance
- Intubation
- Ventilation with 100% FIO_2

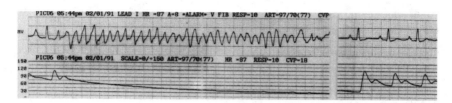

Figure 9.13. Simultaneous recording of ECG (upper panel) and blood pressure (lower panel) in a 12-year-old with cardiomyopathy. A fusion beat initiated VT. Blood pressure fell rapidly; cardioversion successfully restored sinus rhythm and pressure.

Intravenous lidocaine should be administered and repeated if there is evidence of deterioration of the underlying rhythm toward VF. In all instances of VF, however, cardiopulmonary resuscitation and treatment of the arrhythmia by direct cardioversion is indicated. A starting dose of 2 J/kg, followed by doubling until cardioversion occurs, is indicated. As mentioned previously, intravenous bretylium tosylate may be efficacious.

Coarse versus Fine VF Fine VF may mimic an isoelectric ECG and is generally thought to be more difficult to convert than coarse VF. The addition of a potent catecholamine such as isoproterenol or epinephrine and even the use of intravenous calcium may convert a fine ventricular fibrillation or apparent asystole into coarse ventricular fibrillation or VT, which is more amenable to electrical cardioversion. This therapy may be useful in the desperate situation of apparent asystole or fine ventricular fibrillation.

Prolonged Q-T Syndromes Ventricular tachydysrhythmias that occur in prolonged Q-T syndromes may be either pause-dependent (usually acquired or drug induced) or adrenergic-dependent (usually congenital or familial). The former respond to magnesium, pacing, isoproterenol, and even atropine; the latter to β-blockade. In the acute ICU setting, torsade de pointes has been treated with propranolol, lidocaine, and phenytoin, but success with these agents has been poor. Intravenous magnesium sulfate (10 mg/kg) has been reported to be efficacious, especially in acquired prolonged Q-T syndromes.

THERAPEUTICS

Specific Pharmacotherapy

Antidysrhythmics have been classified into four classes (Table 9.7).

Class I. These drugs depress the fast inward sodium ion channels and thus increase the refractory period and delay the return of excitability. Resting membrane potential is generally unchanged in phase 4 and may, in fact, be depressed. Class I drugs are further divided into those agents that shorten total action potential duration (e.g., lidocaine) and those that lengthen it (e.g.,

Table 9.7
Classification of Antidysrhythmics

Class I—sodium channel blockers
A. Quinidine
   Procainamide
   Disopyramide
B. Lidocaine
   Phenytoin
   Mixetelene
   Tocainide
Class II—β-blockers
Propranolol
Timolol
Class III—prolonged repolarization
Bretylium
Amiodarone
Sotalol
Class IV—calcium channel blockers
Verapamil
Nifedipine
Ditiazem

---

quinidine). Their major effect is to slow repolarization and depress spontaneous depolarization. This class of drugs has wide clinical usage.

Class II. These drugs inhibit the catecholamine-dependent spontaneous depolarization of phase 4. Thus automaticity is slowed.

Class III. These drugs, which prolong phase 3 repolarization and thus prolong the effective refractory period, are useful for treating and suppressing ventricular tachydysrhythmias.

Class IV. Drugs that block the calcium channels prolong conduction and increase nodal and bundle of His tissue refractory time. They are, therefore, quite effective in treating reentry-type dysrhythmias.

Electrical Cardioversion

Indications

Direct-current countershock (DCC) is most useful in treating dysrhythmias arising from reentrant phenomena, including atrial flutter, atrial fibrillation, SVT, VT, and ventricular fibrillation (see Chapter 1). The major indication for DCC is life-threatening tachydysrhythmias with hemodynamic compromise. DCC also may be used to convert less threatening dysrhythmias such as atrial flutter and fibrillation. Its use in these cases is considered "elective."

Technique

The electrodes are placed over the fifth intercostal space in the midaxillary line and in the second intercostal space just right of the sternum. Electrode impedance should be reduced by the liberal use of conducting electrode jelly; however, the conducting jelly areas should not be contiguous to avoid "shorting" the circuit. When possible, anterior-posterior electrode placement is used, because smaller currents are then required. A dose of 1 to 4 J/kg is recommended for VT and SVT.

Adequate sedation is mandatory, and in children, a short-acting general anesthetic is probably indicated. In elective DCC, the shock is synchronized with the patient; ECG to avoid the T wave and potential deterioration into life-threatening ventricular dysrhythmias. The rest of the procedure is the same as stated previously. Usually, lower doses are effective for SVT (0.5 to 2 J/kg).

Complications

Complications of DCC are rare but not insignificant. They include:

- Superficial burns
- Bradycardias caused by enhanced vagal tone with heart block
- Sinus exit block (frequently requires atropine)
- Total sinus arrest

Acute cardiac pacing may be emergently required.

PACEMAKERS

Pacemakers are simply controlled pulse generators in which output current (in milliamperes), pulse interval (in milliseconds), and the ability to be inhibited are incorporated. Electrical cardiac pacing can be used not only to cause an asystolic heart to beat but also to convert certain dysrhythmias and to optimize cardiac output in the critically ill child.

Electrodes may be unipolar or bipolar and may be attached to the heart in various fashions. Clearly, both an anode (i.e., positive electrode that causes hyperpolarization) and a cathode (i.e., negative electrode that causes reduction in membrane potential) are necessary to cause a cardiac contraction.

Unipolar Pacemakers

In pacemakers, the anode is not in direct contact with the heart. In temporary pacemakers, the anode is usually a skin wire or electrode patch; in permanent pacemakers, it is usually the generator case itself.

Bipolar Pacemakers

These devices have both an anode and a cathode placed in contact with the myocardium. Transvenous pacemakers are this type.

Briefly, bipolar electrodes sense better, and the pacemaker artifact is less noticeable. In addition, as anodal stimulation is more likely to lead to a ventricular dysrhythmia than is cathodal stimulation, bipolar pacers are more frequently implicated as a cause of ventricular dysrhythmias.

Indications

Symptomatic bradydysrhythmias or anticipation thereof are the major indications for pacemakers in children (Table 9.8). These include both sinus node dysfunction and AV block. The single most common indication for cardiac pacing in children is postoperative heart block. The types of surgery that commonly result in the need for pacing include repair of:

Table 9.8
Indications for Cardiac Pacing

Congenital AV block
1. Ventricular rate < 55 beats/min in a neonate or < 50 beats/min in an older child
2. Atrial rate > 140 beats/min
3. Association with other congenital heart defects
4. Congestive heart failure from low heart rate unresponsive to medical therapy
5. Syncope, history of Stokes-Adams attacks
6. Decreasing exercise tolerance
7. Block located at or below bundle of His in the asymptomatic patient
8. Dizziness associated with arrhythmia or combined with Q-T prolongation
9. Ventricular ectopy refractory to drug treatment
Surgical heart block
1. Complete or second-degree AV block present 2 weeks after surgery and located at or below the bundle of His
2. Symptoms of syncope, low cardiac output, and congestive heart failure no matter what the site of block is
Acquired nonsurgical heart block
If symptomatic or if block is at or below bundle of His
Sinus bradycardia
1. Symptoms of dizziness
2. Sleeping heart rate < 35 beats/min
Sick sinus syndrome
SVT refractory to medical treatment
1. Inability to be treated with surgical ablation and medication causes severe bradycardia
2. Demonstration that slow atrial pacing controls SVT in the catheterization laboratory
3. Surgical destruction of the normal AV conduction system necessary and pacemaker needed to ensure adequate ventricular response
4. Primary treatment for SVT

- TGA
- AV canal
- Tricuspid atresia
- Tetralogy of Fallot
- Complex congenital heart disease with Wolff-Parkinson-White syndrome

The other major cause of bradyarrhythmias is nonsurgical complete heart block, which may be congenital and associated with such disease states as endocardial fibroelastosis, prolonged Q-T interval, myotonic dystrophy, and mesothelioma.

Pacemakers have also been reported as effective therapy for:

- Recurrent, severe vasovagal syncope
- Atrial arrhythmias associated with Emery-Dreifuss muscular dystrophy
- Recurrent VT
- SVT
- Fatal tachydysrhythmias

Temporary Pacing

Indications

Temporary pacing is indicated for patients in the ICU for similar disorders until a permanent pacemaker can be implanted. It is also used to support patients through life-threatening but reversible situations including:

- Profound bradycardias
- Conduction blockade
- SVT
- VT
- Escape rhythms
- Drug toxicity from digitalis, propranolol, or verapamil
- Electrolyte imbalances such as hypokalemia or hyperkalemia
- Immediately after cardiac surgery, for backup and support for the transiently depressed myocardium that may have a rate-dependent output
- Diagnosis of several arrhythmias

Methods of Placement

The pacemaker may be placed through the jugular, subclavian, brachial, or femoral veins. ECG guidance is recommended, and pacemaker operation in the VOO mode will demonstrate capture. Atrial or ventricular pacing is possible.

Temporary pacemakers are either routinely attached to postoperative cardiac patients by surgically implanted wires or used in conjunction with transvenous or transthoracic emergent pacing.

Modes of Pacing

Transthoracic Pacing Transthoracic pacing is readily established by placing a pacing wire into the right or left ventricle via a spinal needle inserted either subxiphoid or through the left fifth intercostal space. These pacemakers provide the most rapid means of pacing the arrested heart and are indicated if time does not allow transvenous insertion.

Transesophageal Pacing This emergency pacing alternative is less invasive. The esophagus is intimately related to the left atrium, and thus electrode placement can be established without surgery or transvenous pacing. This mode of pacing is especially useful for:

- Overdrive suppression pacing of SVT
- Terminating reentrant phenomenon-dependent dysrhythmias
- Atrial flutter and fibrillation conversion

It is of less use for treating ventricular dysrhythmias and not useful at all for managing heart block, since only atrial pacing is achieved.

Its use requires a stronger pulse generator because cardiac tissue is further from the electrode (0 to 40 mA at a pulse width of 0 to 10 ms). A standard bipolar intracardiac pacing catheter can be positioned in the esophagus with ECG guidance. This technique provides a useful approach to atrial dysrhythmias in the pediatric ICU.

Transcutaneous Pacing For this noninvasive method, large pacing electrodes are placed on the chest and back. Special equipment is required. Current is increased until ventricular capture is produced.

Pacemaker Use

The pacemaker rate is set according to the patient's need, and in pediatric patients, this varies widely with age (Fig. 9.1). Once an ECG QRS complex is produced (i.e., capture), the patient's blood pressure should be assessed. If it is not improved, then increasing pacemaker output will not help. An increased rate may help, however. If there is capture without pressure generation, electromechanical dissociation exists and requires appropriate therapy, not more pacing.

Settings for Capture

Tachydysrhythmias are treated either by slow "underdrive" atrial pacing, which may interrupt SVT, or by overdriving the abnormal rhythm with a fast rate and acutely discontinuing pacing. For this reason, the pacemaker must be capable of high rates (200 to 600/minute).

The output current to achieve the threshold potential generally required by a temporary pacemaker is usually below 1 mA, often 0.5 mA or less. The maintenance current should be set two to five times above this threshold to ensure constant capture. The threshold current required should be routinely checked, and the output control adjusted. In an emergency situation when the electrode position is questionable, the pacer can be set to maximum output (i.e., 20 mA) to capture, and the current can then be slowly decreased as proper positioning is obtained.

Synchronous Demand Pacemaking Mode

This method of pacing is provided by using a sensing circuit to inhibit ventricular pacing in the critical period after an intrinsic cardiac contraction. In this mode, the heart is ventricularly paced and sensed, and the pacemaker is inhibited (VVI mode). Competition with the patient's own intrinsic rhythm is prevented and there is less chance of ventricular tachydysrhythmias. Also, in this VVI mode, a backup rate can be set below the patient's intrinsic rate as a safety feature should a sudden bradydysrhythmia occur. The sensing dial should be set with sensitivity to more than 6 mV consistently, and it should be noted that the sensing indicator is being triggered.

In the emergency situation, when there is not intrinsic rhythm, the asynchronous mode is used. The heart is ventricularly paced, not sensed, and there is no response to the patient's intrinsic rate (VOO mode). This mode is not indicated if the patient has an intrinsic rate.

AV Sequential Pacemakers

The physiologic AV sequential pacemaker, especially useful in children with hemodynamic compromise, can pace independently, both atrially and ventricularly (i.e., anode and cathode for each chamber). The operator can set both atrial and ventricular output and set the ventricular rate. In addition, the duration between the atrial impulse and the ventricular impulse (P-R interval) can be varied. These pacemakers thus are double-chamber pacing (i.e., atrial and ventricular) and double-chamber sensing, can have double-mode response (atrial inhibited, ventricular paced), and can be programmed to the universal mode (DDD).

Complications

Complications of cardiac pacing are multiple but clinically uncommon.

- Pericardial bleeding and tamponade, associated with removal of pacing wires inserted temporarily
- Ventricular dysrhythmias and the potential for decreased cardiac output as the result of poorly timed pacing at an inadequate rate
- Failure to capture, caused by either myocardial damage or improper electrode replacement

THE PROBLEM TACHYCARDIA

Suggestive and Distinguishing Features

Narrow complex tachycardias can be atrial, junctional, or even ventricular in origin, especially in children. Wide complex tachycardias are due to either VT or aberrantly conducted SVT. Diagnosis depends on whether or not there is a P wave and its timing, morphology, and relationship to the QRS complexes. In SVT, clear P waves should have a constant relationship to the QRS complex. If AV dissociation is present, the tachycardia has a lower origin (JET or VT). If the frontal plan axis alters, then atrial origin is unlikely.

The presence of aberrantly conducted PACs before the onset of the tachycardia with similar morphology to the tachycardias complexes suggests SVT, but this is not always easy to determine (Fig. 9.14). Detailed 12-lead ECG analysis may reveal the underlying source of the tachycardia (Fig. 9.15).

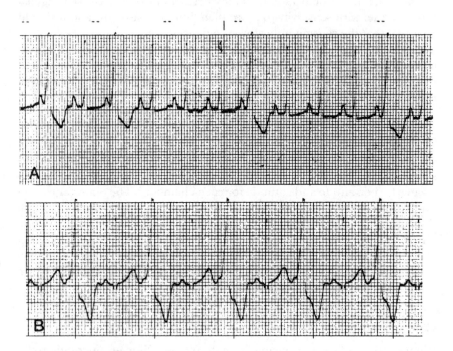

Figure 9.14. Two different examples of wide QRS complexes. Timing is crucial. Is (A) an example of ventricular extrasystoles, fusion beats, or preexcitation with aberrant conduction? The P-P interval is regular (sinus node not reset). The abnormal QRS complexes are premature. The P- R intervals in the first three abnormal complexes are shorter than the last, while QRS morphology is constant. Thus, these are most likely ventricular ectopics occurring before AV nodal conduction has occurred. In (B), the P waves are regular, but every other one is variably lost in the QRS. These have a compensatory pause. In effect, these are more obviously ectopic PVCs than those in A.

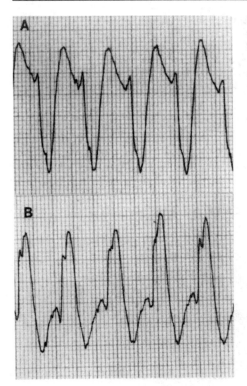

Figure 9.15. Wide complex tachycardia (145 beats/minute, regular). In (A), obvious P waves are absent in lead V_1. By observing lead II (B), clear P waves and a P-QRS 1:1 relationship are seen, identifying this as SVT.

The presence of fusion beats is also critical (Figs. 9.9 and 9.16). Premature beats with a combination of atrial and ventricular characteristics occur when an atrial beat occurs almost simultaneously with an ectopic ventricular beat.

Frequently, vagal maneuvers may slow or convert SVT (Fig. 9.17). Responses to carotid massage, Valsalva maneuvers, or ice to the face (i.e., diving reflex) may demonstrate the atrial origin of the tachycardia and guide further therapy.

Treating Persistent Tachycardia

What should be done if, in consultation with a cardiologist and after several diagnostic ECGs, the rhythm remains undiagnosed and the patient's clinical condition warrants therapy? If the child is hypotensive and in need of urgent therapy, follow these steps:

1. Direct-current countershock, starting at 1 J/kg and increasing to 4 J/kg, will convert both SVT and VT 85 to 95% of the time. QRS synchronization is preferred but may be difficult in wide complex tachycardia. Cardioversion is not indicated in digoxin-induced tachycardias.

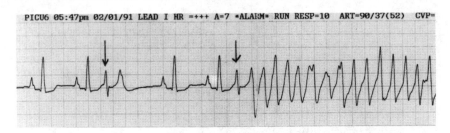

PICU6 05:47pm 02/01/91 LEAD I HR =+++ A=7 *ALARM* RUN RESP=10 ART=90/37(52) CVP=

Figure 9.16. ECG in a 17-year-old with cardiomyopathy. Demonstrating a sinus rhythm (morphologically abnormal P waves, ST depression) with fusion beats (arrows) preceding a fusion R-on-T-initiated VT.

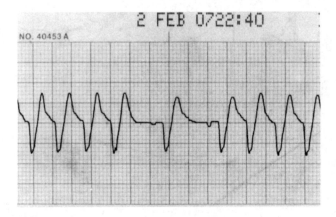

2 FEB 0722:40

NO. 40453 A

Figure 9.17. Wide complex tachycardia that was slowed, with emergence of P waves, by carotid sinus massage. This suggests that the underlying rhythm is SVT.

2. Correct electrolyte abnormalities
3. Ensure volume resuscitation
4. Administer oxygen

If the patient is relatively stable and the rhythm still uncertain, a trial of therapy is indicated. The choice is between drugs and pacing depends on the clinical situation and availability of equipment. Pharmacologic therapy is often more readily available. At this stage, a hunch must be played:

- In wide complex tachycardia, if VT is more likely, lidocaine should be given as many as three times
- In narrow complex tachycardia, a bolus of adenosine has few side effects and will rapidly convert SVT (and possibly JET)
- Esmolol, a short-acting cardioselection β1-agent, may convert SVT and VT in children
- Magnesium may be of help and has few side effects

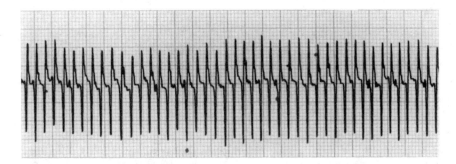

Figure 9.18. An ECG with apparent narrow complex tachycardia at a rate of nearly 600 beats/minute. This is from a 6-year-old child during a prolonged myoclonic seizure who did not respond to adenosine. Valium resolved the rhythm disturbance. Despite the alarming ECG appearance, 1:1 conduction at a rate of 600, or a ventricular rate of 600, is extremely unlikely, if not impossible. This is a neurologic, not a cardiac, problem.

If the rhythm persists and remains unresponsive to therapy, and no clues have been gained, pacing and cardioversion should be considered. Other drugs (e.g., bretylium, digoxin) have significant risks and are best avoided in an uncertain situation, especially after the above agents have been tried. Finally, understanding the child's entire condition and interpreting this with the cardiac status may occasionally resolve the most difficult ECG dysrhythmia problem (Fig. 9.18).

SURGICAL TREATMENT OF DYSRHYTHMIAS

Surgical ablative techniques have progressed from ablation of the AV mode, with resultant third-degree heart block and pacemaker placement, to specific interruption of reentry pathways. The development of percutaneous nonoperative catheter ablative techniques, using either direct-current or radiofrequency ablation, has further increased the potential for nonpharmacologic treatment of cardiac dysrhythmias. Although the major application is for treatment of chronic or relapsing tachydysrhythmias, therapy for refractory life-threatening situations is also possible. Not only may reentry dysrhythmias be treated, but foci of ectopic activity can be ablated. SVT, VT, atrial tachycardia, flutter and fibrillation, JET, and AV nodal reentry phenomena have all been treated by this approach.

This technique requires precise electrophysiologic mapping as well as specialized, interventional cardiology techniques and expertise. In the life-threatening situation, this approach may present a useful option for the refractory tachydysrhythmia.

10.

Shock and Multi-Organ System Failure

Joseph R. Tobin and Randall C. Wetzel

INTRODUCTION

Shock is a clinical syndrome of acute disruption of both microcirculatory and macrocirculatory function, leading to a general insufficiency of tissue perfusion, oxygen use, and cellular energy production that ultimately results in deranged homeostatic mechanisms and irreversible cellular damage.

CLASSIFICATION OF SHOCK STATES

Shock can be etiologically classified into:

- Hypovolemic (lack of blood volume)
- Distributive (altered vascular tone, either primary or secondary to neurologic or neurohormonal alterations)
- Cardiogenic (cardiac pump failure)
- Septic

Septic shock categories that have characteristics of all of the previous types of shock, is important, and has enough unique characteristics to require separate classification are listed in Table 10.1).

It is helpful to consider three stages in shock: compensated, uncompensated, and irreversible. In the early compensated stage, homeostatic mechanisms function to maintain essential organ perfusion. Blood pressure, urine output, and cardiac function may appear normal, although early cellular metabolic alterations already are underway.

In the decompensated stage, circulatory compensation fails because of ischemia, endothelial injury, the elaboration of host-inducible gene products and toxic materials from host and microorganisms, and often the deleterious impact of physiologic compensatory mechanisms. Eventually, cellular function deteriorates and widespread abnormalities occur in all organ systems.

When this process has caused such significant, irreparable functional loss in essential organs that death is inevitable despite temporary support, the terminal or irreversible stage of shock is reached.

Hypovolemic Shock

Causes

Hypovolemic shock results from decreased intravascular volume and, therefore, decreased venous return and myocardial preload. This intravascular fluid depletion may be a result of hemorrhage (e.g., trauma, surgery, gastrointestinal bleeding), water and electrolyte losses (including diarrhea and vomiting, diabetes insipidus, renal losses, heat stroke, intestinal obstruction, burns), or plasma losses (e.g., burns, nephrotic syndrome, sepsis, peritonitis, intestinal obstruction), all of which may be either external or internal (i.e., third space losses).

The major cause of infant mortality is shock resulting from dehydration resulting from the diarrhea and vomiting that accompany infectious gastroenteritis.

Hemorrhagic shock resulting from trauma may occur because of external or internal blood loss.

- Splenic, mesenteric, or hepatic rupture can lead quickly to profound hypovolemic shock and mandates immediate surgery.

Table 10.1
Classification of Shock

Hypovolemic
Dehydration
  Gastroenteritis
  Deprivation
  Heat stroke
Burns
Hemorrhage
Distributive
Anaphylaxis
Neurogenic
Drug toxicity
Septic
Cardiogenic
Congenital heart disease
Ischemic heart disease
  Anoxia
  Kawasaki disease
Traumatic
Infectious cardiomyopathies
Drug toxicity
Tamponade
Obstructive
Pulmonary embolism (air, blood, fat)
Cardiovascular Obstructive Lesions
Dissecting aortic injury or aneurysm
Asymmetric septal hypertrophy/idiopathic hypertrophic subaortic stenosis
Aortic stenosis
Critical pulmonic stenosis
Mitral stenosis
Critical coarctation of the aorta
Interrupted aortic arch
Septic shock
Miscellaneous
Heat stroke
Adrenal insufficiency (congenital adrenal hyperplasia, HIV, autoimmune, steroid use,
  idiopathic)
Pancreatitis
Drug overdose
  Barbiturates
  β-Antagonists
Ca^{++} channel antagonists

- Soft tissue trauma and long bone fractures can lead to less obvious massive blood loss and edema formation.
- Vascular lacerations (or penetrating trauma) and scalp lacerations may bleed profusely and rapidly compromise the circulation.

Gastrointestinal hemorrhage can occur as part of a systemic illness (e.g., coagulopathy associated with leukemia, idiopathic thrombocytopenic purpura, chemotherapy, or disseminated intravascular coagulation), gastrointestinal infection (e.g., salmonellosis, shigellosis), or a gastrointestinal tract primary lesion (Table 10.2).

Clinical Presentation

Flow is diverted away from the skin and splanchnic circulation to preserve central nervous system (CNS), myocardial, adrenal medulla, and central perfusion. Release of antidiuretic hormone (i.e., vasopressin) and stimulation of the renin-aldosterone system tend to restore and preserve intravascular volume. As a result, the patient with early compensated hypovolemic shock presents with:

- Cool extremities
- Decreased peripheral perfusion
- Tachycardia
- Decreased urine output

Table 10.2
Primary Lesions that Cause Gastrointestinal Hemorrhage

Neonates
Hemorrhage diseases of the newborn
Anorectal trauma
Infectious diarrhea
Colitis (milk and soy)
Necrotizing enterocolitis
Volvulus
Gastric ulcer/perforation
Idiopathic
Infants
Intussusception
Gastritis
Esophagitis and varices
Duodenal ulcers
Gangrenous bowel
Gastric ulcers
Children
Colonic polyps
Esophagitis and varices
Gastric and duodenal ulcers
Ulcerative colitis and Crohn's disease
Mallory-Weiss syndrome
Meckel's diverticulum
Intussusception
Henoch-Schönlein purpura

- Normal to reduced filling pressures
- Increased systemic vascular resistance
- Decreased cardiac output
- Normal blood pressure

Distributive Shock

Abnormalities in vasomotor tone can cause maldistribution of normal circulatory volume, which, if severe enough, may lead to shock. Consequent peripheral pooling and vascular shunting lead to a state of "relative hypovolemia." In addition, loss of arterial tone leads to marked hypotension.

Although it may resemble hypovolemic shock clinically, distributive shock generally arises from different causes (Table 10.3).

Neurogenic shock is most familiar after high spinal cord transection, but it may occur in severe brain stem and isolated intracranial injuries. Hypotension accompanying CNS injuries can have grave consequences on the adequacy of CNS perfusion. Spinal shock occurs with cord transections above T1, which cause total loss of sympathetic cardiovascular tone. The result is profound hypotension with systolic pressures of less than 40 mm Hg accompanied by bradycardia resulting from interrupted integrated output conduction of the cardiac accelerator center. Not surprisingly, mentation is affected and urine output is low.

Table 10.3
Distributive Shock

Anaphylaxis
Antibiotics
Vaccines
Blood
Local anesthetics
Iodine contrast media
Insects
Foods
Latax
Neurologic injury
Head injury (brainstem)
Spinal shock
Septic shock
Early phase
Drugs
Barbiturates
Phenothiazines
Tranquilizers
Antihypertensives

Cardiogenic Shock

Cardiogenic shock does not occur frequently in children, but it does account for a large number of admissions to pediatric intensive care units (PICUs). The major cause of cardiogenic shock in the PICU is surgical repair of congenital heart disease (e.g., hypoplastic left heart syndrome). Other major causes of cardiogenic shock include:

- Inflammatory processes (myocarditis)
- Ischemic infarction (as in infants with anomalous left coronary artery, isoproterenol-treated asthmatics, or children with Kawasaki disease)
- Primary cardiomyopathy (obstructive, metabolic, or degenerative)
- Secondary cardiomyopathy (infectious, toxic, and radiation)
- High-output cardiac failure (shunt related, catecholamine-induced)
- Hypoglycemia
- Metabolic abnormalities
- Hypothermia
- Asphyxial episodes
- Various drug intoxications
- Sepsis
- Supraventricular tachycardia in infants
- Junctional escape tachycardia (JET) after surgical repair of congenital heart disease
- Ventricular arrhythmias
- Trauma

Septic Shock

Shock that occurs during sepsis may result from deficient intravascular volume, maldistribution of intravascular volume, impaired myocardial function, and tissue cellular metabolic derangements (e.g., impaired oxygen use, acidosis) that make tissues unable to use whatever substrates are delivered by the compromised cardiovascular system. All of these abnormalities occur at different times during the course of septic shock, but occur earlier in septic shock than in other forms of shock.

Common Causes

The pathogens responsible for initiating or associated with septic shock in children vary with age and are listed in Table 10.4.

Distinctive Clinical Presentation

The early compensated stage of septic shock in humans is characterized by:

- Decreased vascular resistance (distributive shock)
- Increased cardiac output

Table 10.4
Common Pathogens Causing Septic Shock

Bacterial
    Group B β-hemolytic streptococci
    Enterobacteriaceae
    Listeria monocytogenes
    Staphylococcus aureus
    Streptococcus pneumoniae
    Neisseria meningitidis
    Pseudomonadaceae
Viral
    Herpesvirus
    Haemophilus influenzae
    Dengue
    Varicella
    Adenovirus
Rickettsial
    Typhus
    Rocky Mountain spotted fever
Candida albicans
Chlamydia
Malaria

- Tachycardia
- Warm extremities
- Adequate urine output

Coexisting hypovolemia may lead to a decreased output, but overt myocardial depression is not characteristic of the early, hyperdynamic shock secondary to sepsis.

The uncompensated phase is characterized by:

- Intravascular volume depletion
- Myocardial depression
- Cold, listlessness, anuria, and respiratory distress
- High vascular resistance
- Decreasing cardiac output

With ischemic injury added to that caused by endotoxins, irreversible shock is reached when multi-organ and myocardial damage is profound. This final pattern is similar to that seen in other forms of shock.

Sepsis Syndrome

The septic process may result from any infectious process, either as a primary cause of septic shock or secondary to other shock processes, most significantly by translocation of gut bacteria and secondary sepsis. When infection and bacteremia trigger a wide spectrum of host responses, sepsis or the sepsis syndrome occurs (Table 10.5). This pattern of response to sepsis has been characterized as a response in many illnesses as a generalized inflammation and has been termed the Systemic Inflammatory Response Syndrome (SIRS).

The most significant finding in sepsis syndrome is the actual presence or a high suspicion of infection. Other accompaniments include:

- Leukocytosis
- Proteinuria
- Eosinopenia
- Hypoferrinemia
- Liver function abnormalities
- Hyperglycemia
- Further manifestations of CNS injury
- Coagulation abnormalities with thrombocytopenia
- Prolonged prothrombin time (PT) and partial thromboplastin time (PTT)
- Cardiovascular instability and collapse
- Multi-organ system failure (MOSF) in patients with septic syndrome

MOSF syndrome is common to critical care clinicians. Positive identification and isolation of an organism is not necessary for definition of septic syndrome. This broadened definition of sepsis is useful for identifying patients at risk for the development of shock and MOSF.

Obstructive Causes of Shock

Pulmonary Embolism

Although traditionally said to be extremely uncommon in children, pulmonary embolism is increasing in frequency with more invasive, aggressive care. Although venous thromboembolism is the most common embolism, fat and air emboli can occur after trauma and surgery and air embolism can occur as an iatrogenic complication in the care of critically ill children.

Table 10.5
Findings of Sepsis Syndrome

Tachypnea/hyperpnea
Tachycardia
Fever or hypothermia with some clinical evidence of infection
Hyperdynamic circulation followed by hypoperfusion
Altered central nervous system function
Oliguria
Lactic acidemia
Impaired organ system function
Hypoxemia
Renal failure

Thromboembolism Acute massive pulmonary thromboembolism can occur in children after the following:

- Surgery, especially pelvic surgery
- Instrumentation of the heart vessels
- Catheterization (e.g., cardiac, ventriculojugular, pulmonary artery)
- Hemodialysis
- Hyperalimentation
- Trauma, especially to the pelvis
- Hypercoagulopathies (polycythemia, severe thrombocytosis, and antithrombin III, protein C, or protein S deficiency)
- Dehydration
- Heat stroke

Although it is not embolic, sickle cell disease can lead to massive pulmonary artery thrombosis, which has characteristics in common with massive pulmonary embolism.

Acute pulmonary embolism leads to circulatory failure via:

- Total blockage of the pulmonary artery prevents venous return to the left heart, mimics acute hypovolemic shock, and is rapidly fatal.
- Acute right ventricular afterloading with right ventricular failure leads to ventricular septal shift and to decreased left-heart end-diastolic length/volume and performance, preload, and shock.
- Right ventricular failure is due both to mechanical blockage of the pulmonary arteries and to reflex pulmonary vasoconstriction.

Fat Embolism Fat embolism occurs in a wide variety of clinical settings that give rise to bone trauma. Although traumatic fracture is the most common, it may also follow orthopedic surgery and even occur in sickle cell disease. Fat embolism after long bone fracture is rare in children, but it still requires consideration.

In acute massive fat embolism, shock occurs secondary to low output as a result of sudden right ventricular failure. As in pulmonary thromboembolism, fat globules in the pulmonary arteries lead to pulmonary vasoconstriction and pulmonary capillary endothelial damage with resulting shock.

Air Embolism Entry of air into central vessels may be rapidly fatal or may give rise to a shock state. Air emboli can occur when large vessels are lacerated after trauma, during spinal surgery or neurosurgery, and iatrogenically by accidental air entry during intravenous therapy. "Air block" of the right ventricular outflow tract, main pulmonary artery, or distal alveolar arterioles leads to decreased right and left ventricular output and decreased systemic perfusion. Reflex pulmonary vasoconstriction increases right ventricular afterload. In addition, paradoxic systemic emboli may occur, giving rise to CNS signs and myocardial ischemia. Profound hypotension and cyanosis with hyperpnea indicate a grave shock state.

Diagnosis All pulmonary emboli are associated with low output states, hypoxia, and hypercarbia. Aspiration of pulmonary arterial blood—if a catheter is in situ—may reveal air or fat globules. Microscopic urinalysis may reveal fat globules if a fat embolus has occurred, but this is not completely sensitive, and the appearance may be delayed many hours. The final diagnosis of thromboembolism is best performed by a pulmonary ventilation/perfusion scan and, less frequently, a pulmonary angiograph.

Therapy Therapeutic measures consist of hemodynamic support, oxygen, prevention of further embolization, and removal of emboli. Thromboembolus may be dissolved by the use of heparin or by thrombolytic therapy such as streptokinase, urokinase, or tissue plasminogen activator (tPA). Air should be aspirated from the pulmonary artery or right ventricular outflow tract when possible. There are no effective methods of removing fat emboli. Although unusual, pulmonary emboli may lead to shock on their own or may complicate the course of children in shock from other causes.

Obstructive Cardiac and Great Vessel Lesions

Many congenital or acquired structural heart and great vessel lesions are responsible for shock. Newborns and young infants may present in shock from poor cardiac output secondary to valvular stenosis. Critical aortic stenosis, atrioventricular valve stenosis, and pulmonic valve stenosis are tolerated in utero but may present catastrophically in the infant. Myocardial contractility may be normal, but stenotic lesions prevent forward ventricular output and inadequate oxygen delivery to the tissues. Critical pulmonic stenosis presents with cyanosis and shock unresponsive to airway intervention and assisted ventilation. Mitral stenosis prevents pulmonary venous return to the left ventricle, which impairs left-sided output. Elevated pulmonary venous pressures result in pulmonary congestion, edema, and increased right ventricle afterload, reducing the ventricle's performance.

Critical aortic stenosis, subaortic stenosis (i.e., resulting from a subaortic membrane), or idiopathic hypertrophic subaortic stenosis impairs left ventricular output, and the tissues suffer from ischemia. This is also seen in an infant with critical coarctation of the aorta or interrupted aortic arch. Use of PGE_1 (i.e., alprostadil) may save the infant's life by improving pulmonary or systemic circulation because it opens the ductus arteriosus when an obstructive lesion impedes forward flow. Trauma to the aorta may also cause a dissection that results in an obstruction to left ventricular output and shock. These lesions along with pulmonary embolism can be collectively considered etiologies of "obstructive" shock.

Miscellaneous Causes of Shock

Heat Stroke

Cardiovascular collapse secondary to excessive body temperature can result from increased body heat production or decreased body heat dissipation. The former usually occurs in older children after a pyrexial illness or exercise and the latter occurs in younger infants and neonates who may be kept excessively warmed and covered. Elevated body temperature may aggravate shock from other causes. Fever increases oxygen consumption, carbon dioxide formation, and the demand for augmented cardiopulmonary performance that the child may not be capable of generating. Fever may be an appropriate host response to infection, although it is undesirable physiologically in the presentation of heat stroke and should be aggressively managed.

A clinical syndrome of hemorrhagic shock, hyperpyrexia, and encephalopathy has been described in infants and children. Levin et al. described "hemorrhagic shock and encephalopathy syndrome" as a mild prodromal illness progressing to encephalopathy, shock, disseminated intravascular coagulation, and negative bacterial cultures. Fevers ranged from 38° C to 41.5° C or higher. Postmortem examination and microbiologic analysis could not demonstrate either viral or bacterial pathogens.

Acute Pancreatitis

Acute hemorrhagic pancreatitis can give rise to hypotension, hemoconcentration, anuria, hypocalcemia, fever, and acidosis that may require therapy aimed at correcting the shock state. The leading causes of this condition in children are:

- Drug therapy (e.g., thiazides, prednisone, azathioprine)
- Congenital biliary disease
- Mumps
- Idiopathic disease

Pancreatitis is classically divided into interstitial and hemorrhagic forms. Shock is most common in the hemorrhagic form and occurs in 16% of children with pancreatitis.

In pancreatic shock, severe pancreatic damage occurs with widespread liquefaction, thrombosis, and massive peripancreatic edema and occasionally is complicated by massive gastrointestinal bleeding. Metabolic disturbances include hyperglycemia and hypocalcemia.

Septic shock may precipitate or complicate acute pancreatitis. The diagnosis relies on recognizing the clinical constellation and measuring serum amylase and lipase and amylase clearance. Therapy is directed at reversing shock, correcting metabolic abnormalities, and providing respiratory support. Surgery carries an immense risk and should be avoided if at all possible.

Drug Overdose and Poisonings

A shock-like picture is frequently seen in patients after both inadvertent and intentional drug overdoses. Several groups of drugs produce a shock-like picture, including narcotics, barbiturates, tricyclic antidepressants, and β-blockers.

Adrenal Shock

Although infrequent in childhood, adrenal shock should be considered when the etiology of shock is not obvious. Any newborn younger than 30 days of age should be considered at risk for adrenal insufficiency or congenital heart disease as occult etiologies of shock and empiric stress. Glucocorticoid and PGE_1 should be administered until definitive diagnosis is achieved. In older infants and children, adrenal insufficiency is also an infrequent cause of shock, which must be considered and treated until the diagnosis is confirmed or excluded.

DIAGNOSIS OF SHOCK
Historical Information

Early diagnosis of shock requires knowledge of which children are predisposed to it. In addition to considering the child's age, the physician should interrogate the child's parents or other physicians, nurses, and emergency transfer personnel caring for the child. Useful information that affects management and therapy includes the following:

- Maternal history (peripartum fevers, premature rupture of membranes, intrapartum blood loss, fetal distress, lethargy or irritability, and possibly even bacterial cultures)
- Indication of injury severity, amount of blood loss, and status of child before his or her arrival of emergency personnel in cases of trauma
- History of underlying immunodeficiency state (e.g., chemotherapy patients)
- Assessment of development of lethargy, decreased oral intake, apathy, and general responsiveness
- Amount of excessive fluid loss from diarrhea or vomiting is necessary in dehydration
- History of decreased urine output
- Details of environmental exposure, potential drug ingestion, previous medical problems, and allergies

Examination of past records for details of chemotherapy, surveillance cultures, cardiac diagnosis, and other potential problems is necessary.

Physical Findings

The physical examination may demonstrate signs reflecting the underlying physiologic process.

Body Temperature

Body surface temperature is a time-honored, simple, and effective method of assessing adequate tissue perfusion. Cold extremities or increased peripheral-core temperature gradients (greater than 2° C) indicate intact homeostatic mechanisms that have decreased nonessential cutaneous perfusion despite contracted intravascular volume. This efficient system is an early indicator of decreased intravascular volume.

Decreased Capillary Refill

This finding is also a sensitive indicator of tissue perfusion. The exact technique for determining capillary refill must be determined by each physician, because there are no universally recognized standards. The rate of refill following firm compression of soft tissues and nail beds for 5 seconds is related to the site of determination, because of the intricacy of the capillary bed, the temperature, and the amount of circulation through the microvasculature. In general, refill over the face is faster than that over the chest, which is faster than that over the hands and feet. Normally, a blanched area disappears in less than 3 seconds. Capillary refill that takes longer than 5 seconds is clearly abnormal. Although as an indicator of tissue hypoperfusion capillary refill is nonspecific, it is sensitive.

Peripheral Cyanosis

Stasis as a result of peripheral vasoconstriction may lead to peripheral cyanosis. Although peripheral hypoperfusion is the physiologic response to intravascular volume contraction, it does not in itself indicate shock; however, it clearly heralds it. In addition, the physical findings of dehydration may also be present and can indicate the severity of hypovolemia (Table 10.6). Vital organ hypoperfusion can be assumed to occur if oliguria from renal hypoperfusion exists or if altered mentation occurs, indicating CNS hypoperfusion.

Acidosis and Alkalosis

The physical findings of acidosis are primarily respiratory. Tachypnea, hyperpnea, and hyperventilation frequently are seen as early findings in shock states. Respiratory alkalosis is frequently an early accompaniment of all stages of all types of shock.

Autonomic Response to Stress

Peripheral vasoconstriction is an early phase of autonomic response. In children, tachycardia also occurs early. The younger the child, the more dependent the cardiac output is on heart rate in comparison with increases in stroke volume. Extremely rapid heart rates occur before notable alterations

Table 10.6
Clinical Signs of Dehydration in Children

Clinical signs[a]	Mild	Moderate	Severe
Activity	Normal	Lethargic	Lethargic to coma
Color	Pale	Gray	Mottled
Urine output	Decreased (<2–3 mL/kg/h)	Oliguric (<1 mL/kg/h)	Anuria
Fontanel	Flat	Depressed	Sunken (retreated)
Mucous membranes	Dry	Dry	Cracked
Skin turgor	Slight decrease	Marked decrease	Tenting
Pulse	Normal to increased	Increased	Grossly tachycardic
Blood pressure	Normal	Normal	Decreased
Weight loss	5%	10%	15%

[a]Hypernatremic dehydration may occur with only moderate changes in clinical signs.

in mean arterial pressure in infants and small children, although close attention to pulse pressure and pulse intensity by clinical examination reveals early alterations.

Alteration in mean arterial pressure is a late manifestation of hypovolemia in children. Blood pressure is well defended, and only when hemodynamic compromise is severe does mean arterial pressure begin to fall.

Classification of Shock

Classes as defined by the Advanced Trauma Life Support Standards of the American College of Surgeons are outlined in Table 10.7. This classification, based on the amount of blood loss and severity of symptoms, can be used to guide therapy, assess severity, standardize various shock states, and provide a useful basis for information transfer between caretakers of children in shock.

Laboratory Tests

Several laboratory investigations assess the severity and cause of shock states:

- Serum electrolytes, blood cell counts, platelet counts, and hematocrits, which delineate the extent of metabolic disturbance
- Serum calcium levels (hypocalcemia can further compromise respiratory muscle, myocardial, and metabolic function). Calcium replacement is indicated if cardiovascular performance is unacceptable.
- Serum protein, albumin, and colloid oncotic pressure (guide volume replacement and severity of the capillary endothelial defect)
- Arterial oxygen content and carbon dioxide tension (evaluate adequacy of ventilatory function)

Table 10.7
Advanced Trauma Life Support Classification

Class I
15% or less acute blood volume loss
Blood pressure normal
Pulse increased 10–20%
No change in capillary refill
Class II
20–25% loss of blood volume
Tachycardia > 150 beats/min
Tachypnea 35–40 breaths/min
Capillary refill prolonged
Systolic blood pressure decreased
Pulse pressure decreased
Orthostatic hypotension > 10–15 torr
Urine output > 1 mL/kg/h
Class III
30–35% blood volume loss
All of the above signs
Urine output < mL/kg/h
Lethargic, clammy, and vomiting
Class IV
40–50% blood volume loss
Nonpalpable pulses
Obtunded

- pH and base deficit determination (quantify tissue hypoperfusion by the degree of metabolic acidosis). Persistent acidosis indicates inadequate or ineffective therapy and the need for further intervention and investigation. Restoration of normal pulse and blood pressure but with persistence of acidosis mandates further action, cautious monitoring, and therapeutic support.
- Mixed venous oxygen tension, saturation, and content (assess adequacy of tissue perfusion and cardiovascular compensation and performance; guide optimization of oxygen consumption and delivery).

Because a major therapeutic intervention in shock treatment is respiratory support, the arterial blood gas and venous blood gas determinations may be discordant, indicating adequate respiratory support but severe cellular injury, poor cardiac performance, and persistent venous acidosis.

MONITORING OF SHOCK

The purposes of monitoring children who are potentially shocked are to detect alterations in physiologic status and to assess outcomes of therapeutic interventions. The exact type and extent of monitoring depends on the severity and complexity of the child's underlying illness and shock state.

Certain essential minimum requirements for baseline monitoring should be applied to all children who are at risk for shock. All monitoring for children with shock is best facilitated by admission to a PICU.

The most effective and sensitive physiologic monitoring available is the repeated and careful examination of the child's physical status by a competent and experienced clinician. In addition, the minimum monitoring of a child with shock or at risk for shock includes:

- Continuous electrocardiogram monitoring
- Pulse oximetry
- Temperature and blood pressure measurements
- Blood glucose determination (e.g., Dextrostix) in infants
- Intake and output
- Urine production
- Body weight

In all but the most mild cases, blood pressure determination will probably necessitate invasive intra-arterial cannulation. These indwelling arterial cannulae also can be used for continuous monitoring of blood gases. The unstable and potentially catastrophic compromise in circulation requires beat-to-beat continuous blood pressure measurement and display.

Urine output in children is normally 2 to 3 mL/kg/hour, and urine outputs of less than 1 mL/kg/hour are indicative of renal hypoperfusion and activation of homeostatic water and sodium conservation mechanisms in shock states. It is usual for oliguria to occur early in shock states and injury before alterations in mean arterial pressure or development of significant tachycardia. Alterations in urine-specific gravity should be noted.

In patients with severe shock and certainly in children with myocardial compromise, invasive venous and pulmonary arterial pressure monitoring must be considered. Evidence suggests that obtaining "physiologic" cardiac output and cardiopulmonary indices may not be sufficient. There may be some value in attaining supraphysiologic values for many parameters. As it gains further confirmation and acceptance, invasive monitoring may have more widespread use.

Measurements of continuous, mixed venous oxygen saturation allows minute-to-minute assessment of interventions in cardiorespiratory support and resuscitation. An oximetric catheter assists in titration of positive end-expiratory pressure (PEEP), minimizing barotrauma, and assessing changes in mode of ventilatory support.

TREATMENT OF SHOCK

An aggressive multi-modal approach to shock means considering many therapies- often simultaneously. The initial step is to ensure a patent airway and adequate oxygenation. Preload augmentation with intravascular fluid therapy follows and should be considered at every stage of shock therapy and for every type of shock. Therapy directed at the underlying cause, be it instituting antibiotics, converting a cardiac dysrhythmia, or stopping hemorrhage, should occur concurrently. Frequently, oxygenation, ventilation, and fluid therapy are all that is required and, even in severe circumstances, will often delay further deterioration that requires more aggressive therapy. The administration of pharmacologic agents to correct metabolic abnormalities and restoring cardiovascular function is the final step in completing the multi-modality therapy of shock states. Figure 10.1 provides an abbreviated algorithm for shock therapy.

Initial Measures

Correct and Avoid Hypoxemia

The first goal is to increase arterial oxygen content by ensuring 95 to 100% saturation and adequate hemoglobin content for oxygen delivery. All children with compromised circulation should receive supplemental oxygen because the risks of providing it are minimal.

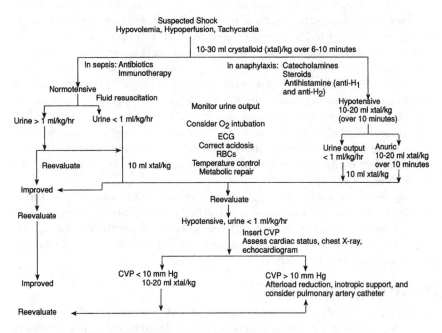

Figure 10.1. Abbreviated algorithm for shock therapy.

Correct Acid-Base Disturbances

The correction of acid-base disturbances allows better cellular function and myocardial performance, allows decreased systemic and pulmonary vascular resistance, and decreases the need for respiratory compensation of metabolic acidosis. A base deficit greater than 6 mEq/L in acute shock states probably should be corrected. Renal compensation and correction may be of help in correcting the acidosis over time, but acidosis in a life-threatening situation requires bicarbonate and volume supplementation.

Bicarbonate

Bicarbonate supplementation can be delivered by repeated slow boluses of sodium bicarbonate of 1 to 2 mEq/kg. In neonates, a solution of 0.5 mEq/mL is used to avoid acute change in osmolarity, which may lead to intraventricular hemorrhage. Frequently, 10 to 20 mEq/kg may be required to correct profound acidosis. The formula required to half-correct acidosis [0.3 (body weight in kg) × (base deficit) = mEq $NaHCO_3$] may serve as a rough guide.

If bolus therapy is not effective or the metabolic acidosis persists or grows more severe, a continuous intravenous sodium bicarbonate infusion may be required. The major limitation in bicarbonate replacement therapy is sodium overload and hyperosmolarity. Close monitoring of serum sodium is required if massive bicarbonate replacement (i.e., more than 10 mEq/kg) is undertaken.

If serum sodium increases more than 150 mEq/L, another method of correcting acidosis may be required. Tromethamine (or THAM) has been recommended; however, serious problems are associated with its use. Carbicarb has also been recommended but has not yet received widespread acceptance.

Volume Supplementation

Peritoneal dialysis may be necessary to remove excess acid, lactate, phosphate, and hydrogen ion; to correct hypernatremia; and to allow further bicarbonate administration. In severe metabolic acidosis with hemodynamic collapse, which may occur in aspirin overdose and with inborn errors of metabolism or sepsis, peritoneal dialysis may be lifesaving because it not only removes excess acid but also alleviates the underlying cause of shock. Adequate peritoneal perfusion is necessary for effective peritoneal dialysis, so initial blood pressure and intravascular volume resuscitation is mandatory.

When correcting acidosis with bicarbonate replacement, other electrolyte abnormalities may be expected.

- Decreased serum ionized calcium can lead to alterations in level of consciousness, tremors, seizures, tetany, hypotension, tachycardia, myocardial depression, and acidosis. Levels of ionized calcium below 0.90 mm should be treated. Either calcium gluconate (100 mg/kg intravenous slow bolus) or calcium chloride (20 mg/kg) will rapidly restore serum ionized calcium.

- Hypokalemia warrants serial serum potassium measurements and urine output monitoring. Potassium therapy should be given prudent consideration and slow administration (0.1 to 0.3 mEq/kg/hour).
- Hyperglycemia frequently accompanies severe stress and shock states in children. Correction of the underlying stress leads to homeostatic control of glucose levels before insulin supplementation is required.
- Hypoglycemia may occur in infants in shock as glycogen reserves are exhausted and homeostatic mechanisms in support of blood sugar fatigue (cortisol, growth hormone, catecholamines, glucagon, and somatostatin). Frequent monitoring is important.

Cardiovascular Support

Rate and Rhythm

Ensuring adequate cardiac rate and rhythm is basic to life support. Heart rates are acceptable within a wide range of normal for age, and monitoring the heart rate is essential in guiding therapy.

Stroke Volume

Preload Augmentation

Volume Replacement Rapid intravascular volume expansion guided by clinical examination and urine output frequently is adequate to restore blood pressure and peripheral perfusion in children with shock. In the case of otherwise-normal cardiorespiratory function, volume overload resulting in pulmonary edema is rare. Standard volume replacement is 10 to 20 mL/kg over 10 minutes, which can be repeated if necessary (Table 10.8). Replacement of losses resulting from excess urine output, stool output, or hemorrhage can be guided by body weight changes, careful monitoring of intake and output, and repeated physical examinations.

When volume resuscitation greater than 50 to 100 mL/kg in the first 1 to 2 hours is required, more invasive monitoring and diagnostic investigations should be considered. Severe third-space losses because of capillary leak can occur, but occult hemorrhage must not go undiagnosed.

Antishock Trousers Another method of increasing venous return and augmenting preload is by application of military antishock trousers, which are manufactured in pediatric sizes. Use in children suffering from severe hypotension may prove lifesaving and provide a means of maintaining blood pressure until more definitive therapy is provided.

Preload augmentation in patients with septic shock, myocardial impairment, or pulmonary disease may require central pressure monitoring.

Cardiac Contractility The use of dopamine, dobutamine, isoproterenol,

Table 10.8
Fluid Therapy Guidelines

	H$_2$O (mL/kg)	Na	K(mEq/kg)	Cl	HCO$_3$
To correct 10% dehydration					
Isotonic	150	7–10	7–10	4–8	8–15
Hypotonic (Na <130 mEq/L)	75	10–15	10–15	5–10	10–20
Hypertonic (Na >150 mEq/L	125	2–5	2–5	2–4	4–10
Maintenance					
Calories					
900/m²/day or by weight:	1–10 kg	—	—	—	—
100 cal/kg	11–20 kg	—	—	—	—
1000 + 50 cal/kg	>20 kg	—	—	—	—
1000 + 20 cal/kg	—	—	—	—	—
Water	100 ml/100 cal/d	Na = 3–5 mEq/kg/d	—	—	—
Electrolytes^a	K = 2–3 mEq/kg/d	Ca$^+$ = 2–5 mEq/kg/d	—	—	

^{a}Balance anion as chloride, bicarbonate, or phosphate guided by laboratory tests.

epinephrine, and other catecholamine pressor agents is well described in both infants and older children (Table 10.9).

Specific Catecholamines

The complexity of the cardiovascular derangement in shock states makes it difficult to predict the response to individual hemodynamically active therapeutic agents. Table 10.9 summarizes key points concerning these agents.

Isoproterenol This catecholamine causes peripheral vasodilatation, as manifested by a fall in diastolic blood pressure, and pulmonary vasodilatation. Also, renal, splanchnic, muscle, and cutaneous flows are increased. The latter may unfortunately lead to perfusion of nonessential vascular beds and a relative "steal" phenomenon.

Isoproterenol is useful in children with right heart failure and elevated pulmonary vascular resistance. It blunts hypoxic pulmonary vasoconstrictor activity and may thus increase intrapulmonary shunting. Hypoxia may be exacerbated secondary to increased V/Q mismatch. Isoproterenol has β-adrenergic metabolic effects causing hyperglycemia, albeit less than that seen with epinephrine (with its α and β actions), and increased release of free fatty acids. Apart from the tendency to aggravate myocardial ischemia, it is also dysrhythmogenic. The clinical use of isoproterenol is best reserved

Table 10.9
Specific Agents

Agent	Site of Action	Dose (μg/kg/m)	Effect
Dopamine	Dopaminergic	0.5–4	Renal vasodilator
	β	4–10	Inotrope
	α > β	11–20	Peripheral vasoconstriction
			Increased PVR
			Dysrhythmias
Dobutamine	β_1 and β_2	1–20	Inotrope
			Vasodilatation (β2)
			Decreases PVR
			Weak α-activity
			Tachycardia and extrasystoles
Isoproterenol	β_1 and β_2	0.05–2.0	Inotrope
			Vasodilatation
			Decreases PVR
			MVO_2
			Dysrhythmias
Epinephrine	β > α	0.05–2.0	Inotrope
			Tachycardia
			Decreased renal flow
			MVO_2
			Dysrhythmias
Norepinephrine	α > β	0.05–2.0	Profound constrictor
			Inotrope
			MVO_2, SVR
Sodium nitroprusside	Vasodilator: arterial greater than venous	0.5–10	Rapid onset, short duration
			Increases ICP
			$\dot{V}/\dot{Q}$ mismatch
			Cyanide toxicity
Nitroglycerin	Vasodilator: venous greater than arterial	1–20	Decreased PVR
			Increases ICP
PGE_1	Complex	0.05–0.2	Vasodilatation
			Open ductus arteriosus
Amrinone	PDE_3 inhibitor	1–20	Inotrope
			Chronotrope
			Vasodilatation

PVR, pulmonary vascular resistance; SVR, systemic vascular resistance; ICP, intracranial pressure; and PDE3, phosphodiesterase inhibitor.

for those situations in which potent inotropic stimulation is required, especially in conjunction with pulmonary vascular dilatation.

Dobutamine Dobutamine is less likely to give rise to ventricular dysrhythmias than either epinephrine or isoproterenol. Dobutamine can enhance myocardial performance under certain circumstances, but if falling blood pressure and increased maximum oxygen consumption (VO_{2max}) occur concurrently, myocardial ischemia is still a serious threat. Dobutamine has little metabolic effect and only 1/45th the α effect of norepinephrine and 1/180th the β_2 effect of isoproterenol. It does not selectively enhance renal perfusion. In summary, dobutamine is the intravenous drug that is at present closest to being a pure inotropic agent.

Dopamine Dopamine remains the most commonly used therapeutic agent in shock states in spite of or perhaps because of its less than pure effects.

- In low doses (0.5 to 4 μg/kg/min), it causes renal and splanchnic vasodilatation, thus serving as a diuretic and protecting renal perfusion.
- In medium doses (4 to 10 μg/kg/min), its increasing inotropic effect produces increased stroke volume and cardiac output.
- In larger doses (more than 10 μg/kg/min), increasing α- vasoconstrictor activity may lead to decreased peripheral and renal perfusion and increased myocardial afterload.

Because the exact degree to which these mixed effects occur in an individual varies, careful monitoring is required.

Tachycardia and extrasystoles may occur but are less of a problem with dopamine than with the previously mentioned agents. Pulmonary vascular resistance may be increased. This effect should be remembered in treating newborns and patients at risk for pulmonary hypertension.

Epinephrine Epinephrine is associated with the following:

- Increased cardiac output, blood pressure, and heart rate
- A hypermetabolic state
- CNS stimulation
- Increased VO$_{2max}$
- Elevated pulmonary and systemic vascular resistances
- Renal ischemia
- Ventricular tachydysrhythmias

Epinephrine can be expected to enhance myocardial contractility and to lead a still heart to beating, but its myriad untoward activities cause its use to be reserved only for dire cases.

Norepinephrine Norepinephrine can elevate myocardial perfusion pressures and enhance perfusion. When peripheral vascular resistance is low, such as during anaphylaxis, in neurogenic shock, and, most remarkably, in septic shock, enhancing peripheral vasomotor tone with norepinephrine may be the most beneficial single therapy. The combination of enhanced contractility and a return to normal peripheral vascular resistance should restore blood pressure and perfusion to multiple vascular beds rapidly. The use of norepinephrine in these circumstances may be beneficial but requires exact hemodynamic diagnosis and careful hemodynamic monitoring.

Amrinone and Milrinone These agents:

- Augment myocardial contractility
- Increase cardiac output
- Decrease left ventricular end-diastolic and pulmonary capillary wedge pressures
- Induce relaxation of vascular smooth muscle, thereby reducing systemic vascular resistance

Amrinione and mildrinone may be used in combination with catecholamines to achieve further increases in cardiac output and a decrease in afterload. These agents are most efficacious in the postoperative period in patients with impaired myocardial performance after cardiotomy. Amrinone is administered intravenously (given in a bolus of 750 μg/kg over 1 to 3 minutes, followed by continuous infusion as listed in Table 10.9). Platelet effects often limit usefulness.

Afterload Reduction

Afterload reduction plays a role in improving myocardial performance in children in cardiogenic shock after surgery, myocarditis, or ischemic heart disease or in the later stages of septic shock with myocardial failure. In the late stage of septic shock, high systemic vascular resistance, poor peripheral perfusion, and decreased cardiac output may respond to afterload reduction. Afterload-reducing agents may also benefit children who require epinephrine or norepinephrine as an inotropic agent to decrease the α-adrenergic effects of increased systemic vascular resistance.

Correction of hypoxia, optimization of respiratory support, and correction of metabolic abnormalities are essential in reducing pulmonary vascular resistance. Unfortunately, no truly specific pulmonary vasodilator is available at the present time. In older children, isoproterenol is the drug of choice, but the use of nitroprusside or nitroglycerin may also be advantageous. Close monitoring and volume augmentation frequently are required when vasodilators are used to decrease pulmonary vascular resistance. Calcium channel-blocking agents such as nifedipine have the potential for decreasing pulmonary vascular resistance, but there is little experience in children at the present time.

Other experimental therapies (i.e., adenosine triphosphate [ATP], ATP-MgCl, adenosine, nitric oxide) continue to be developed, but further characterization of their effects and experience are required before they are recommended for widespread use. Inhaled nitric oxide has been used for many causes of respiratory failure (e.g., sepsis, pulmonary hypertension, meconium aspiration) with promising results.

Steroids

Children and all patients with human immunodeficiency virus (HIV) infection may have a predilection to adrenal failure during sepsis. Adrenal cortical failure is associated with cardiovascular hyporesponsiveness to endogenous mediators and exogenous therapies. Glucocorticoid replacement or stress doses should be considered. Physiologic doses (12.5 mg/m^2/day) or stress doses (50 to 100 mg/m^2/day) of hydrocortisone have not been shown to be detrimental and may be lifesaving in adrenal failure. When adrenal function may be impaired, such as in the Waterhouse-Friderichsen syndrome after meningococcal or *H. influenzae* infection, or in congenital adrenal hyperplasia, glucocorticoid replacement is essential, and mineralocorticoid replacement should be considered.

Immunotherapy

Despite years of extensive research into the use of immunotherapy for critically ill patients, outcomes have not improved significantly and our understanding of the complex immunologic responses in septic shock still is insufficient. Better definition of subpopulations that may benefit from this therapeutic approach is necessary.

Supportive Therapy

The management of the multisystem deterioration with shock states is as important as treating the underlying condition.

Hematologic Abnormalities

Monitoring of PT, PTT, platelet count, fibrinolysis, and observation for excessive bleeding are essential. Replacement therapy specifically designed to replace absent clotting factors is advantageous; use of vitamin K, fresh frozen plasma, and platelet transfusions should correct most coagulopathies. If replacement therapy is ineffective and peripheral gangrene from thrombosis occurs, heparinization may be of value.

Other therapies that have been reported in few patients include the use of regional anesthetic blocks and fibrinolytic therapy. More experience is necessary before these can be widely applied.

Gastrointestinal Tract Disturbances

Hypoperfusion and stress may lead to:

- Bleeding
- Ileus
- Brush border cell and enzyme loss
- Bacterial translocation

Ileus may result from electrolyte abnormalities and may lead to abdominal distention with respiratory compromise. Endothelial damage with diffuse gut edema and ischemia may underlie a host of other problems. Gastrointestinal blood loss from either acute gastritis or peptic ulceration should be prevented by using antacids and/or an H_2-receptor blocker such as cimetidine or gastric mucosal coating with sucralfate. Intensive investigations into metabolic changes in the gastrointestinal tract may reveal important new therapies.

The gastrointestinal tract may not be a functional route for nutrition for some time, and parenteral nutrition will be necessary. However, trophic enteral feedings may play an important role in decreasing gastrointestinal pathology.

Renal Abnormalities

Renal support is essential to avoid prolonged renal shutdown in hypoperfusion states. Volume augmentation and the use of diuretics (e.g., mannitol, furosemide, ethacrynic acid) encourage renal blood flow and maintain tubular function. Low-dose dopamine (0.5 to 4 g/kg/min) improves renal blood flow and may be beneficial in preventing acute renal failure in shock states. Acute renal failure leading to anuria may require treatment with either peritoneal dialysis or hemodialysis. High-output renal failure may occur in shock states without any previous episodes of oliguria. This may falsely indicate adequate renal perfusion and adequate prerenal augmentation at a time when the patient's intravascular volume is, in fact, being depleted. Renal function, therefore, should be assessed by response to current circulatory status and serial measurements of serum creatinine.

Respiratory Support of the Child in Shock

Ensuring optimal oxygen delivery is a major goal. In addition to hemodynamic abnormalities, the child with acute circulatory failure may have ineffective oxygen delivery, because of decreased respiratory muscle function, which causes hypoventilation and hypozemia. Causes of decreased respiratory function include:

- Decreased respiratory muscle perfusion
- Acidosis
- Hypoxia
- Electrolyte abnormalities

Under these circumstances, children may become fatigued rapidly. They will compensate until complete, and sometimes alarmingly rapid, deterioration occurs.

Another cause of respiratory failure in shock is the development of intrapulmonary shunting as a result of noncardiac pulmonary edema (ARDS), which may further aggravate ventilation and perfusion abnormalities. For these reasons, increased inspired oxygen is essential in all children in shock. Furthermore, to ensure the airway provides optimal relief from respiratory muscle fatigue and facilitates provision of positive airway pressure, early intubation of the trachea should be considered.

In children with cardiogenic shock and pulmonary edema, intubation, and mechanical ventilation may improve myocardial function rapidly by relieving deleterious cardiorespiratory interactions. Increased negative pleural pressure leads to increased left ventricular transmural pressure that may have the same deleterious effect on the myocardium as increased afterload. Children can develop negative intrathoracic pressures (-60 cm of H_2O can occur in neonates), which can contribute to myocardial afterload.

Intubation and synchronization of ventilation may improve myocardial function by decreasing this afterload effect. Furthermore, expansion of functional residual capacity, improvement in pulmonary compliance, and a decreased intrapulmonary shunting greatly improve oxygen delivery and decrease pulmonary vascular resistance, improving right ventricular performance.

Mechanical ventilation in children may be provided in both intermittent mandatory ventilation (IMV) mode (volume cycled) or by pressure-controlled ventilation. Close observation of chest movement, ventilator pressures and flows, and arterial blood gases is essential to ensure adequate oxygenation and ventilation. Changes in compliance or obstruction of the endotracheal tube can lead to inadequate alveolar ventilation and oxygenation, and vigilance must be maintained.

The management of ARDS in children is achieved with an increase in PEEP, leading to an increase in end expiratory lung volume, a decrease in intrapulmonary shunt, and improvement in oxygenation. Increasing intrathoracic pressure can impair venous return and may lead to decreased cardiac output and oxygen delivery if cardiac preload is not maintained. For this reason, children in shock with severe ARDS requiring PEEP greater than 15 cm H_2O should have cardiac output, central pressure, and oxygen transport data monitored.

Extracorporeal Circulatory Support

Despite maximal cardiopulmonary support, the shocked child still is at high risk of death and developing prolonged MOSF. Extracorporeal membrane oxygenation (ECMO) has proven useful for neonatal respiratory distress. Neonates and certain older children in shock develop early respiratory distress or ARDS, pulmonary hypertension, and/or heart failure and may be unresponsive to conventional maximal therapies. ECMO has been used successfully to treat infants in septic shock.

Extracorporeal technology (e.g., extracorporeal CO_2 exchange, intravascular oxygenators [IVOX], hemoperfusion) has been used in critically ill adults. Many of these devices have not yet been miniaturized for use in infants and small children. The intra-aortic balloon pump has been used in children, and many children have benefited from continuous arteriovenous hemofiltration for volume overload and renal failure.

MULTI-ORGAN SYSTEM FAILURE

After severe injury, hypotension, or sepsis, each organ is at risk for dysfunction. With initial resuscitation from hemorrhage, hypotension, or sepsis, the restitution of normal perfusion pressure is only an early goal. MOSF results from the initial event and the associated host responses.

Clinical Manifestations

The clinical pattern of MOSF varies. After apparently successful resuscitation from shock, one organ, then another, show dysfunction that slowly worsens over many hours or days. In the acute onset pattern, MOSF is attributable to nutrient and oxygen deficiency and manifests as circulatory, respiratory, renal, hepatic, CNS, and coagulation cascade failure. This overwhelming insult is fatal.

The second pattern of MOSF subacute development occurs after initial successful resuscitation, but over the next few days slowly rising creatinine, hepatic transaminase levels, and hyperbilirubinemia appear. Progressive respiratory or circulatory dysfunction evolve. During this pattern, the host response factors, bacterial translocation or other source of secondary infection, and products of mesenteric ischemia contribute to the development of MOSF.

Table 10.10
Prognostic Indicators[a]

Variable	% Survival in Range	Range
Oxygen consumption	75	>200 mL/min/m^2
Arteriovenous O_2 gradient	71	>5.5 mL/dL
pH	69	>7.4 U
$\dot{Q}_s/\dot{Q}_T$	69	<12%
WEDGE	69	<11.3 torr
Cardiac index	67	3.3–6.0 L/min/m^2
Oxygen extraction	59	>28%
Core temperature	58	>37°C

[a]From Pollack MM, Fields AI, Ruttiman VE. Distribution of cardiopulmonary variables in pediatric survivors and nonsurvivors of septic shock. Crit Care Med 1985;13:454.

WEDGE, pulmonary artery occlusion pressure.

Supportive Care

Each component organ involved in MOSF may require technologic support in addition to meticulous overall clinical care. Respiratory support is also required in MOSF. Airway control and mechanical ventilation usually is essential to maintaining oxygenation and ventilation during the dynamic processes in MOSF. Newer ventilation strategies to diminish barotrauma and volutrauma by allowing hypercapnia and accepting lower oxygenation parameters may affect outcome.

ASSESSING OUTCOMES

In children who survive septic shock, Pollack et al. determined the median levels of multiple physiologic parameters and assessed which of these levels best correlate with outcome. On the basis of this analysis, they have suggested therapeutic goals in children suffering from septic shock (Table 10.10).

11.

Evaluation and Monitoring of the Central Nervous System

Gitte Y. Larsen, Donald D. Vernon, J. Michael Dean, Francis Filloux, and Jeffrey R. Kirsch

THE COMATOSE STATE

The initial approach to a comatose patient involves stabilizing the airway, breathing, and circulation. The degree of neurologic injury, regardless of the etiology, is then addressed to facilitate planning of further evaluations, such as a computed tomography (CT) scan or neurosurgical intervention. Careful monitoring is appropriate to assess further neurologic deterioration and to anticipate possible cerebral edema.

Assessment

The Glasgow coma scale is useful in the emergent setting because the information required for this score is quickly available and places no reliance on patient history. [The components of the score are shown in Table 27.2.]

Etiology of Coma

Common metabolic and infectious causes of coma are listed in Table 11.1.

A metabolic cause for the comatose state should be suspected if the neurologic examination—including physical findings, electrophysiologic studies, and CT scans—cannot be reconciled. For example, any structural lesion that completely eliminates respiration would do so by compression or destruction

Table 11.1
Metabolic and Infectious Causes of Coma[a]

Metabolic Causes

Acidosis
Alkalosis
Hemolytic-Uremic syndrome
Henoch-Schönlein Purpura
Hepatic failure, portosystemic shunts
Hyperammonemia
    Ornithine transcarbamylase deficiency
    Reyes syndrome
Hypercalcemia and hypocalcemia
Hypercapnia (Pickwickian syndrome)
Hypermagnesemia, hypomagnesemia
Hypoglycemia
Hypoxia
Hyperosmolar states
Hypertonic dehydration
Infection
Juvenile rheumatoid arthritis
Kearns-Sayre syndrome
Poisonings
    Anticholinergic eye drops
    Isoniazid toxicity
    Methotrexate/Ara-C therapy
    Organophosphate/carbamate poisoning
    Phenothiazine/Butyrephenone poisoning
    Sertraline overdose
    Tricyclic overdose
Porphyria
Status epilepticus
Hyrotoxicosis
Uremia
Vitamin deficiency or dependency states
    Carnitine deficiency
    Nicotinic acid
    Pantothenic acid
    Pyridoxine
    Thiamine (Leigh's disease)
    Vitamin B_{12}

Infectious Causes

Brain abscess with ventricular rupture
Empyema, epidural, or subdural
    Encephalitis, bacterial
    Myocoplasma
Encephalomyelitis, postinfectious
Encephalitis, viral
    Herpes
    Sleeping sickness

continued

Table 11.1
Metabolic and Infectious Causes of Coma[a]

Metabolic Causes

Typhoid fever
Varicella zoster
Hemorrhagic shock and leukoencephalopathy
Meningitis, bacterial
Meningitis, fungal
  Cryptogenic
Meningitis, tuberculous
Protozoan infections—amebic, malarial, cysticercosis
  Malaria
Severe systemic infection, sepsis

[a]Adapted from Lockman LA. Coma. In: Swaiman K, Manning S, eds. Pediatric Neurology: Principles and Practice. St Louis: Mosby Yearbook Inc., 1994.

of medullary structures, and supramedullary structures would precede in such destruction; therefore, fixed and dilated pupils would be expected.

An infectious cause is considered if the child has fever, meningismus, or a suggestive history. If meningitis is a possibility, a lumbar puncture should be performed when the child is stabilized. Antibiotics should be instituted promptly, before the lumbar puncture, if the child is too unstable. Other infectious etiologies for coma also are outlined in Table 11.1.

CEREBRAL FLOW MEASUREMENT
Radionucleotide Angiography

This qualitative technique identifies regions of the brain with increased or decreased blood flow. After radionucleotide injection into a peripheral vein, brain activity is measured by an externally placed collimated scintillation detector. Resolution is 2 to 3 cm at best. The percent contribution of extracranial circulation cannot be determined.

^{133}Xe Clearance

The validity and accuracy of the ^{133}Xe clearance technique in children is open to question. Erroneous measurements may result from contamination from the extracerebral circulation and failure to correct for isotope recirculation. In addition, the blood-brain partition coefficient probably is not constant with age and across differing disease states, no established normative data exist, and the risks of radiation exposure further limit the frequency with which the technique may be applied to a given child.

Magnetic Resonance Imaging (MRI)

When an MRI with contrast enhancement is undertaken, a paramagnetic contrast agent (e.g., gadolinium) is injected. This agent courses rapidly through normally perfused brain regions, producing a powerful magnetic field gradient in the capillary vasculature and adjacent tissue. This gradient produces a decrease in signal intensity in normally perfused areas. By contrast, ischemic (i.e., unperfused) regions do not manifest a signal change.

Kety-Schmidt Technique

The Kety-Schmidt N_2O technique is safe for use in children and has been modified to make use of smaller blood samples. Continuous monitoring of arteriovenous oxygen extraction also has been described. Because of anxiety associated with catheterization of the jugular bulb for cerebral venous blood sampling, this technique is more successful in children who are paralyzed, sedated, or comatose than who are awake. Swedlow et al., using the N_2O technique, measured cerebral blood flow (CBF) in children with head trauma and Reye syndrome and described the technical problems associated with this method.

Doppler Flow Velocity

Advantages associated with use of Doppler flow velocity include:

- Noninvasive nature
- Modest cost of required equipment
- Portability
- Ability to apply without disturbing the patient

Infrared Technique

Brazy et al. described the infrared method for continuously measuring preterm infants' cerebral oxygenation at the bedside. The near-infrared oxygen sufficiency scope (NIROS-SCOPE) delivers light with wavelengths between 760 and 904 nm to an infant's head. Based on the changes in the light absorbance collected on the other side of the child's head, the relative oxidation-reduction state of cytochrome aa_3, the amounts of oxygenated and deoxygenated hemoglobin, and the hemoglobin volume in the light field can be estimated.

INTRACRANIAL PRESSURE MONITORING

In contrast to serial measurements of CBF that have little application to the routine care of critically ill children, monitoring of intracranial pressure (ICP) is common practice in the pediatric intensive care unit.

The ventricular catheter is considered the gold standard of ICP monitoring methods.

Epidural Devices

A balloon radiotransmitter or a fiberoptic transducer is placed within the patient's epidural space, or the signal is transmitted to an extracranial sensor via an extradural screw. These devices afford easy placement and a low incidence of infection. Major disadvantages include:

- Sensor plate-dura interrelationships
- Signal dampening
- Tendency to overread compared with ventricular pressure
- Inability to measure brain compliance and withdraw excess cerebrospinal fluid (CSF)

Subarachnoid Devices

A subarachnoid catheter or extradural screw is placed in the subdural or subarachnoid space, connected to a fluid-filled manometer system. These devices provide ease of insertion, avoidance of brain puncture, and ability to obtain some information of brain compliance and withdrawal of CSF. Disadvantages include the possible obstruction or leakage of CSF and the risk of infection. Mendelow et al. observed that Richmond and Leeds screws underread in the subdural space at ICP values greater than 20 mm Hg.

Intraventricular Devices

An intraventricular catheter is inserted through a burr hole into the nondominant or nonaffected hemisphere. The tip is then positioned within the frontal or occipital horn of the lateral ventricle and the catheter is connected to a fluid-filled manometer system, with the transducer positioned at the level of the lateral ventricle or external auditory meatus.

Major advantages to its use are:

- Direct measurement of CSF pressure
- Testing for brain compliance by injection of air or contrast media
- Withdrawal of CSF to decrease pressure and/or for sampling purposes
- Regular adjustment of zero drift

Disadvantages include:

- Leakage of CSF
- Infection (1%)
- Intracerebral bleeding
- Difficulty of insertion in patients with small ventricles

Intraparenchymal Devices

Fiberoptic pressure transducers measure changes in light reflected off a pressure-sensitive membrane, which is located at the tip of the fiberoptic device. Such catheters can be designed for insertion into any intracranial compartment (i.e., subdural, intraparenchymal, intraventricular) or for implantation directly into cerebral tissue (i.e., intraparenchymal placement). Proponents claim they are:

- Accurate as the gold standard (intraventricular catheter)
- Easy to implant on a single pass (reducing trauma)
- Safe and rarely associated with infection
- Particularly advantageous because the reference pressure point is at the tip of the catheter, thereby obviating a need for calibration adjustments with changes in head position, etc.
- Subject to minimum drift (cumulative drift of ≤6 mm Hg per 5-day period, although this could be clinically significant)

A disadvantage to intraparenchymal devices is that the fiberoptic catheter itself cannot be used for CSF drainage. The relative risk of such devices is yet to be elucidated.

Waveforms

Normal ICP levels range from 0 to 15 mm Hg or 0 to 200 cm H_2O. Even in the normal patient, however, pressure may rise transiently 30 to 50 mm Hg during a Valsalva's maneuver or coughing without a deleterious effect. Sustained elevations, however, can decrease cerebral perfusion pressure, resulting in parenchymal ischemia.

ELECTRICAL MONITORING OF THE CENTRAL NERVOUS SYSTEM

Standard multichannel electroencephalography (EEG) is not practical to either continuous or frequent intermittent monitoring of the CNS in the intensive care unit setting. Serial EEG recordings, however, are the primary means of evaluating brain electrical activity in critically ill patients. Furthermore, routine EEG continues to be necessary as a complement to actual electrical monitoring systems (i.e., cerebral function monitor [CFM], compressed spectral array [CSA]) available for intensive care use. Finally, understanding the electronic and technical principles of routine EEG is a prerequisite to the comprehension of these newer methods of EEG averaging as well as the theory and use of evoked potentials (EPs).

Routine EEG in Intensive Care

The EEG provides the following:

- Diagnostic and prognostic information during assessment of obtunded, comatose, or seizing critically ill patients
- Means to measure cerebral activity in therapeutically paralyzed or anesthetized patients
- Method to ascertain the effects of various therapeutic interventions

Drawbacks to EEG use in continuous monitoring include its production of volumes of detailed information. Two methods used to condense EEG data include the CFM and CSA.

Cerebral Function Monitor

The simplest form of the CFM provides no information regarding the frequency distribution of the original EEG activity. Subsequent models address this problem by providing simultaneous crude estimates of the percentage contribution of various frequencies (δ, v, α, and β) to the net EEG amplitude. The cerebral function analyzing monitor (CFAM) provides an estimate of percent suppression and presents a continuous readout of muscle artifact and electrode impedance, both representing measures that may aid in artifact identification.

Compressed Spectral Array

This widely used monitoring method retains and depicts a greater amount of detail than the aforementioned CFM. The CSA produces a pseudo three-dimensional image of the temporal evolution of EEG frequency distribution and relative amplitude over time.

Evoked Potentials

Recording of EPs has become a routine adjunct to the clinical evaluation of many neurologic conditions, including circumstances requiring critical care. These measurements are best suited for serial evaluation of certain neurologic conditions, particularly encephalopathies. Three short-latency EPs are used on the basis of the three different sensory modalities that can be activated: visual, auditory, and somatosensory. Their interpretation requires considerable skill, and their presumed advantages over other means of CNS evaluation remain largely unproven.

12.

Status Epilepticus

Robert C. Tasker and J. Michael Dean

INTRODUCTION

Status epilepticus, a condition in which epileptic activity persists for 30 minutes or longer, causes a wide spectrum of clinical symptoms and has a highly varied pathophysiologic, anatomic, and etiologic basis. This medical emergency requires prompt recognition and immediate, vigorous treatment. If patients are left untreated or poorly treated, or if effective treatment is delayed, permanent neurologic sequelae or even death may ensue.

359

CLINICAL PRESENTATION

Clinical Appearance

Seizures associated with status epilepticus in infants and children include a number of forms or types seen only at particular ages (Table 12.1); therefore, the pediatric specialist should not place all clinical emphasis on generalized tonic-clonic episodes, although this is the most common form in children and adults.

Etiology

In pediatric practice, status epilepticus may occur in those children known to have epilepsy or those who have never had a seizure. Among children with epilepsy, the incidence of status epilepticus may approach 8%, and in 50 to 86% of such children, it may be the presenting seizure. Studies indicate that causes differ widely (Table 12.2), probably reflecting factors such as age distribution of the group studied and the referral base of the institution performing the analysis. Certain causes special to infants and children

Table 12.1
Forms of Status Epilepticus in Relation to Age at Presentation

Age	Type of Status Epilepticus	Features
Neonate	Neonatal status epilepticus	Subtle, tonic, clonic, myoclonic, apneic, fragmentary
	Neonatal epilepsy syndromes	
	• early infantile epileptic encephalopathy	Tonic
	• neonatal myoclonic encephalopathy	Erratic, myoclonic
	• benign familial neonatal seizures	Clonic
Infant and child	Febrile status epilepticus	Convulsive or hemiconvulsive (tonic-clonic)
	Infantile spasms (West syndrome)	Salaam attacks
	Status in childhood myoclonic syndromes	Myoclonic ± absence
	Status in benign partial epilepsy	Complex partial seizures
Child and adult	Tonic-clonic status epilepticus	Tonic-clonic, subtle
	Absence status epilepticus	Absence
	Epilepsia partialis continua	Simple partial
	Myoclonic status epilepticus in coma	Myoclonic
	Myoclonic status in epilepsy syndromes	Myoclonic
	Complex partial status epilepticus	Complex partial
	Status epilepticus in mental retardation	Atypical absence, tonic, minor motor

Adapted from classification by Shorvon SD, In: Shorvon SD, ed. Status epilepticus: its clinical features and treatment in children and adults. New York: Cambridge University Press, 1994.

Table 12.2
Causes of Status Epilepticus

Cause	Percentage of Cases by Selected Series					
	Janz 1961	Aicardi and Chevrie 1970	Rowan and Scott 1970	Yager et al. 1988	Phillips and Shanahan 1989	Maytal et al. 1989
Symptomatic	—	14	4	15	14	6
Tumor	25	—	5	4	1	1
Trauma	24	1	26	0	5	4
Cerebrovascular	4	—	7	2	1	2
Infection	3	12	5	19	14	8
Congenital/ asphyxia	3	27	16	23	14	23
Miscellaneous	7	—	2	4	6	9
Unknown	34	52 (28 febrile)	26 (5 febrile)	33 (21 febrile)	45 (29 febrile)	48 (24 febrile)
Total patients	95	239	43	52	218	193
Mortality (%)	7	11	21	6	6	4

may be indicated by the age at presentation (Table 12.3) (e.g., neonatal or infancy) or the form of status epilepticus (Table 12.4) (e.g., infantile spasms, epilepsia partialis continua, and myoclonic status epilepticus in coma). Fever may be the sole precipitating event for recurrent seizures and status epilepticus in children and accounts for approximately 25% of all such episodes.

The largest group of patients with status epilepticus are those with known epilepsy who are suffering from an acute exacerbation of seizures. A second large group consists of nonepileptic patients with acute central nervous system (CNS) lesions precipitating status epilepticus. In these patients, a variety of cerebrovascular diseases, CNS infections, head trauma, neoplasms, anoxic metabolic disorders, and toxins may precipitate status epilepticus.

PROGNOSIS

Mortality

Before 1960, reported mortality rates after convulsive status epilepticus were as high as 50%. Current mortality rates of tonic-clonic status epilepticus in children range from 4 to 6% (see Table 12.2).

Neurologic Sequelae

Twenty-six to 28% of patients are reported to have neurologic sequelae seemingly related to status epilepticus, although estimating neurologic mor-

Table 12.3

Potential "Nonidiopathic" Causes of Status Epilepticus According to Age at Presentation

	Newborn	First 1–2 Months	Later Infancy and Childhood
Acute insult	Hypoxic-ischemic	CNS infection	CNS infection
	CNS infection	Subdural hematoma	Intracranial hemorrhage
	Intracranial hemorrhage	—	Anoxia
Genetic and	Hypoglycemia	Hypoglycemia	Hypoglycemia
metabolic	Hypernatremia	Hypernatremia	Hypernatremia
	Hyponatremia	Hyponatremia	Hyponatremia
	Hypocalcemia	Hypocalcemia	Hypocalcemia
	Hypomagnesemia	—	—
	Hyperbilirubinemia	—	—
	Organic acidemia	Organic acidemia	Lysosomal defects
	Urea cycle defects	Urea cycle defects	Uremia
	Nonketotic	Phenylketonuria	Liver failure
	hyperglycinemia		
	Congenital lactic	Riley-Day syndrome	—
	acidosis		
	Pyridoxine dependency	—	—
Malformation	Neuronal migration	Sturge-Weber	—
	defect	syndrome	
	Chromosome anomaly	Neurofibromatosis	—
		Tuberous sclerosis	—
Other	Toxins	Cocaine toxicity	Febrile convulsion
	Drugs	—	—
	Narcotic withdrawal	—	—
	Epileptic	—	—
	encephalopathies		

CNS, central nervous system.

bidity directly attributable to an episode of status epilepticus is fraught with difficulties.

Motor problems after an episode of status epilepticus include hemiplegia, diplegia, and extrapyramidal and cerebellar disturbance. The status-induced hemiconvulsion-hemiplegia (HH) and hemiconvulsion-hemiplegia-epilepsy (HHE) syndromes seen in children, typically from 6 months to 2 years of age, rarely occur when status is of short duration. Most of these patients (i.e., 80 to 100%) eventually develop a permanent epileptic condition.

Systemic Complications

Systemic changes and complications of status epilepticus are protean, with the involvement of all organ systems (Table 12.5). Leukocytosis is a frequent finding (i.e., 67% of episodes), even in the absence of infection, which may result in some diagnostic confusion. Also, minimal elevation in cere-

Table 12.4
Causes of Specific Forms of Status Epilepticus

Infantile Spasms	Epilepsia Partialis Continua	Myoclonic Status in Coma
Cerebral malformation —neuronal migration defect —neurocutaneous syndrome	**Brain tumors** —astrocytoma —oligodendroglioma	**Hypoxic-ischemic encephalopathy** —cardiopulmonary bypass —postresuscitation syndrome —carbon monoxide poisoning —CO_2 narcosis —subarachnoid hemorrhage
Genetic metabolic disease —phenylketonuria —nonketotic hyperglycinemia —pyridoxine dependency —histidinemia —hyperornithinemia-hyperammonemia —homocitrullinemia —maple syrup urine disease —leucine-sensitive hypoglycemia	**CNS infection** —brain abscess —tuberculosis —viral encephalitis —cysticercosis **Vascular** —cortical vein thrombosis —malformation	**Toxic-metabolic encephalopathy** —hepatic failure —uremia and dialysis syndrome —hyponatremia —heavy metal poisoning —drug toxicity with tricyclic antidepressants, anticonvulsants, penicillin, and opiates —nonketotic hyperglycinemia
Degenerative disease —Leigh's encephalopathy —leucodystrophies —Alpers' disease (neuronal degeneration) —Sandhoff's disease —Tay-Sachs disease	**Trauma** —posttraumatic cyst —chronic subdural —focal gliosis	**Injury** —posttraumatic —heat stroke —lightning
Perinatal or acute insult —hypoxia-ischemia —hemorrhage —infection —trauma		**Inflammatory** —viral encephalitis —subacute sclerosing panencephalitis —postinfectious encephalomyelitis —opportunistic CNS infection —progressive leukoencephalopathy

CNS, central nervous system.

brospinal fluid (CSF) white blood cell (WBC) count (from 5 to 25 WBC/mm³) is attributable to status epilepticus alone.

Physiologic and Organ-System Effects

Autonomic changes can be prominent and may include cardiac tachyarrhythmias, hypertension, apnea, pupillary dilation, hypersecretion, and sweating. In addition, respiration may be compromised by excessive salivation and tracheobronchial secretions (Table 12.6).

Table 12.5
Medical Complications of Status Epilepticus

Interictal coma
Cumulative anoxia
Cerebral and systemic
Cardiovascular complications
Tachycardia, bradycardia
Cardiac arrest
Hypertension
Cardiac failure, hypotension, cardiogenic shock
Respiratory system failure
Apnea
Cheyne-Stokes breathing
Tachypnea
Neurogenic pulmonary edema
Aspiration, pneumonia
Pulmonary embolism
Respiratory acidosis
Cyanosis
Renal failure
Oliguria, uremia
Acute tubular necrosis
Rhabdomyolysis
Lower nephron necrosis
Autonomic system disturbance
Hyperpyrexia
Excessive sweating, vomiting
Hypersecretion (salivary, tracheobronchial)
Airway obstruction
Metabolic and biochemical abnormalities
Acidosis (metabolic, lactate)
Anoxemia
Hypernatremia, hyponatremia
Hyperkalemia
Hypoglycemia
Hepatic failure
Dehydration
Acute pancreatitis
Infections
Pulmonary
Bladder
Skin
Other
Disseminated intravascular coagulation
Multiple organ system dysfunction
Fractures
Thrombophlebitis

Arterial and Cerebral Venous Blood Pressures

At the onset and during the first 25 minutes (phase I) of seizure activity, arterial and central venous pressures increase dramatically with each convulsion; arterial systolic pressures often exceed 200 mm Hg. Within 1 hour, the

Table 12.6
Time-Related Systemic Complications of Status Epilepticus

Parameter	Phase I Early (<30 Min)	Phase II Late (>30 Min)	Complications Observed
Blood pressure	increase	decrease	hypotension
Arterial oxygen	decrease	decrease	hypoxia
Arterial CO_2	increase	variable	increased ICP
Serum pH	decrease	decrease	acidosis
Temperature	increase by 1° C	increase by 2° C	fever
Autonomic activity	increase	increase	arrhythmias
Lung fluids	increase	increase	atelectasis
Serum potassium	increase or normal	increase	arrhythmias
Serum CPK	normal	increase	renal failure
Cerebral blood flow	increase 900%	increase 200%	cerebral bleed
$CMRO_2$	increase 300%	increase 300%	ischemia

CO_2, carbon dioxide; ICP, intracranial pressure; CPK, creatine phosphokinase; $CMRO_2$, cerebral metabolic rate for oxygen.

blood pressure returns to normal or subnormal levels, but the mean arterial pressure did not drop below the level considered adequate for cerebral perfusion (i.e., 60 mm Hg). Because the initial increase in blood pressure can be blocked by phentolamine hydrochloride, it is presumably the result of massive sympathetic discharge.

CLINICAL MANAGEMENT

The clinical approach to management and therapy must include the provision of an appropriate level of care, intervention, supervision, support for vital functions, anticonvulsant treatment, and directed consideration for possible underlying causes that may necessitate and benefit from specific therapies.

Management Priorities

The longer generalized convulsive status epilepticus persists, the harder it is to control, and the greater the likelihood of significant morbidity and the risk of mortality. Planning a sequence of escalating treatment efforts is imperative. An approach such as that outlined in Table 12.7 should be known to everyone administering and supervising emergency care. In this context, the underlying goals are as follows:

1. To stabilize the patient:
   a. By ensuring adequate cardiorespiratory function and oxygenation
   b. By correcting and preventing metabolic imbalance of hydration, electrolytes, glucose, and lactate

Table 12.7

Summary of Standard Emergency Management of Status Epilepticus from Emergency Department to Intensive Care[a]

Immediate

Airway	• Protect—use 100% oxygen and endotracheal tube if necessary
Breathing	• Support and use muscle relaxants if necessary
Circulation	• Verify good blood pressure—support if necessary
	• Establish secure intravenous line
Draw	• Laboratory samples for glucose, blood urea nitrogen, electrolytes, calcium, phosphate, complete blood count, toxicology
Administer	• 2–4 mL of 25% dextrose in water/kg (500 mg/kg)
Anticonvulsants	• See Table 12.8
First-line	• Diazepam (0.2–0.4 mg/kg) or lorazepam (0.1–0.2 mg/kg) administered over 2 minutes, maximum of 10 mg
	OR
	• Phenytoin (15–20 mg/kg) up to 1000 mg (no faster than 25 mg/min)
Second-line	• Phenytoin if not already administered (dose as above)
	• Phenobarbital (10 mg/kg) no more than 30 mg/kg × 2
	Intubate if respiratory depression occurs

Critical care

CNS protection	• Intubate and mechanically ventilate
	• See Tables 12.9 and 12.10
Drugs	• Phenytoin—rebolus and administer according to levels
	• Paraldehyde (0.15 mL of 4% solution/per kg/h) by continuous and intravenous line
	• Anesthesia with short-acting barbiturates

[a]Based on the history, progression to critical care may be appropriate within minutes of presentation.

CNS, central nervous system.

2. To treat the treatable
   a. By stopping clinical and electrical seizure activity as soon as possible, preferably within 30 minutes
   b. By preventing the recurrence of seizures
   c. By preventing or correcting any systemic complications
   d. By evaluating for and treating specific causes of status epilepticus

Stabilizing the Patient

The top priority in the management of patients with status epilepticus is preservation of vital function- airway protection, maintenance of ventilation, assurance of oxygenation, and support of the circulation. The patient should be positioned to avoid aspiration, suffocation, or physical injury. Adequate aeration should be ensured, and a plastic airway may be placed if it can be done easily. The forced use of such an airway or the use of tongue blades or metal objects may cause severe oral injury and should be avoided. The child with poor air exchange should be intubated and mechanically ventilated. The authors also recommend proactive intubation and ventilation for patients in whom seizure activity does not cease after administration of appropriate anticonvulsants. It is wrong to wait long enough for the development of florid systemic complications such as cyanosis, severe acidosis, or hemodynamic instability before proceeding to intubation.

Neuromuscular blockade often is necessary to accomplish intubation. Moreover, because it should be assumed that all such patients have a full stomach and are at significant risk of aspiration, the rapid sequence technique with cricoid pressure is mandatory. After having administered a muscle relaxant, anticonvulsant therapy can no longer be titrated against a clinical endpoint. If clinical parameters for treatment evaluation are used, a short-acting agent is preferable. In some patients with complex multisystem pathology, however, a long-acting agent may be preferable for optimal treatment of their other problems, and alternative monitoring should be used.

After intubation is accomplished, or if it is deemed unnecessary, the child should be receive 100% oxygen to avoid developing hypoxia. Subsequent oxygen therapy should be guided by arterial blood gas measurements and other appropriate oxygen monitoring, with the caveat that a seizure-associated decline in cortical oxygenation may respond to such treatment.

Monitoring

As with any patient receiving neurologic intensive care, clinical surveillance should include regular observations of motor, sensory, and pupillary function; blood pressure, pulse, and electrocardiographic state; and oximetry and temperature. More severely affected patients require more complete and invasive monitoring (e.g., capnography, central venous pressure, Swan-Ganz pulmonary artery pressure monitoring). Given that metabolic abnormalities may cause or result from status epilepticus, it is also important to review serum biochemistry, blood glucose, blood gases, pH, clotting, and hematologic parameters.

Nursing care is also vitally important, because tracheobronchial secretions may be excessive, and bronchial or endotracheal tube obstruction is a significant hazard. If the patient is comatose, all measures applied to standard care (e.g., early tube feeding for nutrition, regular turning to avoid pressure sores, eye care) should be applied.

In the acute setting, fluids and drugs are administered intravenously, preferably in large veins as many anticonvulsants can cause severe phlebitis and thrombosis at the infusion site. When more than one anticonvulsant is used, more than one line or lumen is necessary, mainly because of incompatibilities in mixing or precipitation if added to glucose infusions. Arterial lines, commonly used for monitoring, should not be used to administer anticonvulsants because severe arterial spasm and necrosis may develop. If additional access for administering anticonvulsants is required, the intraosseous or intramuscular route can be used.

Emergency Investigations

In an emergent situation, the following measurements should be obtained:

- Blood gases
- pH
- Blood sugar level
- Renal and liver function
- Calcium and magnesium levels
- Hematologic parameters (including platelet count)
- Anticonvulsant levels

Blood and urine should be kept for toxicologic or metabolic screening at a later time, if this analysis is deemed necessary.

Further investigations depend on the clinical circumstances, whether or not there is a history of epilepsy, and age of presentation (Tables 12.3 and 12.4). When the episode of status is unexplained, focal, or coexistent with an acute illness, cranial computed tomography scanning is warranted. The CSF should be examined only when there is no risk to the patient.

Circulatory Support

When seizures have continued for a significant period, cerebral autoregulation is impaired and cerebral blood flow becomes perfusion pressure dependent (i.e., systemic arterial pressure is a major determinant). Maintaining blood pressure within normal levels, therefore, is of utmost importance.

Although hypertension may occur as a consequence of seizures, hypotension becomes a problem with prolonged seizure activity and may be exacerbated by respiratory failure and intravenous anticonvulsants, with a cardiodepressant effect.

Abatement of hypotension should include attention to general respiratory status, anticonvulsant infusions and levels, and administration of inotropic agents. If necessary, dopamine (5 to 20 µg/kg/min) can be titrated against the desired hemodynamic and renal response. Persistent hypotension that is unresponsive to supportive therapy represents a severe state in protracted seizures and may portend a poor outcome.

Other Physiologic Changes and Management

Status epilepticus may produce a variety of acute metabolic, autonomic, and cardiovascular derangements that require active intervention.

Acidosis Lactic acidosis is common and can contribute to a compromised hemodynamic state. If the patient is in shock, appropriate fluid and pressor therapy should be administered. Rarely, intravenous bicarbonate is necessary, but it can be given to half correct an acidosis when the pH is less than 7.2. In most instances, correction of respiratory abnormalities and cessation of convulsive movements will adequately contain an acquired metabolic problem.

Hypoglycemia Hypoglycemia may cause or be a consequence of status epilepticus. This abnormality should be considered early and, when present, treated with intravenous dextrose, 500 mg/kg stat dose. Appropriate blood and urine investigation also is necessary, because profound hypoglycemia may be a symptom of inherited metabolic disease.

Hypercarbia, Pulmonary Artery Hypertension, and Pulmonary Edema A variety of factors account for these abnormalities, which may be fatal. Treatment should be aimed primarily at optimizing mechanical ventilation; thereafter, diuretics and vasoactive agents may be needed.

Hyperthermia In the patient with uncontrolled seizures, hyperpyrexia may develop. Generally, this response can be limited by neuromuscular blockade, adequate fluid resuscitation, and the use of body-temperature cooling aids (e.g., temperature-controlled water mattresses).

Disseminated Intravascular Coagulation Disseminated intravascular coagulation may develop rapidly and requires appropriate treatment. More importantly, deranged clotting may herald the onset of complicating liver failure or drug toxicity.

Renal Failure Hypotension, severe metabolic acidosis, or rhabdomyolysis may compromise renal function. Oliguria is an important sign. It is important to initiate measures to avoid renal failure, ensuring adequate cardiac output, hydration, and urine flow.

Electrolyte and Fluid Balance Initially, if the patient is hyperthermic and in shock, active fluid resuscitation to achieve a good blood pressure and urine output must be initiated. Thereafter, a balance is achieved, providing enough to avoid renal failure, yet not so much as to compromise pulmonary alveolar-capillary leak and any cerebral edema. Electrolytic abnormalities in potassium and sodium are treated when present.

Cerebral Edema Persistent seizures may result in the development of cerebral edema and increased intracranial pressure. On occasion, seizures may continue unabated, despite seemingly adequate anticonvulsant therapy, until specific cerebral edema therapy is initiated (mannitol 0.25 g/kg stat dose). In patients in whom status is a symptom of underlying brain insult, regular mannitol administration or even neurosurgery may be necessary.

Implementing Drug Therapy

To control status epilepticus quickly and to prevent recurrence, a therapeutic serum concentration of a long-acting anticonvulsant medication must be achieved. The therapeutic endpoint in such cases, however, is not the production of a particular drug concentration, but rather a clinical and/or electrical endpoint. Clinical experience suggests that virtually any antiepileptic drug, sedative, hypnotic, or general anesthetic agent works, but dangerously high concentrations of hypnotics often are needed. It is not the particular choice of drug but rather the timing, route, and vigor of therapy that are major determinants of the duration of status epilepticus and subsequent morbidity. Furthermore, early therapy is far more effective than later therapy, suggesting that vigorous intravenous therapy early in a seizure may abort status epilepticus.

Standard Anticonvulsant Medications

The most common anticonvulsant drugs used in the acute treatment of status epilepticus and their dosages are described in Table 12.8.

Diazepam

Diazepam is the most lipid-soluble drug used to treat status epilepticus, and it has the largest volume of distribution. It gained popularity because of its rapid distribution in the brain (i.e., within 10 seconds) and its relatively low toxicity. In addition, it is effective in virtually all types of status epilepticus, including grand mal, focal motor, absence, myoclonic, and secondarily generalized grand mal status epilepticus. It is, however, associated with an extensive drop in serum concentration during the distribution phase, with limitation of anticonvulsant activity to approximately 20 minutes and a greater than 70% fall in serum concentration within the first 2 hours after administration; this fall may be associated with seizure recurrence.

Lorazepam

The lipid solubility, volume of distribution, and distribution half-life of lorazepam are approximately one half those of diazepam. Like diazepam, lorazepam enters the brain rapidly; the onset of lorazepam and diazepam action in status epilepticus is 3 and 2 minutes, respectively. Unlike diazepam, however, redistribution is minimal, and effective levels persist in the brain several hours after a single intravenous dose. As a result, the anticonvulsant effect is extended but with a somewhat rapid development of tolerance.

Phenytoin

Phenytoin is effective in controlling tonic-clonic status epilepticus in adults and children and in neonates and young infants. Phenytoin has relatively low lipid solubility and therefore enters and equilibrates in the brain slowly. The elimination kinetics are nonlinear, and approximately 30% of children have a degree of saturated metabolism that makes it difficult to adjust phenytoin concentration within the therapeutic range; this also means that a nonlinear relationship exists between clinically relevant doses and concentrations achieved. Whenever phenytoin doses are increased, therefore,

Table 12.8
First-Line Anticonvulsants for Status Epilepticus

Drug	Loading Dose	Route	Blood Level	Side Effects	Idiosyncratic Effects
Diazepam					
Neonatal	0.2–0.4 mg/kg	IV		Sedation, hypotension, respiratory depression, laryngospasm, arrest	Absence status may convert to tonic status, leukopenia (neutropenia, granulocytopenia), agranulocytosis, aplastic anemia, hemolytic anemia, transient decrease in renal function, increased AST (SGOT), ALT (SGPT), LDH, alkaline phosphatase, and total and direct bilirubin
Infant/child	0.2–0.4 mg/kg	IV			
	0.5 mg/kg	PR			
Adult	10 mg	IV			
Lorazepam					
Infant/child	0.1–0.2 mg/kg	IV		As above	As above
Adult	4–8 mg	IV			
Phenytoin			10–20 μg/mL		
Neonatal	20 mg/kg	IV		Hypotension, cardiac conduction defects, less sedation	Blood dyscrasia, lupus-like syndrome, reduced IgA, rash, peripheral neuropathy, hepatotoxicity, lymphoma
Infant/child	20 mg/kg	IV			
Adult	15–20 mg/kg	IV			
Phenobarbital			10–40 μg/mL		
Neonatal	20 mg/kg	IV		Same as diazepam, may set synergistically	Maculopapular rash, hepatotoxicity, toxic epidermal necrolysis, exfoliation
Infant/child	20 mg/kg	IV			

AST, aspartate transaminase; SGOT, serum glutamic oxaloacetic transaminase; ALT, alanine transaminase; SGPT, serum glutamic pyruvic transaminase; LDH, lactic dehydrogenase; IgA, immunoglobulin A.

the serum concentration increases disproportionately. A compounding phenomenon is that the apparent half-life for phenytoin progressively increases as the serum concentration increases.

With a loading dose of 18 to 20 mg/kg, peak brain drug levels may not be reached for 10 to 30 minutes, although the level should have equilibrated by 1 hour and a subsequent therapeutic level maintained for 24 hours. Therefore, when delivering a dose of phenytoin as a second-line drug in status epilepticus, it is important to wait at least 30 minutes before drug failure is concluded. The rate of intravenous administration should be limited to 25 mg/min in older children or 0.5 to 1.0 mg/kg/min in younger children.

Phenobarbital

As the initial agent of choice for many years, phenobarbital is the least lipid-soluble drug used to treat status epilepticus and, therefore, has the slowest onset of action. Its distribution phase lasts 1 hour or more and has a long elimination half-life. During status epilepticus, the entrance of phenobarbital into the brain is enhanced, largely due to changes in blood pH and blood pressure.

Compared with shorter acting barbiturates, such as thiopental, phenobarbital is a much more potent anticonvulsant when related to equal CNS depressant effects. The short and medium half-life barbiturates can be used with more rapid effect, but at the expense of inducing anesthesia.

Therapeutic Strategies

Treatment in Relation to Age

Neonates In newborns, the relationship between drug dose and concentration is highly unpredictable and changing because of a lesser degree of drug protein binding and an evolving ability and capacity to eliminate drugs. The result is an enormous range of required doses, with average doses being of value only as initial treatment.

Phenobarbital and phenytoin are effective for status epilepticus; phenytoin has been effective as an initial drug—dosage not exceed 20 to 30 mg/kg before blood levels are monitored—and phenobarbital is preferable for safer and longer term administration. Benzodiazepines, including diazepam and lorazepam, are effective at all ages in stopping status epilepticus, but high dosages are required. Diazepam has a short duration of anticonvulsant action after bolus dosing and leads to some uncertainty of the actual dose administered when delivered by infusion, and lorazepam becomes progressively less effective because patients develop tolerance rapidly, particularly if used repeatedly for a recurrence within 48 hours.

Infants Infants have the highest relative capacity to eliminate anticonvulsant drugs. The half-life of phenobarbital diminishes from 114 to 45 hours. Phenytoin is eliminated rapidly, and its nonlinear kinetics mean that when phenytoin concentrations are low, the apparent half-life is usually very short, sometimes necessitating the use of maintenance doses as high as 20 mg/kg/day to produce consistent therapeutic levels.

Older Children and Young Adults After infancy, relative drug clearance progressively declines until adult values are achieved at ages 10 to 15 years. Benzodiazepines are extremely effective in stopping status epilepticus. Because diazepam has a short duration of anticonvulsant action, a longer-acting drug should be coadministered to prevent seizures from recurring. Lorazepam has been put forward as a better alternative because it has proved effective (i.e., between 80 and 100%) in a number of studies; thus, the need for early institution of a second anticonvulsant is avoided. In most patients treated with lorazepam, however, a second anticonvulsant must be started in the first 12 to 24 hours after status epilepticus, which in practice would confer little advantage over the coadministration of diazepam with another anticonvulsant. Finally, it should be remembered that benzodiazepines have not been demonstrated to be superior to phenobarbital.

Treatment According to Duration of Seizure

Some anticonvulsants are more appropriate than others as the duration of an individual episode increases. For practical purposes, an unrelenting seizure can be divided into four phases:

1. Prodromal stage. Emergency treatment with diazepam or midazolam usually halts evolution to true status.
2. Initial 30 minutes. Lorazepam and diazepam with phenytoin are potential first-line choices.
3. Status 30 to 60 minutes. The therapeutic objective in this stage changes to cerebral protection and limiting morbidity and mortality. Patients seen for the first time at this stage receive diazepam, lorazepam, or phenytoin, and phenobarbital. Doses of phenobarbital should be increased before additional drugs are administered to patients who do not respond. Other agents that can be coadministered with the above drugs are chlormethiazole, clonazepam, diazepam, midazolam, and paraldehyde (Table 12.9).
4. Resistant status epilepticus lasting longer than 60 minutes. The primary aim in this stage is cerebral protection by suppression of CNS activity and metabolism with the use of anesthetic agents (see subsequent section).

Refractory Status Epilepticus and Treatment Failure

If convulsive status epilepticus has continued for 60 minutes despite treatment, the episode is deemed refractory, and emergency therapy with anesthetic agents is instituted. Initiation of such treatment before 60 minutes has elapsed is often guided by personal experience. It is important to weigh the advantages of rapid suppression of CNS metabolism with induction of anesthesia by short or medium half-life barbiturates or inhalational agents (Table 12.10) against the risks of hemodynamic instability during therapy and difficulties in seizure control during weaning.

Table 12.9
Alternative Anticonvulsants for Refractory Status Epilepticus

Drug	Initial IV Dose	Rate of Infusion	Notes	Side Effects
Paraldehyde	0.15 mL/kg (4% solution)	Divide over 1 h	Give under EEG control and titrate dose against effect. More than 1 mL is rarely needed (use <5–10 mL)	Drowsiness and coma, pulmonary embolus, pulmonary hemorrhage, hepatic toxicity, renal toxicity
		Repeat dose in 1–4 h	Use fresh solution: half-life 6–9 h	
Lidocaine	1–2 mg/kg	2–4 mg/kg/h (neonates 2–6 mg/kg/h)	ECG monitoring for changes such as prolonged PR interval and in QRS complex	Hypotension, heart block, arrhythmia, and CNS toxicity
Clonazepam	0.25 mg neonate 0.5 mg child	Repeat bolus 0.01 mg/kg (10–40 μg/kg/min)	More potent than diazepam in sedation. Long half-life (20 ± 50 h) so infusion not usually used	Hypotension—can paradoxically worsen tonic status
Chlormethiazole	0.08 mg/kg/min or 0.1 mL/kg/min (0.8% solution)	Increase dose every 2 h until seizures abolished	Accumulates— metabolism is affected by changes in hepatic blood flow	Risk of hypotension, heart block, tachycardia, fluid overload, and electrolyte disturbance

EEG, electroencephalogram; ECG, electrocardiogram; CNS, central nervous system.

Anesthesia for Control Suppression of CNS metabolism with short-acting barbiturates such as thiopentone and pentobarbitone can be achieved rapidly with acute control of seizures and status epilepticus. A protocol outlined in Table 12.11 has proven effective, without hemodynamic compromise. Few guidelines exist regarding depth or duration of anesthesia, and although acute seizure control can be achieved, difficulties in control may arise on weaning.

Phenobarbital An alternative to adopting the above protocol of anesthesia is to administer more phenobarbital at an earlier stage. In the controlled environment of the intensive care unit, there does not appear to be a maximum dose of phenobarbital. In a study of a large series of children with refractory status epilepticus, seizures were controlled eventually by repeated bolus doses of 5 to 20 mg/kg, spaced by an adequate time to allow for penetration of the drug into the CNS (i.e., approximately 30 to 60 minutes). Maximum doses administered in 24 hours ranged from 30 to 120

Table 12.10
Anesthesia for Control of Status Epilepticus

Drug	Dose	Notes	Side Effects
Thiopental sodium	See Table 12.11	Saturable kinetics, active metabolite	Hypotension, hypersensitivity—laryngeal edema, bronchospasm, and erythema 1/30,000. Pancreatitis and hepatic dysfunction.
Pentobarbitone sodium	5–20 mg/kg loading 0.5–3 mg/kg/hr infusion (5–20 mg/kg bolus for breakthrough seizures)	Advantage over thiopental: nonsaturable kinetics, no active metabolites, longer duration of action, and GABA-ergic action	Hypotension and cardiac dysfunction Decerebrate posturing and flaccid paralysis during anesthesia, and weakness may persist for weeks.
Isoflurane	End-tidal concentration 0.8–2%—dose titrated to maintain burst suppression	Pupils are rendered small. Isoflurane can be used in liver and renal disease.	Muscle relaxant effect. After prolonged use a transient movement disorder may become evident.
Etomidate	0.3 mg/kg 20 μg/kg/min infusion	Corticosteroid coadministration is required	Hypotension, drug-induced myoclonus, and muscular twitching. Interferes with adrenocorticoid function.
Propofol	2 mg/kg bolus 5–10 mg/kg/h initially then reduced to 1–3 mg/kg/h		Proconvulsant Prolonged infusion results in lipemia and accumulation of inactive gluconuride metabolites with metabolic acidosis—especially in children.

mg/kg (median 60 mg/kg), and the maximum blood levels achieved were 70 to 344 μg/mL (median 114 μg/mL). Despite such a regimen of high dose administration and continuing high serum levels of phenobarbital, many patients were weaned from respiratory support, and there did not appear to be any acute drug-related complications. The authors concluded that such an approach would, in most cases, obviate the need for intubation, mechanical ventilation, and electroencephalogram monitoring. Although these data support the use of higher doses of phenobarbital, further prospective evaluation for such treatment is needed.

In an emergency such as refractory status epilepticus, rapid control of the clinical state is essential. This goal can be achieved with induction of

Table 12.11
Thiopental Infusion Therapy for Status Epilepticus

Aim of therapy
To control the physical effects of seizures
To suppress electrical correlates of seizure activity
To induce burst suppression or electrocerebral silence
To avoid toxic drug levels and complications

Basics of critical care

Mechanically ventilate	
(Muscle relaxation)	Muscle rest (see text)
Maintain physiologic parameters	Normoxia and normocarbia
	Normotension
	Normoglycemia
	Normothermia
Monitor	Blood pressure, ECG, capnography, oximetry, EEG
	Drug levels

Therapy

Loading dose	2–8 mg/kg thiopental in increments of 2 mg/kg under EEG
Infusion	1–10 mg/kg via central intravenous line (giving the minimum necessary to achieve the above aims)

EEG, electroencephalogram; ECG, electrocardiogram.

anesthesia, and there appears to be little advantage in a more delayed approach, given the facility of modern intensive care. Phenobarbital, however, is a better anticonvulsant than pentobarbitone or thiopentone, and it may be effective as long-term maintenance therapy.

Reassessment When the clinical course does not follow an expected pattern of response to therapy and improvement, it is valuable during either the initial hours of treatment or the weaning stage of anesthesia to reassess all the correctable factors systematically:

- Adequacy of drug therapy, both choice of agents and the doses administered.
- Initiation of appropriate maintenance antiepileptic therapy
- Control or exclusion of all systemic and metabolic derangements (see Table 12.5)
- Identification of any treatable underlying structural, metabolic, or infective cause (See Tables 12.3 and 12.4)

Treatment for Nontonic-Clonic Forms of Status Epilepticus

In nontonic-clonic forms of status epilepticus, systemic derangements are generally less evident than in the tonic-clonic forms, and in practice such changes usually result from the unwanted effects of anticonvulsants used. The presence or absence of generalized motor concomitants of status epilepticus should not be the sole determinant of aggressive and prompt treatment, since even nonconvulsive status epilepticus results in a rise in serum neuron-specific enolase, indicating at least a transient neuronal injury.

Intensive care unit management of these patients is complex because they often are receiving a complex anticonvulsant mixture that may be difficult to rationalize. Simply adding or discontinuing an anticonvulsant drug may result in converting one type of seizure into another, more resistant form. In the authors' experience, optimal treatment of these patients can be achieved successfully only with full support from clinical neurophysiologic and neurologic services. The range of preferred treatments for nontonic-clonic forms of status are listed in Table 12.12.

Drug Toxicities

Knowledge of the potential drug toxicities occurring during the treatment of status epilepticus is essential, not least because they usually are iatrogenic (see Tables 12.8 to 12.10). An important distinction must be made between an anticonvulsant-related toxicity and that produced by a drug that has also

Table 12.12
Preferred Anticonvulsants for Nontonic-clonic Forms of Status Epilepticus

Infantile spasms (West's syndrome)	Treat any underlying cause, e.g., hypoglycemia, metabolic disorders, endocrine abnormalities, infection. • ACTH 150 IU/day in two divided doses for 1 week —then 75 IU/day in two divided doses for 1 week —then decrease over 5–8 weeks • Other drugs: benzodiazepines, valproate, vigabatrin, pyridoxine phosphate, gamma globulin
Epilepsia partialis continua	This may remit spontaneously. • First choice anticonvulsants: phenytoin, carbamazepine, phenobarbitone • Other treatment: corticosteroids or gamma globulin, nimodipine, surgery
Status epilepticus in mental retardation	Sedation may worsen all types of seizures. Tonic status is usually resistant to treatment, and occasionally benzodiazepines may worsen the episode. • First choice anticonvulsants: valproate, clonazepam, clobazam, lamotrigine • In emergencies, high-dose ACTH 80 IU/day or corticosteroids 0.3–1 mg/kg/d • Surgery
Status epilepticus in myoclonic syndromes	This is highly resistant to therapy. Urgently treat any fever or infection. • ACTH (as above) • Valproate and ethosuximide • Other drugs: acetazolamide, nitrazepam, corticosteroids
Myoclonic status epilepticus in coma	• Phenytoin or phenobarbitone • Corticosteroids can be tried.

Table 12.13
Drugs that Cause Seizures

Antimicrobials
Isoniazid
Penicillins
Nalidixic acid
Metronidazole
Anesthetics, narcotics, analgesics
Halothane, enflurane
Cocaine, fentanyl, meperidine
Ketamine
Psychopharmaceuticals
Antihistamines
Antidepressants
Antipsychotics
Phencyclidine
Tricyclic antidepressants

induced seizures (Table 12.13). In the latter case, treatment is improved by withdrawal of the implicated agent.

Electroencephalography

Electroencephalography provides not only valuable diagnostic information, but also an observable endpoint for anticonvulsant treatment when this point is not clinically discernable. In status epilepticus, multichannel electroencephalograms present global findings and changes. Disadvantages are evident after several days of use, including large volumes of data and continuous bedside interpretation.

13.

Toxic-Metabolic Encephalopathies

Robert C. Tasker, W. Bradley Poss, and J. Michael Dean

INTRODUCTION

Many metabolic disturbances may produce a fluctuation in level of consciousness or a coma. During the course of an acute illness, whether at presentation or as a secondary complicating factor, these fluctuations may be symptomatic of significant morbidity and even lead to death.

Acute toxic encephalopathy exemplifies this acute encephalopathic progression. Although Reye syndrome is seen infrequently in the wider context of clinical management during toxic-metabolic derangement and nontraumatic coma, it should be considered prototypic. The refined critical care approach to children with Reye syndrome has shaped the practice of pediatric intensive care. Many techniques used for its treatment are beneficial for some cases of overwhelming liver disease, renal disease, hyperammonemia, and inborn errors of metabolism.

ETIOLOGY AND DIFFERENTIAL DIAGNOSIS

A variety of toxic-metabolic disorders may produce an acute depression in level of consciousness (Table 13.1), with some being more common at particular ages. In some patients, etiology may be complex, with more than one known factor being implicated as the cause for coma. For practical application in the context of critical care, two patient presentations may occur:

1. A characteristic history and findings, frequently seen and suggestive of certain disorders, the so-called classic syndromes of critical illness:
   a. Reye syndrome and Reye-like illness (Table 13.2)
   b. Raised intracranial pressure
   c. Hepatic encephalopathy
   d. Fulminant infantile encephalopathy
2. An identified profound biochemical derangement requiring further management (e.g., acidosis, hyperammonemia, hypoglycemia, electrolyte imbalance)

Table 13.1
Causes of Acute Toxic-Metabolic Encephalopathy in Childhood

Acid-base disturbance
Acidosis—diabetic ketoacidosis, organic acidemia, renal tubular acidosis
Alkalosis
Fluid and electrolyte derangement
Dehydration
Adrenal crisis
Water intoxication—inappropriate ADH secretion, psychogenic polydipsia
Hypercalcemia/hypocalcemia
Hypernatremia/hyponatremia
Hypomagnesemia/hypermagnesemia
Deprivation of oxygen, substrate, or metabolic cofactor
Hypoxia/ischemia
Hypoglycemia
(Seizure postictally)
Vitamin/cofactor deficiency—thiamine, niacin, pyridoxine
Diseases of organs other than brain
Liver failure/hyperammonemia—infection, urea-cycle, Reye-like
Renal failure—uremia
Lung—carbon dioxide narcosis
Endocrine—thyroid, parathyroid, adrenal, diabetes
Endogenous (inherited metabolic disorders)
Aminoaciduria
Organic acidemia
Galactosemia
Porphyria

ADH, antidiuretic hormone.

Table 13.2
Conditions Producing Reye-like Illness

Infective conditions
Acute liver failure (viral hepatitis, antituberculous drugs, monoamine oxidase inhibitors, acetaminophen, ischemia)
Severe infection (endotoxic shock)
Inherited disorders of urea cycle
Carbamoyl-phosphate synthase deficiency
Ornithine carbamoyltransferase deficiency
Citrullinemia
Arginosuccinic aciduria
Arginase deficiency (rare)
Organic acidemias
Proprionic and methylmalonic acidemia
Other inherited metabolic disease
Triple H syndrome (hyperammonemia, hyperornithinemia, homocitrullinuria)
Hyperlysinemia
Fat oxidation defects (medium- and long-chain and multiple acetyl-CoA[a] dehydrogenase deficiency)
Toxins and medications
Drugs (salicylates, valproate, warfarin)
Toxins (aflatoxin, hypoglycine, ackee, pteridine, calcium hopantenate, isopropyl alcohol methobromide, lead, margosa oil, diallylacetate)

[a]acyl-CoA, acylocoenzyme A.

Classic Syndromes of Critical Illness

Urea Cycle Disorders

Metabolic acidosis and hypoglycemia are not usually found, but hyperammonemia is present and often severe. The plasma and urine amino acid profiles are abnormal, and urinary orotic acid is elevated in most of these disorders. In the most serious cases, patients are affected in the neonatal period, but there is a wide spectrum of severity, and patients may be affected at any childhood age. The female carrier of the X-linked disorder ornithine carbamylase deficiency, and the homozygous male with partial enzyme deficiency, may present with mild episodic symptoms.

Organic Acidemias

Overriding metabolic acidosis is the main distinguishing feature of organic acidemias. Hyperammonemia, at times as dramatic as that associated with urea cycle disorders, commonly is seen in critically ill neonates, but is less consistently observed in older children. The most common conditions are propionic acidemia, methylmalonic acidemia, and maple syrup urine disease. Although the plasma amino acid profile is diagnostic in the latter, gas chromatography of plasma and urine organic acids is required to establish the diagnosis of most of these disorders.

Disorders of Fat Oxidation

Medium- and long-chain acyl CoA dehydrogenase deficiency may resemble Reye syndrome. Typical clinical findings include:

- Nonketotic hypoglycemia
- Hyperammonemia
- Moderate metabolic acidosis
- Episodes of encephalopathy, often associated with hepatomegaly (due to fatty infiltrates), that tend to become less frequent with time
- Low serum carnitine level

Some children may have primary systemic carnitine deficiency present with a Reye-like illness. The cause of this primary carnitine deficiency is unclear but possibly is caused by a combination of impaired gastrointestinal absorption and renal tubular resorption.

Raised Intracranial Pressure

In the absence of an intracranial space-occupying lesion or hydrocephalus, raised intracranial pressure can result from:

- Increased venous pressure (as in dural sinus thrombosis)
- Increased resistance of arachnoid villi to resorption of cerebrospinal fluid
- Hypersecretion of cerebrospinal fluid (as in certain endocrine abnormalities)
- Cerebral edema

The toxic-metabolic causes are listed in Table 13.3. Early symptoms and signs of raised intracranial pressure are nonspecific (Table 13.4), and the late identification of this problem often is indicated by signs of brain-tissue herniation (Table 13.5).

Pathologic Types of Cerebral Edema Cerebral edema is defined as an increase in brain volume resulting from an increase in its water content. When generalized, it causes raised intracranial pressure. Localized edema, however, may alter cerebral function with no change in fluid dynamics. Cranial imaging aids in diagnosis: computed tomography (CT) scanning may show diffuse or localized low attenuation as a result of high water content; T2-weighted magnetic resonance imaging (MRI) will show an intense signal.

Cerebral edema can result from a variety of brain insults, with specific types of edema being associated with certain pathologic processes. In many instances, more than one process may be implicated.

Vasogenic Edema An increase in cerebral capillary endothelial permeability will result in the exudation of proteinaceous fluid into surrounding cerebral white matter. Whether there is focal or global cerebral edema will be determined by the underlying cause of the change in cerebral vascular permeability:

Table 13.3
Toxic-Metabolic Encephalopathies in which Significant Cerebral Edema Has Been Reported[a]

Inherited metabolic
Aminoacidopathies
Organic acidemias
Hyperammonemia
Porphyria
Nonketotic hyperglycinemia
Organ failure
Uremia
Hepatic failure
Electrolytes, minerals, and vitamins
Hypercalcemia
Hypernatremia
Water intoxication
Lead poisoning
Vitamin A toxicity
Other
Hypoglycemia
Hypoxia/ischemia

[a]This list, rather than being exhaustive, reflects the diversity of disease categories associated with cerebral edema.

Table 13.4
Nonspecific Symptoms and Signs of Raised Intracranial Pressure

	Infant	Child
General state	Poor feeding, vomiting	Anorexia, nausea, vomiting
	Irritability—coma	Lethargy—coma
	Seizures	Seizures
Head/eyes	Full fontanele	False localizing signs (see Table 13.11)
	Scalp vein distention	
	False localizing signs	
Other	Altered vital signs	Altered vital signs
	Hypertension	Hypertension
	Pulmonary edema	Pulmonary edema

- Infection
- Trauma
- Toxins
- Focal seizures
- Hypertension

Cytotoxic Edema All cells within the brain can undergo rapid swelling resulting from membrane ionic pump failure that is secondary to intracellular energy failure. Causes include:

Table 13.5
Clinical Signs of Brain Downward Herniation

	Tentorial	Foramen Magnum

Mechanism	1. Diencephalon and hypothalamus downward and caudally
	  • Optic chiasm stretched and twisted
	  • Infundibulum displaced
	  • Brain stem torsion
	  • Vertebral arteries displaced
	2. Compression of
	  • Cerebral peduncle
	  • Nerve VI
	  • Posterior cerebral artery
	3. Secondary hemorrhage in brain stem
		1. Tentorial downward shift continues to the posterior fossa
		2. Cerebellar tonsils herniate at the side of the cord (may be down to C5)

Signs		
Consciousness	Decreased, tonic seizures	Comatose
Motor	Decerebrate responses	Hypotonia/spinal flexion Brisk flexor withdrawal Tongue fasciculation, bulbar palsy Erb's palsy
Eyes	Nerve palsy III and VI "Sunsetting" Cortical blindness	Absent calorics or doll's eyes response Absent ciliospinal reflex
Respiration	Central neurogenic hyperventilation Cheyne-Stokes respiration	Bradypnea, apnea Laryngeal stridor
Other	Loss of temperature control Cardiac irregularity	Hypotension

- Hypoxic-ischemic insult
- Severe infection
- Toxins
- Status epilepticus
- Low cerebral blood flow

Hypo-osmotic Edema Osmotic dysequilibrium between a low osmolality plasma compartment and higher osmotic pressure within glial cells results in astrocytic water accumulation and brain tissue edema. Causes include:

- Hyponatremia
- Excessive fluid resuscitation for diabetic ketoacidosis
- Dialysis dysequilibrium syndrome

Interstitial Edema In patients with raised intracranial pressure and hydrocephalus, periventricular interstitial edema caused by transependymal resorption of cerebrospinal fluid into the extracellular space may occur.

Hydrostatic Edema Increased intravascular pressure transmitted to the capillary bed prompts a net efflux of water into the extracellular space. Such hydrostatic edema may be seen in states of deranged autoregulation, as occurs in systemic hypertension and hypercapnia.

Benign Intracranial Hypertension Benign intracranial hypertension is characterized by raised intracranial pressure in the absence of focal neurologic dysfunction, intracerebral mass lesion, obstructive hydrocephalus, chronic meningitis, hypertension, and pulmonary encephalopathy. In most cases, the cause and pathogenesis are poorly understood (Table 13.6).

The apparent well-being of these patients distinguishes raised intracranial pressure from cerebral edema. In the intensive care unit, it may be difficult to interpret the clinical significance of elevated intracranial pressure in some patients who have multiple reasons for coma. The conscious patient may demonstrate the following signs:

- Headache (i.e., the most common complaint)
- Nerve VI palsy
- Visual acuity loss
- Papilledema
- Vertical strabismus or other oculomotor abnormalities
- Pupillary abnormalities

Table 13.6
Causes and Differential Diagnosis of Benign Intracranial Hypertension

1. Intracranial venous sinus thrombosis
   Ear infection—related to lateral sinus thrombosis
   After head trauma
   Idiopathic
   Secondary to vena cava and other venous thrombosis and obstruction
2. Endocrine and metabolic disorders
   Corticosteroid withdrawal
   Chronic hypocalcemia (hypoparathyroidism)
   Pseudohypoparathyroidism
   Vitamin D deficient rickets
   Chronic carbon dioxide retention
   Addison's disease
   Obesity
3. Drugs and toxins
   Excess dose of vitamin A
   Nalidixic acid
   Tetracycline and minocycline
   Amiodarone
4. Hematologic disorders
   Iron-deficiency anemia
   Infectious mononucleosis
   Wiskott-Aldrich syndrome

- Facial palsy
- Ataxia

Hepatic Encephalopathy

Hepatic encephalopathy complicates both acute and chronic liver failure and may be caused by potentially reversible metabolic abnormalities. In its extreme form, hepatic encephalopathy can lead to coma and death.

Fulminant Neonatal Encephalopathy

In the first postnatal month and early infantile period, the clinical presentation of metabolic disease may include a combination of biochemical derangement (e.g., glucose, acid base, liver function), and hepatic failure (Table 13.7). The most common causes associated with various constellations of metabolic derangement are shown in Table 13.8. Of particular note with neurologic distress is the neonatal sepsis syndrome and infantile seizure-myoclonic syndromes.

Profound Biochemical Derangement

Hypoglycemia

Hypoglycemia may result from a variety of causes (Table 13.9).

Electrolyte Disturbance

Any central neurologic disturbance in patients hydrated intravenously or by nasogastric tube should prompt the search for an abnormal electrolyte concentration (e.g., sodium, calcium, magnesium).

Vitamin Deficiency

Thiamine (i.e., vitamin B_1), pyridoxine (i.e., vitamin B_6), and vitamin A deficiencies may result in an altered level of consciousness, sometimes rather precipitously.

Thiamine Vitamin B_1 deficiency decreases energy availability. In patients receiving total parenteral nutrition, chronic dialysis, or a high-carbohydrate diet during debilitating illness, Wernicke's encephalopathy may be observed. In these settings, the features are highly variable, ranging from sudden collapse and death or seizure to classic ataxia, confusion, and ocular abnormalities.

Pyridoxine Vitamin B_6 in the form of pyridoxal-5-phosphate is essential for normal brain function. It is particularly necessary for the decarboxylation of glutamic acid to γ-amino butyric acid (GABA), an essential inhibitory neurotransmitter. Pyridoxine deficiency, such as that seen in patients receiving isoniazid or penicillamine, is associated with seizure activity.

Table 13.7
Infantile Encephalopathic Presentation of Metabolic Disease[a]

	Seizures	Acidosis	Renal Dysfunction	Liver Dysfunction	Hypoglycemia	Other
Organic acidemia						
MSUD	+	+	-	-	+	Bone marrow depression, increased lactate, hyperammonemia (applies to *all* organic acidemias)
Propionic acidemia	+	+	-	-	+	
Isovaleric acidemia	+	+	-	-	+	
Methylmalonic acidemia	+	+	-	-	+	
HMG CoA lyase deficiency	+	+	-	-	+	
Urea cycle defects						
CPS deficiency	+	±	-	+	-	
OTC deficiency	+	±	-	+	-	Orotic acid crystals
Citrullinemia	+	+	-	+	-	
Carbohydrate disorders						
Galactosemia	-	+	+	+	+	Jaundice
Hereditary fructose intolerance	+	+	+	+	+	Decreased serum phosphate
Aminoacidopathies						
Hereditary tyrosinemia	-	+	+	+	-	Coagulopathy
Homocystinuria	+	-	-	-	-	
Nonketotic hyperglycine	+	-	-	-	-	Hypsarrhythmia
Endocrinopathies						
Congenital adrenal hyperplasia	+	±	-	-	±	Virilization, hyperkalemia
Congenital diabetes	-	+	-	-	-	Hyperglycemia, ketonemia

[a] Adapted from Nyhan WL. An approach to the diagnosis of overwhelming metabolic disease in early infancy. Curr Prob Pediatr 1977;7:1.

MSUD, maple syrup urine disease; HMG, 3-hydroxy-3-methylglutarate; CPS, carbamyl-phosphate synthase; and OTC, ornithine transcarbamylase.

Table 13.8
Most Common Metabolic Causes of Infantile Coma and Seizures Associated with Various Constellations of Metabolic Derangement[a]

	Biochemical Presentation of Infantile Seizures and Coma			
		Acidemias		
Acidosis	−	+	+	−
Ketosis	+	+	+	−
Hyperammonemia	−	+	−	+
Hyperlactacidemia	−	−	+	−
Most frequent diagnoses	1. Maple syrup urine disease	1. Methylmalonic 2. Propionic 3. Isovaleric	1. Congenital lactic acidosis	1. Urea cycle defects	1. Hyperglycinemia 2. Peroxisomal 3. Sulfite oxidase deficiency 4. Respiratory chain diseases

[a]Adapted from Saudubray JM, et al. Clinical approach to inherited metabolic disease in the neonatal period: a 20 year survey. J Inherited Metab Dis 1989;12(S1):25.

Table 13.9
Causes of Hypoglycemia

Deficient substrate provision
  Ketotic hypoglycemia
  Inadequate infused glucose during total intravenous therapy
Deranged endocrine balance
  Hyperinsulinism: nesidioblastosis, leucine-induced, islet cell adenoma
  Adrenal insufficiency
  Hypothyroidism
  Glucagon deficiency
Inborn errors of carbohydrate metabolism
  Glycogen storage disease types I, III, IV
  Galactosemia
  Fructose intolerance
  Pyruvate carboxylase deficiency
  Phosphoenolpyruvate deficiency
Inborn errors of lipid metabolism
  Medium- and long-chain acetyl CoA dehydrogenase deficiency
Inborn errors of amino acid metabolism
  Maple syrup urine disease
  Methylmalonic aciduria
  Propionic acidemia
  Isovaleric acidemia
Drug-induced hypoglycemia
  Insulin
  Sulfonylureas
  Salicylates
  Acetaminophen
  Propranolol
Hepatic failure

Vitamin A Vitamin A deficiency can result in an increase in intracranial pressure, which may be reversed by replacement.

Diabetes Mellitus

Diabetic Ketoacidosis This condition may result in impaired cerebral blood flow and oxygen uptake by the brain, cerebral edema, and focal neurologic deficit.

Nonketotic Hyperosmolar Coma Affected children experience generalized or focal seizures, ophthalmoplegia, and hemiparesis.

Hypoglycemia The abnormal biochemical state of hypoglycemia may result in a spectrum of clinical findings, ranging from transient focal neurologic signs to coma and focal or generalized seizures.

Renal Disease The encephalopathies associated with underlying renal disease invariably are multifactorial and may be attributable to electrolyte disturbance, hypertension, or specific disease toxins.

Uremic Encephalopathy This neurologic complication of renal insufficiency is characterized by:

- Obtundation
- Hypotonia
- Seizures
- Athetoid movements
- Nystagmus
- Ataxia

Focal cerebral symptoms, hemiparesis, and cortical blindness are more often due to hypertensive encephalopathy.

Dialysis Dysequilibrium Syndrome Failure of urea to establish equilibrium between brain and blood rapidly during dialysis results in a net shift of extracellular water into the brain.

Rejection Encephalopathy In some recipients of renal transplants, encephalopathy that is not caused by electrolyte disturbance, hypertension, steroids, or fever produces a syndrome of coma, cortical blindness, quadriplegia, and seizures. Cyclosporin toxicity has been implicated.

Septic Encephalopathy

An encephalopathy seen in bacteremic patients that is not caused by meningitis, abscess, cerebritis, or emboli has been described in critically ill adults. Mortality and morbidity is high. Causes include:

- Microabscesses in the cerebral cortex (appreciable only at autopsy)
- Metabolic disturbance, such as the ratio of branched-chain to unbranched and aromatic amino acids
- Cerebral microcirculatory dysfunction
- Cerebral edema
- Drug administration

Poisons and Drugs

Drug intoxication is an important cause of encephalopathy in children (Table 13.10).

Other Causes

Neurotoxic processes seen with other common causes of metabolic encephalopathy in patients coming to intensive care are summarized in Table 13.11.

NEUROPATHOLOGY

Specific or selective damage of particular groups of brain cells or regions of the brain is seen in association with a variety of disorders, especially those with a

Table 13.10
Drug Intoxication and Encephalopathy

Drug	Neurology	Eyes	Cardiac	Other Organ Systems
Amphetamines	Depressed consciousness Delirium Agitation Chorea Hyperreflexia	Mydriasis	Cardiac arrhythmia Tachycardia Hypertension	Hyperpyrexia Sweating
Tricyclic antidepressants	Agitation Muscle rigidity Seizures Coma	Mydriasis	Tachycardia	Sweating Vomiting
Antihistamines	Depressed consciousness Hallucinations Tremor Seizures	Mydriasis	Hypotension	Dry mouth Urinary retention
Barbiturates	Ataxia Coma Arreflexia	Miosis	Hypotension	Hypothermia Respiratory depression
Methadone	Depressed consciousness	Miosis	Hypotension	Urinary retention Respiratory depression

predilection for either basal ganglia or cerebellar or cortical disease. Although these areas of damage often are identified macroscopically postmortem, they can be appreciated grossly with modern imaging techniques (Table 13.12).

CLINICAL MANAGEMENT

In the context of a child referred with a presumed or identified metabolic encephalopathy, the priority is not only supportive therapy but also the identification and treatment of treatable problems, which should reduce morbidity and optimize outcome (Tables 13.13 and 13.14).

Prompt therapy and correction of biochemical derangement at an early stage reduce the likelihood of neuronal injury. Despite aggressive management and correction of metabolic upset, however, central neurotoxic processes may continue because of a secondary complication (e.g., cytotoxic cerebral edema and raised intracranial pressure) or a persistent brain neurochemical or transmitter imbalance.

Presentation and Physical Findings

An infant or child with metabolic derangement and encephalopathy may be seen during an apparent prodromal phase of illness, when it is often difficult

Table 13.11
Summary of Pathogenic Mechanisms and Pertinent Clinical Features of Not Uncommon Encephalitic Conditions Seen in Patients Presenting for Intensive Care[a]

	Pathogenesis	Clinical Notes
Renal disease		
Uremia	Chronic progressively worsening uremia produces a spectrum of CNS signs. **A. Implicated** • Imbalance of neurotransmitters (GABA, dopamine, and serotonin) caused by plasma amino acid levels • Increased CSF and brain guanidino compounds that inhibit inhibitory GABA and glycine systems • Increased brain tissue osmolality • Increased gray matter calcium **B. Contributory factors in renal failure** • Hypercalcemia, hypertension, hemorrhage, drug toxicity **C. Noncontributory** • Energy state (normal levels of cerebral ATP and phosphocreatine, secondary reduction of glycolysis)	**Examination** • Sensorium: headache, nausea, vomiting • Motor: tremor, myoclonus, asterixis • Neurology: focal signs often seen • Seizures: focal and generalized
Dialysis dysequilibrium	Occurs during or immediately after hemodialysis or peritoneal dialysis. **A. Implicated** • Brain edema (increased brain tissue water content caused by blood-brain osmotic gradient, idiogenic osmoles) • CNS acidosis	**Examination** • Sensorium: headache, confusion, and heightening of preexisting obtundation and coma • Motor: muscle twitching • Seizures: focal and generalized
Hypercalcemia	Cerebral infarction caused by arterial spasm has been reported. **A. Implicated** • ? Brain parathormone levels • ? CSF citrate and lactate buffering	**Examination** • Neurology: focal findings • Seizures: generalized and focal

Acute electrolyte disturbance

Hyponatremia

B. Contributory
- Azotemia, dehydration

C. Noncontributory
- Normal CSF content of calcium and phosphate

Acute presentation with seizures and obtundation.

A. Implicated
- Cytotoxic cerebral edema with increased brain water

Examination
- Motor: rare asterixis and multifocal myoclonus
  Neurology: occasional focal signs, hemiparesis, monoparesis, unilateral corticospinal tract signs
- Seizures: frequent (Na <115, acute)

Treatment
- Slow/rapid/overcorrection (cf. central pontine myelinosis)
- Hypertonic saline (to correct Na 120–125), water restriction

Hypernatremia

Factors responsible for the obtundation are unclear but:

A. Implicated
- Increased brain tissue osmolality
- Increased osmotically active particles (Na, K, Cl, and "idiogenic osmoles," e.g., urea and amino acids)

Examination
- Motor: tremor, hyperreflexia
- Neurology: focal signs related to hemorrhage (subdural-bridging veins or multiple intraparenchymal)
- Seizures: frequent, often progress to coma

Hypocalcemia

Hypocalcemic states often present with neurologic . manifestations.

A. Implicated
- ? Acute lowering or absolute level of serum calcium
- ? Alteration in neurotransmitter synthesis as well as uptake and release of catecholamines
- ? Brain parathormone levels

Examination
- Sensorium: confusion-coma
- Motor: tetany, movement disorder
- Seizures: generalized and partial complex

continued

Table 13.11

Summary of Pathogenic Mechanisms and Pertinent Clinical Features of Not Uncommon Encephalitic Conditions Seen in Patients Presenting for Intensive Care[a]

	Pathogenesis	Clinical Notes
Hypomagnesemia	Usually associated with other abnormalities, including alkalosis, hypocalcemia, and hypophophatemia. **A. Implicated** • ? Brain parathormone levels	**Examination** • Sensorium: delirium, vertigo • Motor: choreoathetosis • Seizures: generalized and focal
Hypophosphatemia	**A. Implicated** • ? Related to change in RBC metabolism and affinity for oxygen (decreased RBC ATP and 2,3-DPG heightens affinity for oxygen and decreases availability for tissues) **B. Noncontributory** • CSF phosphorus remains constant	**Examination** • Sensorium: stupor-coma • Motor: tremor, ballismus • Seizures: generalized
Glucose **Hyperglycemia**	Hyperosmolality rather than hyperglycemia appears to be associated with depression of sensorium. **A. Implicated** • Rapid water loss by the brain • Increased brain tissue concentration of ions and metabolites **B. Contributory factor** • Focal circulatory impairment	**Examination** • Hyperosmotic hyperglycemic nonketotic • Sensorium: obtunded • Neurology: focal signs • Seizures: focal, (epilepsia partialis continua) Ketotic hyperglycemia is seldom associated with seizures or focal signs.
Miscellaneous **Thyrotoxicosis**	**A. Implicated** • Acute neuronal accumulation of thyroid hormone • ? Altered catecholamine sensitivity	**Examination** • Motor: tremor-chorea/athetosis • Neurology: acute reversible bulbar dysfunction, progressive myelopathy with paraplegia

B. Noncontributory

- Cerebral oxygen consumption not increased
- Brain mitochondria do not undergo changes that occur in other tissues

Intussusception encephalopathy

Intestinal intussusception with the most prominent presenting feature of depressed level of consciousness and reported apparent responses to naloxone.

A. Implicated

- ? Gastrointestinal release of neurotoxins, vasoactive peptides, and neuroactive gut hormones
- ? Age-related pain release of endorphins

B. Contributory

- Blood loss, dehydration, electrolyte imbalance, and sepsis

- Seizures: generalized

Examination

- Sensorium: coma
- Motor: hypotonia, hyporeflexia
- Neurology: miosis

[a]The range of conditions illustrates the diversity of implicated mechanisms.

CNS, central nervous system; GABA, γ-aminobutyric acid; CSF, cerebrospinal fluid; ATP, adenosine triphosphate; RBC, red blood cell(s); 2,3-DPG, 2,3-diphosphoglyceric acid.

Table 13.12
Predominant Region of Involvement Inferred from Computed Tomography Scanning or Magnetic Resonance Imaging of the Head

Primary destructive or calcification abnormality of basal ganglia and brainstem (examples)

Leigh disease	Barbiturate intoxication
Mitochondrial cytopathies	Heavy metals
Hypoglycemia	Carbon monoxide
Hypocalcemia	Cyanide poisoning
Central pontine myelinosis	Methylmalonic acidemia
Sulfite oxidase deficiency	

Primary diffuse myelin (white matter) involvement (examples)
Defects of protein metabolism
• Maple syrup urine disease
• Phenylketonuria

Nonspecific predilection: diffuse changes with or without demyelination, ischemic change, calcification, and hemorrhage (examples)

Hypoglycemia	Nonketotic hyperglycinemia
Organic acidemias	Hartnup disease
Congenital lactic acidosis	Mitochondrial cytopathies

Table 13.13
Hierarchical Approach to the Encephalopathic Child

	Assessment	Action
Vital signs	Respiratory	Maintain oxygenation
	Cardiovascular	Maintain circulation
	? Seizures	Treat and check blood gas, electrolytes,
	? Hypoglycemia	glucose, blood count, toxicology
	? Coagulopathy	(see Table 13.14)
Level of coma	Neurologic	Treat and monitor trends
	? Deteriorating	
	? Raised ICP	
	? Seizures	
Diagnosis	Full history/examination	Specific or supportive therapy
	? CT scan	(see Table 13.16)
	? Neurophysiology	

ICP, intracranial pressure; CT, computed tomography.

to differentiate a cause of irritability, mild pyrexia, and upper respiratory tract symptoms from metabolic disease precipitated or exacerbated by infection. Alternatively, patients may be seen after a seizure, in coma, or occasionally with multiorgan disease that is marked by severe cardiorespiratory impairment.

Evaluation of all organ systems is essential, because some therapies used to manage severely affected children are aggressive, invasive, and dangerous.

Table 13.14

Investigations and Screening in Infants and Children with Suspected Metabolic Cause of Encephalopathy

Primary investigations that will facilitate initial therapy
Blood
- Acid-base balance (arterial)
- Glucose
- Urea, electrolytes, creatinine
- Osmolality
- Full blood count, coagulation screen
- Toxicology screen
Urine
- Sedative and toxic drug screen

Bedside urinary screening tests
Odor
- Maple syrup/burned sugar (MSUD)
- Cheesy/sweaty feet (isovaleric acidemia)
- Cat's urine (multiple carboxylase deficiency, HMG CoA lyase deficiency)
Ferric chloride test: place two drops of 10% ferric chloride in 1 mL of fresh urine; mix and observe color immediately on standing (negative test result does not exclude disease)
- Green (PKU, tyrosinemia, direct hyperbilirubinemia)
- Blue-green (histidinemia)
- Gray-green (MSUD)
- Purple (ketones, salicylates)
Reducing substances
- Galactose (galactosemia, severe liver disease)
- Fructose (hereditary fructose intolerance)
- Glucose
- p-Hydroxyphenylpyruvic acid (tyrosinemia)

Secondary investigations that may provide specific diagnosis
Blood
- Liver function tests
- Ammonia
- Amino acids
- Organic acids
- Ketones
- Pyruvate/lactate, octanoic acid, carnitine, fructose, porphyrins
Urine
- Organic acids
- Amino acids
- Ketones
- Orotic acid
- Carnitine

Further definitive diagnostic tests
Deep-freeze urine and plasma
Initiate fibroblast culture for specific enzyme assay
Obtain liver biopsy for histology and enzyme assay

MSUD, maple syrup urine disease; PKU, phenylketonuria.

Concerning the specific central nervous system features of an encephalopathy found in the infant or child, interpretation of signs and symptoms is influenced by the the child's stage of development and expected normal responses.

Generally, the neurologic findings fall into one of the following categories:

1. A generalized depression of predominantly cerebral hemisphere function: consciousness is depressed, motor tone becomes diminished, pupils are small but reactive, and reflex eye movements are disinhibited. Asterixis, one of the hallmarks of metabolic encephalopathy, may relate to intermittent depression of motor function.
2. A heightened excitability of neural tissue resulting from a direct lowering of the threshold for neuronal excitability or resulting from a selective depression of inhibitory influences on neuronal function: Cheyne-Stokes respiration may result from bilateral hemispheric inhibition, and certain types of seizures from neuronal excitability.
3. Selective vulnerability or focal involvement of a specific brain region to a systemic metabolic insult. This may be due to regional differences in tissue metabolic requirements for oxygen, glucose, or amino acids or, alternatively, regional differences in neurotransmitters and receptors. It is not uncommon for focal findings to remain unexplained (e.g., those occurring during hypoglycemia, hyperglycemia, uremia, and hypercalcemia) or possibly be representative of an anamnestic response to a previous (perhaps occult) neurologic injury.
4. Progressive deterioration with features and signs indicative of raised intracranial pressure and brain-tissue shifts, which may represent a cytotoxic cerebral edema (Tables 13.3 to 13.5).

The clinical examination, electroencephalographic, and CT scans are useful tools to assess the severity of the illness.

Laboratory Investigation

After clinical suspicion of metabolic disease is aroused, general supportive measures and laboratory investigation must be undertaken immediately. The initial approach for investigation is outlined in Table 13.14.

An autopsy protocol (Table 13.15) should be developed so that items such as biopsy needles (e.g., liver, kidney, skin), dry ice, and culture media can be readily available and samples can be stored appropriately at any time.

Specific Clinical Treatment

Therapy ranges from the relatively simple correction of electrolytes or metabolic substrate to the extremely complex neurointensive care of children with more severe complications, such as renal failure, fulminant hepatic failure, or raised intracranial pressure.

Table 13.15

Perimortem Genetic-Metabolic Diagnostic Protocol for Infants and Children with Encephalopathy of Unknown Cause[a,b]

	Samples	Storage and Usage
Body fluids		
Blood	Heparinized	Serum and plasma are separated
	Unheparinized	before freezing at −20° C
	Incubated with	For metaphase chromosome
	phytohemagglutinin	analysis
	Whole blood in	Store at 4° C for up to 5 days, used
	ethylenediamine	to extract DNA from leukocytes
	tetraacetic acid	
Urine	Centrifuge to remove	Stores at −20° C
	blood and debris	
Fibroblast culture		
Skin	Punch biopsy sample fully	Store at 4° C
	immersed in tissue culture	
	media or patient's serum	
Tissue enzyme activity		
Liver	Needle or open biopsy	Snap-freezing: immerse immediately
		in liquid nitrogen or isopentane
		chilled on dry ice
Muscle	Needle or open biopsy	Store at −70° C
Histology		
Liver	Needle or open biopsy	Tissue fixed in formalin for light
		microscopy
Muscle	Needle or open biopsy	Tissue fixed in glutaraldehyde for
		electron microscopy

[a]From Kronick JB, Seriver CR, Goodyear PR, Kaplan PB. A perimortem protocol for suspected genetic disease. Pediatrics 1983;71:960.

[b]Before invasive investigation, appropriate informed consent, according to institutional requirements, should be gained.

General Care Measures

Care rests on the following principles:

- Strict attention to fluid and electrolyte balance
- Adequate oxygenation and perfusion
- Temperature control
- Prevention of infection
- Seizure control

More specific therapy for individual organ system failure and the total care of patients with multisystem disease are described in other chapters.

Ammonia Reduction Therapy

Immediate therapy includes elimination of protein intake and caloric supplementation with hypertonic glucose to decrease catabolism. Concentrated solutions of glucose are infused at 75 to 100 $g/m^2/day$ (2.5–3.5 g/kg/day) plus insulin if hyperglycemia becomes a problem. Acidosis should be corrected with sodium bicarbonate. If this effort is ineffective or if hypernatremia develops, bicarbonate peritoneal dialysis should be instituted.

When removal of ammonia by dialysis is the only effective treatment, it can be undertaken in one of three ways:

Table 13.16
Metabolic Therapies

Agents Activating Alternative or Normal Pathways of Nitrogen Balance

Medication	Metabolic Mechanism of Action	Product and Excretion Rate	Atomas of Waste Nitrogen/Molecule
Sodium benzoate load: 0.25 g/kg IV then: continuous IV 0.25–0.5 g/kg/d	Conjugates with glycine to form hippuric acid	Hippurate Five times glomerular filtration rate	1
Arginine hydrochloride load: 0.8 g/kg IV then: continuous IV 0.2–0.8 g/kg/day	Provides substrate for intact part of urea cycle—ensures ornithine deficiency does not limit detoxification	Citrulline 25% glomerular filtration rate	1
Phenylacetate load: 0.25 g/kg then: continuous IV 0.25–0.5 g/kg/d	Conjugates with glutamine to form phenylacetylglutamine	Phenylacetylglutamine Glomerular filtration rate	2
Phenylbutyrate	Oxidized in vivo to its active metabolite phenylacetate		

Vitamins and Cofactors

Enzyme Deficiency	Medication	Daily Dosage	Other Therapy
Multiple carboxylase deficiency	Biotin	10–20 mg	
Methylmalonic acidemia	B_{12}	1–2 mg or less	L-carnitine[a] 100 mg/kg IV in 6 h, then 100 mg/kg/d
Maple syrup urine disease	Thiamine	5–20 mg/kg	
Multiple acyl-CoA dehydrogenase deficiency	Riboflavin	300 mg	L-carnitine 100 mg/kg IV in 6 h, then 100 mg/kg/d

[a]Carnitine therapy may be beneficial in several organic acidemias to remedy secondary carnitine deficiency.

- Peritoneal dialysis has the advantage of not requiring large intravascular access. This method removes ammonium (albeit slowly, 5–8 mL/min/m^2), and other nitrogen-containing waste molecules (glutamine, glutamate, and alanine).
- Episodic hemodialysis enables clearance of ammonium 10 times higher, but rebound hyperammonemia may occur between episodes.
- Continuous hemofiltration with dialysis avoids such problems, with more rapid clearance rates.

More aggressive extracorporeal techniques, including exchange transfusion, charcoal hemoperfusion, and heart-lung bypass total-body washout are used infrequently.

Metabolic therapies designed to accelerate the detoxification of ammonia or to decrease its rate of production rely in part on the cause of the hyperammonemia (Table 13.16).

Table 13.17
Factors That Affect Ammonia Production and Levels

Source	Action to Limit Ammonia
Gastrointestinal	
Dietary nitrogen	Restrict
Bacterial production	Increase gut motility with cathartics
	Reduce bowel flora with antibiotics
Renal production	Correct metabolic alkalosis
Brain accumulation	
Ammonia diffusion	Correct metabolic alkalosis
	Accelerate ammonia detoxification by providing substrate for brain transamination of α-keto amino acids

Table 13.18
Precipitants of Hepatic Encephalopathy

Drugs	Sedatives
	Tranquilizers
	Narcotics
	Diuretics
Electrolyte imbalance	Hyponatremia
	Hypokalemic alkalosis
Excessive nitrogen load	Gastrointestinal hemorrhage
	Excess dietary protein
	Azotemia
	Constipation
Other	Infection
	Hypoxia
	Hypovolemia

Table 13.19
Treatment of Hypoglycemia

Newborns and infants
• 0.25 g glucose 0.25 g/kg IV followed by increase in maintenance
Repeat if persistent
• Hydrocortisone 5 mg/kg/d
If adrenal insufficiency or hypopituitarism suspected, 20–60 mg/m^2/d
• Glucagon 0.03 mg/kg/d IV or IM up to 1 mg if hyperinsulinemia suspected
• Diazoxide 10–25 mg/kg/d oral or IV in hyperinsulinism
Children
• 0.25 g glucose/kg IV followed by increase in maintenance. Repeat if persistent
• Hydrocortisone 5 mg/kg/d up to 100 mg
• Glucagon 0.03 mg/kg/day IV or IM up to 1 mg
• Diazoxide 10–25 mg/kg/d oral or IV

Hepatic Encephalopathy

Encephalopathy due to acute or chronic hepatic disease requires a variety of measures to affect ammonia production (Table 13.17). It also is important to recognize and treat precipitating factors that may have led to increased ammonia production or poor clearance (e.g., gastrointestinal bleeding, infection, an increase in dietary protein) (Table 13.18).

Raised Intracranial Pressure

Any child with metabolic encephalopathy who is seriously ill and who has an impaired level of consciousness should be assumed also to have raised intracranial pressure. In these patients, careful thought should be given to monitoring their intracranial pressure and instituting standard management. However, although this form of therapy has been used in Reye syndrome, hepatic encephalopathy, and many other types of metabolic derangement, it is unlikely that this form of treatment controls or reverses a cytotoxic edema.

Hypoglycemia

Table 13.19 summarizes the initial management approach for hypoglycemia.

14.

Head and Spinal Cord Injury

*Elizabeth M. Allen, Richard Boyer, W. Bruce Cherny,
Douglas Brockmeyer, and Vera Fan Tait*

INTRODUCTION

Head injury is one of the major causes of morbidity and mortality in children today. Trauma is the leading cause of death in children older than 1 year of age in the United States. Most of these trauma deaths are from head injuries. Injuries lead to more days of hospital care than any disease, cause the highest proportion of discharges to long-term care facilities, and result in the highest proportion of children requiring home health care after being discharged from the hospital.

PRIMARY INJURY
Scalp Injuries

Scalp injuries often are seen in association with traumatic brain injuries. The scalp is composed of five layers, each of which plays a role in the pathophysiologic characteristics of scalp injury and in the physician's considerations for appropriate treatment.

- Skin. As the hair-bearing layer, the skin must be considered when issues of cosmesis arise.
- Subcutaneous tissue. This layer consists mainly of fat in the superficial portion and large blood vessels and nerves in the deeper portion.
- Musculoaponeurotic layer. This layer contains the galea, a fibrous helmet that covers the cranial vault. This noncompliant structure is responsible for most of the tensile strength of the scalp. Any significant scalp closure must include this layer, but it may be the limiting factor when considering closure of scalp defects.
- Areolar layer. This potential space contains the emissary veins. The areolar layer gives rise to scalping injuries, in which large portions of the skull are denuded, and represents possible planes for infection to spread through the emissary veins and the accumulation of other materials (e.g., blood and serous fluid).
- Periosteum. Tightly adherent to the skull, this layer forms a limiting membrane between the skin and the skull. It is vital for bone nutrition and is a source of potential fibroblasts for secondary coverage of the denuding injury.

Blood Loss

The scalp carries a rich blood supply that is interconnected by an extensive network of anastomoses. Blood loss from a laceration can be rapid and extensive enough to result in hypotension, shock, and even death, especially in infants and small children.

Direct digital tamponade at the patient's wound edges provides the best control for bleeding, except when a laceration overlies a depressed skull fracture, in which, case, pressure is applied at the edge of the palpably intact cranial bone. Surgical clamps (e.g., hemostats) should not be placed on the skin except under extreme circumstances, to avoid tissue damage and possible necrosis. Most bleeding subsides with adequate pressure and sufficient time. A pressure dressing with a firm head wrap minimizes further blood loss until the physician can perform primary repair. Especially brisk bleeding can be controlled with a full-thickness figure-of-eight suture around the skin edge at the bleeding vessel or with surgical scalp clips. These methods are temporary until the physician can perform definitive debridement and repair.

Treatment and Repair

When underlying skull and intracranial pathologic lesions have been ruled out, the treatment of scalp injuries usually is straightforward. Uncomplicated subgaleal hematomas and cephalhematomas are treated conservatively. Antibiotics rarely are needed.

Simple lacerations are treated by using conventional general surgical techniques and principles. Adequate anesthesia is mandatory. Close inspection and digital probing are needed before the wound is closed. The physician must look for evidence of a foreign body or bony disruption, which indicates a fracture. A simple one-layer closure is most often used, but the surgeon must take care to include the galea in the closure planes. Because of the rich vascular supply of the scalp, wound infection is rarely encountered. Even so, a grossly contaminated wound may warrant delayed closure.

Tissue Loss and Grafting

Avulsion lacerations with tissue loss of less than 3 to 4 cm often can be closed because of the scalp's compliance. Larger defects, however, require grafting. When the patient's vascular periosteum has been left intact, a split-thickness skin graft can be used. Hair grafting can be undertaken later for cosmetic purposes. If the vascular periosteum is not intact or the blood supply is otherwise uncertain, various forms of skin flaps and pedicle flaps must be used.

The same principles apply in total scalp avulsion cases. Except in rare instances of microvascular reimplantation, the avulsed scalp cannot be replaced. If suitable, however, the scalp may be used as a donor for split-thickness skin grafting or tissue coverage. If the scalp is unsuitable and the periosteum remains normal, grafts from other donor sites may be used.

Burns

Burns of the scalp are treated as are burns elsewhere (see Chapter 28). First-degree burns may be treated by shaving the scalp and applying topical antibiotics (e.g., bacitracin zinc and polymyxin B sulfate ointment [Polysporin] or sulfadiazine). Partial- and full-thickness injuries require skin grafting. Hair grafting may be undertaken later for cosmetic purposes.

Skull Fractures

Types of Fracture

Skull fracture types include linear, comminuted, depressed, and diastatic. Ninety percent of fractures found in children with head trauma are linear. The importance of a linear fracture is twofold. First, the force required to fracture a child's skull is significant; therefore, the potential for underlying brain damage is more likely with fracture. Second, the location of the fracture, such as crossing the path of a known major vascular structure, holds potential for significant intracranial bleeding and subsequent complications. Childhood fractures tend to be more diastatic than their adult counterparts; therefore, their radiographic appearance may be more impressive, although most are uncomplicated.

Interpretation of Symptoms

Most children with skull injuries tend to be symptomatic, but observation is the treatment of a closed simple linear fracture that does not involve a major vascular structure. Children who are completely asymptomatic may be discharged to the home environment with a safe, reliable caregiver. If, however, a child has significant neurologic signs or symptoms (e.g., protracted bouts of nausea and vomiting after occipital or posterior fossa fractures) or worrisome or significant radiographic findings, the patient should be admitted to the hospital for observation. Most of these children recover without sequelae.

Leptomeningeal Cyst

Unique to the pediatric population, the leptomeningeal cyst, or so-called growing skull fractures, consist of resorbing bone edges overlying a dural defect. Interposed between the bone and dural defect are leptomeninges or a porencephalic cyst lined with gliotic brain. Leptomeningeal cysts occur more often in fractures involving the suture line. Cerebrospinal fluid (CSF) pulsations and the active growth and resorption of bone result in a persistently enlarging defect. Growing skull fractures sometimes resolve with age, but surgical intervention may be necessary. Patients with such potential must be observed closely for at least 1 to 2 years.

Open Skull Fracture

If the patient's linear fracture is associated with an overlying laceration, it is, by definition, an open fracture. Because such a fracture is a potential opening to the central nervous system, neurosurgical evaluation is mandatory to decide whether operative repair should be undertaken. If cerebrospinal fluid is leaking from the wound or collecting under the scalp, a dural laceration and operative exploration is indicated.

When managing these wounds, the physician must adhere to routine aseptic principles strictly. If surgical closure is not indicated, the wound should be copiously irrigated and meticulously debrided. The child should be admitted not only for a period of observation, but also for antibiotic coverage, especially in the case of gross wound contamination. In these instances, the rate of infection is low, and the posttraumatic complications are few.

Depressed Skull Fracture

This type of fracture, in which the inner table of the skull is displaced by more than one thickness of the entire bone, usually requires a greater amount of force and thus represents a more severe injury than other skull fractures. The location of depressed skull fractures, in descending order of relative frequency, is the frontal, parietal, temporal, and occipital bones.

Diagnosis Although plain skull radiographs are helpful, computed tomography (CT) scanning with appropriate bone windows clearly shows the location and degree of depression and any underlying cerebral trauma, which provides clues of potential dural laceration or cortical laceration. One third of all depressed fractures are simple, one third are associated with dural laceration, and one third are associated with cortical lacerations.

When the physician has made the diagnosis of depressed skull fracture and has evaluated the lesion radiographically, no further probing or exploration of the wound nor any attempt at removal of bony fragments or foreign objects is justified in the emergency department. Such attempts involve a great risk of removing a fragment that may be tamponing a torn or lacerated blood vessel. Also, further probing may push fracture fragments further into the brain.

Indications for Surgical Intervention Surgical elevation of a depressed skull fracture is appropriate in the presence of the following:

- Cerebral spinal fluid leak
- Probable dural compromise
- Focal neurologic deficits
- Depression in a cosmetically important area
- Segment of depression greater than or equal to the thickness or table width of the skull in that region

Left unrepaired, depressed fractures with significant compression of the cerebral cortex are believed to be associated with an increased incidence of focal neurologic deficits or seizure development.

Open depressed skull fractures are considered relative surgical emergencies, primarily because of the risk of bacterial spread into the central nervous system. With modern broad-spectrum antibiotic therapy and prompt surgical care, however, chronic infections and osteomyelitis of the skull rarely are seen. In general, broad-spectrum antibiotic coverage is administered for at least 72 hours, but under special circumstances, it may be warranted for 10 to 14 days.

Surgical Treatment Definitive treatment measures include meticulous debridement of devitalized scalp, hair, any contaminants, and copious irrigation.

Basilar Skull Fracture

This type of fracture is seen in 6 to 14% of children who sustain head injuries. A tremendous force is required to fracture the base of the skull; thus, this injury is not trivial. In most instances, however, an uncomplicated basilar skull fracture has an excellent prognosis for recovery.

Diagnosis

Clinical Evidence A history of a blow sustained to the back of the head should raise clinical suspicion. There may or may not be an associated loss of consciousness, seizures, or other manifestations of neurologic injury.

On physical examination, certain findings are pathognomonic of basilar skull fracture:

- Retroauricular or mastoid ecchymosis without history or evidence of direct trauma to the area. Battle's sign represents a dissection of blood from the disrupted skull cortex in the occipital and mastoid regions.
- Laceration of the external auditory canal without history or evidence of trauma to the ear or canal, which is the result of a fractured petrous bone. This injury may be complicated further by concomitant laceration or disruption of the facial and auditory nerves.
- Blood behind the tympanic membrane imparting a bluish discoloration and often resulting in a bulging membrane, may be the result of a deeper fracture of the petrous temporal bone. Disruption of facial and auditory nerves also may occur.
- Periorbital ecchymosis without other evidence of trauma to the region (i.e., "raccoon eyes") results from the forward dissection of blood from the disrupted skull cortex into the soft areolar spaces of the periorbital regions.
- Cerebrospinal fluid otorrhea or rhinorrhea, which occurs secondary to disruption of the leptomeninges (see subsequent discussion). Cerebrospinal fluid rhinorrhea is rare during the first decade of life, however, and CSF otorrhea is unusual in children 5 years of age and younger.

Radiographic Evidence The diagnosis of basilar skull fracture often is based on the previously mentioned clinical signs. With the use of CT scanning, however, it is possible to demonstrate the area of fracture and to identify associated brain injury (Fig. 14.1).

Complications

Nausea, Vomiting, and Malaise Patients with a basilar skull fracture are more prone to prolonged symptoms of nausea, vomiting, and general malaise than are individuals with other types of fractures, especially without other evidence for underlying brain injury. The close proximity of the fracture to the emesis and vestibular centers of the brain stem may play a role. Management of these patients involves close observation, intravenous hydration, pain control, and antiemetic agents. Because of the disruption of the cribriform plate, nasotracheal intubation and placement of nasogastric tubes are to be avoided in these patients; orotracheal and orogastric tubes should be placed instead. The course usually is uncomplicated, and an excellent recovery can be expected.

CSF Leak The most significant complication of basilar skull fractures is CSF leak. In 80% of patients, CSF rhinorrhea heals spontaneously within 1 week, and only a few of the remaining unresolved cases require surgical

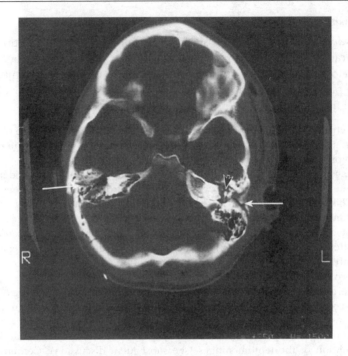

Figure 14.1. Basilar skull fracture. Head computed tomography scan through the petrous temporal bones and skull base displayed in bone window in a child with severe closed head trauma shows a complex basilar skull fracture (arrows) extending in a coronal plane across the petrous portion of both temporal bones. Note that there is fluid opacification (blood or cerebrospinal fluid) in the left middle ear cavity with dislocation of the ossicles (arrowhead).

intervention. As with CSF rhinorrhea, most CSF otorrhea resolves spontaneously. Rarely, the CSF leak persists without resolution and requires surgical intervention. Keeping the head elevated with or without serial lumbar puncture may be sufficient to lower the CSF pressure and allow spontaneous resolution. If surgical repair is necessary, the area of leakage must be identified precisely by using radionuclide cisternography coupled with high-resolution CT scanning.

Meningitis Meningitis occurs in 3 to 25% of patients with CSF rhinorrhea and in approximately 4.5% of patients with CSF otorrhea. Because of the risk of nosocomial infection with antibiotic-resistant agents, the trend is to avoid antibiotics except in actual cases of meningitis or in special situations in which clinical judgment deems it necessary.

Cranial Nerve Injury Cranial nerve injury ensuing from the fractured bone also is a significant problem. Three to ten percent of patients are anosmic at the end of their hospitalization; this deficit tends to be permanent. Ocular nerve palsy develops in 1 to 10% of patients. The order of decreasing frequency is the sixth, third, and fourth cranial nerves. Oculomotor nerve palsies rarely are complete, and 75% of patients make a full recovery. Facial nerve palsies appear in 1 to 12% of patients with basilar skull fractures, and 90% can be expected to make a spontaneous recovery. Dizziness, tinnitus, and sensory hearing loss from eighth nerve injury may also occur. Complete sensorineural hearing loss occurs in approximately 1.5% of cases.

Concussion

Concussion, defined as a transient loss of consciousness that occurs as the consequence of head trauma, is a descriptive term and does not denote any specific anatomic or physiologic abnormalities.

Diagnosis

Because the concussive injury is transient, the results of a patient's neurologic examination often are normal; therefore, the physician's diagnosis of mild concussion is made primarily on the basis of history, which differs in patients of varying age groups.

In infants and very young children, the incidence of benign posttraumatic seizures is higher, but unconsciousness is uncommon. The history often uncovers a syndrome of delayed somnolence and vomiting, which becomes less common as the child gets older.

In older children more able to cooperate with a medical historian, posttraumatic amnesia is an important finding. In general, the length of posttraumatic amnesia is proportional to the severity of the injury. In the older child, more waxing and waning of the level of consciousness occurs without attendant physical damage.

Ahead CT scan is recommended in patients with loss of consciousness and concussion. In most cases of mild concussion, the studies are negative, although in one study, 31% of patients with a score of 12 or more on the Glasgow Coma Scale had abnormal CT findings.

Outcome

Even in patients with traumatic subarachnoid hemorrhage, an excellent recovery can be expected. The patient's neurologic function usually normalizes in approximately 1 week, although for periods of months to a year, the child may continue to have slight behavioral difficulties and some slowness in the acquisition of new knowledge. The child also may experience mild headaches, which are related to postconcussive syndrome and can be expected to resolve completely without significant impact on outcome.

Contusion

A brain contusion is defined as an area of intraaxial posttraumatic bruising or microscopic hemorrhage.

Causes

In the pediatric population, contusions usually are caused by direct injury to the head, with the focal energy being transferred to the underlying brain. Contusions also may occur when the brain strikes skull-base bony protuberances during rapid acceleration or deceleration. Brain contusion often is associated with other forms of brain injury. Normally, it is other concomitant injury that dictates the aggressiveness with which the patient is treated, although the contusion itself has its own clinical consequences.

Management

The clinical course of a child with contusion typically is one of gradual neurologic deterioration caused by progressive local edema, infarction, or late-developing hematomas. Physicians may have to control increased intracranial pressure (ICP). In some instances, the hemorrhage may extend, leading to a late-developing intracerebral hematoma. Surgical intervention may be indicated to relieve significant mass effect. Unless the course is complicated by other neurologic injury, the outcome is favorable.

Epidural Hematoma

Clinical Course

In the event of a head injury of sufficient force to cause separation of dura from the underlying bone, blood accumulates between the skull and the dura. The resulting hematoma usually encounters a limiting border at a suture line, which it rarely crosses unless a concomitant skull fracture is present that disrupts the dural adherence at the suture. A high percentage of patients with epidural hematomas have overlying skull fractures. Depending on the location and vascular structures involved, the hemorrhage may be arterial or venous. The arterial pressure may be sufficient to allow further separation of the dura from the bone, resulting in an enlarging mass.

In general, epidural hematomas of arterial origin reach their peak size by 6 to 8 hours after the injury; those of venous origin may continue to grow for the first 24 hours and possibly longer. Epidural hematomas in the posterior fossa may grow silently and become symptomatic just before the patient's rapid deterioration and herniation.

Clinical Presentation

By history, the initial injury may seem minor, and the associated loss of consciousness may be brief or absent altogether. The classic "lucid interval" between initial loss of consciousness and subsequent rapid neurologic deterioration occurs in 50 to 60% of adult patients with epidural hematomas, but is much less common in pediatric patients.

Without prompt treatment, the patient's condition may deteriorate rapidly, including focal pressure effects leading to a significant mass effect, temporal lobe herniation, and brain stem compression. These events are reflected in the sequential neurologic examination. The patient may be awake initially and complain of headache associated with vomiting and nuchal rigidity. Contralateral hemiparesis may progress to unconsciousness with posturing and ipsilateral pupillary dilatation. Seizures are uncommon. Emergent CT scanning is mandatory, and will reveal a localized, lenticular, high-density lesion with obvious mass effect (Fig. 14.2).

Management and Treatment

Although most epidural hematomas are treated with emergent craniotomy and clot evacuation, up to 20% of them can be treated by conservative

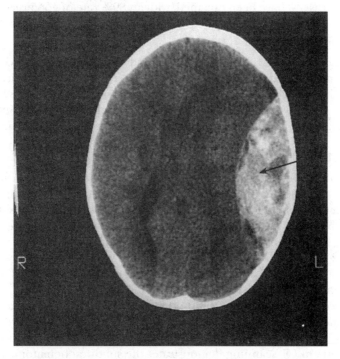

Figure 14.2. Epidural hematoma with subfalcine herniation. Head computed tomography scan of a young child after head injury shows a large epidural hematoma (arrow) compressing the left cerebral hemisphere and shifting the midline to the right (asterisk). In this setting, the anterior cerebral artery on the side of the hematoma is compressed against the free margin of the falx, possibly leading to herniation.

measures alone. Aggressive medical management of intracranial hypertension is important to stabilize the patient's rapidly deteriorating neurologic status while awaiting surgery. Burr-hole evacuation of clotted blood is technically difficult and usually unsuccessful and should not be attempted in the emergency department. Under extreme circumstances, however, burr holes may be of help as a diagnostic procedure in the absence of adequate radiologic evaluation.

Patients managed conservatively should be closely monitored, both clinically and radiographically. Surgical evacuation should be performed immediately if the patient becomes symptomatic or if the hematoma seems to be enlarging on CT scan.

Outcome

The results of surgical evacuation and overall clinical outcome are related directly to the promptness of adequate medical care. The usual mortality is approximately 17%, although of these, approximately 66% of these patients are in a coma from associated brain injury. With prompt intervention, mortality rates as low as 5% have been obtained, with an 89% rate of good recovery.

Subdural Hematoma

A subdural hematoma is a collection of blood located on the surface of the cortex beneath the dura. In most instances, there is associated cortical damage from lacerated vessels or direct cortical contusion, which results in a less favorable prognosis than that seen with epidural hematomas. Subdural hematomas usually are classified as acute and chronic subdural hematomas.

Acute Subdural Hematoma

Acute subdural hematomas usually are traumatic. They arise from bleeding points on the surface of the brain and are not limited by suture lines.

Etiology A great amount of force is required to cause a subdural hematoma, and often the underlying cortical disruption is severe. When subdural hematomas occur secondary to birth trauma, changes are seen within 12 hours of life. The child often is listless and dyspneic, with full fontanelle, anisocoria, and subhyaloid hemorrhages. Emergent CT scanning is mandatory in these patients.

Clinical Presentation The child often presents with profound and progressive neurologic deterioration. The physical examination depends on the severity of the injury, the size of the hematoma, and the time since injury. Emergent CT scanning demonstrates the subdural hematoma as a hyperdense crescentic mass located along the cerebral convexities (Fig. 14.3). A considerable mass effect is evident from the hematoma, underlying contusion, and associated brain edema. In many cases, a significant amount of hemispheric edema already may be present.

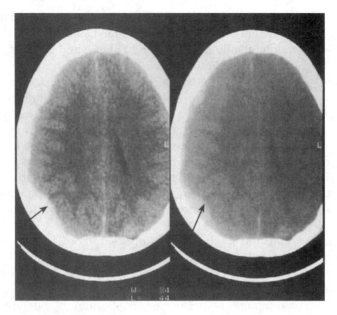

Figure 14.3. Subdural hematoma. Head computed tomography scan at the level of the top of the lateral ventricles in a child with head injury shows a moderately large acute subdural hematoma (arrows) with mass effect on the adjacent hemisphere and effacement of the right lateral ventricle. Note that the blood is better seen in the right image, which is photographed at intermediate windows, because it can be distinguished from the adjacent calvarium. In the left image, photographed at brain windows, the blood blends with the high attenuation of the overlying calvarium and is more difficult to detect.

Management The initial approach to the patient with a subdural hematoma is medical management of intracranial hypertension. Large subdural hematomas should be surgically evacuated without delay. The hematoma is evacuated through an appropriately placed craniotomy, hemorrhage control, and possible resection of badly damaged brain. In some instances, the brain may be so swollen and tense that closure of the dura or replacement of the craniotomy defect is difficult or impossible.

Outcome The outcome of children with subdural hematomas is less favorable than of those with epidural hematomas, primarily because of the frequent association of underlying brain injury. The eventual outcome seems strongly related to the initial presentation of the child.

Chronic Subdural Hematomas

Causes Chronic subdural hematomas are rare in children older than 2 years of age, except in instances of intracranial shunt complications. The usual cause is trauma, although in many instances no history of trauma can be elicited. It is believed that the compliant nature of the infant's skull, with an open fontanelle and pliable sutures, allows the slow accommodation of the subdural fluid. Additionally, many subdural hematomas in this age group arise from long-standing cases of child abuse, and the patient may present a long time after the initial insult.

Clinical Features Chronic subdural hematomas are characterized by seizures caused by cortical irritation from the fluid and by intracranial hypertension. Thus, the clinician sees a poorly thriving, irritable child with evidence of intracranial hypertension. Focal neurologic deficits are unusual. The occipital frontal circumference is enlarged, and the fontanelle often is tense. Retinal hemorrhages are seen in approximately 10% of cases. A significant amount of force is required to produce retinal hemorrhages, and its association with subdural hematoma is almost pathognomonic for child abuse. Young infants may have associated anemia; however, this is usually on a nutritional basis.

Diagnosis Evaluation may be made by ultrasound or CT scanning. Typical CT findings are that of a hypodense collection located over the cerebral convexities in a crescentic shape. Mass effect and midline shift are unusual, but occasionally occur. In fact, the sulci are often widened, as are the CSF spaces. A subdural tap may be performed to determine the nature of the fluid.

Therapy Treatment considerations must include the liquid portion of the chronic subdural hematoma and the subdural membrane. Failure to remove the membrane results in reaccumulation of the subdural fluid. Bilateral subdural tapping alone usually is reserved for relief of intracranial hypertension; however, in many cases, subdural taps alone, singly or in series, result in permanent resolution of the subdural hematoma. When taps alone fail, placement of a subdural shunt is effective. Craniotomy for removal of membrane is not often required but is the definitive treatment of the subdural hematoma and its associated membrane.

Intracerebral Hematoma

Development of a solid blood clot in the brain parenchyma in children is an infrequent complication of head injury-most arise as an extension or late development from cortical contusion. The prognosis of children with intracranial hematoma, especially hematomas in deep locations, is poor because of the association of this problem with injury to the surrounding brain parenchyma. In some cases, however, isolated hematomas in polar locations do not cause significant neurologic deterioration.

Indications for surgical evacuation of the hematoma include:

- Easy accessibility (polar location)
- Progressive neurologic deterioration
- Intracranial hypertension intractable to medical therapy

Penetrating Injury

Evaluation and Detection

Penetrating injuries should be considered neurosurgical emergencies. The penetrating body or bodies should be left in place in the field or the emergency department, because its removal could result in further neurologic injury or uncontrollable hemorrhage. Computed tomography scanning and other studies such as angiography or magnetic resonance imaging (MRI), when appropriate, should be obtained as quickly as possible to guide the surgical approach. Such injuries require prophylactic antibiotics and possibly anticonvulsants if the cerebral cortex is involved.

Treatment

Definitive treatment of a penetrating injury is surgical removal of all accessible foreign bodies and debridement of necrotic and grossly contaminated brain. Missile injuries from gunshot wounds often are especially severe. Patients presenting with a Glasgow Coma Score of 5 or lower after initial resuscitation, with an interhemispheric trajectory of the bullet, have an especially poor prognosis. Injuries to the dominant hemisphere also indicate a poor potential for recovery.

Intraventricular Hemorrhage

Most intraventricular hemorrhage from trauma is minor and resolves spontaneously; however, obstructive hydrocephalus may occur with larger hemorrhages, especially those located at the foramen of Monroe or the aqueduct of Sylvius. In these cases, the hydrocephalus may require external ventricular drainage. Large bilateral intraventricular hemorrhage may require a drain be placed on each side. Posthemorrhagic hydrocephalus may occur secondary to a diminished capacity for normal CSF absorption. The mechanism is a proteinaceous obstruction of the arachnoid villi. Significant, symptomatic hydrocephalus requires shunting. Only a small percentage of patients with intraventricular hemorrhage require a shunting procedure.

Subarachnoid Hemorrhage

Subarachnoid hemorrhage is the most common type of posttraumatic intracranial hemorrhage. Small blood vessels on the cerebral cortex are disrupted, and this bleeding tends to occur on the outer cortical surface or along the falx cerebri or tentorium. Subarachnoid hemorrhage usually does not require specific treatment, but blood in the subarachnoid space is chemically irritating to the meninges, and patients may complain of headaches, nuchal rigidity, fever, restlessness, and nausea or vomiting. Supportive care with acetaminophen often is sufficient to alleviate minor symptoms. Subarachnoid hemorrhage alone usually is not associated with significant neurologic sequelae and rarely causes posttraumatic hydrocephalus.

Diffuse Axonal Injury

Diffuse axonal injury is a disruption of small axonal pathways and results from rapid cranial acceleration and deceleration. This injury often involves the deep hemispheric nuclei, the thalamus and basal ganglia, and the crossing white-matter tracts (corpus callosum), because their weight and angle of momentum are different from the rest of the cerebral cortex. Thus, shear forces tend to preferentially affect these structures.

Initial Findings

Often the patient's initial CT scan shows no significant intracranial pathology despite a severely compromised neurologic state. Occasionally, numerous small petechial hemorrhages may be seen. Evidence of parenchymal swelling also may be present. When an ICP monitor is placed, the initial reading often is normal, but may become elevated later in the patient's hospital course.

Long-Term Care

These patients invariably present in various states of coma and often remain in long-term vegetative states. MRI scanning is a valuable tool to understand underlying anatomic abnormality. Typical findings include high-signal intensity lesions, which are best seen on T_2 or proton density images. The prognosis for full recovery often is poor. Many medical, surgical, and rehabilitative resources are required to care for these patients.

SECONDARY INJURY

Pathophysiology

Secondary insults that occur during the recovery phase, such as hypotension or hypoxia, or intracranial events that occur in response to the primary injury, inhibit the ability of injured cells to survive. Such insults may lead to a widening area of microcirculatory disruption and neuronal damage. This phase of injury evolves across time, beginning immediately after the primary injury and peaking in a matter of several days. The outcome of the patient depends on the extent of the primary and secondary injuries. Most of the medical therapies used in patients with head injury are aimed at reducing or eliminating secondary insults.

Systemic Events

Hypotension

Hypotension, a common concomitant to head trauma, lowers cerebral perfusion pressure (CPP) and leads to cerebral ischemia, especially in the face of impaired autoregulation. Hypovolemia caused by blood loss and vasodilation caused by spinal cord injury are two of the most common causes of hypotension in victims with head injury. Cardiac contusions or arrhythmias may lead to low cardiac output and hypotension. The Traumatic Coma Data Bank found that the mortality of patients with head injury who are hypotensive was 50% compared with 27% in patients with head injury without hypotension.

Hypoxia

Many unconscious victims develop hypoxia secondary to airway obstruction from positioning, vomitus, or blood. Additional causes of hypoxemia include hypoventilation caused by direct brain stem injury, high arterial-alveolar gradient secondary to pulmonary contusion or tension pneumothorax. Early hypoxia is no longer associated with increased mortality, perhaps because modern methods of emergency management and transport of patients with head injury have minimized hypoxia and thereby secondary hypoxic damage. Prompt attention to securing an airway, administering supplemental oxygen, and resolving hypotension have a significant impact on limiting secondary cerebral damage in patients with severe head injury.

INITIAL CLINICAL ASSESSMENT

History

For the clinician to determine the mechanism of injury, anticipate problems, and establish priorities, he or she must obtain an accurate description from available witnesses and emergency personnel that includes the following:

- Type of accident
- Estimated degree of force
- Position of the victim when found
- State of consciousness

Any subsequent deterioration in the patient's level of consciousness indicates decreasing cerebral perfusion and should be acted on promptly. This decrease could be caused by an intracranial process such as an extending hematoma, or could be caused by a systemic effect such as hypotension caused by hemorrhage.

Primary Survey

Many victims of severe head injury also have sustained traumatic injury to other organs. The primary survey consists of a rapid, focused physical examination designed to identify and treat life-threatening injuries quickly.

Airway

The initial maneuver in the resuscitation of any trauma victim is establishing a secure airway, especially in patients with head injury, to prevent hypoxia or hypercarbia, which may lead to secondary brain injury.

The threshold for endotracheal intubation should be low in any child who sustains a head injury. Indications for intubation are listed in Table 14.1.

Intubation Technique The intubation technique should be modified to protect the patient's cervical spine and to minimize the rise in ICP associated with intubation. The patient's neck should be maintained in a neutral position, with axial traction applied by a person whose sole responsibility is to maintain the position of the neck.

Sedation Sufficient sedation to minimize the ICP response to intubation should be administered. All sedatives that lower ICP also have the potential to cause hypotension, especially in hemodynamically unstable trauma victims. Maintaining the blood pressure within a normal range during sedation is essential to avoid hypotension and subsequent impaired

Table 14.1
Indications for Airway Management in the Pediatric Trauma Victim

Upper airway obstruction
   Loss of pharyngeal muscle activity and tone
   Inability to clear secretions
   Foreign body
   Direct trauma
   Seizures
Loss of protective airway reflexes
Abnormalities of respiratory rate and rhythm
Chest wall dysfunction
Respiratory muscle dysfunction
   Fatigue
   Shock states
   Secondary to nerve dysfunction
Pulmonary disease
   Failure of oxygenation
   Failure of ventilation
   Pulmonary hypertension
Intracranial hypertension
Prophylactic

cerebral perfusion. Lidocaine (1 mg/kg) may be given intravenously before muscle relaxants to blunt the rise in ICP during intubation. Although succinylcholine often is used in rapid sequence intubation because of its rapid action, short duration, and reliable muscle relaxation properties, it may raise ICP. This response may be attenuated by defasciculating doses of a nondepolarizing muscle relaxant.

Ventilation

Hypoventilation caused by several pulmonary or neurologic causes is common in head-injured patients. Hypercarbia is a potent cerebral vasodilator, and should be strenuously avoided in these patients. Short-term use of moderate hyperventilation in the immediate resuscitation of any seriously head-injured patient is recommended. Patients with physical findings suggestive of brain stem compression from herniation (r.g., Cushing's triad, dilated and unreactive pupils) should be hyperventilated as soon as possible to lower ICP acutely.

Supplemental oxygen should be provided for all patients with moderate to severe head trauma to prevent hypoxia that may cause secondary brain injury. The patient's oxygen saturation should be monitored with a pulse oximeter and should be maintained 90% or higher.

Circulation

Assessment and optimization of perfusion is the next therapeutic goal. Shock, or an inadequate delivery of oxygen and nutrients to meet the metabolic demands of the tissue, can result from multiple causes. The injured brain is highly susceptible to inadequate perfusion, and unless prompt resolution of shock occurs, secondary injury results. The primary goal should be to restore adequate perfusion, and adequate fluid resuscitation should not be withheld because of concerns about cerebral edema. Isotonic fluid, however, should be used to minimize free water administration.

Hypovolemic shock from blood loss commonly is seen in trauma victims. Except in small infants, it is impossible to lose enough blood in the cranium to cause hypotension; therefore, other sources of blood loss besides head injury should be sought in these patients. Other causes of hypotension besides hypovolemia can occur and should be diagnosed quickly. Cardiac contusions may lead to cardiogenic shock and arrhythmias; inotropic and antiarrhythmic medications are beneficial in these cases. Spinal cord injury may lead to vasodilatation, hypotension, and the loss of sympathetic tone. Although adequate fluid administration is required in these cases, alpha adrenergic agonists to increase systemic vascular resistance often are necessary.

Neurologic Examination

The primary aim of this examination is the diagnosis and treatment of life-threatening intracranial hypertension with incipient herniation.

Pupillary Light Reflex Evaluation of pupillary response to light can be performed quickly and can be helpful in diagnosing herniation. Bilaterally dilated pupils that are unresponsive are an ominous sign, whether caused by bilaterally compressed third nerves or severe cerebral anoxia and ischemia; their presence is an indication for rapid therapeutic maneuvers to decrease ICP.

Hyperventilation and other maneuvers to lower ICP acutely should be instituted immediately if a unilateral or bilateral dilated, unresponsive pupil is found.

Level of Consciousness If possible, the level of consciousness should be rapidly assessed at this stage (Table 14.2).

Secondary Survey

The secondary survey involves a thorough physical examination of the patient and its aim is to identify all traumatic injuries and to begin to prioritize treatment. Areas included in this examination are the head, neck, thorax, and neurologic system.

Laboratory Evaluation

Laboratory studies obtained after the initial physical evaluation of the patient has been completed include:

- Complete blood count
- Platelet count

Table 14.2
Modified Glasgow Coma Score for Infants

Activity	Best Response	Score
Eye opening	Spontaneous	4
	To speech	3
	To pain	2
	None	1
Verbal	Coos and babbles	5
	Irritable cries	4
	Cries to pain	3
	Moans to pain	2
	None	1
Motor	Normal spontaneous movements	6
	Withdraws to touch	5
	Withdraws to pain	4
	Abnormal flexion	3
	Abnormal extension	2
	None	1

- Electrolytes
- Type and cross
- Amylase
- Coagulopathy panel (PT, PTT, fibrinogen level)
- Arterial blood gas, with subsequent placement of a pulse oximeter

Neuroradiologic Evaluation

Computed tomography is the method of choice for urgent neuroimaging of patients with apparently serious head injuries.

Approach to the Head Computed Tomography Scan

Progressively greater attenuation (i.e., brighter intensity) is seen by fat, water, soft tissues, contrast material, bone, and metal. Blood has variable attenuation depending on its age, clotting, and dilution (Fig. 14.4). The dif-

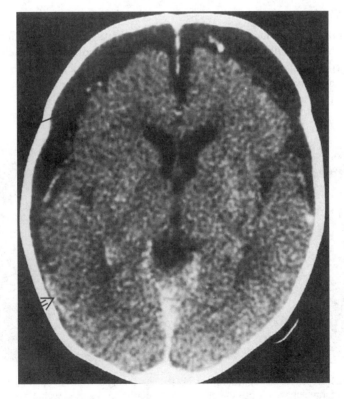

Figure 14.4. Varying attenuation of blood. Head computed tomography scan of an abused child shows both acute (bright) blood (open arrow) and chronic (dark) blood (closed arrow) in the subdural space, indicating multiple episodes of intracranial hemorrhage secondary to nonaccidental head trauma.

ferences in attenuation of these structures allow discrimination of the various intracranial structures and abnormalities.

Bone Windows

Review of bone-window images (if available) reveals soft-tissue swelling (indicating acute injury), fractures, spread sutures, bulging fontanels, foreign bodies, and surgical changes. It is possible to evaluate the skull base, temporal bones, sinuses, mastoids, and maxillofacial-orbital structures. Linear skull fractures that approximate the angle of the scan plane may not be visible on the axial scan images. Coronal scanning may be helpful in this setting. Plain skull radiographs may be necessary to visualize the entire course of a fracture accurately. Reference to the digital radiograph, or scanogram, obtained at the beginning of the CT study may be helpful in visualizing a fracture not seen on the axial images. Diastasis, depression, and fragmentation of fractures are important observations (Fig. 14.5).

Brain Windows

The brain-window images reveal the normal structure and appearance of the brain stem, cerebellum, basal ganglia, cerebral hemispheres, ventricles, basilar cisterns, and convexity extra-axial fluid spaces, as well as such abnormalities as hemorrhage (acute or chronic, parenchymal, intraventricular, or extra-axial); areas of increased attenuation (calcification, foreign body, or

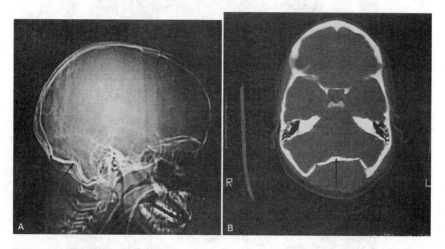

Figure 14.5. Depressed skull fracture. Lateral digital radiograph or scanogram (A) and axial computed tomography scan (B) through the posterior fossa in a child with a direct blow to the occiput show a markedly depressed occipital skull fracture (arrows). Brain-window images (not shown) showed intraventricular hemorrhage and acute hydrocephalus.

tumor); or decreased attenuation (edema, infarction, contusion, cerebritis, abscess, cyst, or tumor). Loss of distinction of the gray-white interface may be an early sign of edema, even before mass effect or shift occurs (Fig. 14.6).

Mass Effect and Shift

Infarction, contusion, hemorrhage, tumor, and abscess cause local mass effect and may lead to shift of the intracranial contents. Cerebral edema, focal or diffuse, also leads to shift. If the mass effect is unilateral in the cerebrum, the shift is from side to side. The midline falx is a relatively rigid structure. There may be injury to the brain or blood vessels as the brain shifts from side to side (i.e., subfalcine herniation). The distal anterior cerebral artery on the side of the mass effect is especially prone to injury or compression in this setting as it impinges on the falx (see Fig. 14.2).

When the mass effect is generalized in the cerebral hemispheres, the shift is downward through the incisural opening of the tentorium (i.e., descending transtentorial herniation) (Fig. 14.7). Pupillary dilation is indicative of compression of cranial nerve III. Less commonly, the mass effect is

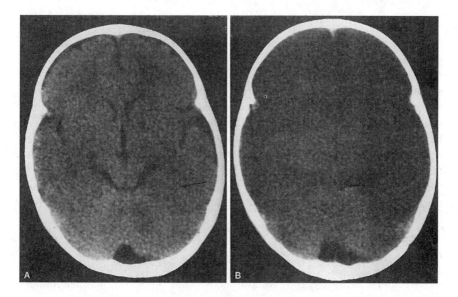

Figure 14.6. Signs of cerebral edema. Head computed tomography scans of a 6-month-old infant with near sudden infant death syndrome event. Initial scan (A) on the day of admission shows only subtle decrease in the normal contrast between gray and white matter structure, best seen in the posterior temporal lobes (arrow). Follow-up scan (B) performed 3 days later shows diffuse low attenuation of the brain indicative of severe cerebral edema. Note effacement of the lateral ventricles and quadrigeminal plate cistern (arrow).

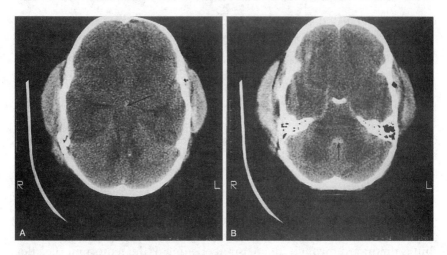

Figure 14.7. Descending transtentorial herniation. Head computed tomography scans of a child with severe closed head injury (same patient as in Figure 14.10) at the level of the tentorial incisura (A) and the fourth ventricle (B) show effacement of the cisterns at the skull base and in the posterior fossa and compression of the brainstem at the incisura. There are also signs of tonsillar herniation. Note the blood in the third (arrow in A) and fourth (arrow in B) ventricles.

in the posterior fossa and the herniation is upward (i.e., ascending transtentorial herniation) (Fig. 14.8).

The relatively rigid margins of the tentorium at the incisura compress vessels adjacent to them when herniation occurs. With descending herniation, the posterior cerebral arteries are compressed against the tentorium, leading to bilateral occipital lobe infarction; in ascending herniation, bilateral cerebellar infarction may occur with compression of the superior cerebellar arteries against the under surface of the tentorium. Downward herniation through the foramen magnum may be difficult to detect on CT studies. A "tight" appearance to the posterior fossa, absence of fluid in the cisterna magna, or posterior displacement of the fourth ventricle may be helpful signs.

Appearance of Ventricles

Changes in the ventricles may be helpful in detecting mass effect and shift.

- A lateral ventricle may be compressed by a mass in the cerebral hemisphere adjacent to it.
- The third ventricle may be compressed or displaced by mass effect deep in the cerebrum (i.e., in the basal ganglia and thalamus).
- The fourth ventricle is displaced or distorted by mass effect in the cerebellum.
- Generalized enlargement may result from developing hydrocephalus secondary to intraventricular hemorrhage, inflammation, or blockage by mass

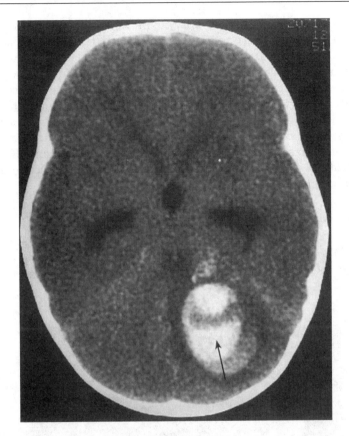

Figure 14.8. Ascending transtentorial herniation. Head computed tomography scan of an infant with hemorrhage (arrow) of a cerebellar vascular malformation shows effacement of the posterior fossa and basilar cisterns and acute hydrocephalus secondary to obstruction of cerebrospinal fluid flow at the level of the aqueduct.

effect or from loss of brain tissue ("ex vacuo dilatation"), especially after the acute phase of a global brain injury resolves.

Serial measurements of head size may be helpful in making this distinction, especially in younger children with more mobile cranial sutures.

Extra-Axial Fluid

Extra-axial fluid may be difficult to evaluate because there is normally some CSF in the subarachnoid space over the convexities of the cerebral hemispheres. This fluid should have identical attenuation to that of normal intraventricular CSF. If the attenuation of an extra-axial collection is greater than that of intraventricular CSF, the fluid contains increased protein or cellular content, most likely secondary to previous hemorrhage or inflammation. It is normal to have an increased volume of the subarachnoid space in infants and toddlers, but the fluid should have normal CSF attenuation.

Because the cortical veins course in the arachnoid membrane, when the subarachnoid space enlarges, the veins are displaced off the surface of the brain (the "cortical vein sign") (Fig. 14.9). Careful inspection of the location of the cortical veins can be helpful in correctly assigning the space of low-attenuation extra-axial fluid. Alternatively, if the veins are closely applied to the surface of the brain with the fluid peripheral to them, especially if the fluid has greater attenuation than normal CSF, the collection is most like a chronic subdural hematoma or hygroma.

Basilar Extracerebral Space

Absence of basilar cisterns containing CSF raises the possibility of brain swelling. These cisterns are best seen in the suprasellar region and around the midbrain above the level of the incisura. One of the early signs of cerebral

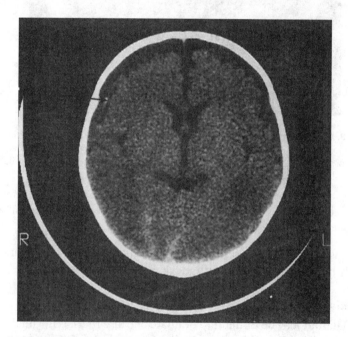

Figure 14.9. Cortical vein sign. Head computed tomography scan of an abused child shows bilateral chronic subdural hematomas. A cortical vein (arrow) can be seen at the interface of the subdural hematoma (peripheral to the vein, which runs in the arachnoid membrane) and the underlying cerebrospinal fluid in the subarachnoid space (between the brain and the cortical vein).

edema is effacement of the normal basilar cisterns. Nonvisualization of these cisterns may be caused by the presence of a lumbar CSF drain or shunt.

Evidence of Hemorrhage

Blood in the subdural compartment may be "isodense" to the brain as it evolves from the phase of increased attenuation (i.e., acute) to decreased attenuation (i.e., chronic) relative to the brain. Careful attention to the displacement of the gray-white junction medially or the "hematocrit effect" caused by layering of cellular and serum elements of blood may be helpful in detecting subtle subdural hemorrhage.

Hemorrhage in the parenchyma of the brain may be subtle and diffuse, as in hemorrhagic infarction or contusion; focal and discrete, as in an hematoma; linear in the cortex, as in laminar cortical necrosis; or punctate at the gray-white interface, as in diffuse axonal injury. Intraventricular hemorrhage usually is caused by trauma, shunt placement, or rupture of an arteriovenous malformation.

A recognized pattern of hemorrhage and extracerebral fluid accumulation is seen in the shaking-impact form of child abuse. In this setting, acute hemorrhage often occurs in the extracerebral compartment (usually subdural) frequently adjacent to the falx or tentorium or the tips of the occipital or temporal lobes. This acute hemorrhage is adjacent to more chronic-looking hemorrhage in the subdural space over one or both convexities. In addition, there may be diffuse brain swelling, indicating cerebral edema caused by diffuse axonal injury or suffocation. The constellation of these findings is highly suggestive of nonaccidental injury to the infant or young child (see Figs. 14.4 and 14.9).

Contrast Enhancement

After intravenous contrast medium administration, the enhancing pattern of the brain, blood vessels, brain coverings, and any abnormal structures is informative.

- Increased parenchymal enhancement may indicate inflammation, tumor, infarction, "luxury perfusion," or other cause of loss of the normal blood-brain barrier.
- Decreased enhancement may indicate infarction, cerebral edema, or nonenhancing tumor.
- Decreased caliber of the vessels at the skull base may reflect spasm, inflammation, vasculitis, or encasement.
- Increased vessel size reveals loss of autoregulation, a vascular malformation, or a high flow tumor.
- Enhancement of the leptomeninges covering the brain may indicate inflammatory change as in meningitis, with development of subdural effusion or

empyema, postoperative inflammation, or spread of tumor to the subarachnoid space or membrane adjacent to a subacute or chronic subdural hematoma.

Other Imaging Methods

Magnetic Resonance Imaging

Magnetic resonance imaging (MRI) is a powerful modality for brain imaging. Its use allows the following:

- Displays the brain in exquisite detail in multiple planes
- Distinguishes soft tissues better than with CT
- Detects various stages of hemoglobin degradation
- Assesses maturity of myelination
- Evaluates hemorrhage in or around the brain

Limitations to its use include:

- Use near a strong magnetic field, including intravenous pumps, most respirators, and other life-support equipment.
- The patient must be still for several minutes at a time.

Magnetic resonance imaging usually is used to clarify findings initially seen on CT or to reveal abnormalities that may escape detection by CT.

Nuclear Medicine Studies

Nuclear medicine studies are of limited value to the head-injured patient. Its most frequent application is to assess cerebral perfusion in the determination of brain death. Using newer isotope formulations, it is possible to obtain both flow and static images of the brain to establish the presence or absence of cerebral perfusion.

Indications for Acute Surgical Intervention/Intracranial Monitoring

Intracranial Pressure Monitoring

Placement of an ICP monitor in head-injured patients is indicated in the presence of:

- A Glasgow Coma Score lower than 8
- Rapid deterioration noted in the patient's neurologic examination
- Loss of the ability to follow the patient's neurologic examination during surgery or while he or she is receiving muscle relaxants or sedatives
- Computed tomography evidence of diffuse cerebral edema in anticipation of intracranial hypertension developing, even though their initial Glasgow Coma Score is higher than 8
- Intraventricular hemorrhage with secondary hydrocephalus that should be drained with a ventricular drain-monitor

Surgical Treatment

Rapidly expanding mass lesions, such as subdural or epidural hematomas, that cause focal compression of the underlying brain, and rapidly increasing ICP, should be surgically decompressed as soon as possible. Prompt surgical resolution of these injuries in patients sustaining no other underlying brain injury has a major impact on morbidity and mortality. Patients who have suffered more diffuse brain injury in addition to hematomas still may have a dismal outcome despite surgical decompression. Smaller focal lesions that seem to be symptomatic also are considered likely to benefit from surgical evacuation. Exceptions include deep contusions or hematomas that require dissection of large areas of the brain to access them, or lesions in eloquent areas of the brain such as the speech or motor cortex.

CLINICAL MANAGEMENT

Pulmonary Management

Neurogenic Pulmonary Edema

Neurogenic pulmonary edema (NPE) is the most dramatic of the pulmonary complications common after serious head injury.

Clinical Presentation

Classically, NPE develops within 2 to 12 hours of the injury, but can be delayed up to several days. Patients present with hypoxia, hyperventilation, and hypocarbia. Radiographic examination reveals diffuse "fluffy" infiltrates. Measurement of wedge pressure by a Swan-Ganz catheter generally are low, suggesting that the origin of the edema is noncardiac and caused by increased pulmonary permeability. Other causes of noncardiogenic pulmonary edema, such as direct chest trauma with contusion or aspiration, should be considered in the diagnosis. The diagnosis of NPE is made by exclusion of these other causes of pulmonary edema in a patient with a compatible history.

Outcome

Generally, NPE resolves if the patient survives. Few, if any, of these patients die of respiratory failure; most succumb from their neurologic injury. If not aggressively treated, however, NPE may lead to prolonged hypoxia and increase the secondary hypoxic damage in the injured brain. Additionally, NPE may complicate the management of these patients. High levels of positive end-expiratory pressure (PEEP) often are necessary to treat hypoxia in these patients; this amount of PEEP may impair venous return from the head, thereby increasing ICP.

Breathing Patterns

Abnormal breathing patterns after head injury are common (Fig. 14.10).

Cardiovascular Management

A hyperdynamic cardiovascular response occurs after head injury, and is directly related to sympathetically mediated elevations of plasma epinephrine and norepinephrine. As with NPE, injury to the medulla and hypothalamus are implicated as the cause of the sympathetic outpouring. This hyperdynamic state can be blocked by beta antagonists. Primary or secondary injury to the brain stem also may cause an increase in vagal tone.

All patients admitted to the pediatric intensive care unit after head injury should have continuous electrocardiographic monitoring. The incidence of arrhythmias after head injury is unknown, but may be more common than previously appreciated in children.

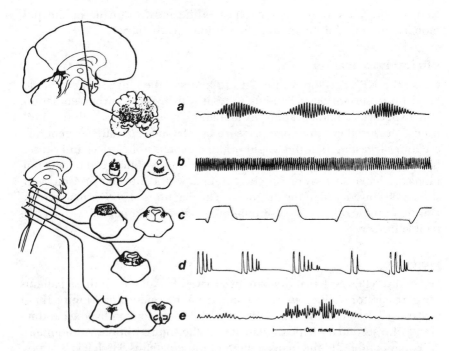

Figure 14.10. Injury to different portions of the brain leads to distinctive abnormal breathing patterns that may help localize the area of injury. A prolonged abnormal respiratory pattern may interfere with oxygenation and ventilation. (Reprinted with permission from Mettler FA. Neuroanatomy. St. Louis: CV Mosby, 1948:816.)

Hematologic Support

Approximately one third of pediatric patients have disseminated intravascular coagulopathy (DIC) after head injury. Because brain tissue is a potent stimulator of DIC, the severity of hematologic abnormalities correlate with the severity of the head injury. Because of concerns about excessive bleeding, the presence of DIC complicates potential surgical procedures, including the placement of intracranial monitoring devices. Additionally, DIC has been associated with delayed and recurrent intracerebral hematomas. For these reasons, DIC should be treated aggressively with replacement factors.

Nutritional Support

A hypermetabolic response occurs shortly after any traumatic injury, including head injury, and can last for several weeks. An increase in sympathetic tone leads to a sudden increase in plasma catecholamine concentrations, which causes an increase in oxygen consumption. Abnormalities in temperature regulation may lead to fever or hypothermia with shivering, which also increases metabolic demands. Excessive muscle activity such as seizures or posturing can increase oxygen consumption.

Early nutritional support can improve outcome in head-injured patients. The goals of nutritional support should be to provide adequate calories to support cellular metabolism, prevent catabolism, and promote healing. A positive nitrogen balance is optimal, but often difficult to achieve in these patients.

Seizure Control

Posttraumatic seizures occur in 6.5 to 10% of children.

Early Seizures (Within 1 Week of Injury)

Children are more prone than adults to develop early seizures, given the same degree of injury. Early convulsions occur in 5% of children with minor head injury and 35% of children with severe head injuries. Predisposing factors include a depressed skull fracture, dural or cortical laceration, hematomas, and posttraumatic amnesia longer than 24 hours.

Late Seizures (More than 1 Week after Injury)

Children are less prone to late-onset seizures than adults. The risk of late epilepsy in children sustaining early or impact seizures is 15%.

After Effects of Seizure Activity

Convulsions may interfere with effective oxygenation and ventilation, thereby potentially worsening secondary hypoxic brain injury and causing cerebral vasodilatation with a concurrent increase in ICP. Even if oxygenation and ventilation are maintained, the metabolic demands of the injured brain are increased.

Anticonvulsant Therapy

Convulsions should be treated aggressively with standard anticonvulsants. Lorazepam (0.1 to 0.3 mg/kg) usually is effective in stopping seizure activity; its half-life is short, however, and long-acting agents such as phenytoin or phenobarbital should be administered. Phenytoin has some advantage over phenobarbital because of its nonsedating qualities.

CEREBRAL PERFUSION PRESSURE MANAGEMENT
Positioning

Traditional practice has been to maintain the head at a 30 degree angle and in a midline position to improve cerebral venous drainage. This drainage lowers cerebral blood volume, thereby lowering ICP, especially when cerebral compliance is low. Some investigators question the effect of head elevation on cerebral perfusion pressure and blood flow.

Sedation/Paralysis

Agitation and muscular activity increases ICP; presumably, increased respiratory tone interferes with cerebral venous return. Patients with an altered mental status and agitation after a head injury may injure themselves or medical staff. Therefore, muscle relaxants or sedatives or both are commonly used in head-injured patients.

Fluid and Osmolality Therapy
Euvolemia

Maintaining adequate filling pressures helps to ensure a normal cardiac output, thereby optimizing systemic blood pressure and cerebral perfusion. Overaggressive administration of fluid, especially hypotonic solutions, should be avoided. Placement of a central venous or pulmonary arterial catheter may be indicated in some patients to guide fluid administration.

Use of Diuretics

Loop and osmotic diuretics frequently are used in head-injured patients to maintain euvolemia, although both types of diuretics have actions on the injured brain independent of their ability to remove excess fluid via the kidney. The loop diuretic, furosemide, has been shown to decrease CSF production, which may be beneficial when cerebral compliance is low. Mannitol lowers blood viscosity and thereby improves cerebral blood flow. Its effects on reducing cerebral edema remain unproved.

Cerebrospinal Fluid Drainage

Cerebrospinal fluid is one of the three normal components of intracranial volume. The volume of CSF may be small when compared with brain and cerebral blood volume, especially in patients with hyperemia and cerebral edema after head trauma; however, patients with low intracranial compliance may experience a large change in ICP even with small changes in intracranial volume. Removal of CSF often improves intracranial hypertension in these patients.

Hyperventilation

Prolonged hyperventilation is no longer the mainstay therapy in patients with head injury. Most patients initially retain their cerebrovascular responsiveness to changes in $PaCO_2$ after head injury, making it possible to reduce cerebral blood volume by lowering $PaCO_2$. Ideally, intracranial hypertension should be corrected using the methods just outlined, reserving hyperventilation for use to treat acute, severe rises in ICP that impair cerebral perfusion.

Corticosteroids and Barbiturates

Multiple studies have shown that corticosteroids are ineffective in reducing intracranial hypertension in head-injured patients, and the use of barbiturates in treating intracranial hypertension is controversial. The cardiodepressant effect of barbiturates makes their use in head-injured patients especially challenging because of concerns about lowering blood pressure and, thereby, cerebral perfusion pressure. At most, barbiturate therapy should be reserved for patients with intractable intracranial hypertension.

SPINAL CORD INJURY

Primary Injury

It is possible for bony or ligamentous injuries or both to occur without injury to the spinal cord. Alternatively, spinal cord injury without radiographic evidence of bony or ligamentous injury can occur, especially in the pediatric population. Identified by the acronym SCIWORA, or Spinal Cord Injury Without Radiographic Abnormality, this type of injury occurs when the excessive flexibility and elasticity of the pediatric osseoligamentous complex allows transient segmental subluxation followed by spontaneous reduction.

Bony Injury

Stable Fractures Stable fractures, which involve nonarticulating surfaces or bony elements anterior to the spinal cord, such as the vertebral bodies and the transverse and spinal processes, do not result in abnormal movement of spinous elements. Although the stability of the spine is not jeopardized, the possibility of bony fragments or disk material being forced into the spinal canal still exists.

Unstable Fractures Unstable fractures result in the potential for abnormal movement of the spinal column, with resultant spinal cord trauma. Because the posterior osseoligamentous complex is crucial in the stability of the spinal column, fractures involving the posterior articulating elements, the pedicles or facets, often are unstable.

Supporting Structure Injury

The accessory supporting or shock-absorbing structures of the spinal column also can be injured. Pure ligamentous injury can occur and lead to spinal instability. Similarly, traumatic disk herniation in the absence of a bony fracture can occur and lead to neural compression syndromes. Disk herniation in an anterior or posterior position occurs because of excessive flexion or extension. These injuries often are recognized initially by neurologic examination because the initial plain radiographs may be normal.

Pediatric Considerations

Cervical Cord Injuries Children are more likely to sustain a cervical cord injury; thoracic and lumbar spinal injuries are more common in adolescents. Additionally, of all children sustaining cervical cord injuries, younger children are more prone to have high cervical injuries, and older children are more likely to have lower cervical spine injuries. Minor trauma may lead to cervical cord injury in children with abnormalities of the bony structures such as juvenile rheumatoid arthritis or achondroplasia, or ligamentous complex such as Down's syndrome.

Subluxation Injuries Nondisplaced bony fractures occur more commonly in adolescents and adults, but children seem to have more subluxation injuries without bony fractures. The pediatric spine is hypermobile because of factors mentioned above. Increased ligamentous laxity and immature paraspinal musculature also contribute to the hypermobility. While ligamentous laxity protects the bony spine from fractures, it also allows for a high chance of ligamentous injury in children. Transient subluxation can lead to SCIWORA syndrome in children.

Initial Clinical Assessment

Primary Survey

Immobilization For any injured patient, appropriate precautions to prevent further spinal injury should be taken by emergency personnel at the scene. These precautions include meticulous attention to immobilization of the cervical spine during extrication, mobilization, and transportation. If injury to the thoracic or lumbar spine is suspected, the patient should be immobilized on a backboard.

Adequate Respiration Similar to head-injured victims, the primary survey should focus on airway, breathing, and circulation. Similar indications for establishing an airway and positive pressure ventilation apply. Protection of the cervical spine during intubation in any injured patient should always occur. Spinal injury above the level of the fourth cervical vertebrae results in paralysis of all the muscles involved in respiration. These patients have poor to absent spontaneous respiratory effort. Injuries to the lower cervical spinal cord spare the diaphragm but abolish some of the accessory muscle strength, resulting in decreased vital capacity and retention of secretions. Although these patients have adequate respirations initially, they may develop respiratory failure over time as the diaphragm fatigues.

Neurogenic Shock

Interruption of the sympathetic outflow in patients with spinal injury above the level of the fourth thoracic vertebrae can result in neurogenic shock, with vasodilatation, decreased systemic vascular resistance, and hypotension. This form of shock may be difficult to differentiate from hypovolemia in patients with multiple injuries. The presence of a relative bradycardia considering the patient's age and hypotensive state can help to diagnose neurogenic shock; most hypovolemic patients have a compensatory tachycardia. Restoration of blood volume alone may not improve patients with injury-induced vasodilatation, and alpha-adrenergic agents such as dopamine or epinephrine, as well as military antishock trousers, may be needed to raise systemic vascular resistance and blood pressure.

Secondary Survey

The patient's other injuries should be identified and treated during a secondary survey. Although other injuries sustained may be life-threatening and, therefore, take precedence over identification of a spinal injury, precautions to immobilize the patient's spine to prevent further damage should occur during this time.

Evaluation of Bony Spine When feasible, the entire spine should be examined carefully. The patient should be logrolled to perform this examination. Ecchymoses indicate trauma, and should be noted. The spinal column should be palpated, and widening of the spaces between adjacent spinous processes, malalignment of the spine, or stepoff of the spinous processes may indicate underlying distraction or dislocation.

Functional Integrity of the Cord Sensory and motor examinations are performed (see previous section). The sensory level is described according to the lowest dermatome in which sensation is normal (Fig. 14.11). The motor level is defined as the lowest segment in which muscle strength is assessed as able to move and hold in an antigravity position. Key muscles for determination of motor level are shown in Table 14.3.

Superficial reflexes such as the abdominal, cremasteric, and anal reflexes are helpful in localizing the level of injury in patients with spinal injury. Absent or diminished superficial reflexes suggest corticospinal lesions above the segmental innervation of this reflex. Complete loss of sensation, segmental reflexes, and motor function below a given level indicates a complete lesion. Retention of any function below the level of injury indicates an incomplete lesion. The function classically retained is that of the sacral nerves. Thus it is imperative that perianal sensation and reflexes be tested and documented. A rectal examination should be performed to evaluate anal sphincter tone. An incomplete lesion has the potential for improvement.

Patterns of Incomplete Lesions The Brown-Sequard syndrome consists of ipsilateral motor weakness, decreased position, and vibratory sensation, and contralateral diminution of pain sensation below the level of injury. This syndrome results from lateral damage to the spinal cord, especially in penetrating injuries.

The anterior cord syndrome consists of absent motor function and pain sensation with preservation of position and vibratory sensation. This syndrome results from injury to the anterior spinal artery that supplies motor tracts, the central gray matter, and the spinothalamic tracts, and may be seen in fractures involving displacement of intervertebral disk into the spinal cord.

The central cord syndrome consists of bilateral arm weakness with relative sparing of lower extremity function and perianal functions and is caused by injury to the central portions of the cord from compression.

The presence of a spinal cord injury above the seventh thoracic vertebrae may mask the tenderness normally associated with an intra-abdominal injury. A high index of suspicion is needed in these patients to diagnose intra-abdominal bleeding. Ongoing physical examinations to evaluate increasing abdominal distention and rapid radiologic examination of the abdomen are helpful in diagnosis.

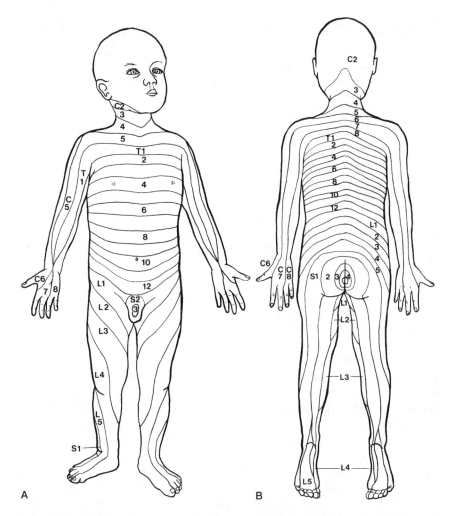

Figure 14.11. Segmental dermatomes are reproducible and helpful in identifying the level of spinal cord injury.

Neuroradiologic Evaluation

Contrary to neuroimaging of the head, in which CT is the modality of choice, plain film radiographs are preferable for evaluation of the cervical spine. Interpretation of these radiographs is often difficult, especially in children. The simple mnemonic ABC'S is useful in approaching a radiograph of the cervical spine: A, alignment; B, bones; C, cartilage (disks); and S, soft tissues.

Table 14.3
Key Muscle Groups and Reflexes

Nerve Root	Muscles and Function	Reflexes
C-4	Diaphragm: inspiration	
C-5	Deltoid: shoulder flexion and abduction	Biceps (C-5, C-6)
	Biceps: elbow flexion	
C-6	Extensor carpi radialis: wrist extension	
C-7	Triceps: elbow extension	Triceps (C-7, C-8)
C-8	Flexor digitorum superficialis: finger flexion	
T-1	Interossei: finger abduction and adduction	
T-2–T-7	Intercostals: expiration, forced expiration	
T-8–T-12	Abdominals: expiration, trunk flexion	Superficial abdominals
L-2	Iliopsoas: hip flexion	Cremasteric (L-1, L-2)
L-3	Quadriceps: knee extension	Knee (L-3, L-4)
L-4	Tibialis anterior: foot dorsiflexion	
L-5	Extensor hallucis longus: great toe extension	Hamstring (L-5, S-1)
S-1	Gastrocnemius: foot plantar flexion	Ankle (S-1, S-2)
S-2–S-4	Anal sphincter: fecal continence	Anal wink, bulbocavernosus

From Massagli T, Jaffe K. Pediatric spinal cord injury: treatment and outcome. Pediatrician 1990;17:246, published by S. Karger, AG, Basel.

Alignment A lateral radiograph should be obtained as soon as it is clinically feasible. The radiograph must show the entire cervical spine from skull base to upper thoracic spine. The clinician should follow the anterior body line, the posterior body line, and the laminar junction line, which is formed by the union of the lamina in the posterior arch of each cervical vertebra (Fig. 14.12). With the spine in neutral position, these lines form a gentle curve reflecting the normal lordosis of the cervical spine. This curve may be straightened by the presence of a cervical collar or by muscle spasm from trauma or inflammation.

Flexion and extension lateral radiographs of the cervical spine may be used to supplement the neutral position films. These films require the supervision of a qualified member of the neurosurgical or critical care team in a patient with impaired level of consciousness. Ligamentous instability and subluxation that is not present on the neutral views may be apparent on these films.

Bones and Cartilage The bones are evaluated for fracture (i.e., trauma), destructive change (i.e., histiocytosis, tumor, infection), and congenital malformation (i.e., achondroplasia, dysplasias, segmentation, fusion anomalies). It is important to evaluate the height of the cartilage (i.e., disk) spaces. Loss of the normal disk space may reflect a congenital malformation, disk herniation, or inflammatory change.

Soft Tissues Swelling in the prevertebral space of the upper cervical spine may be caused by trauma (i.e., ligamentous injury, fracture, penetrating injury), inflammation (i.e., retropharyngeal abscess, osteomyelitis, diski-

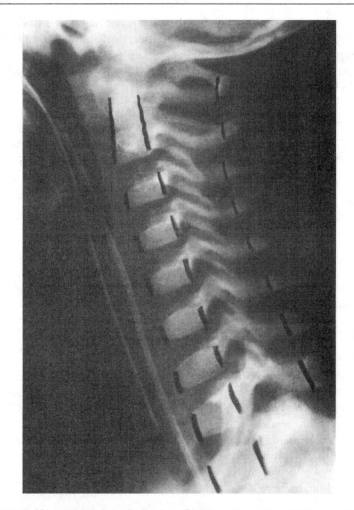

Figure 14.12. Normal lateral cervical spine alignment. A portable lateral cervical spine radiograph obtained in the emergency department on an injured child must show all seven cervical vertebra and the cervicothoracic junction. Three curvilinear lines are followed in assessing alignment. These are, from anterior to posterior, the anterior body line, the posterior body line, and the laminar junction line (each marked on the radiograph with a wax pencil).

tis), or tumor. Assessment of airway compromise from inflammatory or neoplastic mass may be possible.

Other Imaging Methods

Computed Tomography Computed tomography is used to evaluate fractures, especially at the craniocervical junction, or ring fractures of the vertebral bodies and posterior elements. Sagittal and coronal reconstructions of thin, overlapping scans obtained in the axial plane may have sufficient spatial resolution for diagnostic purposes when cervical spine injury precludes positioning for directly obtaining these projections.

Magnetic Resonance Imaging Magnetic resonance imaging is the technique of choice for:

- Assessment of the cervical spinal cord in the setting of trauma (i.e., contusion, laceration, hematoma, penetrating injury, infarction), inflammation (i.e., myelitis, abscess), demyelination (i.e., multiple sclerosis, postviral encephalomyelopathy) and congenital abnormality (i.e, syringohydromyelia, split cord syndromes, Chiari's malformations)
- Detecting hemorrhage or inflammation in the extra-axial (usually epidural) space of the cervical canal
- Demonstrating vertebral body and disk abnormalities secondary to inflammatory or neoplastic disease

Angiography Angiography of the carotid and vertebral arteries is indicated when the clinical findings and other imaging studies suggest injury or other abnormality of one or more of these vessels as a result of penetrating injury, skull base or cervical fracture, dissection, stroke, tumor, or retropharyngeal abscess.

Clinical Management

Spinal Cord

Immobilization and Traction The first step in preventing further spinal cord damage from compression or laceration is immobilization. If subluxation is present, the bony vertebrae are realigned and the spinal cord is decompressed with cervical traction by gentle manipulation under fluoroscopic control or using Gardner-Wells tongs with weights. Halo braces and various external fixation devices also are used to maintain long-term immobilization while allowing vertebral column fractures to heal.

Surgical Intervention Acute surgical indications include:

- A penetrating wound with an associated cerebrospinal leak or hematoma
- Failure of closed reduction
- Nerve root impingement
- Spinal cord compression from bony fragments
- Initial fixation of some unstable fractures
- Partial spinal cord injury and progressive neurologic deficit
- Need for bone grafting and rigid internal fixation to maintain stability of the vertebral column and to facilitate rapid remobilization

There is no evidence that surgery results in an improved neurologic outcome in patients with a stable neurologic examination.

Steroids Evidence shows that patients who receive intravenous corticosteroids shortly after partial or complete spinal cord injury have an improved long-term physiologic outcome. Methylprednisolone, 30 mg/kg followed by a 23-hour infusion of 5.4 mg/kg/hour, should be administered to any patient with suspected spinal cord injury as soon as possible.

Pulmonary Management

Pulmonary complications are the leading cause of death in hospitalized patients with spinal cord injuries, primarily secondary to pneumonia. Patients with injuries above the fourth cervical vertebrae have an impaired respiratory effort secondary to muscle weakness, and initially often require intubation and positive pressure ventilation. Unless lung disease coexists with muscle weakness, these patients usually are easily oxygenated and ventilated using moderate conventional ventilator settings. Adequate pulmonary toilet to minimize atelectasis is essential. Patients with a loss of sympathetic tone may develop profound bradycardia during suctioning because of the unopposed parasympathetic tone; atropine should be administered to these patients before suctioning. The use of kinetic beds to improve pulmonary toilet has been suggested.

Cardiovascular Management

Neurogenic shock with sympathetic interruption is associated with hypotension, hypothermia, and bradycardia. These patients may not mount a tachycardic response to hypovolemia, so aggressive monitoring of the intravascular space is required. For this reason, appropriate fluid resuscitation may require the placement of a central venous catheter. Vasopressor support also may be required. Bradycardia is generally responsive to atropine, but prolonged infusions of epinephrine or isoproterenol may be necessary. A transvenous pacemaker may also be considered.

Although neurogenic shock eventually resolves, the patient may experience prolonged dysautonomia, with postural hypotension. Close attention should be paid to blood pressure changes associated with position changes in these patients.

TRAUMATIC BRAIN INJURY REHABILITATION
Team Approach

Rehabilitation of traumatic brain injury consists of an transdisciplinary team of professionals who coordinate the treatment and recovery of the patient with his or her family (Table 14.4).

Medical Management

Rehabilitation can begin early in a child's hospitalization. Preventive and therapeutic intervention should begin in the intensive care unit during the acute stages of the recovery process. Rehabilitation nursing is crucial in all stages of recovery.

Table 14.4
Rehabilitation Transdisciplinary Team

Patient	Social worker
Family	Nutritionist
Primary care physician	Audiologist
Neurologist	Psychologist
Physiatrist	Child life specialist
Consultants	Financial assistant
Nurses	Neuropsychologist
Occupational therapist	Teacher
Physical therapist	School personnel
Speech language pathologist	Educational specialist
Recreational therapist	Orthotist
Adaptive equipment specialist	Discharge planner
Case manager	Respiratory therapist

Skin Care

Decubiti are decreased by careful observation of the patient, with frequent turning and appropriate skin care. Special skin precautions are necessary when splints, casts, or braces are used.

Bowel and Bladder Function

Bowel and bladder problems must be anticipated and treated. Urinary tract infections are common, because many of the children are catheterized when in the intensive care unit. Occasionally a more complete urologic evaluation, including a cystometrogram, is necessary for appropriate bladder treatment and "retraining."

Hydrocephalus

Posttraumatic hydrocephalus must be considered if clinical deterioration occurs in the patient. Symptoms of hydrocephalus (or shunt malfunction) often include decreasing responsiveness or increased agitation, headache, vomiting, or increasing spasticity. A comparative CT scan usually is diagnostic; however, often the radiographic changes are subtle, so neurosurgical consultation is critical.

Spasticity

Spasticity may be difficult to manage, even with intense therapy and medications. Other movement disorders requiring treatment may include dystonic posturing, ataxia, choreoathetosis, or tremor.

15.

Pediatric Drowning and Near-Drowning

Mark E. Rowin, David Christensen, and Elizabeth M. Allen

INTRODUCTION

Submersion events include both drowning and near-drowning episodes. Drowning is death from asphyxia, caused by submersion in water. Death is usually at the time of the submersion event or within a 24-hour period. Near-drowning is defined as an immersion event of sufficient severity to require medical treatment in which the patient survives for at least 24 hours, regardless of eventual outcome. Outcome following near-drowning may not be predicted reliably in the emergency department, so aggressive resuscitation should be performed.

PATHOPHYSIOLOGY

Decreased Tissue Oxygenation

Decreased oxygen delivery to tissues, specifically the central nervous system (CNS), is the most important consequence of near-drowning, although hypoxemia affects all organ systems to some degree. It is the magnitude of the hypoxic insult, as well as the body's ability to endure and recover from oxygen deprivation, that ultimately affects the patient's chances for survival and ensures good neurologic outcome. Early reinstitution of tissue oxygenation is the current hallmark of therapy and is the best regimen available to improve neurologic outcome.

Hypervolemia

Systemic fluid overload may be secondary to fluid absorbed through both the pulmonary and gastric circulations. The exact volume of fluid in the pulmonary tree varies from victim to victim but generally is less than 5 mL/kg. However, 80 to 90% of near-drowning victims will swallow large volumes of water into their stomachs. Not only will this potentially cause systemic fluid overload, but it often causes gastric distention and increases the risk of vomiting and aspiration during resuscitation. Additionally, overzealous administration of intravenous fluids during the early phases of resuscitation may contribute to fluid overload.

Hypovolemia

More often, near-drowning victims exhibit hypovolemic shock. Hypovolemia is most likely due to excessive capillary permeability secondary to endothelial damage from hypoxia and resultant loss of protein-rich fluid into the third space.

Hyperglycemia

Hyperglycemia noted after the stress of a near-drowning episode is believed to be secondary to excessive endogenous catecholamines. Hyperglycemia may potentiate neurologic damage in an ischemic brain. In children with severe neurologic insult, blood glucose levels of greater than 250 mg/dL have been associated with an increased likelihood of death or poor neurologic outcome when compared to children with similar injuries who were normoglycemic. Similarly, rats treated with insulin after a hypoxic-ischemic event to maintain normoglycemia demonstrated an improved neurologic outcome when compared to hyperglycemic controls.

Hypoglycemia

Hypoglycemia produced by the use of insulin also may have neurologic effects. Hypoglycemia has been shown to increase cerebral blood flow as much as 300%, which can change can increase intracranial pressure (ICP) dramatically in a patient with cerebral edema from hypoxia. There is also evidence that hypoglycemia may cause direct neuronal injury. The exact blood glucose levels at which neuronal injuries occur is unknown.

Pulmonary Effects

Hypoxia and Hypercarbia

During the breath-holding portion of a near-drowning event, the lung's functional residual capacity is the only source of gas exchange for the pulmonary capillaries. As oxygen uptake and carbon dioxide elimination are compromised, hypoxia and hypercarbia rapidly develop. A mixed metabolic and respiratory acidosis subsequently develops. If the victim is rescued before fluid aspiration, this hypoxia and acidosis tend to resolve rapidly because lung damage and pathophysiologic changes are minimal.

Fluid Aspiration

Aspiration of fluid into the airway triggers a cascade of pathophysiologic events. The primary effect is to increase ventilation-perfusion mismatching, resulting in hypoxemia. The effect of both salt and fresh water on pulmonary surfactant alters the surface tension properties of the alveoli and results in atelectasis, decreased lung compliance, and increased intrapulmonary shunting. This increased intrapulmonary shunting may take days to return to normal, even in children who are no longer hypoxemic and otherwise appear clinically well.

Secondary Pulmonary Edema

Secondary pulmonary edema may develop in response to water aspiration during drowning. Inhalation of water leads to an intense inflammatory reaction that may result in the destruction of alveolar pneumocytes. The alveolar capillary membrane is disrupted, leading to an outpouring of a plasma-rich exudate into the alveolus.

Secondary Drowning

In a subset of patients who initially respond well to pulmonary management but demonstrate significant respiratory deterioration 3 to 72 hours after rescue, surfactant loss can continue. This loss of surfactant ultimately leads to significant alveolar collapse, known as secondary drowning, probably occurs in less than 5% of survivors. It is defined as the occurrence of respiratory deterioration after "successful" resuscitation because of primary alveolar membrane dysfunction.

Other causes of postrescue pulmonary deterioration include:

- Bacterial pneumonia
- Barotrauma
- An inflammatory response to a foreign body aspiration (e.g., sand, mud, debris)
- Hypoventilation from neurologic deterioration
- Oxygen toxicity
- Adult respiratory distress syndrome

Cardiovascular Effects

The pediatric heart is remarkably tolerant of hypoxic-ischemic insult, and electrical activity often can be generated after a prolonged period of oxygen deprivation. Electrocardiographic changes usually mimic those seen in primary respiratory arrest (i.e., bradycardia that progresses to asystole).

Although it is often possible to obtain cardiac electrical activity after aggressive resuscitation, cardiogenic shock after near-drowning is common. Hemodynamic effects noted in all near-drowning victims, regardless of the tonicity of the water, include:

- Poor contractility after hypoxic insult
- Increased capillary permeability as a result of anoxia leading to intravascular hypovolemia
- Elevated systemic vascular resistance

Inadequate tissue perfusion because of ongoing cardiogenic and hypovolemic shock may continue the ischemic damage to the heart and other organs, especially the CNS.

Renal, Hepatic, and Gastrointestinal Effects

Renal dysfunction is a common sequela of hypoxic ischemic insult. Manifestations include:

- Albuminuria
- Hemoglobinuria
- Hematuria
- Oliguria
- Anuria

The cause of the dysfunction is believed to be anoxic injury to the kidney itself, resulting in acute tubular necrosis.

Liver Dysfunction

The liver also is susceptible to anoxic injury. Manifestations include:

• Elevated bilirubin levels
• Elevated transaminase levels
• Impaired production of procoagulant factors

Liver dysfunction undoubtedly plays a role in the disseminated intravascular coagulation seen after near-drowning.

Gastrointestinal Injury

The intestinal mucosa is sensitive to anoxic injury and often will slough after a hypoxic-ischemic event. The patient passes large quantities of foul-smelling, bloody, mucus-filled stools. These patients are at risk for bacterial translocation, or, in severe cases, perforation of the gastrointestinal tract. These complications can be severe, although with supportive care, they rarely pose a threat to overall survival in an otherwise salvageable patient.

Neurologic Effects

Acidosis and hypercarbia are undoubtedly important in cerebral injury, but it is irreversible hypoxic-ischemic damage to the brain that ultimately determines the outcome in the majority of near-drowning patients. Secondary cerebral injury may occur as a result of hypotension associated with cardiogenic shock, hypovolemia, and hypoxia that follows fluid aspiration and subsequent pulmonary dysfunction.

As a result of primary and secondary injuries, cerebral edema usually develops within 24 to 72 hours of a severe near-drowning event.

Hypothermia and the Diving Reflex

Two theories have been proposed to explain how children survive prolonged submersions in extremely cold water with good neurologic outcome: hypothermia and the diving response.

Heat Loss

Hypothermia develops rapidly after submersion in cold water. Heat loss presumably occurs both through the skin and with cold-water ingestion and aspiration. Ethanol may potentiate heat loss because of its vasodilatory properties. Children have larger surface areas and decreased insulation from fat than adults and can lose heat much more rapidly.

Changes in Cerebral Metabolism

When the brain is cooled rapidly, cerebral metabolism is depressed: oxygen consumption is 50% of normal at 28° C and 25% of normal at 20° C, and blood flow decreases 6 to 7% per 1° C temperature drop. If cerebral oxygen consumption decreases at an equal or greater rate than oxygen delivery, the brain is able to withstand longer periods of hypoxia.

Diving Reflex

This oxygen-conserving adaptation noted in many marine mammals appears to be triggered by breath-holding and cold stimulation. Cardiovascular changes that conserve oxygen for those tissues most sensitive to hypoxia include:

- Reduced cardiac output
- Peripheral and mesenteric vasoconstriction, which shifts blood away from the skeletal muscles, skin, gut, and kidneys
- Reduced coronary blood flow (to approximately 10% of predive level)

Systemic oxygen consumption and metabolic rates decrease, but cerebral blood flow and oxygen delivery are maintained.

INITIAL MANAGEMENT AND RESUSCITATION EFFORTS

The goal in the setting of near-drowning is to improve tissue oxygen delivery as rapidly as possible to minimize cerebral hypoxic-ischemic damage. Improving oxygen delivery optimally begins at the scene and continues during transport to a medical facility.

At the Scene

The rescuer follows the following steps:

- Begin mouth-to-mouth resuscitation as soon as the victim reaches the surface of the body of water.
- Anticipate gastric distention and an increased risk of regurgitation and aspiration related to attempted ventilation.
- Assess the hemodynamic status. If the victim is pulseless, start closed chest compression after the victim is on solid ground.
- Arrange and activate emergency medical services and transport to a medical facility.

Initial Assessment

Airway/Breathing

The patient with adequate respiratory effort requires only supplemental oxygen. A weak respiratory effort may not allow adequate oxygenation and ventilation. The threshold for endotracheal intubation should be low in these patients (Table 15.1).

After the patient arrives at the hospital, initial resuscitation should continue to focus on stabilizing the respiratory system. The goal of airway management should be maintaining sufficient arterial oxygen saturation to maximize oxygen delivery to tissue beds, especially the CNS. Aspirated water can cause significant intrapulmonary shunting due to distal airway obstruction and alveolar collapse that may not respond to increasing the FiO_2. Positive end-expiratory pressure (PEEP) may be necessary. PEEP improves oxygenation and ventilation by alveolar recruitment and increasing functional residual capacity of the lungs, thus decreasing ventilation-perfusion mismatching.

Circulation

Arrhythmias Arrhythmias can occur in the drowning patient, especially if he or she is hypothermic. Common rhythms include bradycardia and asystole (i.e., in warm-water drownings) and atrial and ventricular fibrillation (i.e., in cold-water drownings). Electrocardiographic monitoring initiated by emergency medical personnel should continue.

Perfusion The goal of initial cardiovascular stabilization is return of end-organ perfusion. Indications of poor perfusion include:

- Prolonged capillary refill
- Mottled appearance of the skin
- Poor pulses
- Cool extremities
- Small urine output
- Altered sensorium

The hypovolemia and vasoconstriction seen in near drowning that makes detection of distal pulses extremely difficult warrants judicious intravenous fluid administration. Large volumes of hypotonic fluid are contraindicated because of the lack of effective volume expansion and free water in hypotonic

Table 15.1
Indications for Endotracheal Intubation in Near-Drowning

- Loss of airway protective reflexes as a result of a depressed level of consciousness
- A deteriorating neurologic examination
- Severe respiratory distress or severe hypoxia despite administration of supplemental oxygen
- Cardiorespiratory arrest
- Severe hypothermia (core temperature less than 30° C)

fluids may worsen cerebral edema and cause hyponatremia, thereby lowering the seizure threshold. A central venous or pulmonary artery catheter may be needed to monitor fluid administration.

Intravenous fluids should not be withheld because of concerns regarding cerebral edema, because optimizing cerebral perfusion is one of the most important goals of cardiovascular management. If poor perfusion continues after intravascular volume has been expanded adequately, the use of inotropic agents to improve cardiac contractility should be considered.

Neurologic Examination

After reestablishing respiratory and circulatory stability, a brief but thorough neurologic examination is performed.

Information from serial neurologic examinations can distinguish intact survivors from those with a poor neurologic outcome as early as 24 hours after the accident. The neurologic evaluation involves the assessment of the level of consciousness using the Glasgow Coma Scale (GCS) and the evaluation of brainstem reflexes.

Brainstem Reflexes This evaluation may aid in determining the extent of cerebral damage and has been shown to have some prognostic value.

In evaluating the pupillary response to light, unilateral pupillary dilation and unresponsiveness generally indicates an increased ICP with transtentorial herniation causing compression of the blood supply to the brainstem. Bilaterally unresponsive pupils indicate severe cerebral dysfunction from the hypoxic-ischemic injury or bilateral uncal herniation. These findings warrant immediate initiation of hyperventilation and other means to lower ICP.

Other brainstem reflexes to be assessed include: corneal, gag, oculovestibular, and oculocephalic reflexes and spontaneous respiratory effort.

Associated Injuries Closed-head injuries that can occur in diving into shallow water may cause intracranial accumulations of blood that rapidly raises ICP. Injury to the cervical vertebrae and spinal cord may also occur.

Other Systems

Intra-abdominal trauma should be considered if abdominal bruising is present and the story of the injury is consistent (i.e., diving accident or possible child abuse). When the index of suspicion of child abuse is high, possible fractures or evidence of previous injury should be evaluated.

Laboratory and Radiographic Evaluation

Initial laboratory assessment should include:

- Arterial blood gas, to evaluate the degree of acidosis and hypoxia and the effectiveness of ventilation

- Serum electrolyte levels
- Initial blood glucose levels, which may predict eventual outcome after near-drowning in children
- Toxicologic tests, when appropriate

Chest radiography is needed for all intubated patients to check the location of the endotracheal tube, assess the degree of pulmonary edema, and evaluate possible barotrauma.

Hypothermia

Rewarming

Efforts at rewarming should begin as soon as possible. Wet clothing should be removed to prevent continued conductive heat loss.

Mild Hypothermia

Active external (i.e., surface) rewarming should be instituted in patients with core temperatures greater than 30° C. Methods include convective heaters, hot water bottles, warm bedding, and radiant heat sources.

Severe Hypothermia

For near-drowning victims with core temperatures less than 30° C, active internal rewarming is needed. Core rewarming can be accomplished by warmed intravenous fluids, warmed humidified oxygen, gastric or rectal lavage with warmed fluids, peritoneal lavage, and cardiopulmonary bypass.

External rewarming of the markedly hypothermic patient is problematic:

- Rewarming the peripheral circulation first increases the risk of cardiac collapse, and by-products of anaerobic metabolism that circulate back to the heart may contribute to worsening cardiac function.
- Poor peripheral circulation from vasoconstriction or a cardiogenic source does not adequately dissipate the heat emitted from localized sources increasing the risk of severe localized burns at the sites of rewarming.

Initial Clinical Assessment

The patient may appear clinically dead because of decreased cardiac and neurologic activity from the hypothermia itself. As the patient becomes normothermic during resuscitation, hypoxic injury to organ systems becomes more readily apparent. Often, the injury is too severe and the organs will not recover function. Many clinicians, however, report remarkable recoveries after prolonged submersions. Unless a drowning victim is clearly dead with no hope of responding to appropriate resuscitative efforts, he or she should not be declared legally dead until the core temperature is 32° C or greater.

Resistance to Defibrillation

The hypothermic heart is extremely irritable and prone to ventricular fibrillation. Attempts at electrical defibrillation are not likely to be successful if core temperature is less than 30° C. If ventricular fibrillation persists after three attempts to defibrillate, cardiopulmonary resuscitation should be continued, the patient should be aggressively rewarmed, and defibrillation should be repeated as body temperature increases. Cardiotonic medications should be used with caution in hypothermic patients. Hypothermia slows renal and hepatic excretion of drugs so routine doses of such drugs as epinephrine, lidocaine, and procainamide may accumulate to toxic levels if used repeatedly. It is best to administer a single dose of lidocaine or bretylium to a hypothermic patient in ventricular fibrillation, holding subsequent doses until the patient's core temperature is greater than 30° C.

PEDIATRIC INTENSIVE CARE UNIT MANAGEMENT

The degree of organ dysfunction related to near-drowning tends to correlate with the severity and length of hypoxia and ischemia. The primary aim of modern therapy is directed toward cerebral resuscitation and protection. Intensive care unit management attempts to minimize secondary neurologic damage from hypoxia, ischemia, acidosis, seizure activity, and fluid/electrolyte abnormalities.

All near-drowning patients admitted to the pediatric intensive care unit (PICU) require:

- Continuous electrocardiograms
- Pulse oximetry
- Arterial and central venous pressure monitoring in unstable patients
- Flow-directed pulmonary artery catheter placement
- Monitoring of urine output as a measure of end-organ perfusion

Respiratory Management

Monitoring

Spontaneously breathing patients must be watched closely for the development of the following:

- Tachypnea
- Retractions
- Decreased breath sounds
- A change in level of consciousness
- Other signs of respiratory distress

Serial examinations also are important in intubated, mechanically ventilated patients to ensure adequacy of the ventilatory assistance provided and to observe any deterioration of the respiratory system (see previous discussion of secondary drowning).

Hyperventilation

A moderate degree of hyperventilation may be helpful in patients who show evidence of cerebral edema. A $PaCO_2$ in the 30 to 35 mm Hg range is adequate. Excessive hyperventilation may induce vasoconstriction so that cerebral perfusion is impaired. Additionally, the efficacy of prolonged hyperventilation is questionable.

Resolving Hypoxia

When conventional ventilatory methods are ineffective in resolving hypoxia, it is possible to use high-frequency jet ventilation or extracorporeal membrane oxygenation (ECMO).

Drug Therapy

Replacement of inactivated surfactant with artificial surfactant is one of several new therapies directed toward increasing pulmonary function after near-drowning.

Prophylactic use of corticosteroids in this setting has shown no benefit and is uniformly discouraged. The use of prophylactic antibiotics has not been shown to improve survival, and there are concerns that their use will select out antibiotic-resistant organisms.

Cardiovascular Management

Anoxic and ischemic injury to the heart after a near-drowning episode can occur. The electrocardiogram may show nonspecific ST- and T-wave changes, and levels of cardiac isoenzymes may be elevated.

The goal of cardiovascular management is to maintain adequate cardiac output and organ perfusion. Persistent cardiac dysfunction often is due to hypoxic cardiomyopathy. Ensuring adequate intravascular volume helps cardiac function and ensures improved end-organ perfusion. Excessive administration of intravascular fluids may increase symptoms of left-sided heart failure and worsen cerebral edema. Poor cardiac function may need to be augmented by inotropic support. In patients with significant hypoxic organ injury, a flow-directed pulmonary artery catheter may be useful in assessing cardiac function and oxygen delivery.

Neurologic Management

Cerebral Resuscitation

Aggressive brain-preservation techniques aimed primarily at controlling cerebral edema, treating elevated ICPs, and decreasing cerebral metabolic requirements are no longer considered of benefit in preventing secondary CNS damage after hypoxia-ischemia. It appears that cerebral edema and resultant intracranial hypertension is a direct result of the original hypoxic cerebral injury and not a manifestation of a reversible process.

Current neurologic intensive care is directed at conservative management, and attempts to decrease possible secondary injury to the brain. Cerebral resuscitation therapy consists of the following:

- Rapid restoration and stabilization of oxygenation and cerebral circulation
- Correction of acid-base and electrolyte abnormalities
- Maintenance of normoglycemia and normothermia is optimal
- Avoidance of hyperthermia
- Control seizure activity
- Control suspected intracranial hypertension

Recommended therapies include:

- Mild hyperventilation
- Sedation
- Elevating the head of the bed
- Avoiding fluid overload
- Limiting potential noxious stimuli
- Neuromuscular blocking agents, when necessary to improve ventilation status in severe pulmonary dysfunction

Assessment of Neurologic Insult

Because use of neuromuscular blockade and/or sedation prevents an accurate neurologic examination, a number of radiologic techniques, neurophysiologic tests, and laboratory studies have been evaluated as adjuncts in determining the extent of neurologic damage and eventual outcome.

Computed Tomography (CT) Whereas a normal head CT scan after anoxic cerebral injury is poorly predictive of outcome, an abnormal scan in the initial 36 hours after the near-drowning event usually is associated with a dismal prognosis. A common finding in this setting is the reversal sign, a diffusely decreased density in the cerebral cortical gray and white matter, with a loss of the gray/white interface and relative increased density of the thalami, brainstem, and cerebellum.

Electroencephalographic Monitoring (EEG) Relevant EEG findings associated with a poor prognosis are:

- Low amplitude activity
- Isoelectric tracings
- Burst-suppression patterns
- Uninterrupted seizure activity
- Alpha activity in the presence of clinical coma (termed alpha-coma)

EEG tracings must be interpreted with caution, however, as they can be influenced by hypothermia, illegal drug use, and barbiturate therapy.

Brainstem Auditory-Evoked Responses (BAER) BAER are useful in differentiating survivors from nonsurvivors after near-drownings, often within 6 hours of admission. They are less useful in differentiating survivors with neurologic deficits. Patients in persistent vegetative states normalize some aspects of their BAER, but cannot be completely differentiated from neurologically intact survivors until day three of hospitalization.

Cerebrospinal Fluid (CSF) Analysis In one study, measurements of creatine kinase, the BB fraction of creatine kinase, and lactate dehydrogenase (isoenzymes 1-n-3) peaked 76 hours after a hypoxic-ischemic cerebral insult in all patients who either died or were disabled neurologically. Patients who recovered normally had no change in their cerebrospinal fluid analysis. A difference could be seen between these groups as early as 28 hours after resuscitation.

PROGNOSTIC EVALUATION

An ability to prognosticate accurately the eventual outcome of a patient early in the hospital course would allow physicians to counsel parents more appropriately. A number of studies have attempted to predict what variables affect a near-drowning victim's outcome, although no system has proven to be entirely accurate.

Predictive Variables

- Arrival at an emergency department with no heart rate (i.e., requiring ongoing CPR): death or a persistent vegetative state is common
- Submersion time longer than 10 minutes in nonicy water and CPR duration greater than 25 minutes: death or severe neurologic impairment is likely to occur
- Submersion time of 5 minutes or less and less than a 10-minute duration of CPR: good outcome is more likely
- Sinus rhythm, reactive pupils, and neurologic responsiveness at the scene: good outcome is likely
- Need for cardiotonic medications: death in 70% of patients and severe neurologic impairment in the remaining 30%

It is important to note, however, that some reports document full neurologic recovery in normothermic pediatric near-drowning patients who arrived at the emergency department without vital signs, required prolonged CPR, and received cardiotonic medications.

Limiting Resuscitation

Because there is no practical medical index or score that will predict with 100% certainty which patients will and will not survive a near-drowning accident neurologically intact, when to limit resuscitation of a near-drowning victim is controversial. Our approach is to provide aggressive initial resuscitative attempts and then consider withdrawing life support within a few days if neurologic improvement is not seen.

OUTCOME

With improvements in cardiovascular and pulmonary intensive care, pulmonary insufficiency is no longer a significant cause of death in the hospitalized near-drowning patient. After the near-drowning patient is stabilized successfully, the main determinant of morbidity and mortality is the degree of posthypoxic encephalopathy.

16.

Brain Death, Organ Donation, and Withdrawal of Life Support

Donald D. Vernon, Mary Jo Grant, and Nancy A. Setzer

CORROBORATIVE TESTING

The use of corroborative tests to obtain "objective" verification of brain death is controversial and variable and are used most often when there is diagnostic uncertainty or confounding factors such as hypothermia or barbiturate administration (Table 16.1).

Electroencephalography

Isoelectric electroencephalography (EEG) predicts nonsurvival in comatose patients with clinically absent brain stem function. The advantage of

Table 16.1
Corroborative Studies for Brain Death

Electroencephalography
Cerebral angiography
Radionuclide flow studies
Transcranial Doppler studies of carotid artery/middle cerebral artery flow
Contrast-enhanced or xenon computed tomography
Echoencephalography
Contrast-enhanced magnetic resonance imaging
Measurement of cerebral perfusion pressure
Multimodality-evoked potential studies
    Brain stem auditory-evoked responses (i.e., BAER)
    Somatosensory-evoked potentials
    Visual-evoked potentials

EEG is that, as a portable procedure, it is easily and safely performed at the bedside. Limitations to its use include:

- Susceptibility to electrical artifact at the highly sensitive settings necessary to confirm electrocerebral silence
- Cortical (not brain stem) activity is reflected and suppressed in such clinical settings besides brain death as circulatory shock, hypothermia, and particularly drug intoxication. Isolated electrical cortical activity can occur in a patient with clinical brain stem death and no clinical evidence of central nervous system (CNS) function.
- Unreliability in very young and premature infants, showing return of neuronal function and EEG activity after electrocerebral silence

Despite these shortcomings, an isoelectric EEG in the absence of sedative drugs still represents hard evidence of absent cortical function (Fig. 16.1) and remains a useful confirmatory test for brain death.

Cerebral Angiography

Because absent cerebral blood flow is incompatible with neuronal survival, it is considered the best confirmation of brain death. Two mechanisms likely responsible for this absence of perfusion in brain death are massive cerebral edema (i.e., intracranial pressure greater than mean arterial pressure prevents arterial flow) and progressive cerebral vascular endothelial swelling that results in absence of flow.

One of two angiograph patterns is seen in brain death: total absence of intracranial circulation or the cessation of circulation at the level of the circle of Willis. Currently, cerebral angiography is not widely used to confirm brain death because of its inconvenience (i.e., transport to the radiology suite) and the invasive nature of the examination.

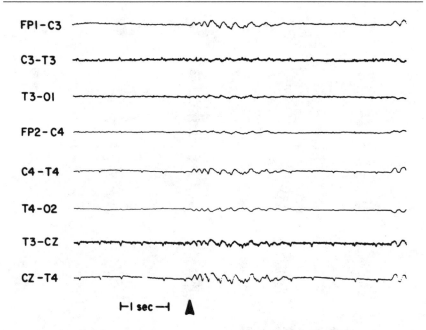

Figure 16.1. Isoelectric electroencephalogram obtained from 9-year-old girl who was brain dead. Solid arrowhead indicates artifact produced by mechanical ventilator. (From Setzer N. Brain death: Physiologic definitions. Crit Care Clin 1985;1:375.)

Radionuclide Flow Studies

Radionuclide flow studies with intravenous 99Tc (Figs. 16.2 and 16.3) are relatively noninvasive, technically easier than four-vessel angiography, and often can be performed in the intensive care unit using a portable scanner. Several studies have correlated absent flow on these scans with brain death as diagnosed by clinical examination and EEG in adults and children, and with absent cerebral flow on four-vessel cerebral angiography.

Most patients show no evidence of cerebral blood flow; others demonstrate late filling of the sagittal sinus only, which is thought to represent venous drainage of extradural perforating arteries. Radionuclide flow studies appear to have limitations, however, at least in infants; persistent cerebral blood flow has been identified in babies clinically brain dead, and values of cerebral blood flow too low to be detected by radionuclide flow studies possibly are consistent with neuronal survival in young infants.

Multimodality Evoked Potential Studies

Evoked potentials measure cerebral electrical responses to a given clinical stimulus (e.g., auditory click, electrical shock, visual pattern). These re-

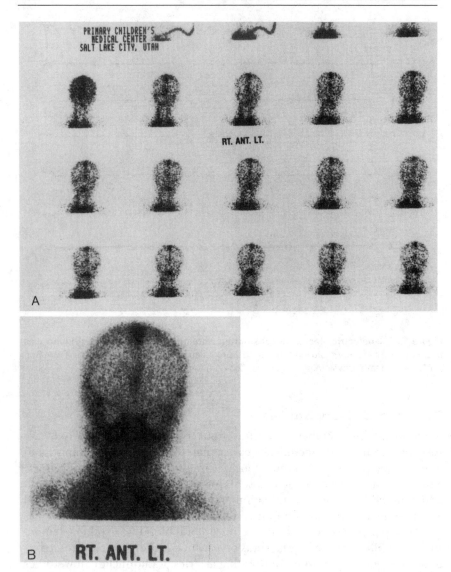

Figure 16.2. A. Dynamic 99Tc scan showing normal cerebral blood flow. Dynamic images were taken at 2-second intervals immediately after radionuclide injection. **B. Static 99Tc scan showing normal cerebral blood flow.** Image was taken 5 minutes after radionuclide injection.

sponses expend extremely small microvoltage amounts and ordinarily are hidden among normal cerebral electrical activity. These reponses may be detected only by repetitive stimulation and measurements, which are computer recorded, summed, and averaged to produce the final wave pattern.

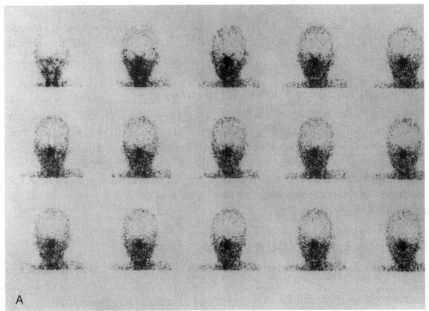

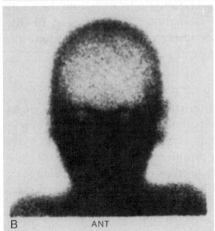

Figure 16.3. A. Dynamic 99Tc scan showing complete absence of cerebral blood flow. Dynamic images were taken at 2-second intervals immediately after radionuclide injection. **B. Static 99Tc scan showing complete absence of cerebral blood flow.** Image was taken 5 minutes after radionuclide injection.

Unlike routine EEG analysis, evoked potentials are not suppressed by sedative anesthetic drugs, including barbiturates, but can only measure activity along specific anatomical pathways and do not represent global cortical or brain stem activity.

The types of clinically used sensory evoked responses (i.e., brain stem auditory, somatosensory, and visual) measure function across different pathways; all of these evoked potentials have been evaluated in the clinical setting of brain death.

Brainstem Auditory Evoked Responses

Physicians evoke brainstem auditory evoked responses (BAER) by using a click stimulus that shows only a wave I (indicating auditory nerve activity) or no waves at all in brain dead individuals (Fig. 16.4A). A totally flat response may also be seen, however, in a patient with auditory nerve failure (as occurs with certain types of deafness and middle ear trauma or fluid). BAER testing is used to confirm absent brain stem function; it is not, by itself, diagnostic of brain death.

Somatosensory Evoked Potentials

Somatosensory evoked potentials show no cortical waves after peripheral nerve electrical stimulus in patients who are brain dead, although a single negative deflection may be detectable over the upper cervical brain with a mean latency of 14 to 15 msec. This wave is thought to arise from the lower medulla or cervical cord near the cervicomedullary junction (Fig. 16.4B). Absent cortical waves may be seen after severe cerebral trauma, however, and are not specific indicators of brain death.

Visual Evoked Potentials

Visual evoked potentials, which measure cortical responses to flashing light stimuli, are uniformly flat in brain dead patients. Flat responses are not specific for brain death, however, because interruption from the retina, optic nerve, or optic radiation pathways may produce a similar pattern.

Evoked potentials are infrequently used as corroborative evidence of brain death, although they are useful in detection of CNS failure during therapeutic drug coma.

Reliability of Test Results

From the discussion, it is clear that no corroborative test is foolproof and that both false-positive and false-negative results may occur. Fackler and Rogers described a clinically brain dead child who had small amounts of both EEG activity and cerebral blood flow observed through angiography (although not on radionuclide scan). Rigid insistence that certain corroborative tests be performed to "prove" brain death in every case inevitably will lead to confusion and anguish, especially for the families of patients.

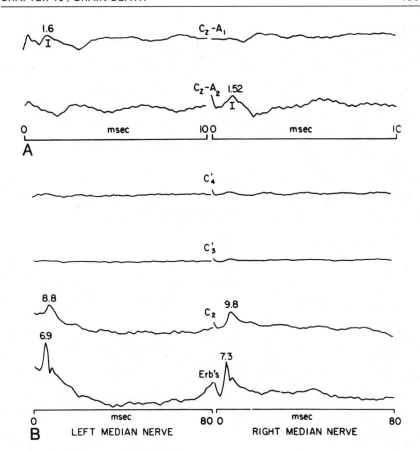

Figure 16.4. A. Brainstem auditory evoked potential tracing obtained in a 2-year-old boy who was brain dead. Note the preservation of wave I only, indicating peripheral auditory nerve activity. **B. Short-latency somatosensory evoked potential after median nerve stimulation in a 2-year-old child with brain death diagnosed.** Electrical activity is recorded over Erb's point (brachial plexus and C2 [cervicomedullary junction]. This latter wave has been identified in the majority of brain-dead adults; here the latency is shorter because of the shorter nerve length in children. There is no cortical activity recorded (C3', C4'). (From Setzer N. Brain death: Physiologic definitions. Crit Care Clin 1985;1:375.)

BRAIN DEATH CRITERIA FOR CHILDREN

Guidelines

In 1987, the Task Force on Brain Death in Children was organized and proffered its *Guidelines for the Determination of Brain Death in Children* (Table 16.2). These guidelines differ from criteria used for adults in several important areas:

Table 16.2

Guidelines for the Determination of Brain Death in Children—Report of the Task Force for the Determination of Brain Death in Children

1. Coma and apnea must coexist
2. Absence of brain stem function:
    Pupils unreactive to light (midposition or dilated)
    Absence of eye movement spontaneously and in response to oculocephalic and
      oculovestibular (caloric) testing
    Absence of corneal, gag, cough, sucking, and rooting reflexes, as well as of
      spontaneous movement of bulbar musculature
    Absence of spontaneous respiratory effort
3. Normal blood pressure and temperature
4. Flaccid muscle tone, absence of spontaneous movements (spinal reflexes acceptable)
5. Examination consistent with brain death throughout the period of testing and
      observation; observation periods and testing are specific for age groups
6. Observation and testing according to age:
    Age 7 days to 2 months:
      Two examinations and EEGs separated by 48 hours
    Age 2 months to 1 year
      Two examinations and EEGs separated by 24 hours, except that repeat examination
      and EEG are unnecessary if radionuclide brain blood flow study demonstrates
      absence of cerebral perfusion
    Older than 1 year:
      Corroborative testing not required if an irreversible cause is identified. An observation
      period of 12 hours is recommended, except that when assessment of extent and
      irreversibility of brain damage is difficult, specifically after hypoxic-ischemic insults,
      an observation period of at least 24 hours is recommended (may be shortened by
      use of EEG or radionuclide flow study).

From Report of special task force. Guidelines for the determination of brain death in children. American Academy of Pediatrics Task Force on Brain Death in Children. Pediatrics 1987;80:298.

EEG, electroencephalogram.

1. They specify that, at least for perinatal insults, 7 days must pass before neurologic assessment is valid (i.e., brain death cannot be diagnosed in infants younger than 7 days).
2. Different criteria are specified for children of different ages.
3. At least for infants, a longer period of observation (i.e., 48 hours) is specified than in other criteria.
4. A specific test (i.e., EEG) is a requirement for the declaration of brain death, at least in the younger age groups.

Although the task force's intent was to clarify the issue of brain death for children, it does not appear to have achieved this goal. The American Academy of Pediatrics, one of the sponsoring bodies of the task force, specifically stated that its official position is not represented by these guidelines. Criticisms of these guidelines include the following:

- Issue of declaration of brain death in premature infants is avoided
- Tests for brain blood flow are considered optional

- Appropriateness of prolonged periods of observation suggested for the youngest infants

These criteria are associated with several respected academic bodies and, as such, may become accepted as standard guidelines despite the lack of evidence or consensus that they are superior to other brain death criteria. Other proposed brain death criteria sets differ in several respects, such as specifying shorter observation periods, placing less reliance on the EEG, and making less of age-related differences.

Studies have shown that the need for special pediatric brain death criteria similar to those used for adults (clinical brain death persistent for 24 hours and one flat EEG) adequately identify brain death in children older than 3 months. In newborns and, especially, premature infants, however, it has been proposed that clinical determination of brain death (i.e., as determined by clinical history and physical examination) can reasonably diagnose brain death in the newborn, with the proviso that observation periods of at least 2 days (for term infants) and 3 days (for preterm infants) are necessary.

Validity and Applicability

Several studies have examined the validity and applicability of brain death criteria in children; a few children have been included along with adults in most of the large prospective studies of brain death criteria. In one retrospective evaluation of children who had absent cortical and brain stem function and an isoelectric EEG, all eventually developed cardiovascular collapse despite aggressive support. Unfortunately, validation of brain death for children may not be as clear-cut as it appears to be for adults, as demonstrated in a report describing a 3-month-old girl who appeared clinically brain dead and had two isoelectric EEG readings but who subsequently regained some cortical and brain stem function and survived on the ventilator for more than a month before dying.

DECLARATION OF BRAIN DEATH

Prerequisites

Brain death can be established only after continuous observation of a comatose patient in a stable environment (i.e., after admission to the intensive care unit), where evaluation can proceed in an orderly fashion. The physician should determine the following prerequisites:

- Cause of coma
- Irreversibility of the lesion
- Patient's medical history and the presence of coexisting disease that might complicate neurologic evaluation

- Possibility of child abuse, if questions regarding the circumstances under which the injury occurred are unresolved. Appropriate authorities are contacted at the time of admission.

Clinical Examination

The physician performs neurologic testing and physical examination when the patient is normothermic (i.e., core temperature of at least 35°C) and hemodynamically stable in the absence of neuromuscular blockade or sedation. Residual blockade (from use of muscle relaxants) can be assessed using a peripheral nerve stimulator, and nondepolarizing agents may be reversible by cholinesterase inhibitors such as edrophonium or neostigmine. These agents should be administered with a vagolytic agent such as atropine or glycopyrrolate to prevent severe bradycardia.

Reflex Testing

The brain dead child should have no spontaneous movements; there should be no purposeful or posturing response to noxious stimuli. Cranial nerve and brain stem function are evaluated by appropriate cephalic reflex testing:

- Pupils should be fixed and dilated, with no response to light
- Pupillary constriction, as part of a iliospinal reflex, should be absent
- Cerebral reflexes, including decorticate and decerebrate posturing, should be absent
- No eye movement with oculocephalic (i.e., doll's eyes) or oculovestibular (i.e., cold caloric) testing
- No pharyngeal reflexes or gagging
- No cough response to tracheal suctioning

Apnea Testing

After preoxygenation with 100% oxygen, mechanical ventilation is discontinued, and oxygen is insufflated passively through the endotracheal tube. The patient then is observed for any respiratory activity for at least 5 minutes. If the physician ensures that the initial $PaCO_2$ is at least 40 torr, then 5 minutes of apnea should yield a $PaCO_2$ of roughly 60 torr, which should elicit at least some ventilatory effort in any patient who is not brain dead. Passive oxygen insufflation is necessary during testing to prevent hypoxemia, and ongoing monitoring of oxygenation should be done. Hemodynamic changes may occur during apnea testing (e.g., hypotension was noted in 39% of 61 comatose individuals during testing despite normoxia).

Spinal Stretch and Deep Tendon Reflexes

At least 50% of brain dead patients exhibit spinal stretch and deep tendon reflexes. Specific spinal reflexes present only in brain dead patients are an ipsilateral flexion withdrawal after noxious stimulation in the L3–L4 dermatome (i.e., 79% of cases) and an ipsilateral extension-pronation response after arm or upper chest stimulation (i.e., 33% of cases). Stereotyped movements of the extremities and extensor posturing seen in patients who are clearly brain dead are termed "the Lazarus sign."

Period of Observation

Once the physician has demonstrated that the clinical examination is consistent with brain death, irreversibility is demonstrated by the persistence of the findings over a 6-hour to 48-hour period of observation. Many centers in the United States require some sort of corroborative test of brain death, most commonly by EEG or radionuclide cerebral blood flow study.

Other Characteristic Findings

Several other findings are characteristic of brain death, although they are not part of the usual diagnostic criteria:

- Diabetes insipidus is common although not universal
- Slowing of metabolism, manifested by low CO_2 production, low glucose requirement, and falling body temperature occurs
- Absence of intracranial blood flow but presence of carotid pulses because of preservation of blood flow through the external carotid system is observed
- Absence of cardiac accelerator response to atropine is noted
- No bradycardia with vagal maneuvers is detected
- Diminished beat-to-beat heart rate variability noted on EEG tracing is indicated
- Incision in brain-dead organ donors elicits a hypertensive response associated with an outpouring of both epinephrine and norepinephrine and increase in systemic vascular resistance
- Absence of cold pressor response to dipping the hand in ice water, which is a central brain stem cardiovascular response

Therapeutic Barbiturate Coma

Pentobarbital blood concentrations greater than 20 to 30 g/dL suppress neurologic function and negate the clinical examination. Barbiturate-induced suppression of electrical activity (electrical silence on EEG is possible and has been described as the therapeutic goal) eliminates the ability of the EEG to evaluate cortical activity. Brain death can be diagnosed during barbiturate coma only with the demonstration of absent intracranial circulation.

BRAIN DEATH AND THE LAW

Brain death is an accepted legal concept in the United States. The general message of most laws and statutes is: brain death is synonymous with death of the person. Furthermore, these laws identify brain death in functional terms (i.e., irreversible cessation of function of the entire brain). They do not require demonstration of anatomic destruction of the brain, define medical criteria by which brain death is determined, or require specific tests. Rather, they specify that brain death has occurred when a physician or physicians have determined that irreversible cessation of function of the entire brain has occurred. Indeed, the variation between brain death laws among states, or even the lack of such laws in a few states, appears to have had little impact on the approach to the diagnosis of brain death across the United States. The selection of criteria by which brain death is declared has thus been left to hospital governing.

BRAIN DEATH AND ORGAN DONATION

Informed Consent

Consent for organ donation may be more readily obtained for the pediatric age group than for adults. In one study series, consent for organ donation was obtained from all families, and the authors attributed this high rate to the empathy that families of brain dead children may have with other families who are awaiting organs for their chronically ill children. Organ donation has also been cited as a factor that helps parents and families with the grieving process.

Maintenance of Organ Donors

Physicians intending to support pediatric organ donors should be prepared to treat the characteristic attending physiologic problems (i.e., coexisting metabolic derangements, hemodynamic disturbances, endocrine abnormalities) for the several hours required to mobilize the surgical team and locate potential transplant recipients. The mean donor maintenance time for pediatric patients is 10.5 ± 6.7 hours. Organ donation should be considered even when high levels of support are necessary for adequate blood pressure and perfusion, because it appears that such care can maintain donor organs in good condition for transplantation.

General Nursing Care

Intensive nursing care measures include:

- Turning the patient to avoid decubitus ulcers
- Maintaining sterility for invasive procedures to decrease the risk of infection
- Lubrication of the patient's eyes
- Frequent airway suction
- Placement of the patient's nasogastric tube on intermittent suction to prevent aspiration of gastric contents

- Insertion of a Foley catheter to measure urine output
- Monitor the patient's body temperature, serum electrolytes, glucose level, hematocrit, and arterial blood gases

Hemodynamic Status

Hemodynamic instability, the most common physiologic derangement noted in pediatric organ donors, results from loss of central neurohumoral regulatory control of vasomotor tone and intravascular volume abnormalities (perhaps related to diabetes insipidus) and myocardial dysfunction related to the original insult. The most important determinant of organ viability is the maintenance of an adequate systemic perfusion pressure; therefore, constant attention to hemodynamic status is essential to preserve donor organ function. The kidneys are especially sensitive to low perfusion levels, and adult studies have demonstrated an increased incidence of acute tubular necrosis and allograft failure when the donor systolic blood pressure is less than 80 to 90 mm Hg.

Invasive monitoring using central venous and arterial catheters is necessary for ongoing assessment. Swan-Ganz catheters may be helpful with this assessment. Suggested therapeutic goals include systolic blood pressure of 70 to 80 mm Hg for patients younger than 6 years, with adolescent parameters similar to those of adult normals.

Initial management should include intravascular volume repletion with isotonic crystalloid or colloid solutions and monitoring of central venous pressure. Catecholamine administration is occasionally necessary to maintain organ perfusion in the organ donor, although adequate intravascular volume must be assured first. Vasoconstriction may compromise organ perfusion, so a vasopressor level with significant α-adrenergic effects, such as epinephrine and norepinephrine, should be used with caution. If additional inotropic treatment is necessary, dobutamine is preferred to isoproterenol because of isoproterenol's potential to increased myocardial oxygen demand.

Cardiac Dysrhythmia

The incidence of bradycardia and asystole is higher in the pediatric than adult population. Significant dysrhythmia affecting blood pressure requires treatment. Transient bradyarrhythmias may be seen in the early phase of brain herniation, but atropine sulfate has no chronotropic effect on the brain dead patient. If the patient's heart is being considered for donation for transplantation into another patient, an electrocardiogram, echocardiogram, and cardiac isoenzyme level may be evaluated to assess function. Hemodynamic support with catecholamines does not limit the viability of the organ for transplantation.

Hypertension

In the early phase of brain herniation, centrally mediated hypertension may occur in association with histologic evidence of microinfarctions in the heart. Adrenergic blocking agents are effective in controlling centrally mediated hypertension and tachycardia. Esmolol hydrochloride or labetalol hydrochloride may be used; because both are short acting and can be administered by an easily titrated continuous infusion.

Pulmonary Insufficiency

The goal of pulmonary support is maintenance of normocarbia and end-organ oxygen supply, achieved in the standard fashion with positive-end expiratory pressure and supplemental oxygen. Hemoglobin oxygen saturation should be maintained higher than 95% if possible. If high positive-end expiratory pressure is used to maintain oxygenation, careful attention must be given to evaluation of cardiac output to ensure organ perfusion. An alveolar-arterial oxygen difference greater than 400 mm Hg may exclude the lung from donation.

Fluid Abnormalities

The patient's maintenance fluid should contain dextrose, though as noted earlier, cerebral metabolism of glucose is nil in the brain dead patient. Potassium and sodium regulation are frequently impaired secondary to free water loss from both diabetes insipidus and diuretics. Ninety percent of brain dead patients develop hypokalemia; however, 39% of these patients also became hyperkalemic in one study.

Hypothermia

Hypothermia, which results from lack of hypothalamic control of body temperature, is found in 53% of pediatric donors. Extreme hypothermia decreases tissue oxygen delivery and predisposes the patient to sepsis by affecting neutrophil function and release. The patient's temperature should be managed with warming blankets, radiant warmers, warmed inspired gases, and intravenous fluids.

Central Diabetes Insipidus

Uncontrolled central diabetes insipidus, noted in 38 to 87% of patients with brain death from trauma or global brain ischemia, leads to massive fluid and electrolyte losses. Treatment can be instituted reasonably when the patient becomes polyuric and his or her serum sodium concentration rises above 150 mEq/L. In the intensive care setting, a continuous intravenous infusion of aqueous vasopressin (0.5 mU/kg/hour to start) is doubled every 30 minutes and titrated to achieve the desired urine output, generally 2 to 4 mU/kg/hour.

Alternative approaches include hormone replacement with desmopressin given intravenously or intranasally, but its long duration of action (i.e., 12 hours) makes it difficult to titrate therapy in the intensive care patient.

Coagulopathy

The donor's hematocrit level is maintained at 25 to 35%. Disseminated intravascular coagulopathy is present in up to 88% of patients with lethal head injuries. Severe coagulopathy should be corrected before organ procurement. Blood products should be administered judiciously to allow pretransplantation serologies to be obtained before transfusions.

Management in the Operating Room

Simply transferring the brain dead patient to the operating room may cause hemodynamic instability. The anesthesia team should anticipate an initial increase in blood pressure and heart rate, as well as a possible reaction of spinal reflexes, after the surgical incision for procurement. The source of this response may be humoral, such as adrenal medullary stimulation by a reflex spinal arc. Hypertension frequently is followed by a significant decrease in systemic vascular resistance. The large incision needed for multiple organ procurement leads to a rapid decline in core temperature in a cold operating room; therefore, the temperature in the operating room should be regulated.

BRAIN DEATH DECLARATION: APPROACH TO THE FAMILY

The first meeting with the family of the brain dead patient usually occurs shortly after admission and includes the family members who accompanied the child to the hospital. In addition to acquiring information about the circumstances of the accident or the patient's previous medical problems, this meeting also should be used to provide information to the family and to begin to support them. All meetings should be unhurried and take place in a quiet room away from the patient's bedside. Communication should involve attending intensive care staff throughout the process; involvement of the social worker is highly desirable.

Definition of Brain Death

Because the public tends to confuse the distinction between patients who are brain dead and those who are permanently vegetative, the physician must clearly and explicitly state that brain death represents the cessation of all CNS function and not just cortical areas governing consciousness, thinking, feeling, and the other functions that make up human behavior. When brain death is determined according to hospital protocol and criteria, death is pronounced, the family is informed, and a death certificate filed.

Discussion of Organ Donation

The family should be approached about organ donation for transplantation only after death has been determined; frequently, they have been discussing this among themselves and may have already reached some decision. In those cases involving accidental death, the medical examiner's or the coroner's office may need to give permission for organ donation. When a death certificate has been filed, the body should be removed from the ventilator or brought to the operating room if organ donation is planned.

Choice to Continue Care

When parents refuse to accept the concept of brain death, family and intensive care staff conferences may be helpful. Should the parents adamantly insist on continued care for their brain dead child, the situation becomes difficult for medical and nursing staff members. Although there is no medical reason to continue supportive care, physicians usually are reluctant to remove supportive care over parental objections.

Special Family Circumstances

Special circumstances exist when brain death is the result of child abuse or homicide. Although usual hospital brain death criteria are applied, early involvement of the hospital or community social services staff may help with family difficulties and in facilitating police, family, and medical communication.

CESSATION OF SUPPORT

Declaration of brain death is not a necessary prerequisite to the discontinuation of supportive care. The major reason for formal brain death declaration is the issue of organ transplantation. In all other cases, there is little reason to subject the parent and the child to the process of brain death determination or to a possibly prolonged period of waiting for brain death to manifest itself.

Motives to Extend Care

The issue of determining the proper limits of medical care for hopelessly ill patients has gained the attention of the general public and the legal profession. Intensive care specialists often are criticized for "doing too much" by continuing to provide high-technology, invasive, and expensive care to patients for whom the prognosis is hopeless.

Factors that might induce physicians in intensive care to "do too much" include "technologic imperative" (i.e., the tendency for a technology to be applied simply because it is available); fear of litigation; diffusion of responsibility among the several specialists often involved with each patient in intensive care—although the intensive care specialist is the logical person to assume the lead in this area; and reticence not only to accept futility and inform the family there is no more to be done, but also to assume the responsibility for making such a weighty decision as the removal of life-support technology with the specific intent of allowing a person to die.

Legal Issues and Risk to Health Care Providers

Confusion about the legal status of decisions to limit or withdraw life-support care for pediatric patients may result from a conflict between federal statutes and state case law. Federal law operant in this area is known as the Federal Child Abuse Amendments, which were specifically written to mandate medical care for even severely handicapped infants, the goal being to prevent discrimination against such children. According to these amendments, decisions concerning withdrawal of support should be largely made by physicians on the basis of perceived prognosis without much influence from the patient's family and other considerations such as quality of life.

Given this situation, then, what is the legal reality for physicians surrounding issues of withdrawal and limitation of life support? Certain celebrated cases might give one pause, however; in California, two physicians involved were indicted for murder after withdrawing support (with consent of the patient's family) from a man in a vegetative state. In truth, however, the legal risk is exceedingly small, and no record exists of any criminal conviction of any physician involved in a withdrawal-of-support decision, including several cases wherein decision making might appear questionable. Generally, the courts have held that the criminal law does not exist to regulate the conduct of physicians attempting to make reasonable decisions.

Deciding to Discontinue Support

When the physician concludes that further care of the patient is futile, the family should be told, with compassion, that their loved one cannot possibly recover and that further aggressive supportive care can be of no benefit to him or her. A decision to discontinue supportive care or to possibly institute do-not-resuscitate status can be made at that time. Decisions are best made in a cooperative fashion between the physician and the family, as well as others involved in the child's care. Current standards call for such a decision to be made largely by the patient's family. The physician, however, must have substantive input into what is fundamentally a medical decision, while at the same time avoiding paternalism.

Steps in Withdrawing Support

Institution of do-not-resuscitate status may be a temporary step while the family considers more active withdrawal of life support or whether they are reluctant to take that course. Cardiopulmonary resuscitation has limited utility in the pediatric intensive care unit.

When a decision is made to withdraw life support, there appears to be wide variation in therapies undertaken, ranging from endotracheal extubation to "terminal weaning," to discontinuation or reduction in dose of catecholamine infusions, to "do not escalate therapy" orders. Mechanical ventilation is the most important and invasive life-support technology, but some families (and physicians) may find its abrupt discontinuation too dramatic and rapid a step.

Role of the Ethics Committee

A withdrawal-of-support decision by itself does not represent an ethical dilemma. Ethics committees should be convened, however, to assist with resolution of conflicts or differences of opinion.

17.

The Critically Ill Child with Human Immunodeficiency Virus Infection

John J. Farley, Robert Englander, Randall L. Tressler, and Peter E. Vink

EPIDEMIOLOGY

Perinatal transmission of human immunodeficiency virus type 1 (HIV-1) from infected mother to infant accounts for 86% of acquired immunodeficiency syndrome (AIDS) cases in children younger than 5 years of age reported through 1994. Transmission of HIV infection through contaminated blood, blood products, and coagulation factors is responsible for most of the remaining cases.

In children with vertically acquired HIV-1 infection, phases of disease progression are observed but are abbreviated compared to HIV-infected adults. Although some children undergo the acute influenza-like illness and primary viremia of HIV-1, many go through a protracted asymptomatic phase that is similar to that seen in adults; however, the length of time is shorter than the estimated 10-year average observed in adults.

DIAGNOSIS OF HUMAN IMMUNODEFICIENCY VIRUS INFECTION

In the pediatric intensive care unit (PICU), the polymerase chain reaction (PCR) test offers the highest sensitivity with the most rapid (i.e., 1 to 2 days) result.

Criteria for definitive diagnosis of HIV infection in children have recently been revised by the Centers for Disease Control and Prevention (Table 17.1). Two positive nonserologic HIV detection tests (e.g., HIV culture, PCR, p24 antigen) are required to make the diagnosis in a child younger than 18 months of age. An infant younger than 18 months of age born to an HIV-infected mother with an AIDS-defining condition (see Table 17.2) meets the criteria without further laboratory testing.

CLINICAL MANIFESTATIONS
Disease Progression

Among infected children perinatally, the earliest clinical findings include:

- Lymphadenopathy
- Hepatosplenomegaly
- Hypergammaglobulinemia
- Skin disease, including candidal dermatitis and/or seborrhea

As the disease progresses, two distinct patterns emerge. Some children develop severe symptomatology in the first year of life, including:

- *Pneumocystis carinii* pneumonia (PCP)
- Symptomatic cytomegalovirus (CMV) infection
- Wasting syndrome
- Encephalopathy

Another group of children have a more indolent course. Clinical problems noted initially include:

- Lymphoid interstitial pneumonitis
- Lymphadenopathy
- Hepatosplenomegaly
- Parotid gland enlargement

Disease progression among children infected by blood transfusion is slower than among those infected perinatally.

Table 17.1
Diagnosis of Human Immunodeficiency Virus (HIV) Infection in Children[a]

Diagnosis: HIV Infected

a) A child <18 months of age who is known to be HIV seropositive or born to an HIV-infected mother **and:**
  - has positive results on two separate determinations (excluding cord blood) from one or more of the following HIV detection tests:
  —HIV culture,
  —HIV polymerase chain reaction,
  —HIV antigen (p24),

or

  - meets criteria for acquired immunodeficiency syndrome (AIDS) diagnosis based on the 1987 AIDS surveillance case definition.

b) A child ≥18 months of age born to an HIV-infected mother or any child infected by blood, blood products, or other known modes of transmission (e.g., sexual contact) who:
  - is HIV-antibody positive by repeatedly reactive enzyme immunoassay (EIA) and confirmatory test (e.g., Western blot or immunofluorescence assay [IFA]);

or

  - meets any of the criteria in a) above.

Diagnosis: Perinatally Exposed (Prefix E)

A child who does not meet the criteria above who:
  - is HIV seropositive by EIA and confirmatory test (e.g., Western blot or IFA) and is <18 months of age at the time of test;

or

  - has unknown antibody status, but was born to a mother known to be infected with HIV.

Diagnosis: Seroreverter (SR)

A child who is born to an HIV-infected mother and who:
  - has been documented as HIV-antibody negative (i.e., two or more negative results of EIA tests performed at 6–18 months of age or one negative result of EIA test after 18 months of age);

and

  - has had no other laboratory evidence of infection (has not had two positive viral detection test results, if performed);

and

  - has not had an AIDS-defining condition.

[a]From Centers for Disease Control. 1994 Revised Classification System for Human Immunodeficiency Virus Infection in Children Less than 13 Years of Age. MMWR 1994;43:RR-12.

Classification System

Using the classification system for HIV infection in children less than 13 years of age that was revised by the Centers for Disease Control and Prevention (CDC) in 1994, clinical categories are based on signs, symptoms, or diagnoses related to HIV infection (Table 17.2). Conditions in category C, and lymphoid interstitial pneumonitis from category B, meet the AIDS surveillance case definition. These clinical categories are then combined with

Table 17.2

Clinical Categories for Children with Human Immunodeficiency Virus Infection (HIV)[a]

Category N: Not Symptomatic

Children who have no signs or symptoms considered to be the result of HIV infection or who have only one of the conditions listed in Category A.

Category A: Mildly Symptomatic

Children with two or more of the conditions listed below but none of the conditions listed in Categories B and C.

- Lymphadenopathy ($\geq$0.5 cm at more than two sites; bilateral = one site)
- Hepatomegaly
- Splenomegaly
- Dermatitis
- Parotitis
- Recurrent or persistent upper respiratory infection, sinusitis, or otitis media

Category B: Moderately Symptomatic

Children who have symptomatic conditions other than those listed for Category A or C that are attributed to HIV infection. Examples of conditions in clinical Category B include but are not limited to:

- Anemia (<8 g/dL), neutropenia (<1000/mm^3), or thrombocytopenia (<100,000/mm^3) persisting $\geq$30 days
- Bacterial meningitis, pneumonia, or sepsis (single episode)
- Candidiasis, oropharyngeal (thrush), persisting (>2 months) in children > 6 months of age
- Cardiomyopathy
- Cytomegalovirus infection, with onset before 1 month of age
- Diarrhea, recurrent or chronic
- Hepatitis
- Herpes simplex virus (HSV) stomatitis, recurrent (more than two episodes within 1 year)
- HSV bronchitis, pneumonitis, or esophagitis with onset before 1 month of age
- Herpes zoster (i.e., shingles) involving at least two distinct episodes or more than one dermatome
- Leiomyosarcoma
- Lymphoid interstitial pneumonia (LIP) or pulmonary lymphoid hyperplasia complex
- Nephropathy
- Nocardiosis
- Persistent fever (lasting > 1 month)
- Toxoplasmosis, onset before 1 month of age
- Varicella, disseminated (complicated chickenpox)

Category C: Severely Symptomatic

Children who have any condition listed in the 1987 surveillance case definition for acquired immunodeficiency syndrome (AIDS), with the exception of LIP (Box 3).

Category C: Severely Symptomatic

Serious bacterial infections, multiple or recurrent (i.e., any combination of at least two culture-confirmed infections within a 2-year period), of the following types: septicemia, pneumonia, meningitis, bone or joint infection, or abscess of an internal organ or body cavity (excluding otitis media, superficial skin or mucosal abscesses, and indwelling catheter-related infections)

- Candidiasis, esophageal or pulmonary (bronchi, trachea, lungs)
- Coccidioidomycosis, disseminated (at site other than or in addition to lungs or cervical or hilar lymph nodes)

continued

Table 17.2
Clinical Categories for Children with Human Immunodeficiency Virus Infection (HIV)[a]

- Cryptococcosis, extrapulmonary
- Cryptosporidiosis or isosporiasis with diarrhea persisting >1 month
- Cytomegalovirus disease with onset of symptoms at age 1 month (at a site other than liver, spleen, or lymph nodes)
- Encephalopathy (at least one of the following progressive findings present for at least 2 months in the absence of a concurrent illness other than HIV infection that could explain the findings): a) failure to attain or loss of developmental milestones or loss of intellectual ability, verified by standard developmental scale or neuropsychological tests; b) impaired brain growth or acquired microcephaly demonstrated by head circumference measurements or brain atrophy demonstrated by computerized tomography or magnetic resonance imaging (serial imaging is required for children <2 years of age); c) acquired symmetric motor deficit manifested by two or more of the following: paresis, pathologic reflexes, ataxia, or gait disturbance
- Herpes simplex virus infection causing a mucocutaneous ulcer that persists for >1 month; or bronchitis, pneumonitis, or esophagitis for any duration affecting a child >1 month of age
- Histoplasmosis, disseminated (at a site other than or in addition to lungs or cervical or hilar lymph nodes)
- Kaposi's sarcoma
- Lymphoma, primary, in brain
- Lymphoma, small, noncleaved cell (Burkitt's), or immunoblastic or large cell lymphoma of B-cell or unknown immunologic phenotype
- *Mycobacterium tuberculosis*, disseminated or extrapulmonary
- *Mycobacterium*, other species or unidentified species, disseminated (at a site other than or in addition to lungs, skin, or cervical or hilar lymph nodes)
- *Mycobacterium avium* complex or *Mycobacterium kansasii*, disseminated (at site other than or in addition to lungs, skin, or cervical or hilar lymph nodes)
- *Pneumocystis carinii* pneumonia
- Progressive multifocal leukoencephalopathy
- Salmonella (nontyphoid) septicemia, recurrent
- Toxoplasmosis of the brain with onset at >1 month of age
- Wasting syndrome in the absence of a concurrent illness other than HIV infection that could explain the following findings: a) persistent weight loss >10% of baseline **OR** b) downward crossing of at least two of the following percentile lines on the weight-for-age chart (e.g., 95th, 75th, 50th, 25th, 5th) in a child ≥1 year of age **OR** c) < 5th percentile on weight-for-height chart on two consecutive measurements, ≥30 days apart **PLUS** a) chronic diarrhea (i.e., at least two loose stools per day for ≥30 days) **OR** b) documented fever (for ≥30 days, intermittent or constant)

[a]From Centers for Disease Control. 1994 Revised Classification System for Human Immunodeficiency Virus Infection in Children Less than 13 Years of Age. MMWR 1994;43:RR–12.

a determined immunologic status (age-specific CD4+ T lymphocyte count or CD4+ percent of total lymphocytes) to form a grid that is then used for the classification (Table 17.3). Children are not reclassified to a less severe category regardless of subsequent CD4+ determinations or resolution of clinical symptomatology.

Table 17.3
Pediatric Human Immunodeficiency Virus (HIV) Classification[a]

	Clinical Categories			
Immunologic Categories	N: No Signs/ Symptoms	A: Mild Signs/ Symptoms	B:[b] Moderate Signs/ Symptoms	C:[b] Severe Signs/ Symptoms
1. No evidence of suppression	N1	A1	B1	C1
2. Evidence of moderate suppression	N2	A2	B2	C2
3. Severe suppression	N3	A3	B3	C3

[a]From Centers for Disease Control. 1994 Revised Classification System for Human Immunodeficiency Virus Infection in Children Less than 13 Years of Age. MMWR 1994;43:RR–12. Children whose HIV infection status is unconfirmed are classified by using the above grid with a letter E (for perinatally exposed) placed before the appropriate classification code (e.g., EN2).

[b]Both Category C and lymphoid interstitial pneumonitis in Category B are reportable to state and local health departments as acquired immunodeficiency syndrome.

Adolescents with HIV infection are classified using the 1993 Revised Classification System for HIV Infection and Expanded Surveillance Case Definition for AIDS Among Adolescents and Adults. A similar grid combining immunologic with clinical categories is used (Table 17.4). With publication of this system, the surveillance case definition for AIDS was broadened to include:

- Mycobacterium tuberculosis infection (any site)
- Recurrent pneumonia
- Invasive cervical cancer
- CD4+ T lymphocyte count less than 200 cells/mL^3 or CD4+ percent less than 14

MEDICAL COMPLICATIONS OF HIV INFECTION
Pulmonary Complications

Pulmonary disease occurs in almost 70% of HIV-infected children, frequently necessitates intensive care for respiratory failure, and often is the cause of death. A wide variety of diseases, both infectious and noninfectious, affect these children (Table 17.5). Some of these infections are truly opportunistic, whereas others also affect normal children.

P. carinii Pneumonia

P. carinii pneumonia is a common opportunistic infection that affects approximately 50% of pediatric AIDS patients and has been the initial HIV-related illness in 72% of children who develop AIDS in the first year of life.

Table 17.4

Classification System for HIV Infection and Expanded AIDS Surveillance Case Definition for Adolescents and Adults[a]

CD4+ T-Cell Categories	Clinical Categories[b]		
	(A) Asymptomatic, Acute (Primary) HIV or PGL[c]	(B) Symptomatic, Not (A) or (C) Conditions	(C) AIDS-Indicator Conditions
1. ≥500/μL	A1	B1	C1
2. 200–499/μL	A2	B2	C2
3. <200/μL AIDS-indicator T-cell count	A3	B3	C3

[a]From Centers for Disease Control. 1993 Revised Classification System for HIV Infection and Expanded Surveillance Case Definition for AIDS Among Adolescents and Adults. MMWR 1992;41:RR–17.

[b]Persons with AIDS-indicator conditions (Category C) and those with CD4+ T-lymphocyte counts <200/μL (Categories A3 or B3) are reportable as AIDS cases in the United States and Territories, effective January 1, 1993.

[c]PGL, persistent generalized lymphadenopathy. Clinical Category A includes acute (primary) HIV infection.

Table 17.5

Pulmonary Diseases in Children with AIDS

Infectious
1. Parasitic
   Pneumocystis carinii, Toxoplasma gondii, Stronglyoides stercoralis
2. Viral
   Respiratory viruses: respiratory syncytial virus, influenza virus, parainfluenza virus, adenovirus
   Measles
   Opportunists: cytomegalovirus, herpes simplex, varicella zoster virus
3. Bacterial
   Streptococcus pneumoniae, Haemophilus influenzae, Staphylococcus aureus
   Nosocomial: enteric bacilli, *Pseudomonas aeruginosa*
   Actinomycetes: *Nocardia* species
   Mycobacterial: *M. tuberculosis, M. avium-intracellulare*
4. Fungal
   Cryptococcus neoformans, Histoplasma capsulatum, Coccidioides immitis, Candida sp., *Asperidillus* sp.
Noninfectious
1. Lymphoid diseases
   Pulmonary lymphoid hyperplasia
   Lymphocytic interstitial pneumonia
   Polyclonal polymorphic B-cell lymphoproliferative disorder
2. Bronchiectasis
3. Kaposi's sarcoma

Clinical Presentation The physiologic disturbance in PCP is characterized by:

- Ventilation-perfusion mismatch
- Decreased pulmonary compliance
- Alveolar capillary block
- Hypoxia
- Elevated alveolar-arterial oxygen gradient

Therefore, patients with PCP usually manifest the tetrad of:

- Nonproductive cough
- Fever
- Dyspnea
- Tachypnea

Diagnosis Although the physician can make a presumptive diagnosis of
PCP on the basis of tachypnea, hypoxia, and diffuse alveolar infiltrates, definitive diagnosis still depends on the demonstration of organisms in pulmonary tissue, respiratory secretions, or lung fluid.

The following methods may be used to obtain appropriate specimens
of pulmonary fluid for definitive diagnosis:

1. Induced sputum technique
2. Deep tracheal suction or tracheobronchial lavage through an endotracheal tube
3. Bronchoalveolar lavage

The induced sputum technique is the least invasive, but broncheolar lavage
is used most widely.

Specimens obtained by these methods are then subjected to cytologic
(e.g., methenamine silver nitrate, toluidine blue O, Giemsa) and microbiologic (e.g., Gram stain and bacterial culture, acid-fast bacilli stain and culture, fungal and viral cultures and rapid tests) studies.

Treatment The treatment of PCP consists of:

- Supportive care
- Antimicrobial therapy
- Coricosteroids
- Oxygen therapy
- Continuous positive airway pressure
- Mechanical ventilation

Trimethoprim-Sulfamethoxazole Trimethoprim-sulfamethoxazole (TMP-
SMX) is recommended for the initial treatment of PCP. It is first administered intravenously (TMP 20 mg/kg/day and SMX 100 mg/kg/day in three
to four equal doses), but the drug may be given orally after clinical improvement has occurred. Therapy should be continued for a total of 21

days. At the completion of therapy, the dosage is reduced and prophylactic use TMP-SMX is continued indefinitely.

Common adverse effects related to TMP-SMX include:

- Cutaneous eruptions
- Bone marrow suppression
- Fever
- Hepatic transaminase elevation

Unless the cutaneous rashes are characteristic of a type 1 hypersensitivity reaction, toxic epidermal necrolysis, or Stevens-Johnson syndrome, therapy should not be discontinued.

Alternate Therapy For patients who cannot tolerate TMP-SMX or do not respond to this therapy, other therapeutic options include the following:

- Pentamidine isethionate (4 mg/kg/day intravenously in a single dose for 21 days), although systemic use of this drug is associated with a wide variety of side effects, including pancreatitis, hypo-glycemia and hyperglycemia, neutropenia, thrombocytopenia, azotemia, and sterile abscesses (i.e., in intramuscular injection).
- Corticosteroids in anti-inflammatory dosages as an adjunct to antimicrobial therapy
- Methylprednisolone (1 mg/kg every 6 hours for 7 days followed by a 1 week taper). Doses as high as 4 mg/kg as initial therapy are in common usage.

Prophylaxis Guidelines for CD4+ T lymphocyte count monitoring and thresholds for primary prophylaxis are outlined in Table 17.6. Because CD4+ T lymphocyte counts lack sensitivity among infants less than 12 months of age, revised guidelines call for administering prophylaxis to all infants less than 12 months of age born to HIV-infected mothers regardless of CD4+ T lymphocyte counts until HIV infection can be excluded reasonably, based on viral diagnostic tests (e.g., culture or PCR). All children with a previous episode of PCP should receive lifelong prophylactic therapy, regardless of CD4+ T lymphocyte measurement.

For prophylaxis, patients should receive 150 mg TMP/750 mg SMX/m^2/day, in two daily doses, 3 days/week on either consecutive or alternate days. Children intolerant of TMP-SMX should receive dapsone, 2 mg/kg/dose once daily (maximum dose 200 mg). Aerosolized pentamidine can be used in older children. Pentamidine may be administered intravenously every 2 to 4 weeks in younger children intolerant of both TMP-SMX and dapsone.

Viral Pneumonia

Common pediatric respiratory pathogens that cause viral pneumonia in children with HIV infection include:

Table 17.6
Recommendations for *Pneumocystis carinii* pneumonia (PCP) Prophylaxis and CD4+ Monitoring for HIV-Exposed Infants and HIV-Infected Children[a]

Age	PCP Prophylaxis	CD4+ Monitoring
Birth to 4–6 weeks	No prophylaxis	1,3,6,9,12 months of age
4–6 weeks to 4 months	Prophylaxis for all	
4–12 months HIV-infected or indeterminate	Prophylaxis for all	
HIV infection reasonably excluded[b]	No prophylaxis	None
1–5 years, HIV-infected	Prophylaxis if CD4+ count <500 or CD4+ percent <15%[c,d]	Every 3–4 months[e]
6–12 years, HIV-infected	Prophylaxis if CD4+ count <200 or CD4+ percent <15%[d]	

[a]From Centers for Disease Control. 1995 revised guidelines for prophylaxis against *Pneumocystis carinii* pneumonia for children infected with or perinatally exposed to human immunodeficiency virus. MMWR 1995;44:RR–4.

[b]≥2 negative HIV diagnostic tests (culture or polymerase chain reaction, both of which are performed at ≥1 month of age and one of which is performed at ≥4 months of age, or ≥2 negative HIV IgG antibody tests performed at >6 months of age in a child who has no clinical evidence for HIV disease.

[c]Children 1–2 years of age who were on PCP prophylaxis and had a CD4+ count 50 or percent <15% in the first year of life should continue on prophylaxis.

[d]Prophylaxis should be considered on a case-by-case basis for children who may otherwise be at risk for PCP, such as children with rapidly declining CD4+ counts or percents or with Category C conditions.

[e]More frequent monitoring (e.g., monthly) is recommended for children whose CD4+ counts or percents are approaching the threshold for prophylaxis.

- Respiratory syncytial virus (RSV)
- Influenzavirus
- Parainfluenza virus
- Rhinoviruses
- Caronaviruses
- Adenovirus

Viral pneumonia may also be a manifestation of disseminated infection with:

- Measles
- Herpes simplex viruses types 1 and 2 (HSV-1, HSV-2)
- CMV
- Varicella zoster virus (VZV)

Viral pneumonia may be superimposed on a patient's respiratory system that already is compromised by lymphocytic interstitial pneumonitis. In addition, children may be coinfected with viruses and *P. carinii* or bacteria.

Bacterial Pneumonia

Bacterial pneumonia in HIV-infected children may progress to respiratory failure. Although bacterial pneumonia usually is considered in the differential diagnosis when lobar consolidation is observed, diffuse and patchy infiltrates also may have a bacterial origin. The most common bacterial causes of pneumonia in children with AIDS are *Streptococcus pneumoniae*, *Haemophilus influenzae*, and *Pseudomonas aeruginosa*.

Mycobacterial Pneumonia

The most important mycobacterial infections to consider in HIV-infected children are those caused by *Mycobacterium tuberculosis* and the *Mycobacterium avium-intracellulare* complex (MAC).

Clinical Manifestations The clinical findings in patients with tuberculosis include:

- Fever
- Weight loss
- Cough
- Hilar lymphadenopathy
- Localized pulmonary infiltrate, diffuse patchy infiltrates, and lobar consolidation

Cavitation, a common finding in adults, is unusual in children.

Symptoms associated with disseminated MAC infection include:

- Fever
- Night sweats
- Malaise
- Weight loss
- Anemia
- Neutropenia

Pneumonia because of MAC infection alone is rare.

Diagnosis Establishing the diagnosis of tuberculosis remains very important. Tuberculin skin testing, along with appropriate controls consisting of two additional antigens (e.g., *Candida*, mumps, tetanus toxoid) should be administered by the Mantoux method to HIV-infected children suspected of having tuberculosis.

Treatment The treatment of tuberculosis in AIDS patients is generally the same as in immunologically normal patients, with the exception that therapy for pulmonary infection should be given for at least 9 months (i.e., as opposed to 6 months), or for 6 months after sputum cultures results are negative. Therapy should consist of isoniazid, rifampin, and pyrazinamide daily for the first 2 months, with only isoniazid and rifampin administered daily from the remainder of therapy. Because of the increased frequency of multidrug-resistant tuberculosis, planned revised guidelines will recommend a four-drug regimen (i.e., isoniazid, rifampin, pyrazinamide, streptomycin or ethambutol) as initial therapy for new cases of tuberculosis until sensitivity is known.

Resistance is particularly problematic in treatment of disseminated MAC infection. Although multiple drug regimens may increase intolerance and toxicity, most experts recommend that treatment of MAC bacteremia should include at least two antimycobacterial agents, one of which should be a macrolide.

Fungal Pneumonia

Although uncommon, pulmonary manifestations of fungal infections occur among HIV-infected children. Meningitis is the most common presentation of cryptococcosis in this population, but pulmonary infiltrates have been noted.

Amphotericin B (0.5 to 1.5 mg/kg every 24 hours) is the treatment of choice for each of these pathogens. Chronic administration of amphotericin B can be complicated by azotemia, hypokalemia, anemia, and weight loss.

Lymphoid Diseases of the Lung

The lungs of approximately 25 to 40% of children who acquire HIV perinatally are affected by lymphocytic infiltrations that form overlapping clinical and pathologic disorders, namely, pulmonary lymphoid hyperplasia (PLH) and lymphocytic interstitial pneumonia (LIP). The interstitial process results primarily in restrictive lung disease with hypoxia and hypocapnia, whereas peribronchial disease may result in obstructive lung disease.

Clinical Manifestations After the first year of life, children PLH and LIP usually demonstrate the following:

- Cough
- Tachypnea
- Wheezing
- Digital clubbing
- Generalized lymphadenopathy
- Hepatosplenomegaly
- Parotid enlargement

Diagnosis The clinical features just described are suggestive of the diagnosis, particularly when supported by radiologic findings of a diffuse reticulonodular pattern, with nodules of 1 to 5 mm in diameter and frequently associated mediastinal lymphadenopathy that persists for several months without evidence of other opportunistic infections.

If clinical deterioration occurs, further diagnostic studies that should be performed include:

- Oxygen saturation monitoring
- Radiographic imaging
- Analysis of respiratory secretions

Lung biopsy may become necessary to obtain specimens for analysis.

Treatment Because there is no known specific therapy, general supportive measures include:

- Attention to nutrition and anemia
- Immunization against respiratory pathogens
- Aggressive management of respiratory infections
- Appropriate monitoring of pulmonary function

In some children, bronchodilators and oxygen may be necessary. Patients with PLH/LIP have symptomatic HIV infection and should receive antiretroviral therapy. The use of systemic corticosteroids such as prednisone (2 mg/kg/day for 4 to 12 weeks with subsequent gradual dose reduction) has been found to be of value.

Cardiac Complications

Children with HIV may be admitted to a PICU with severe life-threatening congestive heart failure or arrhythmias. The etiology of HIV-associated cardiac disease is probably multifactorial, involving HIV; other viral infectious agents (i.e., CMV, Epstein-Barr virus, or coxsackie virus); fungal, bacterial, or protozoan infections; an abnormal host response; and drug toxicity.

Clinical Presentation

Cardiac involvement in HIV-infected children includes:

- Dilated cardiomyopathy
- Myocarditis
- Pericarditis
- Endocarditis
- Arrhythmias
- Conduction disturbances
- Vascular disease

Dilated cardiomyopathy is the most frequent form of heart disease in the HIV-infected child. Early on, such affected children may be asymptomatic clinically, with only echocardiographic evidence of dysfunction. More severe involvement is characterized by cardiomegaly, with ventricular hypertrophy and dilation and poor contractility and signs of overt congestive heart failure.

Diagnosis and Treatment

Echocardiography remains the single most useful diagnostic method with which to assess ventricular function and structure, pericardial disease, and cardiac vascular disease. The electrocardiograph and Holter monitor are used to assess rhythm disturbances.

Congestive heart failure is treated conventionally with inotropic agents (e.g., digoxin, dopamine), diuretics, and afterload reducing agents (e.g., captopril). Class IA antiarrhythmics (i.e., quinidine, procainamide) should be avoided in children with prolonged QTc interval. The therapeutic roles of immunoglobulin treatment, steroids, or micronutrient replacement remain to be clarified.

Renal Complications

Renal disease in HIV-infected patients falls into three categories:

1. Acute renal failure secondary to acute tubular necrosis, related to ischemia from volume depletion and septic shock or to nephrotoxicity complicating therapeutic use of aminoglycosides, acyclovir, pentamidine, or amphotericin B
2. Glomerular disorders referred to as HIV-associated nephropathy
3. Miscellaneous parenchymal lesions, including drug-related interstitial nephritis and an uncommon form of HIV-associated hemolytic uremic syndrome

Routine screening of HIV-infected children by urinalysis, creatinine levels, and blood urea nitrogen screens facilitates early identification and may result in reduced morbidity from renal disease. A urinalysis positive for blood and/or protein suggests glomerulonephropathy and warrants further investigation.

General aspects of treatment of nephrotic syndrome, nephritis, hypertension, electrolyte abnormalities, and renal failure are outlined elsewhere.

Hematologic Complications
ANEMIA

Anemia is the most common hematologic disorder observed in HIV-infected children. Contributing factors include:

- HIV-induced bone marrow suppression
- Iron deficiency from enteric blood loss and poor nutrition
- Reduced endogenous erythropoietin
- Coombs-positive autoimmune hemolysis
- Zidovudine therapy

In addition to iron replacement therapy when indicated, treatment of chronic anemia may include erythropoietin (150 U/kg given subcutaneously 3 days/week).

Neutropenia and Thrombocytopenia

Neutropenia, defined as an absolute neutrophil count (ANC) less than 1500 cells/mm^3, has been reported in 43% of previously untreated children with HIV infection. Thrombocytopenia, when severe, may produce a bleeding diathesis.

Neurologic Complications

Cryptococcal Meningitis

The organism *Cryptococcus neoformans* enters the body through the lungs and spreads hematogenously to cause disseminated or focal infections, the most common of which is meningitis. Cryptococcal meningitis may develop insidiously. The diagnosis is confirmed by:

- Cerebrospinal fluid features of chronic meningitis
- Observation of organisms with an India ink stain
- Presence of cryptococcal antigen
- Positive culture result

Initial treatment involves amphotericin B (0.5 to 1.0 mg/kg/day for 6 to 8 weeks), with or without flucytosine (50 to 150 mg/kg/day in four divided doses).

Toxoplasmosis

Most cases of congenital toxoplasmosis that occur in infants born to mothers infected with both *Toxoplasma* and HIV are not evident at birth. Symptoms that develop in the first few months of life include:

- Chorioretinitis
- Cerebritis with intraparenchymal calcifications
- Pneumonitis
- Myocarditis
- Lymphadenopathy
- Hepatosplenomegaly

Diagnosis is based on symptomatology with supportive serologic testing. The standard regimen for treatment is pyrimethamine (15 mg/m^2/day) in double doses for the first 2 days, sulfadiazine (85 mg/kg/day) two to four times daily, and folinic acid (5 mg) every 3 days. These patients should continue the treatment regimen indefinitely because of the high frequency of relapse.

Gastrointestinal Complications

Malnutrition

Nearly 95% of all HIV-infected children will develop malnutrition before death. Factors that contribute to the malnutrition associated with pediatric HIV/AIDS include:

- Inadequate caloric intake
- Maldigestion
- Malabsorption and subsequent diarrhea
- Increased nutrient requirements

Standard pathogens should be ruled out. *Cryptosporidium* should be considered in cases of large volume secretory diarrhea that is associated with malabsorption, anorexia, and weight loss. *Mycobacterium avium-intracellulare* should be considered in cases of diarrhea, weight loss, and recurrent fevers.

Esophageal Candidiasis

Esophageal candidiasis is a diagnostic indicator disease for AIDS. Dissemination of disease is rare. Treatment options include ketoconazole (5 to 10 mg/kg/day orally in one or two doses), fluconazole (3 to 6 mg/kg/day orally), or amphotericin B intravenously.

Pancreatitis

HIV-infected children frequently manifest symptoms consistent with pancreatitis, accompanied by elevation of amylase and lipase levels. Pancreatitis in these patients may be caused by:

- Dideoxyinosine (ddI), developing as long as 8 months after starting therapy
- Pentamidine, which can cause fatal acute pancreatitis
- Trimethoprim-sulfamethoxazole
- Dapsone
- CMV
- Mycobacteria

Abnormal Hepatobiliary Function

Although hepatic dysfunction is not a common manifestation of HIV disease, many factors contribute to hepatocellular injury or cholestasis in HIV-infected children:

- Sulfonamides (mixed hepatocellular-cholestatic reaction)
- Zidovudine (cholestasis)
- Amphotericin B (mild hepatitis)
- Ketoconazole (mild hepatitis)

- ddI (mild hepatitis)
- Hepatitis A, B, and C
- Mycobacterium avium-intracellulare
- CMV
- Cryptosporidium
- Pneumocystis carinii
- Toxoplasmosis
- Histoplasmosis

Bacteremia

Bacterial infections are a significant cause of morbidity among HIV-infected children. In two studies of infections in children with AIDS, bacteremia occurred in 24 and 46%, respectively, caused by *S. pneumoniae, H. influenzae, Staphylococcus aureus,* and *Salmonella* species.

After the health care provider has obtained appropriate cultures from a patient with suspected bacteremia, meningitis, or bacterial pneumonia, antimicrobial therapy should be instituted. In the absence of a focus of infection or material for Gram's stain, antimicrobial therapy should be directed at *S. pneumoniae, H. influenzae,* and *Salmonella* species.

The most suitable agents are third-generation cephalosporins (i.e., cefotaxime, ceftriaxone). If an organism has been cultured and its antimicrobial susceptibilities have been determined, narrower spectrum antimicrobial therapy should be used to reduce the likelihood of the child developing a superinfection, particularly with *Candida* species.

ANTIRETROVIRAL THERAPY

Therapeutic options for antiretroviral therapy are outlined in Table 17.7. ZDV is available commercially as a syrup. Dosing every 6 hours is recommended.

The development of resistant virus through mutations in the reverse transcriptase gene is an increasing problem and has been associated with

Table 17.7
Currently Approved Antiretroviral Agents

	Dose	Side Effects
Zidovudine	180 mg/m²/dose every 6 h	Anemia, neutropenia, nausea, headache, liver function elevation, myositis
Didanosine BSA m²		
1.1–1.4	100 mg every 12 h	Pancreatitis, peripheral
0.8–1.0	75 mg every 12 h	Neuropathy, retinal
0.5–0.7	50 mg every 12 h	Depigmentation
≤0.4	25 mg every 12 hr	

Table 17.8
Universal Precautions[a]

1. Use appropriate barrier precautions to prevent skin and mucous membrane exposure to blood and body fluid:
   Use gloves for venipuncture or any vascular procedure.
   Use gowns, masks, and protective eyewear for procedures that may produce droplets of blood or secretions (i.e. endotracheal suctioning, transfer of blood from syringes to vacuum tubes).
2. Strict handwashing should be employed after gloves are removed or after inadvertent exposure to body fluids.
3. Do not recap, bend, or manipulate needles in any way after use. All disposable sharp items should be discarded in a conveniently located, puncture-proof container.

[a]From Centers for Disease Control. Recommendations for prevention of HIV transmission in health care settings. MMWR 1988;361(suppl 2):229.

poor clinical outcome. Clinical trials of new agents and combination therapies are ongoing.

HUMAN IMMUNODEFICIENCY VIRUS TRANSMISSION PRECAUTIONS IN THE PEDIATRIC INTENSIVE CARE UNIT

HIV has been detected in many body fluids:

- Blood
- Semen
- Vaginal secretions
- Urine
- Tears
- Cerebrospinal fluid
- Pleural fluid
- Pericardial
- Synovial fluid
- Breast milk

Epidemiologic evidence suggests, however, that blood is the single most infectious medium for HIV in the medical setting.

In 1987, the CDC recommended that all patients should be treated as potentially contagious for bloodborne pathogens, and proposed that blood and body fluid precautions be adopted for all patients regardless of HIV antibody status. These precautions are presented in Table 17.8.

18.

Overwhelming Sepsis

Joshua P. Needleman and Alice D. Ackerman

INTRODUCTION

This chapter highlights diseases of infectious nature that may have such severe expression as to require admission of the patient to a critical care area.
For the most part, these disorders carry a high risk of mortality if unrecog-
nized and untreated. They are illnesses that also tend to result in an unfavorable outcome even when specific antimicrobial therapy is administered
appropriately.

APPROACH TO LIFE-THREATENING INFECTIONS

Treatment of the life-threatening aspects of any disease process must always
take precedence over specific therapy aimed at the underlying illness. The
responsibility of making an etiologic diagnosis and instituting specific therapy must follow or be concurrent with establishment of an adequate airway,
gas exchange, and cardiac output, for these are the processes that potentially will save the patient's life.

Choice of Antibiotics

The initial antibiotics chosen for the treatment of overwhelming sepsis are
dictated by the likely offending organism. This, in turn, depends primarily
on (a) the patient's age, (b) the coexistence of any premorbid condition
leading to impaired immune defenses, and (c) the presenting signs and
symptoms. The initial antibiotic regimens outlined in this section reflect the
authors' preferences and cannot be applied to all situations. Local patterns
of antibiotic resistance by common infecting organisms also must be considered. In all cases, however, the overriding objective is to use the antibiotic or antibiotic combination most likely to eradicate the infection while
minimizing the risks of superinfection or emergence of resistant organisms.
Finally, these recommendations assume that after the first dose of antibiotic, the child will be further assessed, renal or hepatic impairment may be
noted, and the advice of infectious disease consultants will be sought. Thus,
the ongoing therapy may differ from that recommended here. Nonetheless,
what follows represents a reasonable starting point.

Neonates

During the first 7 days of life, the common offending organisms are:

- Group B streptococcus (GBS)
- *Escherichia coli*
- *Listeria monocytogenes*
- *Staphylococcus aureus*
- *Streptococcus epidermidis*
- Herpes simplex virus (HSV)

Recommendations for initial therapy in neonates younger than 7 days of age are outlined in (Table 18.1). Cefotaxime cannot be used as a single agent in this age group; its use with an aminoglycoside is recommended.

In the normal, full-term infant with no prior illness, the possibilities include late-onset GBS disease and *L. monocytogenes,* and therapy with ampicillin, gentamicin, and cefotaxime or ceftriaxone are appropriate (Table 18.2). If the baby has been in the intensive care unit, the likely infecting organisms include:

- *S. aureus* or *S. epidermidis* infections (presence of central lines)
- *Pseudomonas aeruginosa* (endotracheal intubation)

Table 18.1
Initial Antibiotics for Sepsis in Neonates Who Are Younger than 7 Days of Age

Focus	Antibiotics	Dose
Irrelevant at this age	Ampicillin	100 mg/kg/d divided q 12 h
	Gentamicin or tobramycin	2.5 mg/kg/dose administered q 12–24 h depending on gestational age
	Cefotaxime	100 mg/kg/d divided q 12 h
	Acyclovir[a]	30 mg/kg/d divided q 8 h

[a]Only to be used if herpes simplex virus infection is suspected, see text.

Table 18.2
Initial Antibiotics for Sepsis in Neonates Who Are Older than 7 Days of Age

Focus	Antibiotics	Dose
None, respiratory or central nervous system in previously healthy baby	Ampicillin and one of the following:	200 mg/kg/d divided q 8–12 h
	Gentamicin	2.5 mg/kg/dose administered q 8–18 h depending on gestational age and renal function (follow levels)
	or	
	Ceftriaxone	100 mg/kg load, then 100 mg/kg/d divided q 12 h
	or	
	Cefotaxime	100 mg/kg/d divided q 12 h
None, respiratory or central nervous system in baby with central line	Add vancomycin to above	10–15 mg/kg/dose administered q 8–18 h (follow levels)
As above, but with endotracheal tube	Consider Ticarcillin/ Clavulanate	300 mg/kg/d divided q 8 h
Suspected necrotizing enterocolitis	Add Metronidazole	15 mg/kg load, then 7.5 mg/kg/dose administered q 8 h
	or	
	Clindamycin	15–40 mg/kg/d divided q 6–8 h

- Fungal superinfections (previous treatment with broad-spectrum antibiotics)
- Anaerobic and aerobic enteric organisms (risk factors for necrotizing enterocolitis)

Older Children

Major factors determining which organisms are responsible for a particular
infection beyond the first month of life are the focus of that infection and
the presence or absence of a premorbid condition, such as malignancy, or
prolonged intravascular catheterization. The antibiotic regimen we use to
treat the previously healthy child is outlined in Table 18.3.

The empiric management of the child with sepsis and malignant disease
depends on the degree of neutropenia. If the neutrophil count exceeds
$1000/\mu L$, then the child may be managed as outlined in Table 18.3. If the
count is under $1000/\mu L$, then broad-spectrum therapy with a combination
such as vancomycin, ticarcillin clavulonate, and amikacin or ceftazidime
and amikacin are initiated. Conditions other than malignancy may prompt
the physician to initiate a broader spectrum of antibiotics for overwhelming
sepsis while awaiting culture results (Table 18.4).

Table 18.3
Initial Antibiotics for Sepsis in Previously Healthy Children

Focus	Antibiotic	Dose
None, respiratory, or urinary tract infection	Ceftriaxone or Cefotaxime	100 mg/kg load, then 100 mg/kg/d divided q 12 h
Central nervous system	Add Vancomycin	15 mg/kg dose q 8–18 h (follow levels)
Genitourinary or gastrointestinal	Add metronidazole to the above regimen	15 mg/kg load, then 7.5 mg/kg/dose administered 6 h (max 4 g/d)

Table 18.4
Initial Antibiotics for Sepsis in Previously Ill Children

Focus	Antibiotics	Dose
None, in an immunocompromised host	Ceftazadime or Ticarcillin/Clavulanate and Gentamicin or Amikacin and Nafcillin	150 mg/kg/d divided q 8 h 300 mg/kg divided q 4–6 h 2.5 mg/kg/dose q 8 h 15 mg/kg/d divided q 8 h 150–200 mg/kg/d divided q 4–6 h
None, but with a central line	Same as in Table 18.3, but add Nafcillin or vancomycin	

Nosocomial Infection

In the presence of a nosocomial infection, therapy is broadened to cover *Pseudomonas* or other organisms recently identified as colonizing either the child in question or other children in the unit. This approach usually leads us to a combination of either ticarcillin/lavulonate or Ceftazidime with an aminoglycoside and nafcillin or vancomycin, depending on the likelihood of catheter sepsis. Ceftazidime alone should be avoided because the likelihood of resistant organisms developing is high.

Resistant Organisms

If the child receiving this broad-spectrum regimen is deteriorating or the organism is resistant to the usual broad spectrum antibiotics, other expanded spectrum antibiotics may be useful. The imipenem-cilastatin combination is effective against Gram-negative rods including *Enterobacter* and *Klebsiella* species and *P. aeruginosa,* in addition to various Gram-positive organisms and some anaerobes like *Bacteroides.* We reserve its use for patients who have developed sepsis while being treated with broad-spectrum antibiotics or who are unresponsive to the usual broad-spectrum regimen. In patients being treated with such broad-spectrum antibiotics, it is important to maintain vigilance for superinfection with resistant organisms, the health care provider must culture all sites frequently and be acutely alert for fungal superinfection, which can prove disastrous.

OVERWHELMING SEPSIS

Neonate

The pediatric intensive care specialist must be attuned to presenting signs and symptoms and to the likely infectious agents in premature and full-term infants. It is also necessary to recognize the spectrum of nosocomial illnesses seen in the neonatal intensive care unit (NICU). Babies colonized with multiple-resistant Gram-negative organisms in the NICU may excrete them for up to a year after discharge from the NICU.

Clinical Presentation

The symptoms and signs of sepsis in the neonate are nonspecific, because the newborn possesses few means through which to manifest illness. The primary signs are:

- Respiratory distress
- Apnea
- Abdominal distention
- Vomiting
- Diarrhea

- Jaundice
- Loss of tone
- Lethargy
- Seizures
- Abnormal body temperature (fever or hypothermia)

Specific skin lesions, such as petechiae or pustules, may be present, but mottling as a result of decreased perfusion and changes in both cardiac output and peripheral vascular resistance are more common. The presentation of these signs may be subtle or fulminant. Fulminant signs usually indicate that an infectious disease is a diagnostic possibility. When only one or two of the signs are present, and the baby looks well, it is possible to overlook a potentially fatal microbiologic disease.

Laboratory Tests Numerous attempts to refine diagnostic evaluation of sick neonates have employed a variety of specific laboratory tests. Although a markedly elevated white blood count (WBC) or an increased ratio of band forms to more mature neutrophils may be helpful in diagnosing bacterial disease, it is the septic babies with normal or low leukocyte counts who have the poorest outcomes, presumably because of a limited bone marrow reserve. A normal WBC is not necessarily reassuring therefore.

An elevated erythrocyte sedimentation rate or C-reactive protein is nonspecific and also relatively insensitive. A platelet count of less than 80,000 and findings of toxic granulations within polymorphonuclear leukocytes also provide indirect, suggestive evidence of infection. A large number of WBCs and bacteria in the gastric aspirate may be indicative of amnionitis, and examination of the Gram's stain may provide a clue to the predominant organism, but these findings do not differentiate the bacteremic newborn from one without systemic infection.

Lack of Diagnostic Criteria In short, there are no hard and fast diagnostic criteria of sepsis in the neonate; therefore, the practitioner must depend on a high level of suspicion and proceed to make a specific etiologic determination by obtaining samples of blood, urine, and spinal fluid for culture. The availability of rapid bacterial diagnostic testing such as latex agglutination or countercurrent immune electrophoresis has made this process somewhat easier and less time-consuming. One to 10 babies of every 1000 live births will acquire a bacterial infection, and 20 to 75% of those infected will die or have long-term neurologic damage; therefore, good neonatal medical practice will likely entail a fair amount of overtreatment.

Stages of Disease Onset Neonatal sepsis has been classified into two categories, depending on whether presentation occurs during or after the first week of life.

Early-Onset Sepsis Early-onset disease most commonly presents as a fulminant process in the first 24 hours of life and is related to maternal risk factors, such as prolonged rupture of membranes, premature labor, chorioamnionitis, and occurrence of maternal fever in the immediate post-partum period. Organisms implicated in early-onset sepsis generally are related to contaminants of the maternal birth canal. It has a high mortality rate ($\geq 50\%$) and is frequently associated with pneumonia.

Late-Onset Sepsis Late-onset disease that is of community origin (not nosocomial) does not correlate with maternal risk factors. The baby usually is infected with organisms that colonize the mother. Later onset of sepsis generally carries a lower risk of mortality, ranging from 10 to 20%, although a higher percentage of these babies have associated meningitis. Premature babies who remain hospitalized beyond the first week of life are at high risk to develop nosocomial infections.

Common Pathogens Group B streptococci and *E. coli* are the most common perinatal infections, whereas *S. epidermidis* and *S. aureus* are the most common nosocomial pathogens. *S. epidermidis* is the most commonly implicated organism in neonatal indwelling catheter colonization. *Pseudomonas*, other Gram-negative rods, and *Candida* also account for a significant number of episodes of nosocomial neonatal sepsis.

Reports of outbreaks of other organisms, such as *H. parainfluenzae, L. monocytogenes,* and *Flavobacterium meningosepticum,* are a reminder that statistical information cannot replace information regarding local patterns of microbiologic disease. HSV is an important cause of neonatal sepsis syndrome. Immune compromise should be considered in the baby who fails to respond to appropriate therapy for the most common pathogens, an unusual organism, or a new pattern of antimicrobial resistance.

Group B β-Hemolytic Streptococci

Early-Onset Disease

Clinical Occurrence Neonates who develop GBS in the first several days of life most often have a fulminant acute course, characterized by apnea, respiratory distress, hypotension, poor perfusion, and other nonspecific signs of neonatal illness (Table 18.5). GBS primarily is a disease of premature babies of less than 35 weeks gestation and weighing less than 2500 g at birth. Other risk factors include:

- Young maternal age
- Maternal rupture of membranes of longer than 12 hours
- Intrapartum fever
- Prematurity
- Urinary tract infection during pregnancy
- Twin gestation
- Low Apgar scores at 1 and 5 minutes

Persistent antepartum tachycardia is an additional independent predictor of neonatal GBS sepsis. Other factors that correlate with development of disease

Table 18.5
Early-onset Group B Streptococcus

	Clinical Characteristics
Age at onset	Less than 7 days; majority first 48 h
Presentation	Apnea usually
Clinical appearance	Severely ill
	Cardiovascular collapse
	Persistent fetal circulation
	Persistent apnea
	Lung disease indistinguishable from RDS
	Low birth weight (<2500 g)
	Low Apgar scores
Associated maternal obstetrical complications	Maternal fever
	Premature labor (≤35 weeks)
	Ruptured membranes >12 h
	Twin gestation
Mortality	Approximately 50%

RDS, respiratory distress syndrome.

include heavy colonization of infants (i.e., growth of GBS from at least three separate surveillance sites, such as auditory canal, umbilicus, nose or throat, and anus) at or shortly after birth, and finding Gram-positive cocci on a stained smear of gastric aspirate.

Predicting Outcome A scoring system to predict short-term outcome in early-onset disease is presented in Table 18.6. Scores are calculated by adding the products of each of the six variables and their respective weighting coefficients.

Progression of Disease Nearly 30% of infants with early-onset GBS develop meningitis, of whom another 30% are reported to have seizures. Further, in some cases, GBS organisms have been documented in the meningeal space on autopsy, when the patients had normal cerebrospinal fluid during life; this is particularly true of the babies with overwhelming infection that occurs immediately after birth.

Therapeutic Measures Most babies with early-onset GBS require intensive therapy, especially premature infants and those in the high-risk, poor prognostic group. Specifically:

- Ventilatory assistance and supplementary oxygen for hypoxemia or apnea unresponsive to stimulation
- Fluid administration or pressor agents for hypotension
- Usual intensive care approach to postischemic infants for babies with low 5-minute Apgar scores
- Platelets, fresh frozen plasma, or cryoprecipitate for thrombocytopenia accompanied by frank disseminated intravascular coagulation (DIC) and clinical evidence of bleeding

Table 18.6

Discriminant Analysis: Weighting Coefficients and Relative Discriminating Power for Early-Onset Gram B Streptococcus Disease[a]

Variables	Weighting Coefficient	Relative Discriminating Power	Code
Gestational age	1.64	1.0	Weeks
Presence of shock	−10.82	0.93	Yes = 1: no = 0
WBC count	5.37	0.87	≥6000 = 2
			5999 to 3000 = 1
			≤3000 = 0
ROM (>12 h)	−8.34	0.77	Yes = 1; No = 0
Delayed treatment (>12 h)	−8.30	0.71	Yes = 1; No = 0
5-min Apgar score	1.66	0.67	Same

[a]From Lannering B, Larson LE, Rojas J, Stahlman MT. Early onset group B streptococcal disease: seven year experience and clinical scoring system. Acta Paediatr Scand 1983;72:597.

WBC, white blood cell; ROM, rupture of membranes.

Late-Onset Disease The incidence of late-onset GBS ranges from 0.2 to 1.5 /1000 live births. For those babies who develop disease, there is no strong correlation between maternal colonization or perinatal complications. Premature infants who develop late-onset disease generally have been home, eating, gaining weight, and developing nicely when they become ill. The onset is less fulminant, mortality is lower (6 to 20%), and, when death occurs, it does so later in the hospital course (50 hours versus 15 hours) than with early-onset GBS. Approximately 75% of neonates with late-onset disease develop purulent meningitis, and most infants have high cerebrospinal fluid protein (200 mg/dL), low glucose, and elevated white blood cells.

Predicting Outcome Factors predictive of poor prognosis (death or severe neurologic morbidity) include:

- Presence of coma at hospital admission
- Absolute neutropenia (less than $1000/mL^3$)
- Cerebrospinal fluid protein greater than 300 mg/100 mL
- Poor peripheral perfusion

The variables generally contributing to poor outcome in meningitis are discussed in Chapter 19.

Diagnosis The physical signs or symptoms of GBS sepsis are nonspecific, and routine laboratory tests are not helpful when trying to differentiate GBS from other causes of overwhelming sepsis in the neonate or infant. The differential diagnosis of the 10- to 14-day old baby who presents in shock with metabolic acidosis also includes noninfectious entities, such as coarctation of the aorta. If femoral pulses are absent or diminished, the infant should be treated with a continuous prostaglandin infusion, in addition to antimicrobial agents, until a definitive diagnosis is made.

Although the gold standard of diagnosis remains isolation of bacteria in culture, rapid diagnostic methods for differentiating the predominant neonatal organisms has aided clinical judgment. The sensitivity of latex agglutination to test for GBS antigen in concentrated urine samples approaches 100% in bacteremic patients and ranges from 67 to 88% in patients with negative blood and cerebrospinal fluid cultures but clinical evidence of GBS disease. Measurements of sensitivity range from 67 to 88%. Specificity of the test has been measured at 93%. Typing of the GBS organisms provides important epidemiologic information.

Therapy Although once thought to be universally sensitive to penicillin, GBS is more difficult to treat than initially appreciated. Several factors regulate the relative sensitivity of the microorganism to penicillin in the living host. The most important is probably the individual's organism load. Others include determination of the minimal inhibitory concentration (MIC) of the antibiotic of interest against the particular strain of microorganism, and the development of penicillin-tolerant strains of GBS.

Initial Antibiotic Therapy The combination of ampicillin and an aminoglycoside is effective against the majority of organisms encountered in the first month of life. Some evidence suggests that the ampicillin/gentamicin combination has a synergistic killing effect against the GBS organism. The use of ampicillin and either cefotaxime or ceftriaxone probably is appropriate, although the killing time of GBS is slightly delayed when the combination is used in vivo. The addition of chloramphenicol to ampicillin has been shown to be antagonistic because of the bacteriostatic effects of the former drug.

Adjunctive Measures Adjunctive measures may be useful for the critically ill neonate who is experiencing shock and is at risk for dying within the first several hours of hospitalization. These approaches have been devised because of the relative inability of the neonate's immune system to handle GBS.

Granulocyte transfusions are associated with an apparent improvement in short-term outcome. A similar response has been noted after double-volume exchange transfusions with whole blood collected less than 24 hours previously. This procedure is thought to provide complement, antibody, and other plasma components in addition to white blood cells. Simple blood transfusion has also been associated with improved survival. Granulocyte colony-stimulating factor, granulocyte-macrophage colony-stimulating factor, intravenous immunoglobulin, hyperimmune globulin, and human anti-GBS monoclonal antibody all have been evaluated in the therapy of this disease. Because most babies with GBS are born to mothers who do not possess an antibody against the infecting strain, and opsonization is essential in the killing of encapsulated bacteria, including GBS, passive immunization techniques have a great potential to change the outcome of this often catastrophic neonatal infection.

Protective measures, such as active or passive immunization of pregnant women or chemoprophylaxis of colonized mothers and/or babies, holds some promise, but will probably not be as effective as the combination of aggressive antimicrobial and adjunctive therapy of the infected neonate.

L. Monocytogenes

The bacterium *L. monocytogenes* is a facultative anaerobic Gram-positive rod. Populations at risk for infection with this bacterium include:

- Neonates
- Pregnant women
- The elderly
- Immune-compromised hosts
- Patients with reticuloendothelial malignancies
- Individuals receiving exogenous corticosteroids

Adults *Listeria* infection in previously healthy adults has been reported. Disease in adults typically manifests as meningitis, often with associated sepsis. Mortality worsens with advancing age and debilitated preinfection status.

Neonates *Listeria* infection in neonates has a bimodal presentation similar to that of GBS. Most disease appears to be sporadic, with occasional outbreaks and epidemics. Many cases of so-called early-onset disease may actually represent congenital infection with the offending organism.

Early-onset Listerial Sepsis Early-onset disease generally occurs within the first 3 days of life. Babies, often born prematurely, manifest such signs as respiratory distress, fever, and a pustular and petechial rash. Laboratory findings in neonates with early-onset disease have not been reported consistently. An associated anemia is found in 60% of patients and leukopenia in 20%, but the WBC is elevated in 50% of affected newborns.

Symptoms in mothers of affected infants include such consitutional signs as fever, headache, abdominal pain, myalgias, and diarrhea.

Babies with respiratory symptoms generally have chest radiographic findings of patchy areas of pulmonic consolidation. It has been suggested that listerial pneumonitis may be caused by aspiration in utero of infected amniotic fluid.

Late-Onset Listerial Sepsis Less common than early-onset listerial sepsis, late-onset disease occurs primarily in healthy full-term babies, is associated with meningeal infection, has a better prognosis, and is more often caused by type 4b. Mean age at onset is 1 to 2 weeks, with almost all cases occurring by 30 days of age.

Mothers of affected babies are generally asymptomatic, although other family members may have a mild febrile illness. The mechanism of infection appears to be through fecal-oral spread. Long-term sequelae, although infrequent, include postmeningitic hydrocephalus.

There are no specific clinical or laboratory findings that separate neonatal listerial meningitis from that caused by GBS, *E. coli,* or other pathogens. Only a small proportion of patients have a mononuclear predominance of cells in the cerebrospinal fluid at presentation, although this probably changes with duration of infection, and babies may or may not have organisms demonstrable on Gram's stain of the fluid. Other manifestations of disease include: bacteremia, pneumonitis, otitis media, and oculoglandular infection with purulent conjunctivitis. Rash is not a prominent finding in late neonatal infections; likewise, hepatosplenomegaly and evidence of miliary disease are usually lacking.

Therapy and Prevention Antimicrobial therapy for the mother at the onset of febrile illness is effective in preventing overt disease in the neonate or in significantly limiting its severity. Postnatal treatment of the severely affected neonate may not be effective, because disease is generally widespread with disseminated granuloma formation (i.e., granulomatosis infantisepticum) at the time of delivery. As described previously, a number of those infected in utero are stillborn.

Recommended Agents Ampicillin is the first drug of choice for most listerial infections. Most experts recommend initial therapy with the gentamicin and ampicillin for 10 to 14 days, followed by another 7 days of ampicillin alone, if the organism is sensitive. Trimethoprim-sulfamethoxazole (TMP-SMX), a bactericidal drug used successfully in adults, has excellent central nervous system penetration and acceptable MICs against most strains of *Listeria.*

Drugs to Avoid Tetracycline is an effective antimicrobial agent but its use during gestation and infancy is associated with well-described adverse effects on developing teeth and bones. The use of chloramphenicol, alone or in combination with penicillin or ampicillin, has resulted in high mortality in adults and is, therefore, contraindicated. Third-generation cephalosporins are not active against the organism.

Disseminated Herpes Simplex Virus Infection

Introduction and Epidemiology HSV types 1 and 2 are the etiologic agents in most human disease reported to be herpes. Other members of the human herpes virus group include cytomegalovirus (CMV), Epstein-Barr virus (EBV), varicella zoster virus (VZV), and human herpes virus type 6 (HHV-6, formerly known as roseola).

HSV infection is acquired most commonly during delivery (natal infection). Most infections in which a source is identified are related to maternal genital infection at the time of delivery. Likelihood of the neonate contracting disease in this manner is correlated with rupture of membranes of longer than 6 hours in a mother with active genital infection. Premature babies are more likely to become infected, although it may be that active infection predisposes to premature onset of labor. Babies born to women with a primary herpes infection are at a much greater risk than those born to women with reactivation of the disease.

Delivery of babies by cesarean section less than 4 hours after rupture of membranes is to a great extent protective. Approximately 70% of isolates from infected neonates are type 2. Isolation of type 1 virus does not exclude infection through the genital route, because 10 to 20% of adult genital disease may be caused by type 1.

Clinical Manifestations

Initial Findings Neonatal HSV disease generally presents within the first week of life, but an incubation period of up to 21 days has been documented. The early course of disseminated infection is similar to that of acute bacterial sepsis and cannot be distinguished on clinical grounds. Mucosal or skin vesicular lesions are present in only 20 to 30% of affected babies. Meningoencephalitis occurs in approximately 50% of affected babies, but cerebrospinal fluid analysis may be normal in the early stages of disease.

When actively sought, the virus generally is recoverable by culture or fluorescent antibody technique in secretions from the baby's trachea, nasopharynx, gastrointestinal and genitourinary tracts, and from the bloodstream. Recently, the polymerase chain reaction has been used to isolate HSV DNA from cerebrospinal fluid and serum of patients.

Outcome The clinical features and associated rates of mortality are presented in Table 18.7.

Table 18.7
Clinical Features and Mortality Rates of Neonatal Herpes Simplex Virus Disease

Disease	Clinical Features
Disseminated Herpes simplex virus	Apnea
	Respiratory distress
	Liver failure
	Hypotension
	Disseminated intravascular coagulation
	Superinfection common
	Mortality 92%
Central nervous system disease	Seizures
	Lethargy or coma
	Elevated intracranial pressure
	Mortality 40%

Babies who have disseminated disease resulting from infection with HSV-2 have a poorer outcome than those infected with type 1 virus. One reason is the apparently increased rate of pneumonitis and DIC associated with type 2. Another reason is that HSV-2 is less susceptible to treatment with acyclovir.

Prevention Such a grim outlook for HSV infection makes prevention essential and early recognition and initiation of therapy paramount. As mentioned previously, cesarean section in the first few hours after rupture of membranes may be effective in preventing most perinatally acquired infections when the mother has active genital herpes. Mothers with genital lesions should be instructed in frequent hand washing, but need not be isolated from their babies. In the presence of active oral lesions, it may be wise to separate the mother and neonate until the skin has returned to normal and viral shedding has stopped. The risk of nosocomial spread of the virus is decreased by isolating neonates with suspected or proven infection and requiring that care providers wear gloves and engage in vigorous hand washing after contact with the infants' secretions.

Therapy The drug of choice for specific therapy of HSV is acyclovir (ACV) (30 mg/kg/day in three divided doses, administered every 8 hours). In regard to presumptive therapy of babies at risk, we recommend treating any neonate with sepsis with ACV if they do not respond to empiric bacterial coverage, or if there is evidence of disseminated disease or isolated pneumonitis.

Older Infant and Child

Clinical Presentation

Beyond the first month of life, the spectrum of etiologic agents responsible for overwhelming sepsis changes. Gram-negative enteric organisms in the immune competent host are replaced by *S. pneumoniae, N. meningitidis,* and *H. influenzae* type b. Sepsis resulting from β-hemolytic streptococcus and *S. aureus* is uncommon, except in certain situations.

Infants and children younger than 2 years of age are often febrile, and may develop occult bacteremia, although the mere presence of bacteria in the bloodstream (most often pneumococci) does not usually lead to overwhelming sepsis or the need for intensive care. Of greater interest to the pediatric critical care practitioner, however, is symptomatic bacteremia, which results in serious systemic manifestations of disease and may be particularly fulminant, leading to death in a short time; it will be the major subject of discussion here. *H. influenzae* type b, although most often associated with meningitis, is in reality a bloodborne disease that may result in localized infection in a number of areas and, therefore, will also be addressed in this section. Other bacteria, as well as rickettsia and some viruses, can cause a similar picture of overwhelming sepsis in the older infant and child but are not as common as the first two microorganisms mentioned. They include *S.*

aureus, β-hemolytic streptococcus, tularemia, brucellosis, plague, Rocky Mountain spotted fever, and viral hemorrhagic fevers.

Meningococcemia

Overwhelming sepsis in the normal host may be primary (with no apparent localized source) or secondary to infection at a particular site. Meningococcemia is the classic infection in children without a source.

N. meningitidis, a Gram-negative coccus that usually grows in pairs or tetrads, causes a wide range of clinical disease. Noninvasive forms of infection may cause genitourinary and gastrointestinal disease, as well as conjunctivitis and pharyngitis. Categorization of invasive systemic disease depends on whether the infection predominantly causes septicemia or meningitis and has implications regarding therapy and prognosis.

Clinical Manifestations Initial symptoms of systemic infection usually consist of:

- Upper respiratory complaints
- Fever
- Joint pains
- Myalgias
- Rash
- Headache
- Vomiting

Physical findings include:

- High fever (greater than 40°C in 60%)
- Macular, petechial, or purpuric rash
- Meningeal signs, when meningitis predominates
- Diffuse muscle tenderness
- Shock (hypotension, tachycardia, diminished perfusion, and cool skin/elevated core temperature)

When petechiae are present (50 to 60%), they are more pronounced on the trunk and extremities. When purpura develops, the lesions are distinct from the petechiae and are usually a harbinger of severe disease. In the 80% of patients who have signs of meningeal involvement, alterations in level of consciousness and abnormal pupillary responses may occur, suggesting the presence of elevated intracranial pressure.

Prognosis Laboratory findings vary with the severity of disease and have been correlated with prognosis in some situations. Five factors, when present, indicate an unfavorable prognosis (Table 18.8).

The purpose of identifying which patients are most likely to die with conventional therapy is to make the clinician more aware of the need for

Table 18.8
Unfavorable Prognostic Factors in Meningococcal Disease per Niklasson et al.[a]

1. Absence of meningitis (less than 100 WBC/mm^3 in cerebrospinal fluid).
2. Presence of low blood pressure (less than 70 in children younger than 14 y of age)
3. Presence of petechiae for less than 12 h before admission
4. Presence of marked hyperpyrexia (rectal temperature 40° C or above)
5. Absence of marked leukocytosis (less than 15,000 WBC/mm^3 of blood)
6. Presence of thrombocytopenia (less than 100,000 platelets/mm^3 of blood)

[a]Adapted with permission from Niklasson P, Lundbergh P, Strandell T. Prognostic factors in meningococcal disease. Scand J Infect Dis 1971;3:17.

rapid therapeutic action in patients who present with an unfavorable score. The intensive care specialist will be more likely to institute invasive monitoring techniques and support of vital functions in anticipation of potential acute deterioration.

Causes of Death Death from meningococcal disease generally is caused by intractable shock, even in patients with meningitis. Acute fulminating meningococcemia usually results in death within hours from the time of admission. There is also a group of patients who die of profound neurologic deterioration, which may be attributed to elevated intracranial pressure, with or without herniation.

Fulminant Meningococcemia (Waterhouse-Friderichsen Syndrome)

Fulminant meningococcemia is nearly always fatal and represents a hyperacute form of disease. Petechiae are universally present, purpura generally develops, and the patient's shock may or may not respond to the fluids and pressor agents generally employed.

Primary myocardial failure is an attractive explanation of failure of the patient to respond to many therapies generally employed in shock caused by other organisms. The belief that the intractable shock was related to adrenal cortical failure led to attempts at treating this infection with exogenous corticosteroids. Although large studies have not demonstrated an effect on mortality, sporadic reports of success continue to appear in the literature.

Differential Diagnosis The differential diagnosis of acute meningococcemia includes endotoxin-producing bacterial diseases, such as *E. coli*, as well as other infectious diseases listed in Table 18.9. Noninfectious diseases, such as Henoch-Schonlein purpura, DIC of any cause, and idiopathic thrombocytopenic purpura, are also included in the differential diagnosis.

Evaluation of the Patient Diagnostic testing must proceed rapidly and concurrently with initiation of therapy if the patient has the greatest chance to survive.

Table 18.9
Infectious Diseases Associated with Petechiae

N. meningitidis
H. influenzae type b
N. gonorrhoeae
S. pneumoniae
S. pyogenes
Enteroviruses
Rubella
Rickettsiae
Mycoplasma
Epstein-Barr virus
Cytomegalovirus
Colorado tick fever
Arboviruses
Rat-bite fever
Y. pestis

Laboratory Testing Evaluation for possible bacterial pathogens is imperative. This evaluation should include blood cultures and rapid antigen diagnostic testing (countercurrent immune electrophoresis or latex agglutination) when available. The demonstration of Gram-negative diplococci on blood smear or buffy coat smear as well as in scrapings from purpuric lesions may be helpful. Appropriate laboratory tests include WBC with differential, erythrocyte sedimentation rate, platelet count, and evaluation for possible DIC with determination of prothrombin time, partial thromboplastin time, fibrinogen, and fibrin degradation products.

Intensive Care Protocol The remainder of the patient's evaluation should follow usual intensive care procedures. The patient's airway may be inadequate if mental status is diminished. Additionally, oxygenation may be impaired by adult respiratory distress syndrome, pulmonary edema, or pneumonia. Increased metabolic demand of the patient in shock may make an otherwise normal level of gas exchange inadequate for the situation. Arterial blood gases and chest radiographs are required elements of this assessment.

Central Nervous System Evaluation

ALTERED FUNCTION The cause of an abnormal mental status must be determined. Although it is important to examine the cerebrospinal fluid for evidence of meningeal irritation, and to obtain cultures, other causes of altered neurologic function should be considered, some of which preclude the performance of a lumbar puncture. Neurologic dysfunction in a child with meningococcemia may be caused by direct effects of local infection and inflammation, diffuse cerebral edema with intracranial hypertension, or diminished cerebral perfusion resulting from the generalized shock state.

LUMBAR PUNCTURE If the child's Glasgow Coma Scale score is 7 or less, ongoing bedside measurement of intracranial pressure should be considered, and if indicated, should be instituted before the lumbar puncture is performed. If the child's condition allows it, a computed axial tomography (CAT) scan should be obtained before placement of an intraventricular catheter or subarachnoid screw. If the patient cannot be moved safely to the radiology department, a subarachnoid screw may be placed based on clinical findings alone.

If the patient's intracranial pressure reading is less than 20 mm Hg, and there is no evidence of mass effect on CAT scan or physical examination, a spinal tap may be performed. If the patient's intracranial pressure is high, but the ventricles are visible on the scan, a ventricular catheter may be substituted for the screw, and a sample of cerebrospinal fluid obtained in that manner.

CONTRAINDICATIONS TO LUMBAR PUNCTURE Contraindications to lumbar puncture in these children include markedly abnormal clotting studies, thrombocytopenia, irreversible shock, and/or an unstable airway.

Therapy Emphasis must be placed on early recognition, treatment, and prevention as well as multivalent immunizations in high-risk populations.

Antibiotic Treatment Specific antibiotic therapy traditionally has consisted of high-dose penicillin, although some isolates of *N. meningitidis* are relatively resistant to penicillin. Because identification of the organism and antibiotic sensitivities are not available at the time of patient admission, it is inappropriate to use penicillin alone in the treatment of sepsis. A single daily dose of ceftriaxone (100 mg/kg/day) appears to be safe, efficacious, and without significant side effects, even when used for a short course (i.e., 4 days). Simultaneous use of an aminoglycoside (gentamicin) if there is any reason to suspect an enteric Gram-negative organism, and an antipseudomonal cephalosporin if *Pseudomonas* is a strong possibility, should be considered.

Corticosteroids There is neither definitive evidence that corticosteroids are of benefit in changing the outcome of this disease nor contraindication to its use. Because steroids are of some theoretical benefit to possibly borderline adrenal function in the presence of circulatory failure, it is reasonable to use very high septic shock doses of methylprednisolone (30 mg/kg) followed by maintenance doses of steroids once meningococcemia is documented.

Heparin Some researchers think heparin is of value, because the hemorrhagic findings of purpura fulminans are associated with abnormal coagulation. Its benefit has not been conclusively demonstrated, however.

Inotropic Drugs The efficacy of various inotropic and antihypotensive medications has not been documented in shock states related to meningococcal infection. The drug most widely used initially was norepinephrine, which has been sporadically beneficial even when adrenocortical extract was not. Milrinone, with its combined inotropic and afterload reducing effects, might be of significant benefit in this disease. Inotropic agents, however, singly or in various combinations, have not altered the inevitable fatal outcome for some of these patients.

Hemodynamic Support Plasma expansion is the first order of business, and large volumes may be necessary in the presence of endotoxic shock as it occurs in meningococcal infection. Beyond that, an inotropic agent may be of benefit. In the presence of myocardial failure and diminished peripheral perfusion, the combination of dobutamine for inotropy and nitroprusside for afterload reduction, with maintenance of adequate preload through the use of volume expansions, may be effective. Nitroprusside infusion is contraindicated in the patient with elevated intracranial pressure, however, because it leads to preferential cerebral vasodilation and may diminish perfusion pressure by increasing intracranial pressure and, potentially, by diminishing arterial blood pressure.

Appropriate therapy for cardiovascular perturbations is more readily achieved with the aid of invasive hemodynamic monitoring. Placement of a pulmonary artery catheter allows the clinician to measure central venous and pulmonary capillary occlusion pressures, as well as cardiac output. Adequacy of therapy may be assessed by calculating oxygen delivery and consumption.

Pulmonary Edema Pulmonary edema resulting from acute myocardial failure or acute respiratory distress syndrome occurs with varying frequency in septicemic individuals. It may be severe and require intubation and high levels of end-expired pressure. Because of the bleeding tendency of many of these children, any procedure, but especially intubation, should be approached with extreme care. The patient must be appropriately sedated or paralyzed to reduce the risk of trauma to soft tissues and subsequent bleeding complications. When possible, the procedure should be completed by an experienced anesthetist or intensive care specialist. Additionally, it is probably wise to avoid the nasotracheal route, with its increased hazards of bleeding from adenoidal beds in patients with DIC. Overzealous attempts at placing nasogastric tubes should likewise be avoided.

Increased Intracranial Pressure If acute changes suggestive of impending uncal herniation are present, therapy may need to commence before the pressure can be measured. The therapy consists of the following:

- Acute hyperventilation through an endotracheal tube
- Administration of furosemide and/or mannitol
- Fluid restriction
- High doses of barbiturates

Because some of these maneuvers may not be possible in the patient who also has concomitant septic shock, knowledge of intracranial pressure, perfusion pressure, and the left atrial filling pressures is essential to guide rational management decisions. The patient who appears at risk for elevated intracranial pressure in this setting, therefore, should have the airway controlled, a subarachnoid screw or intraventricular catheter, and a central venous or more preferably a pulmonary artery catheter in place. Presence of any of these monitoring devices will not make the infection more difficult to treat.

Purpura Fulminans The use of continuous sympathetic block through caudal or lumbar epidural catheters has been reported in children with this disorder. Local vasodilation may be more efficacious than systemic afterload reduction in the child with marginal cardiovascular status, and has not led to hypotension in the children in whom it has been reported. When left untreated, significant purpura results in loss of the affected limb(s) because of progressive ischemia and eventual gangrene.

Complications Patients who survive the first several days of the infection remain at risk for certain complications of meningococcemia: arthritis, deafness, gastroenteritis, pneumonia, and pericarditis-myocarditis. The last named are the most important to the pediatric intensive care specialist. Generally, clinically evident myocarditis occurs 4 to 7 days into the course of the illness, is probably a hypersensitivity reaction, and is noted in 3 to 5% of all patients. Myocardial involvement may lead to sudden death from a dysrhythmia.

Rifampin prophylaxis of household and day care center contacts is indicated. The dose is 20 mg/kg/day administered twice daily for 2 days. Many pharmacies will make a special suspension for use in young children. This recommendation may change as rifampin resistance emerges.

Haemophilus Influenzae

The *H. influenzae* bacterium is a Gram-negative pleomorphic coccobacillus.

Epidemiology *H. influenzae* is transmitted by person-to-person spread and is carried in the nasopharynx. Isolation of the infected patient is essential, as is treatment of the index case and all close contacts with rifampin to reduce carriage; nosocomial spread to adult hospital staff has been reported. Immunization does not rapidly diminish carriage and, therefore, does not obviate prophylaxis and isolation.

Clinical Manifestations The most common clinical presentation of *H. influenzae* type b is acute meningitis, followed by epiglottitis. Pneumonia caused by *H. influenzae* type b is not dramatically different from that caused by other microorganisms and requires the same general approach as any other acute lower respiratory infection. Acute sepsis secondary to *H. influenzae* type b may mimic meningococcemia.

H. influenzae type b versus Meningococcemia The incidence of meningitis, myocarditis, pneumonia, otitis media, and osteomyelitis is similar with respect to these two types of infection. There are no absolute clinical clues on which to base a microbiologic diagnosis in the patient who has petechiae or purpura accompanying fever and shock. Gram's stain may be helpful, as may be determination of a presumed diagnosis by rapid antigen detection. Until the bacteriologic diagnosis is confirmed, however, the patient with overwhelming sepsis must be treated expectantly for both meningococcemia and *H. influenzae* type b.

Therapy Initial therapy of overwhelming sepsis caused by *H. influenzae* type b is not different from that of meningococcemia. At least 25% of all *H. influenzae* type b isolates throughout the United States, however, are resistant to ampicillin. The current drug of choice is a third-generation cephalosporin, such as ceftriaxone. Chloramphenicol is also efficacious, and may be useful in the child with combined penicillin-cephalosporin allergy. There have been occasional reports of chloramphenicol-resistant *H. influenzae* type b, primarily from the United Kingdom. Multiple-resistant strains also exist.

Prevention Successful immunization is the most effective prevention available. In addition, close household and day care center contacts, both adults and children, should receive chemoprophylaxis with rifampin at a dose of 20 mg/kg/day for 4 days, regardless of results of nasopharyngeal cultures. The index case deserves rifampin therapy as well, because systemic administration of ampicillin and/or chloramphenicol does not eradicate nasopharyngeal carriage of the organism. Rifampin reduces the carriage rate and the rate of secondary infection. It also alters chloramphenicol levels, and so it is reasonable to administer rifampin at the conclusion of the acute course of therapy, if the patient is being treated with chloramphenicol.

19.

Meningitis, Infectious Encephalopathies, and Other Central Nervous System Infections

Ivor D. Berkowitz, Frank E. Berkowitz, Charles Newton,
Rodney E. Willoughby, and Alice D. Ackerman

516

INTRODUCTION

The central nervous system (CNS) can be affected by many kinds of infectious processes that are caused by a multitude of organisms. This discussion concentrates on those that are most common, not only in the United States, but also worldwide, and that are most devastating to the child.

BACTERIAL MENINGITIS

Epidemiology and Bacteriology

The overall incidence of acute hematogenous meningitis in the United States is approximately 5/100,000 persons with a higher incidence in infants. The incidence may increase considerably during epidemics of meningococcal infection.

The predominant organisms in different age groups are outlined in Table 19.1. *Streptococcus pneumoniae, Neisseria meningitidis,* and *Haemophilus influenzae* type b account for at least 80% of culture-proven cases and are the predominant organisms causing acute hematogenous meningitis in children 2 months to 4 years of age. Anatomic abnormalities, surgical procedures, neurologic trauma, or immune deficiency often underlie meningitis caused by other agents (Table 19.2). The bacteriology of these infections varies over time and geographic location. Tuberculous (TB) meningitis is rare in the child, but with the resurgence of tuberculosis, TB meningitis also is increasing in incidence.

Any of the other organisms listed in Tables 19.1 and 19.2 must be considered in the child with underlying risk factors or the previously healthy youngster who fails to respond as expected to the administered antibiotics.

Pathophysiology

Elevated Intracranial Pressure

Intracranial pressure (ICP) is a crucial determinant of cerebral perfusion pressure and is important in the outcome of bacterial meningitis in children. Clinical studies have demonstrated that morbidity and mortality is highest in children with cerebral perfusion less than 30 mm Hg. Analysis of these studies suggests that a decrease in cerebral perfusion pressure was related more to elevation of intracranial pressure than reduction in arterial blood pressure.

Several studies in adults and children demonstrate that ICP frequently is elevated in patients with clinical meningitis, and elevated ICP usually is el-

Table 19.1
Usual Causes of Acute Hematogenous Bacterial Meningitis in Children in Different Age Groups

Age	Organism
0–2 mo	*Streptococcus agalactiae* (Group B)
	Enteric bacilli (*Escherichia coli, Klebsiella Proteus, Citrobacter*)
	Listeria monocytogenes
2–4 mo	*S. agalactiae*
	S. pneumoniae
	Haemophilus influenzae type b
	Neisseria meningitidis
4 mo–5 y	*S. pneumoniae*
	N. meningitidis
	H. influenzae type b
>5 y	*S. pneumoniae*
	N. meningitidis

Table 19.2
Common Microbial Causes of Meningitis Associated with Different Underlying Conditions

Underlying Condition	Organism
Basilar skull fracture	*Streptococcus pneumoniae*
	Haemophilus influenzae type b
	Neisseria meningitidis
	Staphylococcus aureus
	S. pyogenes (Group A)
	Gram-negative bacilli
Postneurosurgery	Coagulase-negative *staphylococci*
	S. aureus
	Gram-negative bacilli
Cerebrospinal fluid shunt	Coagulase-negative *staphylococci*
	S. aureus
	Gram-negative bacilli
	coryneforms (diphtheroids)
	Propionibacteria acnes
	Bacillus species
Nosocomial	*S. aureus*
(not postsurgery)	*Candida* species
	Gram-negative bacilli
Immune Deficiencies	
hyposplenism (e.g., sickle	*S. pneumoniae*
cell disease)	*H. influenzae*
	N. meningitidis
cell-mediated deficiency	*Listeria monocytogenes*
	Salmonella species
	Nocardia species
	Cryptococcus neoformans
	Dimorphic fungi (e.g., *Histoplasma capsulatum,*
	Coccidioides immitis)
neutropenia	*S. pneumoniae*
	L. monocytogenes
	Gram-negative bacilli
	enteric bacilli
	Pseudomonas aeruginosa
terminal complement	*N. meningitidis*
component deficiencies	

evated maximally within the first 24 to 48 hours after diagnosis. Substantial experimental evidence suggests that elevated ICP develops in all experimental models of meningitis.

The major causes of elevated intracranial pressure in bacterial meningitis include cerebral edema, hydrocephalus, and cerebral hyperemia. Other complications that can contribute to increased ICP include subdural effusions and empyema, brain abscess, and cerebral infarction.

Cerebral Edema

Cerebral edema may occur because of vasogenic, cytotoxic, and interstitial mechanisms. Vasogenic edema, distributed mainly in cerebral white matter, is characterized by increased permeability of the capillary endothelial cells. Increase in blood-brain barrier permeability has been demonstrated in experimental models of bacterial meningitis in response to inoculation of bacteria, cell wall components, and cytokines.

Cytotoxic edema is caused by cellular swelling secondary to cell injury. This affects neurons, glial and endothelial cells, and reflects failure of adenosine triphosphatase (ATPase)-dependent sodium exchange.

Interstitial edema is caused by increased cerebrospinal fluid (CSF) hydrostatic pressure associated with hydrocephalus that often accompanies bacterial meningitis.

Hydrocephalus

Hydrocephalus, with attending ventricular dilation and enlargement of the subarachnoid space as demonstrated on CT (computed tomography) or magnetic resonance imaging (MRI) scan, is present in up to 80% of children with bacterial meningitis. Serial scanning of these patients demonstrates that CSF volume is greatest within the first 72 hours of hospitalization, which also is the period of greatest ICP elevation. The relative contribution of increased CSF volume to elevated ICP is unclear but likely has some significant role, particularly when accompanied by cerebral edema and cerebral hyperemia.

Hypoglycorrhachia

Low levels of glucose in CSF is almost an essential element of bacterial meningitis.

Clinical Manifestations

Clinical presentation of acute bacterial meningitis is variable and differs according to infectious etiology, age, resistance factors of the host, and length of time between onset of illness and first evaluation by a physician.

Signs and Symptoms

Most patients have:

- Fever
- Irritability
- Mental status changes
- Vomiting
- Loss of appetite
- Headache
- Neck rigidity 12 to 24 hours into the illness

Neonates and infants younger than 4 months of age may not show signs of meningismus, but rather show nonspecific signs of systemic illness, which may include apnea, convulsions, and other signs of sepsis.

Seizures

Older children also may develop seizures as an early manifestation of acute bacterial meningitis. Convulsions may be confused with febrile seizures if the patient's spinal fluid is not evaluated for presence of cells or microorganisms. Convulsions occur in at least 30% of patients with meningitis at some point in their illness and may be focal or generalized. Focal seizures are more likely to occur with a localized infarction or in the presence of a subdural effusion. Generalized seizures may be the result of diffuse irritation from inflammation, diffuse ischemia, or hyponatremia that accompanies the development of the syndrome of inappropriate secretion of antidiuretic hormone (SIADH). Patients who have convulsions within the first 48 to 72 hours of illness generally have a better prognosis and are less likely to require long-term anticonvulsant therapy than those that occur later in the course of disease.

Duration of Symptoms

The duration and progression of symptoms depend on the peculiarities of the infecting organisms. Meningococcal sepsis and meningitis often progress rapidly and, in some cases, result in death several hours after the onset of illness. Although some cases of *H. influenzae* type b meningitis are fulminant in the same manner as *N. meningitidis,* the course of haemophilus meningitis is usually less rapid. Pneumococcal meningitis may begin as bacteremia, and the child who is destined to develop acute bacterial meningitis is difficult to distinguish in the initial phases of illness from the child who may be considered to have benign or "occult" pneumococcal sepsis.

Diagnosis

History

Evaluation of the child with suspected meningitis begins with a history, particularly exposure to another child with meningococcal or haemophilus meningitis, because these diseases tend to cluster. Day-care arrangements should be explored fully, because children younger than 5 years of age are more likely to develop haemophilus meningitis even in the absence of a documented case. Day care and household information also is important after the diagnosis is made to determine the need for chemoprophylaxis of contacts. If a child has been fully immunized against *H. influenzae* type b, meningitis caused by this organism is unlikely.

Physical Findings

The diagnostic subtleties may not be so pronounced for the pediatric intensive care specialist as for the emergency or primary care physician. If the child requires intensive care, he or she generally is comatose, is having seizures, or is in a state of hemodynamic instability.

The physician evaluates vital functions, and gives specific attention to the basic ABCs of life support before making a search for etiologic clues. Abnormalities clearly present on the physical examination usually include meningismus, or pain associated with neck flexion, and limitation of movement of the neck (Kernig and Brudzinski signs). These signs may disappear with progression of illness and development of deep coma.

Examination of the patient's pupils and retinae are important. Abnormalities in the pupillary response to light may occur because of direct irritation of the third cranial nerve as it leaves the base of the brain. Limitations of ocular movement may result from irritation of the third and sixth nerves. Fourth-nerve involvement is less common but does occur. It is important to determine the cause of such findings, because the subsequent course will be different if the signs are caused by elevated ICP rather than by localized inflammation.

Papilledema is not a reliable sign in determining the presence or absence of elevated ICP, but if it is observed, chances are greater that intracranial hypertension exists. It may also be a helpful sign in the differential diagnosis. Because papilledema that develops within the first day or two of illness is more likely caused by a ruptured brain abscess, subarachnoid extension of an intracranial extradural abscess, or other mass-type lesion. Patients who have tuberculous and cryptococcal meningitis are more likely to have focal signs and papilledema than patients with meningitis caused by the usual bacteria.

The retinae should be evaluated for the presence of possible hemorrhages, because their presence may be helpful in making the diagnosis of cortical vein and sagittal sinus thrombosis, abnormalities of blood clotting mechanisms, and certain types of trauma and child abuse leading to coma or seizure activity. In young infants, elevated ICP may be manifested by a bulging fontanelle. Anterior fontanelle herniation of brain tissue has been reported.

Differential Diagnosis

The clinical differential diagnosis of acute bacterial meningitis is listed in Table 19.3. The differential diagnosis varies with age and other host factors. It includes conditions that cause changes in mental status and those that cause pain on neck flexion.

Indications for Admission to the Pediatric Intensive Care Unit

Most patients with suspected bacterial meningitis are evaluated in the emergency department where the diagnosis is considered, and initial therapy is instituted. Intensive care is required for the following:

Table 19.3
Differential Diagnosis of Meningitis According to the Patient Clinical Syndrome

Clinical Syndrome	Differential Diagnosis
Encephalopathy (disturbed level of consciousness, seizures)	Hypoglycemia, electrolyte disturbance, hypoxia, intoxication, head injury, stroke, vasculitis, inborn error of metabolism, focal intracranial suppuration, encephalitis, Reye syndrome
Raised intracranial pressure	Intracranial hemorrhage, focal intracranial suppuration, tumor, hydrocephalus
Neurological signs with neck-stiffness	Posterior fossa tumor, herniation
Fever with neck-stiffness	Pneumonia (especially right upper lobe), neck infections, cervical lymphadenitis, retropharyngeal abscess, cervical arthritis, spinal epidural abscess

- Infant or child who arrives comatose with abnormal motor response to stimulation, abnormalities of the pupillary response to light, obvious cranial nerve involvement, or other signs of elevated ICP (i.e., bradycardia, hypertension)
- Child with signs of poor perfusion, obvious shock, cutaneous manifestations of disseminated intravascular coagulation (DIC) (e.g., petechiae, purpura), or irregularities of respiratory pattern
- Laboratory data includes significant metabolic acidosis, hypoxemia, hypercapnia, neutropenia, significant hyponatremia, anemia, or evidence of renal or liver dysfunction
- Child who does not appear critically ill, but needs greater level of observation than can be offered on a general pediatric floor
- Child whose course has been particularly rapid before presentation, because he or she is more likely to develop signs of septic shock or intracranial hypertension and to require higher levels of support than generally available on the usual pediatric floor

We recommend, therefore, that in any complicated or severe course, whether from a systemic or neurologic aspect, the child be admitted to the pediatric intensive care unit (PICU) at least until the course can be determined, the first several doses of antibiotics administered, and a tentative bacteriologic diagnosis made. It is only through early recognition of complications, such as shock or elevated ICP, that effective therapy can be initiated in a timely fashion and can potentially alter the outcome of fulminant meningitis.

Lumbar Puncture in the Critically Ill Child

The physician makes the definitive diagnosis of meningitis by recovery of organisms from culture of the CSF, but the lumbar puncture (LP) procedure is not without risks.

Contraindications to Lumbar Puncture

Contraindications to this procedure include:

- Cardiorespiratory instability
- Raised ICP
- Coagulopathy
- Skin infection in the lumbar area
- Such severely elevated ICP that removal of fluid from the lumbar space may result in cerebral herniation
- Active DIC, because of the risk of developing a catastrophic spinal epidural hematoma, a catastrophic complication

For the patient who manifests abnormal clotting parameters, fresh-frozen plasma (FFP) or platelets can be administered immediately before the procedure.

Antimicrobial Therapy

When a patient is suspected strongly of having bacterial meningitis, the physician should institute antimicrobial therapy immediately in the absence of a definitive diagnosis. Most cases of community-acquired acute bacterial meningitis occur because of a limited number of different bacteria; therefore, the physician can institute empiric antimicrobial therapy directed against the most likely organisms. If lumbar puncture is then performed, the CSF might be sterile, although a microbiologic diagnosis might be determined on the basis of blood culture—which frequently yields the pathogen—or by antigen detection. The empiric therapy of nosocomial meningitis is more difficult because there is a much greater variety of potential pathogens and of antimicrobial resistance patterns.

Transfer of Care

The critical care physician often must accept a child with suspected meningitis and mental status abnormalities from another institution. A common question is whether the lumbar tap must be done before transfer. The same guidelines for performing a lumbar tap should be considered when the physician is deciding whether the tap should be done before the patient is transferred. Any procedure that delays antibiotic administration or the child's transfer to an appropriate facility should be deferred and completed at the receiving hospital if the child is stable on arrival. Administration of antibiotics should *never* be postponed because of a proposed transfer, regardless of the ability of the referring physician or hospital to obtain appropriate cultures.

Opening Pressure

The physician must measure an opening pressure (OP) when a lumbar puncture is performed in patients with suspected meningitis. The normal

OP in the adult and older child is up to 180 mm H_2O. For the neonate, the normal value is assumed to be between 90 and 110 mm H_2O.

Laboratory Diagnosis

Cerebrospinal Fluid Analysis

The definitive diagnosis of meningitis is made by recovery of organisms from CSF, although culture results may take 24 to 48 hours or more. Other information derived from CSF examination can help make a presumptive diagnosis of bacterial meningitis within an hour or two.

Leukocyte Count Meningitis is suspected if the patient's CSF is grossly cloudy. Even when the spinal fluid appears clear, determination of the cell count is essential. Normal CSF findings in infants and children are a maximum of 5 white blood cells (WBCs)/mm^3, all of which should be mononuclear. The normal CSF cell count values for neonates are noted in Table 19.4. In newborn babies, polymorphonuclear leukocytes may comprise up to 60% of the total white cell population and still be considered normal.

In meningitis, the CSF white cell count generally is elevated. Spinal fluid will continue to appear clear with up to 500 WBCs/mm^3. Infrequently, in the early stages of meningitis, CSF leukocytosis may not occur in spite of a positive CSF culture. In bacterial meningitis, granulocytes usually make up 80 to 90% of the total number of leukocytes. Table 19.5 outlines the range of CSF values occurring in various forms of meningitis.

Glucose and Protein Concentrations In acute meningitis, the CSF glucose and protein concentrations typically are deranged. The glucose value is generally much lower than the accepted normal of 50 to 60% of the serum glucose (in newborns, the norm is considered to be at least 75% of serum value), and the absolute value may be as low as 0 to 20 mg/dL (Table 19.4 outlines normal ranges of CSF glucose in neonates). Under any circumstances, CSF glucose less than 40 mg/dL is considered hypoglycorrhachia unless the preceding hypoglycemia was severe.

Cerebrospinal fluid protein concentration in bacterial meningitis may increase to greater than 100 mg/dL, although normal CSF protein values also vary with age. In the adult and older child, values of spinal fluid protein up to 45 mg/dL are considered within the normal range; normal values for full-term and premature infants are outlined in Table 19.4. The presence of erythrocytes may raise the protein concentration by approximately 15 mg/dL for every 1000 RBCs/mm^3 of spinal fluid.

Gram Stain A sample of CSF also must be sent to the microbiology laboratory for Gram's stain, culture, and sensitivity determination. The Gram stain is the simplest, quickest, and most useful rapid test for confirming a diagnosis of bacterial meningitis. Although its sensitivity is only approximately 80%, it can be performed within only a few minutes. Occasionally, however,

Table 19.4
Composition of Normal Cerebrospinal Fluid According to Patient Age

	Total WBC/mm³ Count		ANC		% of Neutrophils		Glucose (mg/dl)		CSF-Blood Glucose Ratio		Protein (mg/dl)	
	Mean	Range	Mean	Range	Mean	Range	Mean	Range	Mean	Range	Mean	Range
Premature newborn	9.0	0–29	NR	NR	7.0	0–66	50	24–63	0.74	0.55–1.05	115	65–150
Term newborn	8.2	0–22	NR	NR	61	NR	52	34–119	0.81	0.44–2.48	90	20–170
0–4 weeks	11.0	0–50	0.40	0–7.5	2.2	0–15	46	36–61	NR	NR	84	35–189
4–8 weeks	7.1	0–50	0.18	0–2.1	2.9	0–42	46	29–62	NR	NR	59	19–121

NR, not reported; ANC, absolute nucleated cell count/mm³; WBC, white blood cell; CSF, cerebrospinal fluid.

From Bonadio WA. The cerebrospinal fluid: physiologic aspects and alterations associated with bacterial meningitis. Pediatr Infect Dis J 1992;11:423–432.

Table 19.5
Usual Cerebrospinal Fluid Findings in Different Types of Meningitis

Meningitis Type	Leukocyte Count (cells/mm^3)	Protein Concentration (mg/dL)	Glucose Concentration (mg/dL)
Acute bacterial	Hundreds—thousands, neutrophils predominate	100–500	5–40
Viral	Up to few hundred, initially neutrophils then lymphocytes predominate	<100	Normal
Tuberculous	25–100, rarely >500, lymphocytes predominate	100–200 or even higher	Reduced
Cryptococcal	<50, lymphocytes predominate	20–500	Reduced
Syphilis	Average 500, lymphocytes predominate	100 (mean)	Normal

Adapted form Fishman RA. Cerebrospinal fluid in diseases of the nervous system 1992; 2nd ed., W.B. Saunders, Philadelphia pp 253–343.

the CSF is turbid because of large numbers of bacteria. Gram-negative bacilli also may be confused with pneumococci.

Other Tests Other tests of CSF that assist in the rapid differentiation between bacterial and viral meningitis include the Limulus amebocyte lysate test for the presence of endotoxin and determination of C-reactive protein, fibronectin, and lactate concentrations. These tests, however, are inadequately specific to accomplish their goal.

The antigen detection tests are of value in specific circumstances only. Most of these tests use latex agglutination as the method for antigen detection from *S. agalactiae; S. pneumoniae; H. influenzae* type b; *N. meningitidis;* serogroups A, C, W 135; and *E. coli* type K1. These tests are costly and their sensitivity and specificity are inadequate for complete clinical reliability. Because patients with meningitis should be treated with antibiotics against all likely pathogens until culture results are available, those antigen detection tests that are costly should not influence initial therapy. If the cultures subsequently prove to be negative, these tests might be appropriate if it can be predicted that the results will influence the patient's management.

Nonspecific Laboratory Findings

Most patients exhibit a striking leukocytosis with shift to the "left," although, as with overwhelming sepsis, neutropenia may occur, especially in the neonate. The WBC response may not be striking early in the course of disease, so a normal count, without a predominant concentration of polymorphonuclear leukocytes, should not dissuade the clinician from making the presumptive diagnosis of bacterial meningitis.

Diagnostic Problems in Meningitis

Bloody Cerebrospinal Fluid

To differentiate between a traumatic (bloody) tap and true bleeding into the CSF pathway resulting from an intraventricular or subarachnoid hemorrhage or bloody CSF associated with an infection (e.g., herpetic encephalitis), CSF is collected soon after LP in three or more sequential tubes. If the blood becomes more dilute in successive tubes, as determined by macroscopic examination, hemoglobin estimation, or red cell count, it is most suggestive of a traumatic tap. Blood that does not clear is more suggestive of true pathologic bleeding into the CSF.

The CSF leukocyte:erythrocyte ratio also is helpful in distinguishing a bloody tap from pathologic CNS hemorrhage. This ratio in a traumatic tap is much the same as that in a peripheral blood sample obtained concurrently and is usually between 1:500 to 1:1000. A leukocyte:erythrocyte ratio significantly higher in CSF than in peripheral blood suggests a CSF pleocytosis; this supports a diagnosis of meningitis. In a traumatic tap, the expected number of CSF leukocytes equals the number of CSF erythrocytes × (number of blood leukocytes/number of blood erythrocytes). A ratio or CSF leukocyte count significantly higher than expected suggests CSF pleocytosis.

Partially Treated Meningitis

As many as 50% of children with meningitis receive antibiotics in some form before diagnosis, most as outpatients because of presumed respiratory infection or possible occult pneumococcal bacteremia. These children generally are administered some form of oral penicillin in a relatively low dose compared with standard meningitis doses.

Such treatment primarily affects:

- Length of patient's illness before hospital admission or spinal tap
- Number of bacteria present in the CSF
- Rapid diagnosis of CSF by microscopic observation
- Growth of meningococcus in culture

Despite treatment, most patients with purulent meningitis will still have a predominance of neutrophils, a low glucose level, and elevated protein. Bacteriologic diagnosis of pneumococcal or *H. influenzae* meningitis does not appear to be adversely affected, at least by oral administration of penicillin or ampicillin. This might be different when prior treatment had been in the form of intramuscular ceftriaxone, which has become a common practice.

To improve the likelihood of an etiologic diagnosis, a latex agglutination test may be performed on CSF, blood, and especially urine to detect antigen from the bacterial capsule. Antigen does not disappear rapidly, even with killing of the bacteria, and may persist for up to 5 days in the presence of adequate therapy.

Although diagnosis may not be hampered by prior treatment with antibiotics, neither clinical course nor outcome is improved. Patients have the same number of complications and long-term sequelae whether they are pretreated with oral antibiotics. The symptoms and extent of illness at admission, as well as cell count and glucose and protein values, are unchanged.

Complications

Complications of meningitis are diverse and vary according to the age of the patient, infecting organism, rapidity and adequacy of antibiotic therapy, and other parameters not yet defined. Adverse effects of disease may be acute and temporary or may result in permanent residua.

Long-lasting complications in children include:

- Profound or mild mental impairments
- Visual and auditory defects
- Persistent convulsions
- Communicating hydrocephalus
- Behavioral abnormalities
- Impairment of hypothalamic function
- Long tract signs, such as hemiparesis or quadriparesis

Temporary problems include development of:

- SIADH
- DIC
- Septic shock
- Acutely elevated ICP
- Cerebral vasculitis
- Recurrent fevers

Of course, there is some overlap in the two groups of complications, with some problems, such as seizures, hypothalamic injuries, as well as raised ICP, causing acute management problems and long-lasting sequelae. Seizures and increased ICP have been discussed previously.

SIADH

The incidence of SIADH is unknown but has been noted in at least 4 to 88% of patients at the time of hospital admission. The syndrome is clinically defined as serum hyponatremia and hypo-osmolality in the presence of normovolemia, with a less than maximally dilute urine, and excessive urinary sodium loss in the absence of renal disease (see Chapter 23).

The standard recommendation for fluid therapy in young children and infants with meningitis is to provide approximately two-thirds of calculated maintenance water requirements while providing a normal sodium intake. Not every child with low serum sodium will have SIADH, however; the assumption that a child does may lead to inappropriate restriction of volume in some patients.

Diabetes Insipidus

Of the less common forms of dysfunction of the hypothalamic-pituitary axis that may complicate meningitis, including diabetes insipidus (DI), loss of temperature control, hyperphagia, and precocious puberty, DI is the only entity of major concern during the acute stages of meningitis. The excretion of large amounts of dilute urine creates problems to the opposite extreme as those of SIADH. The patient with DI may rapidly become hypovolemic, with marked hypernatremia and seizures. The pathogenesis involves severe ischemia to the hypothalamus or pituitary and generally occurs only in severely ill patients with a poor prognosis. Therapy of DI consists of replacement of urine water losses when the disorder is mild, proceeding to supplementation of antidiuretic hormone as a continuous infusion, titrated to control urine output and serum sodium and osmolality values.

Focal Neurologic Signs

Focal neurologic signs, including hemiparesis or quadriparesis, may develop in the first few days of illness but are more common later. Although numerous causes for localization of the neurologic examination need to be considered (e.g., effects of vasculitis, vasospasm, inflammation), evaluation of the child is essential for conditions that may require acute neurosurgical intervention (e.g., subdural effusions, brain abscesses).

Subdural Effusions Subdural effusions most likely occur beyond the first week of illness but may be noted at any time, including on admission. Up to 30 to 50% of infants and children have been noted to develop this complication, which is more common in *H. influenzae* type b meningitis than in infection, because of other bacteria.

Effusions usually resolve spontaneously without specific interventions. Indications for drainage of a subdural effusion include the presence of significant and persistent neurologic symptoms (e.g., seizures, paresis, elevated ICP, evidence of subdural empyema).

Brain Abscess Intracerebral abscess also must be considered in a child with worsening focal signs, usually with persistent fever. An abscess develops subsequent to cerebritis, usually in an area of compromised vascular supply.

Other Causes Hemiparesis or other focal signs may result from development of stroke, or relative ischemia, caused by vasculitis, arterial spasm, or venous thrombosis, which may lead to an infarction.

Neurologic Evaluation The evaluation of focal neurologic signs in the course of pyogenic meningitis must include careful documentation of changing neurologic findings.

- Neurologic and neurosurgical consultation is recommended with evidence of progression, worsening of signs or symptoms, presence of papilledema, elevated ICP, decline in Glasgow Coma Scale score, or unexplained cause of symptoms
- CT scan or MRI neuroimaging studies are helpful in evaluating the causes of focal neurologic signs (e.g., infarction, effusion, abscess)
- Doppler studies define flow abnormalities in major cerebral vessels even in adult patients; angiography is rarely indicated
- Radionuclide scanning can provide information relating to blood flow and presence of discrete lesions, such as abscesses, infarctions, or effusions, but has been replaced largely by the previously mentioned neuroimaging techniques
- Electrophysiologic studies, such as electroencephalography (EEG), reveal diffuse evidence of cerebral involvement when neurologic signs are worrisome but are not helpful regarding the cause of the lesion

Fever

Duration Fever that lasts beyond the tenth day is generally considered persistent or prolonged, whereas fever that recurs after at least 24 hours of apyrexia is considered a secondary or recurrent fever. The percentage of children who remain febrile or develop a secondary fever varies from 16 to 47%. The hospital day when patients first become afebrile depends on the bacterial agent. On the fifth day of appropriate antibiotic therapy, more than 85% of children with *S. pneumoniae* or *N. meningitidis* will be afebrile, but only 68% of those with *H. influenzae* meningitis will be free of fever. In addition, up to 80% of children with *H. influenzae* type b will develop a secondary febrile episode.

Etiology The most common cause of recurrent fever is nosocomial in origin, caused by either phlebitis at an intravenous or cutdown site or a hospital-acquired viral respiratory infection. The differential diagnosis of nosocomial illness in a child whose treatment in the PICU has included assisted ventilation or ICP monitoring includes:

- Acute ventriculitis
- Sinusitis
- Mastoiditis
- Subdural effusions
- Drug fevers
- Subdural empyemas

- Disseminated foci of disease, leading to septic arthritis, osteomyelitis, or pericarditis, especially in children with *H. influenzae* type b and group B streptococcus infection

It is unusual for fever to be caused by actual persistence of the organism in the leptomeninges, but antibiotic failure does occur particularly with the emergence of antibiotic resistant bacteria and may result in persistent meningitis or the development of an intracerebral abscess.

In patients in whom fever persists beyond the tenth hospital day, the most likely causes, in descending order of frequency, are:

- Subdural effusion
- Drug fever (most often in response to ampicillin)
- Arthritis
- Brain abscess
- Nosocomial infections

Therapy

Nonspecific Supportive Care

The level of supportive care provided for the neonate, infant, or child with meningitis will vary with the severity of illness exhibited by the patient. For the child in the PICU with acute suppurative meningitis, the necessary care may entail the most sophisticated levels of support, including assisted ventilation, invasive hemodynamic monitoring and control, measurement and therapy of elevated ICP, therapy of any acute seizure activity, and complicated manipulations of fluids and electrolytes. In addition, the youngster will require high levels of nursing care, with meticulous attention paid to the neurologic examination and Glasgow Coma Scale, control of fever, and provision of a comfortable environment and soothing atmosphere. The child with suspected or proven bacterial meningitis requires respiratory isolation for 24 hours of antibiotic therapy after which time he or she is considered to be noninfectious.

Maintenance of Cerebral Perfusion

Rarely, a patient will have overwhelming sepsis, Waterhouse-Friderichsen syndrome with massive adrenal hemorrhage, and acute adrenal failure, which is not a common cause of hypotension.

The clinician must initiate management of dehydration and shock rapidly with adequate volume replacement of either crystalloid or colloid, if necessary guided by invasive hemodynamic monitoring. Despite much attention to SIADH and its therapy by fluid restriction, it is mandatory that hypovolemia and dehydration be corrected and hypotension be avoided before fluid restriction is considered. Restoring normal blood pressure with careful fluid administration is more important than the concern of aggravating cerebral edema with volume infusion.

Management of Elevated Intracranial Pressure ICP monitoring is not instituted routinely in children with meningitis. The clinician should consider monitoring when there are clinical or neuroimaging signs of moderate or severe elevation in ICP.

The conventional means of managing elevated ICP in meningitis include mannitol, other diuretics, hyperventilation, barbiturates, and CSF drainage.

Mannitol Mannitol is effective in reducing elevated ICP in conventional doses in bacterial meningitis. Its efficacy may be reduced because of blood-brain barrier disruption and the passage of mannitol into the brain interstitium, reducing the interstitial to intravascular osmotic gradient.

Hyperventilation The cerebral vasoconstrictive effects of hypocapnia results in decreased cerebral blood volume and reduced ICP. This method is only effective, however, if the cerebral vasculature retains its responsiveness to hypocarbia. Because autoregulation is impaired, CO_2 responsiveness may be similarly compromised.

By reducing cerebral blood flow to levels that can induce ischemia, hyperventilation in meningitis patients could extend the area of vascular compromise. Other ICP therapeutic methods (e.g., mannitol, barbiturates, hypothermia) might play a role in decreasing intracranial hypertension without extending the area of the infarct in these patients. Such therapies, however, have not been proven valuable and indeed may present risks themselves.

Reduction of Cerebrospinal Fluid Volume Patients with increased ventricular and subarachnoid space fluid without evidence of intracranial pressure elevation require no specific therapy since these changes respond with medical management of meningitis. CSF drainage must be considered if clinical or neuroradiographic evidence indicates elevated intracranial pressure, and ventriculostomy may be necessary because removal of CSF by the lumbar route is hazardous. Increased CSF fluid can be medically managed with drugs that decrease CSF production (i.e., acetazolamide, digoxin), but their efficacy is unproven.

Fluids In anticipation of possible SIADH, the well-hydrated child often is placed on a restricted water intake of two-thirds maintenance fluids made up in a solution containing approximately half-normal saline and dextrose as needed. This management plan is controversial since it has not been demonstrated that fluid restriction will actually prevent SIADH.

Anticonvulsants A child who has had at least one seizure during the course of his or her early therapy, although potentially at low risk for ongoing seizures, is best treated with an anticonvulsant drug such as phenobarbital while in the PICU.

The child whose neurologic or cardiorespiratory status is tenuous should be spared the additional metabolic demands and ischemic insults that may accompany seizures.

Antimicrobial Therapy

Although host defenses play a major role in the pathogenesis of bacterial meningitis, they play a limited role in eliminating the infection; therefore, administration of bactericidal antibiotics is necessary.

The empiric treatment of patients with meningitis should be directed against likely organisms, taking into account their possible resistance patterns. A combination of ampicillin and cefotaxime is recommended for neonates. For infants, toddlers, and older children, a combination of a third-generation cephalosporin (i.e., cefotaxime or ceftriaxone, but not ceftazidime) and vancomycin is recommended. Recommendations for treatment of patients with meningitis caused by an organism of known identity and antimicrobial susceptibility are shown in Tables 19.6 and 19.7.

Patients with proven or suspected pneumococcal meningitis should be treated as if they could be infected with a resistant strain until the causative organism has been isolated and its antimicrobial susceptibilities determined. Such therapy should consist of vancomycin in addition to cefotaxime or ceftriaxone until the susceptibility to penicillin and the third-generation cephalosporins is known.

If a patient with pneumococcal meningitis does not respond to therapy or yields an isolate resistant to cefotaxime or ceftriaxone, a lumbar puncture should be performed. Patients with such resistant isolates should be treated for at least 10 days.

Table 19.6
Recommended Antimicrobial Therapy for Meningitis

Microorganism	Therapy	Alternative Therapy
Haemophilus influenzae	Cefotaxime, ceftriaxone, ampicillin[a]	Chloramphicol
Neisseria meningitidis	Penicillin	Cefotaxime, chloramphenicol
Streptococcus pneumoniae	Penicillin, cefotaxime[a] vancomycin (see text)	Imipenem
Streptococcus agalactiae	Penicillin or ampicillin ± gentamicin	Vancomycin, cefotaxime
Enteric bacilli	Cefotaxime, ceftriaxone, ceftazidime	Imipenem ciprofloxacin, aminoglycoside
Listeria monocytogenes	Ampicillin ± gentamicin	Vancomycin, trimethoprim-sulfamethoxazole
Pseudomonas aeruginosa	Ceftazidime or piperacillin + aminoglycoside	
Staphylococci	Nafcillin[a] or oxacillin[a] ± rifampin, vancomycin ± rifampin	

[a]Can be used alone only if susceptibility demonstrated.

Table 19.7
Daily Dosages of Antimicrobial Agents for Treatment of Meningitis in Pediatric Patients[a]

Drugs	Neonates 0–7 d	Neonates 8–28 d	Infants and Children
Amikacin[b,c]	15–20 div q 12 h	20–30 div q 8 h	20–30 div q 8 h
Ampicillin	100–150 div q 12 h	150–200 div q 8 h or q 6 h	200–300 div q 6 h
Cefotaxime	100 div q 12 h	150–200 div q 8 h or q 6 h	200 div q 8 h or q 6 h
Ceftriaxone[d]			80–100 div q 12 h or q 24 h
Ceftazidime	60 div q 12 h	90 div q 8 h	125–150 div q 8 h
Chloramphenicol[c]	25 once daily	50 div q 12 h	75–100 div q 6 h
Gentamicin[b,c]	5 div q 12 h	7.5 div q 8 h	7.5 div q 8 h
Methicillin or nafcillin	100–500 div q 12 h or q 8 h	150–200 div q 8 h or q 6 h	200 div q 6 h
Penicillin G	100,000–150,000 div q 12 h	150,000–200,000 div q 8 hr or q 6 h	250,000 div q 6 h or q 4 h
Ticarcillin	150–225 div q 12 h or q 8 h	225–300 div q 8 h or q 6 h	300 div q 6 h
Tobramycin[b,c]	4 div q 12 h	6 div q 8 h	6 div q 8 h
Vancomycin[b,c]	20 div q 12 h	30 div q 8 h	40–60 div q 6 h

[a]In milligrams per kilogram (units per kilogram for penicillin G) per day divided (div), every (q) 12, 8, 6, or 4 hours(h).

[b]Smaller doses and longer intervals of administration especially for aminoglycosides and vancomycin, for low birth weight neonates may be advisable.

[c]Monitoring of serum concentration is recommended to ensure safe and therapeutic values.

[d]Use in neonates is not recommended because of inadequate experience for neonatal meningitis.

From: Feigin RD and McCracken GH Jr., Klwin JO. Diagnosis and management of meningitis. Pediatr Infect Dis J 1992;11:784–814.

The usual therapy for meningitis caused by *N. meningitidis* has been penicillin. Strains with reduced susceptibility to penicillin, minimum inhibitory concentrations greater than 0.06 μg/mL have been reported from many countries, including the United States, Canada, Spain, Israel, and Sweden. Such strains have remained highly susceptible to third-generation cephalosporins.

Corticosteroids

Only dexamethasone as adjunctive therapy has been studied in clinical trials in patients. These controlled double-blind trials examined the frequency of hearing loss and other neurologic sequelae of bacterial meningitis in children older than 2 to 3 months who were treated with dexamethasone or placebo in addition to antimicrobial therapy.

Efficacy In areas of the world in which *H. influenzae* type b conjugate vaccines are widely used, meningitis caused by this organism is uncommon, and most cases of hematogenous meningitis are now caused by *S. pneumoniae* or *N. meningitidis*. Since penicillin-resistant and third-generation cephalosporin-resistant strains of *S. pneumoniae* are becoming more prevalent, vancomycin should be used in the empiric therapy of bacterial meningitis.

Use in Viral Meningitis Clinicians have raised concerns that steroids might have an adverse effect on the outcome of children with viral meningitis incorrectly diagnosed as having bacterial meningitis after preliminary evaluation of CSF. Studies have revealed no adverse effects of such treatment. A complication of steroid use in meningitis is gastrointestinal hemorrhage, but this is an uncommon event.

Dexamethasone Therapy in Bacterial Meningitis In patients with meningitis likely caused by *H. influenzae*—those not immunized against this organism or those whose CSF shows Gram-negative bacilli—dexamethasone should be administered at the same time as or shortly after the first dose of antibiotic. The dosage is 0.15 mg per kg per dose, intravenously, and every 6 hours for four days.

Although dexamethasone appears to be beneficial in patients with pneumococcal meningitis in some studies, its use might be detrimental in patients in whom attaining a high level of vancomycin in the CSF is critical. The weight of the potential benefits versus the probability of this disadvantage will vary from case to case.

Immunotherapy

Certain bacterial organisms in some groups of children may be more effectively treated by adding passive immunization in the form of human intravenous immunoglobulin (i.e., group B streptococcus) or, when available, monoclonal antibodies. This type of adjunctive therapy is particularly important for children who have immunoglobulin deficiencies and neonates whose immunologic capacities are limited.

Infection Control

Patients with meningitis caused by *H. influenzae* or *N. meningitidis* should be placed in respiratory isolation until they have received effective antimicrobial therapy for 24 hours. People in close contact with patients with hemophilus infections should be offered chemoprophylaxis with rifampin, depending on the ages of the children in the family, and their immunization status. A dosage of 10 to 20 mg/kg (maximum of 600 mg) daily for 4 days should be used. Individuals given rifampin should be informed of adverse effects, drug interactions, and contraindications. All close contacts of patients with meningococcal infections should be offered chemoprophylaxis with rifampin either 10 mg/kg (maximum of 600 mg) per dose every 12 hours, for 2 days, or according to the same schedule as recommended for prophylaxis against hemophilus infection. It is important to emphasize to contacts that chemoprophylaxis is not a guarantee against infection, and that they should see a physician if symptoms develop.

OTHER FORMS OF MENINGITIS AND THEIR ANTIBIOTIC MANAGEMENT

Neonatal Meningitis

Etiology

Meningitis in the neonate is frequently caused by bacteria acquired from the mother's birth canal (i.e., *Streptococcus agalactiae,* enteric bacilli such as *Escherichia coli,* and *Listeria monocytogenes*). Many cases also are hospital-acquired, especially in premature infants receiving intensive care management. The causative organisms in such cases include enteric bacilli (i.e., *Citrobacter, Enterobacter*), other Gram-negative bacilli (i.e., *Pseudomonas aeruginosa, Flavobacterium meningosepticum*) enterococci, and staphylococci, all of which may be resistant to antimicrobial agents.

Treatment

The recommendations for antimicrobial therapy are provided in Tables 19.6 and 19.7. Empiric therapy of a neonate with meningitis should consist of ampicillin or penicillin plus a third-generation cephalosporin or an aminoglycoside. Baker et al. recommend higher doses of ampicillin (300 to 400 mg/kg/day) or penicillin (500,000 U/kg/day) than are outlined in Table 19.7.

In patients with infections caused by highly resistant organisms, imipenem-cilastatin (20 to 25 mg/kg/dose every 12 hours) may be necessary. This combination therapy should not be used routinely for treating patients with meningitis, but may be indicated. In certain circumstances, such as infection caused by *Flavobacterium meningosepticum,* ciprofloxacin has been used (5 to 10 mg/kg/day divided every 12 hours in premature infants and 15 to 20 mg/kg/dose every 12 hours in full-term neonates).

Chronic Meningitis

Chronic meningitis should be suspected in any individual with global or multifocal neurologic deficits, or who has symptoms of meningitis for more than a few days. Although untreated acute bacterial meningitis may become chronic, chronic meningitis is usually caused by infections or diseases that are chronic by nature:

- Tuberculosis
- Syphilis
- Lyme disease
- Fungi, in particular cryptococcal infection

Tuberculous meningitis is perhaps the most important cause because it is rapidly fatal if untreated, and its diagnosis has important public health implications.

Tuberculous Meningitis

Tuberculous meningitis is difficult to diagnose because its progression is insidious. The diagnosis depends on physical findings, contact history, chest radiograph, Mantoux test, and characteristic abnormalities in CSF (see Table 19.5).

Antituberculous Therapy

Initiation of treatment should not depend on the demonstration of *Mycobacterium tuberculosis* on smear or by culture. The mainstay of therapy is antituberculous chemotherapy, which consists of isoniazid (10 mg/kg/day, maximum of 300 mg) rifampin (10 mg/kg/day, maximum of 600 mg), pyrazinamide (35 mg/kg/day, maximum 2 g), and streptomycin (20 to 40 mg/kg/day, maximum of 1 g). All four drugs are used for 2 months, after which pyrazinamide and streptomycin are discontinued. Although the usual duration of antituberculosis treatment is 6 months, the recommended duration for tuberculous meningitis is 12 months. Alternative therapy is required in cases of drug-resistant tuberculosis.

Nosocomial Meningitis

Table 19.2 outlines the most common microbiologic causes of meningitis in a hospitalized immunocompromised patient.

Ventricular Shunt Infections

Most cerebrospinal fluid shunts are ventriculo-peritoneal (VP) or, less commonly, ventriculoatrial (VA). The frequency of shunt infections varies from 2% to 30% and is influenced by numerous factors such as age and skin flora.

Etiology

The most common microbial causes of shunt infections are:

- Coagulase-negative staphylococci
- *Staphylococcus aureus*
- Coryneforms

- Enterococci
- Gram-negative bacilli

The infection is usually introduced at the time of surgery, although infection of the peritoneal end of VP shunts by bowel organisms, especially Gram-negative bacilli, may account for some cases.

Clinical Features

Although the presenting clinical features often are nonspecific (e.g., fever, irritability), some might represent evidence of shunt malfunction, including lethargy, anorexia, and vomiting. Because infected VP shunts discharge organisms into the peritoneal cavity, resulting in peritonitis and the formation of adhesions, patients with these infections may have abdominal pain or features of shunt obstruction. Inflammation may be evident at the surgical wound or along the track of the shunt. Patients with VP shunt infections usually have symptoms within two weeks of shunt insertion, but may have symptoms weeks or months later.

Because infections of VA shunts are not usually associated with shunt malfunction, patients with these infections tend to have symptoms later, and often with nonspecific features of infection and features similar to those of subacute infective endocarditis, such as splenomegaly, hematuria, and arthralgia.

Diagnosis

VA shunt infections are sometimes associated with bacteremia, whereas rarely with VP shunt infections. Examination of ventricular fluid is the usual method by which VP shunt infections are diagnosed, but this fluid may be normal even in the presence of infection. Removing fluid from the shunt does not introduce infection. CSF eosinophilia is frequently associated with shunt infections, and its persistence is associated with an increased risk of a requirement for shunt revision.

Management

Initial shunt removal is advocated by some authors, whereas others advocate removal only if the infection is severe or refractory to initial management. Because these patients require CSF diversion, shunt removal necessitates external ventricular drainage. The external drain may also be used for the instillation of intraventricular antibiotics, such as vancomycin (10 to 20 mg daily). External drainage is associated with the potential for a new infection, which becomes progressively more likely with increased duration of external drainage.

Therapy

Because most shunt infections involve coagulase-negative staphylococci, initial antibiotic therapy should consist of vancomycin (60 mg/kg/24 hours, divided every 6 to 8 hours, intravenously). If the shunt is not removed, the addition of rifampin (20 mg/kg/24 hours, divided every 12 hours orally) should be considered. If the Gram-stain or cultures of the CSF reveal other causes, alternative therapy should be used, such as a third-generation cephalosporin for Gram-negative bacillary infections.

VIRAL ENCEPHALITIS
Etiology
Neonates

Encephalitis in the neonate is often part of a multiorgan disease that resembles other systemic diseases (e.g., inborn error of metabolism). This may explain, in part, the lower success rate in elucidating the cause of encephalitis in the first year of life.

Herpes simplex virus (HSV) encephalitis, usually caused by HSV type 2 virus, is the most common cause of encephalitis in neonates (Table 19.8).

Table 19.8
Frequent Causes of Neonatal Encephalitis and Differential Diagnosis

	Diagnosis		
	Culture	Serology available	PCR[a]
Acute infections			
Herpes simplex virus	Y	Y	Y
Enterovirus[b]	Y		Y
Adenovirus	Y		
Meningitis[c]	Y		
Congenital infections			
Cytomegalovirus	Y	Y	Y
Toxoplasmosis		Y	
Syphilis		Y	
Herpes simplex virus	Y	Y	Y
Rubella	Y	Y	
Metabolic disorders[d]			
Primary central nervous system disorders			
Ischemia			
Hemorrhage			
Neuronal migration disorder			

[a]Polymerase chain reaction often available in larger clinical microbiology laboratories.

[b]Includes aseptic meningitis.

[c]Especially Group B streptococcus, Listeria monocytogenes, Citrobacter spp.

[d]Propionic acidemia, methylmalonic acidemia, urea cycle defects, maple syrup urine disease.

Infants and Children

Encephalitis in the older infant or child can be infectious or reflect an aberrant immunologic response to a previous infection (e.g., postinfectious encephalitis) (Tables 19.9 and 19.10). Infectious encephalitis is usually mild and often occurs in association with viral aseptic meningitis. Enteroviruses and some arthropod-borne viruses (arboviruses) are the most common causes of mild encephalitis (see Table 19.9). Herpes simplex virus infection is the leading cause of severe encephalitis throughout infancy and childhood.

Ehrlichia causes encephalitis much less commonly. Lyme disease occurs in the East, the upper Midwest, and the Pacific Northwest, although its geographic range is spreading. Most infections are asymptomatic. Approximately 15% of untreated patients can develop late neurologic sequelae, including meningitis, encephalitis, chorea, or neuritis.

Table 19.9
Common Etiologies of Acute Encephalitis in Childhood

	Frequency		Diagnosis		
	Infectious	Postinfectious	Culture	Serology Available	PCR[a]
Virus					
Enterovirus	++++[b]		Y		Y
Arthropod borne viruses	++++			Y	
Herpes simplex virus	+++		Y	Y	Y
Epstein-Barr virus	++			Y	Y
Adenovirus	+		Y		
HIV-1	+		Y	Y[c]	Y
Measles[d]	+	+	Y		
Mumps[d]	+	+	Y		
Rubella[d]	+	+	Y		
Varicella-zoster virus	+	++	Y	Y	
HHV-6	+	++	Y	Y	
Influenza virus	+	+	Y		
Nonspecific respiratory or gastrointestinal disease	+++				
Bacteria[e]					
Borrelia burgdorferi	++			Y	Y
Bartonella henselae	++				
Rickettsia rickettsii	++			Y	
Mycoplasma pneumoniae	+	+++		Y	
Vaccines		+			

[a]Polymerase chain reaction may be available in larger clinical microbiology laboratories.

[b]++++ frequent; +++ common; ++ infrequent; + rare.

[c]Insensitive during seroconversion.

[d]Rare in U.S. vaccinated population.

[e]Consider pyogenic bacteria, tuberculosis.

Table 19.10
Rare Causes of Encephalitis

Viruses	Fungi
Mumps virus	*Cryptococcus*
Parainfluenza virus	*Histoplasma capsulatum*
Influenza virus	*Blastomyces dermatitidis*
Respiratory syncytial virus	*Coccidioides immitis*
Hepatitis A virus	**Protozoa**
Hepatitis B virus	*Naeglaria fowleri*
Rabies	*Plasmodium falciparum*
Bacteria	
Treponema pallidum	
Leptospira spp.	
Brucella spp.	
Myocobacterium tuberculosis	
Nocardia spp.	
Listeria monocytogenes	
Whipple's disease	

In immunodeficient patients, the course of infectious encephalitis is frequently subacute or chronic (Table 19.11).

Clinical Manifestations and Differential Diagnosis

Neonates

Encephalitis should be considered in any infant with:

- Fever
- Signs of poor feeding
- Irritability
- Lethargy
- Sepsis
- Seizures or apnea
- History of maternal fever in the peripartum (presages neonatal enterovirus or adenovirus infection)
- History of maternal genital herpes
- HSV skin lesions

Evaluation of suspected neonatal sepsis should include cerebrospinal fluid culture for both bacteria and viruses. Abnormal liver function tests, consumptive coagulopathy, and acidosis are clues to disseminated disease.

Acyclovir is administered empirically to ill infants with a compatible history and signs of neonatal herpes infection. Management of less ill infants is individualized. Prolonged vomiting, hypoglycemia, and either severe acidosis or alkalosis with hyperammonemia in a young infant should lead to prompt evaluation and treatment for metabolic disorders.

Table 19.11
Encephalitis and Immunodeficiency

Immunodeficiency	Culture	Serology Available	PCR[a]	Blood Metabolites
Humoral				
Chronic enteroviral meningoencephalitis	Y		Y	
CMI (including transplantation)[b]				
PML[c]			Y	
Subacute HSV encephalitis	Y	Y	Y	
Subacute measles panencephalitis		Y		
Progressive rubella panencephalitis	Y	Y		
Cytomegalovirus	Y	Y	Y	
Toxoplasma gondii		Y	Y	
Adenovirus	Y	Y		
Varicella-zoster virus	Y	Y	Y	
Human herpesvirus 6		Y	Y	
Reaction to OKT3 infusion[d]				
AIDS[e]				
Toxoplasma gondii		Y	Y	
Cytomegalovirus	Y	Y	Y	
Cryptococcus neoformans	Y	Y		Y[f]
HIV-1 encephalopathy	Y	Y	Y	Y[g]

[a]Polymerase chain reaction may be available in larger clinical microbiology laboratories.

[b]Cell-mediated immunity.

[c]Progressive multifocal leukoencephalopathy (JC virus).

[d]Anti-lymphocyte globulin and anti-thymocyte globulin.

[e]Acquired immunodeficiency syndrome.

[f]D-arabinotol.

[g]Quinolinic acid.

Infants and Children

Clinical Findings Clinical manifestations of the inflammatory response are initially subtle and diverse. Some features of acute encephalitis are similar to those found in aseptic meningitis and include headache, stiff neck, photophobia, fever, vomiting, and irritability. The hallmark of the disease is alteration of higher cerebral function, evidenced by change in level of consciousness, with psychiatric and behavioral abnormalities, or seizure activity. Predominant cortical involvement may lead to disorientation and confusion, basal ganglia involvement to movement disorders, and brainstem involvement to cranial nerve dysfunction. In some cases, spinal cord involvement (i.e., myelitis) may accompany the encephalitis, and flaccid paraplegia with abnormalities of the deep tendon reflexes may be the presenting signs of the illness.

Distinguishing Encephalitides The various types of encephalitides cannot be distinguished on the basis of clinical signs or laboratory findings alone in most cases, although the presence of neurologic signs that localize to the temporal or frontal areas is suggestive of herpes simplex encephalitis.

Fever and Disease Onset Infectious encephalitis frequently begins with a prodrome of fever, headache, personality change, or irritability lasting from hours to days. Lethargy follows and is the extent of progression in most cases. In more severe cases of encephalitis, lethargy may progress rapidly to autonomic instability, coma and, in some cases, death.

The onset of postinfectious encephalitis is characteristically sudden. Convulsions, focal neurologic deficits, ataxia, movement disorders, and meningismus (with little pleocytosis) occur with both. Diagnosis of postinfectious encephalitis is more likely when onset of symptoms occurs one or more weeks after an upper respiratory illness or as fever or an exanthem subsides.

The diagnostic distinction between infectious and postinfectious encephalitis may be difficult when the infectious agents can cause both forms of encephalitis. Mumps encephalitis can precede parotitis by several days; infectious or postinfectious encephalitis can occur as parotitis wanes.

Predisposing Factors to Encephalitides

- Postinfectious encephalitis: antecedent respiratory illness, exanthem, or vaccination
- Epstein-Barr virus encephalitis: history of severe pharyngitis and fatigue in the older child
- *Bartonella henselae* (cat scratch) encephalitis: exposure to kittens
- Rocky Mountain spotted fever, Lyme disease, or encephalitis caused by an enterovirus or arbovirus: encephalitis in warm months, history of travel, or contact with ticks or mosquitoes
- Infectious meningitis: Foreign travel

Suggestive Physical Findings A careful physical examination of the patient is mandatory. The clinician should perform neurologic evaluation including global assessment, such as Glasgow coma scale, and examination of the patient's focal sensory, motor, and cerebellar function.

Prominent bulbar involvement can be suggestive of rabies infection. Documentation of specific findings should replace generalities such as lethargy. Infectious and postinfectious encephalitis may involve the brainstem predominantly. Discrete, localized involvement (e.g., Miller-Fisher syndrome,Birkenstaff's encephalitis) may be so extensive as to mimic brain death transiently. Postinfectious encephalitis typically involves multiple levels of the CNS, and the patient may have symptoms that demonstrate predominantly as cerebellar ataxia (especially after chicken pox), transverse myelitis, or optic neuritis. Lyme disease, which may include optic neuritis, cranial nerve palsies, and radiculitis, also involves multiple areas of the nervous system. *Listeria monocytogenes* rarely causes acute brainstem encephalitis without meningitis.

Careful examination of the skin may reveal a suggestive rash as is found in cases of Rocky Mountain spotted fever, Lyme disease, enteroviral, arboviral, and varicella infections. The rash of Rocky Mountain spotted fever is frequently subtle and present at the wrists, ankles, and axillae; rash of the palms and soles is an inconstant finding. Herpetic skin or mouth lesions in a child with encephalitis does not necessarily indicate causation. Parotitis, pharyngitis, or lymphadenopathy may suggest specific viral origins. Respiratory signs are present in less than 50% of patients with mycoplasma encephalitis.

Differential Diagnosis Hemorrhagic shock with encephalopathy is an idiopathic syndrome of cerebral edema and encephalopathy, profound shock, coagulopathy, and diarrhea. There is substantial overlap of the syndrome with heat stroke and malignant hyperthermia. Rectal temperature is usually greater than 39° C, and the onset of the encephalopathy is sudden. Brain infarction may occur. The coagulopathy appears after the hypotension; diarrhea may become bloody. The diagnosis requires the exclusion of septic shock, toxic shock syndrome, Reye syndrome, and hemolytic-uremic syndrome.

The patient who has Reye syndrome may have a prodrome of nausea and vomiting, followed by encephalopathy. Patients are usually afebrile and have hepatomegaly. Elevated blood ammonia is present in the majority of cases, but hypoglycemia and elevated liver transaminase levels are more variable. Although hemorrhagic shock with encephalopathy and Reye syndrome are not true examples of encephalitis, they must be considered in the differential diagnosis (Table 19.12).

Diagnosis

Cerebrospinal Fluid Analysis

The CSF is clear and colorless but it may be xanthochromic when blood has been present in the CSF for some time. CSF cell count and protein are frequently normal or slightly elevated, and the glucose concentration remains normal.

Viral Isolation and Identification

Viral agents are identified by rapid diagnostic technology, or by demonstration of a rise in specific antibody titer. In only 15 to 70% of cases is an etiologic agent identified. The disease is often inferred from the isolation of pathogens at anatomic sites other than the CNS or by serology.

Most HSV isolates from CSF are identified by tissue culture in 2 to 3 days. Isolation of enteroviruses, cytomegalovirus (CMV), or other viruses may be significantly slower. Many agents remain difficult to culture.

Rapid diagnostic technology augments diagnosis by tissue culture. Shell

Table 19.12
Differential Diagnosis of Acute Encephalitis

Infectious
  Bacterial meningitis
  Viral meningitis
  Tuberculosis meningitis
  Crytococcal meningoencephalitis
  Rocky Mountain spotted fever
  Brain abscess
Toxic
  Drug intoxication
  Lead encephalopathy
  Carbon monoxide poisoning
  Pertussis
  Shigellosis[a]
Metabolic
  Reye syndrome
  Hepatic coma
  Uremia
  Hypoglycemia
  Hypo, hyperosmolar states
  Organic acidemias
  Amino acidopathies
  Urea cycle defects
  Fat oxidation defects[b]
  MELAS syndrome[c]
  Acute intermittent porphyria
Primary brain abscess
  First presentation of epilepsy
  Neoplasms
  Cerebrovascular accidents
Vasculitis
  Systemic lupus erythematosis
  Polyarteritis nodosa
Other
  Pseudotumor cerebri
  Trauma
  Acute confusional migraine
  Postinfectious encephalopathies

---

[a]Also caused by Campylobacter jejuni, Salmonella spp., Yersinia spp.

[b]Medium and long chain acyl-CoA dehydrogenase deficiency.

[c]Mitochnodrial encephalopathy, lactic acidosis, stroke syndrome.

vial assay with fluorescent antibody staining may detect CMV within 24 hours with a sensitivity of approximately 60% of the standard tissue culture. PCR assays can detect DNA from HSV, enterovirus, cytomegalovirus, Epstein Barr virus, varicella-zoster virus, JC polyoma virus, *B. burgdorferi,* and *B. henselae.* Interpretation of polymerase chain reaction (PCR) results must include an awareness of the potential for false positives by cross-contamination of laboratory specimens, as well as false negatives caused by either the anatomic distance of the infectious encephalitis process from the meninges and CSF or the presence of inhibitory factors in CSF. Viral genomic material remains in the CSF from weeks to months, a potentially helpful factor in the elucidation of the cause of post-infectious encephalitis.

Table 19.13 outlines the laboratory evaluation of acute encephalitis.

Brain Biopsy

Before the clinical introduction of acyclovir, a drug without serious side effects, brain biopsy for histologic examination, viral culture, and fluorescent antibody staining was a diagnostic option. This procedure is rarely undertaken for the specific diagnosis of encephalitis.

Imaging Methods

Magnetic Resonance Imaging Magnetic resonance imaging detects brain inflammation and edema in the cerebral cortex, gray-white matter junction, basal ganglia, or cerebellum in infectious encephalitis. Postinfectious en-

Table 19.13
Laboratory Evaluation of Acute Encephalitis

Lumbar Puncture
  Opening pressure
  Routine studies
  Cerebrospinal fluid culture: virus, bacteria
  Consider PCR panel
  Consider specific antibody tests
  Consider myelin basic protein
Other cultures
  Blood culture: bacteria
  Virus isolation: nasopharynx and stool
  Consider virus isolation: blood buffy coat, urine
Metabolic screen
  Serum electrolytes, calcium
  Blood glucose
  Blood pH[a]
  Plasma ammonia[a] and amino acids
  Urine organic acid
  Toxicology screen: urine, serum
Magnetic resonance imaging
  Consider electroencephalogram if herpes simplex virus encephalitis suspected
Collect acute serum specimen
  Consider cold agglutinins
Contact local health epidemiologist

[a]Plasma for amino acids and urine for organic acids are collected and frozen immediately, and sent for assay if blood pH or ammonia are abnormal.

HANDBOOK OF PEDIATRIC INTENSIVE CARE

cephalitis is associated with foci of demyelination in the semilunar white matter, basal ganglia, brainstem, or spinal cord. Demyelination is best detected in T2-weighted images. Postinfectious encephalitis often involves multiple areas of the brain and spinal cord and tends to be symmetric. Lyme disease and multiple sclerosis may also involve diverse areas of brain, brain stem, and spinal cord.

Use of gadolinium contrast improves the sensitivity of MRI for vasculitis and cerebral abscesses. Gadolinium also confirms that the multifocal areas of demyelination in postinfectious encephalitis are all of the same stage; however, this is in contrast to multiple sclerosis, which rarely appears explosively in children.

Computed Tomography and Electroencephalogram Magnetic resonance imaging may be insensitive in detecting encephalitis early, especially in neonates with higher brain water content. The sensitivities of CT and MRI for HSV encephalitis outside of the neonate are 60 and 80%, respectively. EEG is equally sensitive as MRI (80%); the information is complementary to neuroimaging. CT scanning is superior to other methods for detecting intracranial calcifications caused by congenital CMV and toxoplasmosis, HIV infection, and some metabolic diseases.

Therapy

Need for Early Pediatric Intensive Care Unit Treatment

Most children with evidence of acute encephalitis and altered consciousness should be admitted to the PICU for initial evaluation and supportive care, especially in the early phases (i.e., the first 24 to 48 hours), when the differential diagnosis includes other possibilities, such as cerebrovascular accidents and poisoning. It is essential to monitor the course closely and to follow the neurologic examination meticulously. Severe encephalitis can lead to:

- Perivascular infiltrates
- Diffuse cerebral edema
- Elevation of ICP and cerebral herniation
- Seizures that are difficult to control
- Neuronal destruction, particularly of the brainstem, leading to respiratory compromise or hemodynamic instability

Medications

The use of corticosteroids is of no documented value and may prove harmful by causing dissemination of HSV. No recommendations can be given concerning the use of barbiturate coma as an adjunctive measure to control intracranial hypertension in this disease because no systematic studies of this problem have been reported.

Specific antiviral therapy has been of documented benefit only in therapy for herpes simplex infections.

Herpes Simplex Encephalitis

Neonates

Diagnosis Clinical diagnosis of herpes simples encephalitis is difficult unless skin vesicles are present. Cultures of conjunctivae, nasopharynx, and rectum obtained by single swab, in this order, at 48 to 72 hours of age may detect early infection of an exposed infant. Laboratory evidence of hepatocellular disease or coagulopathy may indicate disseminated viral sepsis. MRI, CT, and EEG findings are nonspecific. HSV can be isolated from CSF in approximately 50% of neonates with encephalitis or HSV sepsis, whereas isolation of the virus from older children and adults is uncommon. PCR is often used to diagnose HSV encephalitis.

Therapy Acyclovir and vidarabine are equally effective in treating neonatal HSV encephalitis. Cerebral necrosis may continue for several days after virologic cure. Virologic failures complicate 2% of cases and relapses may occur in 8% of patients after 10 days of acyclovir therapy at a dose of 30 mg/kg/day. Possible treatment regimens include acyclovir at a dose of 45 mg/kg/day for 3 weeks. Recurrences and relapses of HSV-2 have prompted some experts to consider oral prophylaxis with acyclovir for 3 to 6 months after neonatal infection. The 15 to 30% oral bioavailability of acyclovir requires large oral doses administered four to five times daily.

Famciclovir, a more bioavailable agent with longer half-life may be useful in the future in settings of prolonged therapy or secondary prophylaxis. Ganciclovir and foscarnet are active against herpes simplex, and new antiviral agents are in clinical trials.

Infants and Children

Pathogenesis HSV encephalitis in older children may result from primary and recurrent HSV infection. Approximately 70% of HSV encephalitis cases are the result of reactivation, whereas the remaining 30% represent primary infection.

Clinical Manifestations The clinical course in older children is similar to that in adults. In young children and infants, historic information does not generally result in strong support for the specific viral agent, unless gingivostomatitis or skin lesions are also present.

Encephalitis may begin suddenly or after a brief influenza-like prodrome. Children then manifest:

- Fever
- Headache

- Vomiting
- Behavioral changes
- Speech difficulty
- Decreasing consciousness
- Generalized and focal seizures (focal seizures are prominent)
- Neck stiffness
- Focal neurologic signs

In one series, all patients with biopsy-proven HSV encephalitis had evidence of focal CNS disease by clinical or neurodiagnostic assessment. Brain stem abnormalities develop that reflect effects of inflammation or cerebral edema and may be accompanied by papilledema and other signs of elevated ICP, including transtentorial herniation and cardiorespiratory instability.

The clinical syndrome consistent with herpes encephalitis may also be caused by human herpes virus 6, enteroviruses, metabolic disorders such as MELAS syndrome, acute hemorrhagic leukoencephalitis, or systemic vasculitis.

Herpes simplex virus encephalitis does not appear to be more common in immunosuppressed individuals. In some patients, the course is more indolent, with a paucity of inflammation and progression of neurologic deficits over weeks. Despite the high prevalence of seropositivity to HSV, CNS dysfunction in AIDS is correlated with CMV disease or other causes.

Diagnosis Laboratory findings in herpes encephalitis are nonspecific. When SIADH occurs, these patients may have hyponatremia, but otherwise, the electrolyte pattern is unremarkable.

Cerebrospinal Fluid Analysis Evaluation of CSF is essential. Abnormalities consistent with the diagnosis of encephalitis include:

- Pleocytosis, usually less than 200 WBC total and polymorphonuclear
- Progresses to a predominantly mononuclear cell count beyond first 24 to 48 hours of illness
- Xanthochromic fluid
- Elevated numbers of red blood cells
- Mean protein concentration of 80 mg
- Sensitivity of 82%
- Protein levels not exceeding 200 mg/100 mL
- Glucose content usually normal

The laboratory findings in the CSF may remain abnormal for several months. Opening pressure should be measured but will probably be low initially. A sample of spinal fluid should be sent for bacteriologic and viral culture, although it is exceedingly unlikely that herpes simplex will be isolated from the CSF, even during the acute phase of infection. PCR is helpful in the diagnosis of HSV.

Diagnostic Studies The particular predilection of the virus for the temporal or frontal lobes has been used in various ancillary diagnostic studies, which include EEG, CT scan, radionuclide brain scan, MRI scan, and brain biopsy.

The EEG demonstrates temporal region localization in approximately 80% of patients with characteristic paroxysmal localizing epileptiform discharges (PLEDS) in 65% of biopsy proven cases. Only approximately 50% of patients exhibit the classic EEG findings. Others may have nonspecific electrical activity on admission with lateralization occurring later in the course. Similar EEG findings may also occur in nonherpetic encephalitides, such as that resulting from infectious mononucleosis; therefore, EEG may provide evidence to support the diagnosis or point to an area of focal damage that could be biopsied, but it is not specific for HSV encephalitis.

Therapy Acyclovir is the treatment of choice for HSV encephalitis in patients older than 6 months. Treatment (30 mg/kg/day for 10 days) reduced mortality to approximately 30% from approximately 70% in untreated individuals. Relapse may occur in up to 5% of patients. Vidarabine (15 mg/kg/day for 10 days) reduces mortality to 44 to 54%; limited solubility of vidarabine requires its administration in fluid volumes of at least twice the daily basal metabolic requirement for water potentially complicating the management of cerebral edema and elevated intracranial pressure. Ganciclovir is active against most human herpes viruses but is associated with more toxicity.

Acyclovir, ganciclovir, vidarabine, and famciclovir are all prodrugs requiring virion-mediated phosphorylation for activation. Foscarnet and vidarabine do not require virion-enhanced phosphorylation for activity, and may be useful in rare instances or resistant (TK⁻) viruses. It is unclear whether corticosteroid or other immunomodulatory therapies attenuate the disease process of postinfectious encephalitis.

BRAIN ABSCESS

Although uncommon, brain abscesses are the most frequently encountered form of localized intracranial infection in children. Approximately 25% of all brain abscess occur in children younger than 15 years of age. Only recently has the almost uniformly fatal nature of the disease process been halted by a combination of new neurodiagnostic methods, rational use of antimicrobial agents, and appropriate surgical intervention. Death usually results from rupture of the abscess into the ventricular system with ensuing pyogenic ventriculitis or transtentorial herniation secondary to the mass effect of abscess and surrounding edema.

Pathogenesis

The infecting organism causing brain abscess may gain access to the CNS by one of several routes:

- Direct spread from a contiguous-infected extracranial site
- Hematogenous spread from an extracranial site of infection
- Inoculation of organism into brain parenchyma by penetrating trauma
- Spread from meningitis

Table 19.14 outlines the conditions predisposing to brain abscess in children, noting changes in epidemiology during the past 50 years.

The causative organism and the specific location of the abscess generally reflect the etiologic factors related to the abscess formation (Table 19.15). The microbial etiology of brain abscess in immunocompromised patients is also noted in Table 19.15.

Clinical Manifestations

The clinical course of brain abscess before diagnosis depends on the disease-causing organism, the pathogenic mechanism, the location of the abscess, and the presence or absence of meningitis or ventricular rupture.

The progression of the disease may be insidious, lasting many weeks or even months, or else relatively fulminant with rapid deterioration particularly if there is a rupture into the ventricular system with ventriculitis and meningitis. Most brain abscesses are diagnosed within 2 weeks of the onset of symptoms.

Table 19.14
Conditions Predisposing to Brain Abscess in Children

Predisposing Condition	Western Countries		Developing Nations
	Mid-1940s to 1960*	1960s to Present+	1960s to Present++
Congenital cyanotic heart disease	14.5%	35.5%	25.8%
Ear, nose, throat infection	43.9	23.1	23.9
Ear infection	36.2	9.3	21.6
Sinusitis	7.6	12.6	6.1
Head trauma	9.0	6.6	7.6
Neurosurgery	NR	3.3	1.7
Ventricular shunt	NR	2.6	2.2
Pulmonary infection	3.6	0.7	2.0
Dental infection	0.5	0.7	0.8
Bacterial meningitis	1.4	2.2	13.5
Tuberculosis	NR	1.5	NR
Other	11.3	9.5	4.8
Unknown	15.6	14.3	24.2

From Woods CR. Brain abscess and other intracranial suppurative complications. Adv Pediatr Infect Dis 1995;10:41–80.

*n = 221,+ n = 273,++ n = 356 cases from several published series; NR, not reported in these series.

Table 19.15
Relationship of Predisposing Condition to Site of Brain Abscess and Microbial Isolates

Predisposing Condition	Site of Abscess	Usual Microbial Isolates
Contiguous site		
Otitis media or mastoiditis	Temporal lobe or cerebellum	Streptococci (anaerobic or aerobic), *Staphylococcus aureus*, *Bacteroides fragilis*, *Proteus* spp., and other Enterobacteriacese *Haemophilus* spp., *Pseudomonas aeruginosa*
Frontoethmoidal sinusitis	Frontal lobe	Predominantly streptococci; also *Bacteroides*, Enterobacteriaceae, *S. aureus*, *Haemophilus* spp.
Sphenoidal sinusitis	Frontal or temporal lobe	Same as frontoethmoidal sinusitis
Dental infection	Frontal lobe	Mixed *Fusobacterium* spp., *Bacteroides* spp. streptococci
Primary infection		
Penetrating cranial trauma or postsurgical infection	Related to the site of the wound or surgery	*S. aureus*, streptococci (including pneumococci), Enterobacteriaceae, *Clostridium* spp.
Distant infection site		
Congenital cyanotic heart disease (CCHD)	Middle cerebral artery distribution common, can occur at any site; multiple abscesses common	Viridans, anaerobic, and microaerophilic streptococci, *Haemophilus* spp.
Lung abscess, other pulmonary lung infections	Same as in CCHD	*Fusobacterium, Antinomyces,* streptococci, *Nocardia* spp.
Bacterial endocarditis	Same as in CHHD	*S. aureus*, streptococci
Compromised hosts	Same as in CHHD	*Toxoplasma gondii*, *Nocardia* spp., fungi, Enterobacteriaceae

Adapted from Wispelwey B, Dacey RG, Scheld WM: Brain abscess, in Sheld WM, Whitley RJ, Durack DT: Infections of the Central Nervous System. New York, Raven, 1991, p. 459. From Woods CR. Brain abscess and other intracranial suppurative complications. Adv Pediatr Infect Dis 1995;10:41–80.

Neonates

Because brain abscess in neonates usually originates as a complication of meningitis, this entity should be suspected when the course of meningitis, particularly when caused by *Proteus mirabilis* or *Citrobacter diversus*, is complicated by persistently positive CSF cultures, enlarging head circumference, evidence of increased ICP of focal neurologic findings.

Older Children

The clinical manifestations of brain abscess include symptoms and signs of infection, raised ICP, and focal neurologic symptoms and signs that depend on the site of the abscess (Table 19.16).

Differential Diagnosis

The differential diagnosis of brain abscess is presented in Table 19.17.

Laboratory and Radiologic Diagnosis

Routine laboratory results usually do not eliminate or confirm the diagnosis of brain abscess:

- Elevated WBC count
- Elevated erythrocyte sedimentation rate
- Sterile blood cultures
- CSF pleocytosis
- Elevated CSF protein
- Low CSF glucose concentration
- Negative Gram's stain in the absence of ventriculitis or meningitis
- Negative bacterial culture
- Normal CSF in approximately 15% of patients with brain abscess

Because intracranial pressure is elevated in most patients with brain abscess and information gleaned from CSF examination is of little diagnostic or therapeutic use, a *spinal tap should not be performed* before neuroimaging studies if

Table 19.16
Signs and Symptoms of Children with Brain Abscess: Compilation From 13 Series of Pediatric Patients Encountered from 1945 to 1990

Manifestation	%
Headache	65
Fever	55
Vomiting	53
Papilledema	48
Focal neurologic deficit	47
Mental status changes	43
Meningeal signs	36
Seizure	34

From Woods CR. Brain abscess and other intracranial suppurative complications. Adv Pediatr Infect Dis 1995;10:41–80.

Table 19.17
Differential Diagnosis of Brain Abscess

Infectious	Vascular disorders
Meningitis	Venous thrombosis
Bacterial	Cerebral hemorrhage
Viral	Subarachnoid hemorrhage
Tuberculosis	Cerebral infarction
Encephalitis	Migraine headache
Empyema	**Others**
Subdural	Collagen-vascular disease
Epidural	Multiple sclerosis
Cranial osteomyelitis	Cholesteatoma
Mycotic aneurysms	Cerebral contusion
Brain tumors	Congenital hydrocephalus
Primary	Subdural effusion
Metastatic	

abscess is strongly considered. Approximately 25% of brain abscess patients develop signs of transtentorial herniation within several hours after a tap.

Definitive diagnostic studies are CT scanning, MRI, and radionuclide scanning of the brain, which have replaced arteriography and ventriculography for brain abscess diagnosis.

Therapy

The optimal management of most patients with pyogenic brain abscess requires both antibiotic and surgical drainage or excision. Surgical drainage of associated sinus or otologic suppurative disease may also be required.

Antimicrobial Agents

The choice of antibiotics is empiric, because there have been no controlled antibiotic trials. The choice of antibiotics reflects the likelihood of specific organisms in a given clinical setting and the ability of various antibiotics to penetrate the abscess.

- Penicillin, in combination with either chloramphenicol or metronidazole, penetrates the abscess cavities well and is bactericidal for most nonenterococcal streptococci and most anaerobes except *B. fragilis*.
- Chloramphenicol also has good abscess penetration and is bactericidal against most abscess causing organisms, apart from *S. aureus* and Enterobacteriaceae.
- Nafcillin or vancomycin has good abscess penetration and is indicated for *S. aureus* infections.
- Metronidazole is highly active against anaerobes.
- Third-generation cephalosporins are drugs of choice for most Enterobacteriaceae.

In general, aminoglycosides are not drugs of first choice because of poor penetration into abscess cavities and inactivation by low pH in pus.

A broad-spectrum combination of agents must be used. Two widely used combinations are (1) penicillin and chloramphenicol and (2) metronidazole and cefotaxime. For any antibiotic chosen, the highest recommended dose should be used in the therapy of brain abscess, and continued for 6 to 8 weeks. More specific antistaphylococcal therapy with a semisynthetic penicillin such as nafcillin or vancomycin, if methicillin resistance is suspected, should be used in patients whose abscess follows surgical or accidental trauma. Patients who are immunosuppressed should be evaluated for the presence of fungi or parasites, and antifungal therapy may be started if clinical response to broad-spectrum antibiotics fails. Table 19.18 lists suggested initial empirical regimens for brain abscess therapy according to predisposing underlying disease.

Corticosteroids

Although corticosteroids reduce edema surrounding the abscess and may be lifesaving when there is elevated ICP and clinical deterioration, these agents may decrease antibiotic penetration into the abscess cavity. There is no evidence, however, of delayed bacteriologic response to antibiotics when steroids are used.

Table 19.18
Suggested Initial Empirical Antimicrobial Regimens for Brain Abscess in Children According to Predisposing Condition

Underlying Condition	Antimicrobial Regimen
Congenital cyanotic heart disease[a]	Penicillin + chloramphenicol
Sinusitis or head trauma	Nafcillin[b] + chloramphenicol
Otitis/mastoiditis	Nafcillin[b] + ceftazidime + metronidazole
Ventricular shunt infection	Vancomycin + ceftazidime
Meningitis	Third-generation cephalosporin ± aminoglycoside
Unknown	Nafcillin[b] + third-generation cephalosporin + metronidazole
Immunocompromised host	Nafcillin[b] + ceftazidime + metronidazole with consideration of amphotericin B

From Woods CR. Brain abscess and other intracranial suppurative complications. Adv Pediatr Infect Dis 1995;10:41–80. Adapted from Sáez-Llorens XJ, Uman MA, Odio CM, et al: Pediatric Infect Dis J 8:455, 1989.

[a]Children with brain abscess and congenital cyanotic heart disease who have recently undergone corrective heart surgery should probably be treated similarly to children with ventriculoperitoneal shunt-related infections.

[b]Vancomycin should be substituted for nafcillin or other semisynthetic antistaphylococcal penicillins if a gram-positive organism with significant potential for resistance to these agents is suspected. A vancomycin dosage of up to 60 mg/kg/day given intravenously is indicated for intracranial infections. Peak concentrations should be monitored to ensure efficacy.

Surgical Drainage

Surgical intervention provides the definitive treatment of cerebral abscess, but must be timed appropriately to achieve optimal results. Aspiration of the abscess or excision are the surgical techniques available and debate continues as to their relative roles. Opinions for each of these techniques is supported in the literature but neither technique has been proven superior.

The brain abscess patient with depressed neurologic state requires admission to a neurointensive care environment. Measurement of ICP in the child with hydrocephalus accompanying the abscess or who has significant edema surrounding the abscess may help guide therapy directed toward reducing intracranial hypertension and diminish the risk of herniation.

Rupture

Rupture of a brain abscess into the ventricular system is a life-threatening event with a mortality that exceeds 50% and with high morbidity. Manifestations of rupture include:

- Shock
- High fever
- Altered sensorium
- Meningeal signs
- CSF leukocytosis in excess of 50,000 cells/mm^3
- Severe hypoglycorrhagia

Therapy must include surgical drainage and antibiotic therapy.

SUBDURAL EMPYEMA

The presence of pus in the subdural space is an acute life-threatening emergency constituting approximately 20% of focal suppurative intracranial lesions, and carries a mortality of 10 to 20%. Some authors claim it is the most neglected and least understood of the focal intracranial infections, and all agree it represents an important neurosurgical emergency.

Clinical Manifestations

Subdural empyema may take an acute or subacute course, and generally the patient has signs of intracranial hypertension, meningismus, and cerebral dysfunction-symptoms in the older child that are similar to those of brain abscess.

Signs and symptoms include:

- Headache
- Vomiting
- Obtundation
- Herniation

- Fever
- Stiff neck
- Focal neurologic signs (hemiparesis, hemiplegia, or seizures)
- Ocular, brainstem, or cerebellar signs
- Increasing head size in young infants
- Bulging fontanelle
- Irritability
- Lethargy
- Poor feeding
- Vomiting

The organisms responsible for the localized parameningeal infectious process are similar to those causing brain abscesses and depend on the pathogenic mechanisms and the age of the child. In the child and young adult, the most common organisms are the various aerobic streptococci, especially *S. pneumoniae. Staphylococcus epidermidis* and *S. aureus* follow closely. In the infant, the organisms most closely resemble the spectrum of agents seen in neonatal and infantile meningitis.

Laboratory and Radiologic Diagnosis

Laboratory findings are similar to those of brain abscess.

Computed Tomography Scanning

The CT scan usually defines the subdural process but may not document the presence of the infected mass. The usual appearance on CT scan is that of crescent-shaped lesion, which is hypodense, occasionally with visible loculations, and mass effect with shift of midline structures away from the side of the mass. Enhancement of the area immediately adjacent to the dura often occurs when contrast material is injected.

Magnetic Resonance Imaging

Magnetic resonance imaging is the diagnostic imaging procedure of choice. Advantages of MRI over CT scanning include the lack of bone artifact, the ability to detect smaller extracranial fluid collections, and the improved ability to differentiate extracranial fluid collection from cerebritis, cerebral edema, and venous thrombosis.

Treatment

Eradication of the infectious focus requires a combined medical and surgical approach, although the most appropriate or efficacious surgical intervention remains unclear in infants with subdural empyema complicating meningitis. Diagnostic paracentesis and possibly repeated subdural taps and antibiotic therapy is usually adequate.

Management Approach

Empyema secondary to otic or sinus infection requires surgical drainage either through burr holes or more usually through craniotomy. Whatever the surgical approach, high-dose antibiotic therapy, control of intracranial hypertension, and miscellaneous supportive measures must be part of the ongoing care provided in the PICU. Antibiotics are continued for 3 to 6 weeks, and the progression of the lesion should be followed with serial CT or MRI scans.

Medications

The choice of antibiotics before obtaining cultures and sensitivity results depends on the source of the infection. The appropriate treatment for meningitis (i.e., use of third-generation cephalosporin) can continue if the empyema complicates meningitis. Empirical antimicrobial therapy for other forms of subdural empyema is the same for brain abscess (see Table 19.18).

SPINAL EPIDURAL ABSCESS

Acute spinal epidural abscess is a distinctly uncommon entity, particularly in children. Although the disease is rare and diagnosis is difficult, the complications of the disease are tragic and extreme because the victim may become paraplegic. Prompt diagnosis and treatment before paralysis is complete is crucial and increases the likelihood of a favorable outcome.

Clinical Manifestations

The clinical presentation of spinal epidural abscess is related to patient age. The first of four classically described phases are back pain, hyperesthesias and other sensory deficits, limb paresis, and then total paraplegia.

Infants present with fever and irritability but because of the nonspecificity of the symptoms and the difficulty in making the diagnosis, are usually admitted with established severe neurologic deficits. Table 19.19 outlines the common signs and symptoms of 55 pediatric cases of spinal epidural abscess.

Differential Diagnosis

The differential diagnosis of spinal epidural abscess includes:

- Vertebral osteomyelitis
- Diskitis
- Herniated disk
- Spinal cord tumor
- Transverse myelitis
- Meningitis

Table 19.19
Signs and Symptoms in 55 Cases of Spinal Epidural Abscess

Signs and Symptoms	%
Fever	64
Back pain	54
Paralysis	45
Rigor	44
Sphinteric disturbance	38
Paresis	33
Spinal tenderness	27
Sensory level	24
Radicular pain	20
Irritability	16
Paraspinous mass	16
Headache	11
Nausea and vomiting	9
Lethargy	5
Paresthesia	5
Papilledema	2

From Rubin G, Michowiz SD, Ashkenasi A, Tadmor R, Rappaport ZH. Spinal epidural abscess in the pediatric age group: case report and review of the literature. Pediatr Infect Dis J 1993;12:1007–1011.

Diagnosis

Magnetic resonance imaging is the imaging method of choice, particularly with gadolinium contrast to enhance the images. If an MRI scan is not available, a CT scan may be helpful, but is only diagnostic in 30% of cases. The entire spine should be imaged because occasionally multiple abscesses are present.

Treatment

Surgical decompression with laminectomy with or without an epidural drain is the treatment of choice supplemented by appropriate antibiotic administration. Performing a laminectomy over many levels may cause concern because of the risk of instability and spinal deformity.

Appropriate cultures of pus are made at the time of drainage, and antibiotic therapy should be tailored to the culture results. Because of the high incidence of *S. aureus* as the cause of spinal epidural abscess, initial therapy should consist of a penicillinase-resistant penicillin together with a third-generation cephalosporin for Gram-negative coverage. Antibiotic therapy should be continued for at least 4 weeks.

CEREBRAL MALARIA

Cerebral malaria is a clinical syndrome characterized by CNS dysfunction associated with *Plasmodium falciparum* infection. Although it is one of the major causes of death in children in sub-Saharan Africa, it is rarely seen in developed countries. With the increase in international travel, however, the incidence of severe falciparum malaria, including cerebral malaria, in developed countries is likely to increase.

Pathophysiology

Pathophysiologic findings associated with cerebral malaria include the following:

- Seizures are an important presenting feature of cerebral malaria, especially in African children, and are associated with a poor outcome. Focal motor and generalized tonic-clonic convulsions are most common, but subclinical seizures (evident on EEG) are also present.
- Hypoglycemia is a common complication of severe falciparum malaria, particularly cerebral malaria.
- Lactic acidosis is a prominent feature of cerebral malaria in nonimmune adults and African children.
- Hemolytic anemia resulting from the destruction of parasitized erythrocytes is an inevitable consequence of a falciparum malaria infection. Severe anemia is one of the life-threatening complications of *P. falciparum* in African children, either in the presence or absence of cerebral malaria or acidosis.

Clinical Manifestations

World Health Organization criteria for the diagnosis of cerebral malaria include:

1. A patient is unable to localize a painful stimulus (such as pressure on the sternum) at least one hour after last seizure
2. Asexual parasites are present in the peripheral blood
3. Other causes of encephalopathy (e.g., meningitis, encephalitis, hypoglycemia) are excluded.

Table 19.20
Indications for Admission of a Patient with Cerebral Malaria to the Intensive Care Unit

Any pertubation of consciousness, more than 1 hour after seizure
Parasitemia > 5% erythrocytes
Hb < 5.0 g/dL or massive intravascular hemolysis
Repeated episodes of hypoglycemia
Severe metabolic acidosis: pH < 7.2
Spontaneous bleeding
Renal failure
Pulmonary edema

Table 19.21
Antimalarial Therapy

Primary antimalarial therapy

Quinidine (6.2 mg base = 10 mg gluconate salt	6.2 mg base/kg IV infusion over 1–2 h, followed by 0.012 mg/kg/min for 72 h or until patient can swallow.
Quinine (12.5 mg base = 15 mg dihydrochloride salt)	12.5 mg base/kg (loading dose) diluted in isotonic fluid by IV infusion over 2 h, then 8.4 mg/kg over 2 h until patient can swallow.

Drugs used to achieve complete cure

Quinine sulfate	25 mg/kg/d tid for 3–7 d.
Sulfadoxine + pyrimethamine (Fansidar)	Single dose of: <1 y: ¼ tablet 1–3 y: ½ tablet 4–8 y: 1 tablet 9–14 y: 2 tablets >14 y: 3 tablets
Clindamycin	20–40 mg/kg/d tid for 3 d

Although this definition is suitable for research purposes, any child with *P. falciparum* infection and disturbed consciousness should be treated for cerebral malaria.

Treatment

Antimalarial Therapy

Any child with severe falciparum malaria should be admitted to the PICU (Table 19.20) and begin a regimen of parental antimalarial therapy (Table 19.21).

Supportive Treatment

Close monitoring is essential. Blood glucose and fluid balance are measured every 6 hours, parasitemia and hematocrit every 12 hours. Electrolytes, renal function, albumin, calcium, phosphate, and blood gases are determined at least daily during the acute stages.

20.

Specific Infectious Diseases of Interest to the Intensivist

Alice D. Ackerman

Because almost all organisms, including those that usually are benign, may lead to life-threatening diseases or complications under special circumstances, it would be impossible to include a discussion of all the infections

563

the pediatric intensivist may be called on to treat. This chapter contains a selection of diseases that may be of interest to the pediatric intensivist.

TETANUS

Bacteriology and Epidemiology

Tetanus is a major cause of disease and death worldwide, despite the fact that immunization provides almost complete protection. Approximately half of the 500,000 annual deaths from tetanus occur in neonates.

Epidemiologically, tetanus has been divided into numerous types based on the method or source of contamination, including:

- Accidental
- Umbilical or neonatal
- Obstetrical
- Otogenic
- Surgical

Accidental tetanus, by far the most common type, occurs after contamination of a wound with *Clostridium tetani* spores. Under appropriate anaerobic conditions facilitated by the formation of pus or an abscess, a retained foreign body, or diminished blood flow to the area, the spores germinate into the vegetative forms (Fig. 20.1) capable of producing toxin. Although

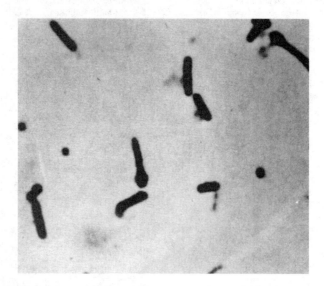

Figure 20.1. Typical drumstick appearance of *C. tetani* from a patient with tetanus. (From Finegold SM. Anaerobic bacteria in human disease. New York: Academic Press, 1977. With permission.)

deep wounds heavily contaminated with dirt or organic material may be more prone to develop clinical tetanus, any wound, abrasion, infection, burn, or ulceration must be considered suspect. Dental infections are relatively frequent but often overlooked sources of infection.

Action of Tetanus Toxin

Tetanospasmin, the toxin responsible for producing disease, is secreted only by vegetative forms of the organism. *C. tetani* exists in soil and animal excreta in the spore form. Toxin production requires induction of the vegetative state, which occurs only when the organism is introduced into a tissue that has a low redox potential and low partial pressure of oxygen. These conditions exist in tissue that has been damaged by injury, foreign body, or local production of pus. Toxin thus produced must then travel to the central nervous system (CNS).

Clinical Presentation

Symptomatology

Symptoms of tetanus develop after an incubation period of from 24 hours to several months after the injury. The usual incubation period is from 3 to 21 days. Symptoms are varied and include:

- Stiffness and crampy pain in the wounded muscle
- Neck and jaw stiffness
- Trismus (i.e., lockjaw) (75% of cases)
- Backache
- Muscular rigidity
- Lower extremity pain
- Facial paralysis
- Unexplained irritability
- Sensory changes
- Psychologic disturbances
- Mental status changes

Generalized Hypertonia

The patient with lockjaw, or trismus, presents with difficulty opening the mouth because of masseter spasm (Fig. 20.2) and is, therefore, unable to chew. As the other facial muscles become hypertonic, the facial features become somewhat contorted into the classic risus sardonicus (Fig. 20.3). The muscles of the trunk become involved next, which leads to rigidity in the paravertebral muscles, resulting in thoracic kyphosis and lumbar lordosis. The involvement of these muscles may result in opisthotonus (Fig. 20.4). The tenseness of abdominal muscles makes it difficult to eliminate peri-

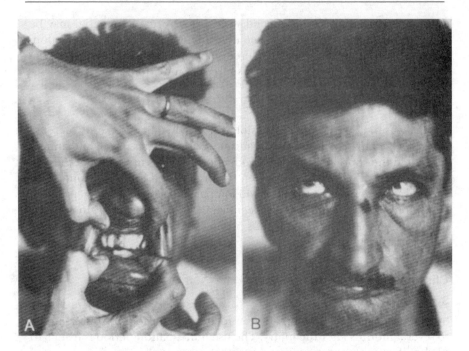

Figure 20.2. Trismus in a patient with tetanus. (From Veronesi R, ed. Tetanus: Important new concepts. Princeton, NJ: Excerpta Medica, 1981. With permission.)

tonitis or an abdominal source of the infection by clinical examination. The limb muscles are involved next, followed by the muscles of respiration. The upper limbs are flexed and the lower limbs extended.

Spasms

As tetanus progresses, the patient develops tetanic convulsions, which actually are rhythmic spasms of sometimes frightening intensity and which may be quite painful. Depending on the severity of the disease, such spasms may occur several times per day to as often as once a minute. When the spasms involve the glottis and respiratory muscles, apnea occurs and may be followed quickly by death if it does not resolve rapidly or is not treated aggressively with muscle relaxants and respiratory support. Pharyngeal spasms result in severe dysphagia, which makes eating impossible. Clinically, tetanus has been divided into three general grades: benign, moderate, and severe (Table 20.1).

Neonatal Tetanus

Neonatal tetanus is almost always generalized and usually severe. The median time of onset is at 6 to 7 days of life. Symptoms include difficulty sucking and

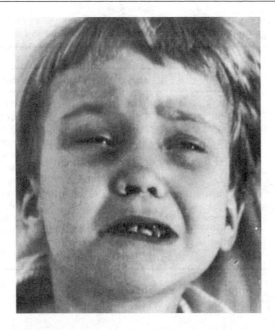

Figure 20.3. Risus sardonicus in a young girl with tetanus. (From Veronesi R. ed. Tetanus: Important new concepts. Princeton, NJ: Excerpta Medica, 1981. With permission.)

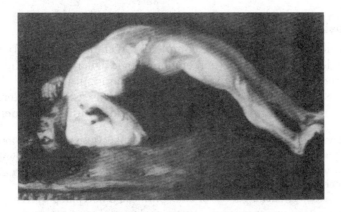

Figure 20.4. Portrait by Sir Charles Bell of a British soldier with tetanus. (From Finegold SM. Anaerobic bacteria in human disease. New York. Academic Press, 1977. With permission.)

swallowing (stiffness of the jaw and pharyngeal muscles) followed by generalized hypertonicity and tetanic spasms. Apnea is commonly a result of spasm of the respiratory muscles, and vomiting occurs because of increased abdominal tone, frequently resulting in pulmonary aspiration of gastric contents.

Table 20.1
Grades of Tetanus Severity[a]

	Grade		
Factor	Benign	Moderate	Severe
Incubation period	>20 days	10 to 20 days	<10 days
Spasms	Absent	Present	Frequent and severe
Fever	Absent	Present	>39° C
Dysphagia	Absent	Present	Severe
Muscle rigidity	Mild: generalized or localized	Intense; upper body most affected	Intense, generalized without relief
Other signs		Cough—inhibited	Apnea, sympathetic overactivity, tissue hypoxia
Therapy	Observation ± sedation	Sedation ± neuromuscular blockade	Sedation, paralysis ± treatment of autonomic dysfunction

[a]Data from Veronesi R, Focaccia R. The clinical picture. In: Veronesi R, ed. Tetanus: important new concepts. Princeton, NJ: Excerpta Medica, 1981:183. With permission.

If the child survives, the spasms generally subside by the end of the second week of illness. Swallowing returns by the end of the fourth week, and relaxation of the hypertonic muscles may take another 2 weeks.

Diagnosis

The diagnosis of tetanus is made completely on clinical grounds. Diagnosis can be aided by obtaining certain epidemiologic data regarding the nature of a preceding injury and a history of previous immunization.

There are no serologic tests to document the disease, and bacteriologic cultures often are negative. Nonspecific laboratory findings include:

- Elevated total white blood cell count with leukocytosis and lymphopenia
- Alterations in the serum protein electrophoretic pattern, with elevation in the $\alpha 2$- and γ-globulin fractions
- Decreased concentrations of $\alpha 1$- and β-globulins
- Increased circulating levels of epinephrine and norepinephrine, as well as a high rate of urinary excretion of metabolites of these compounds
- Elevated plasma creatine phosphokinase levels

Differential Diagnosis

Diagnosis often is difficult or delayed in the patient with early tetanus, who presents with no clear evidence or history of injury and with localized neck stiffness or trismus. Meningitis is easily eliminated because, at this stage, fever does not generally manifest and the child has no mental status changes. The cerebrospinal fluid (CSF) may be mildly abnormal, especially with elevated protein content. Trismus has many causes, and youngsters who arrive in the emergency department unable to open their mouths most likely have a peritonsillar abscess, temporomandibular joint disease, or abscess of the alveolar ridge. Patients suffering from an acute phenothiazine reaction show torticollis in addition to trismus, making that entity easily eliminated.

Other diseases that may mimic tetanus are hypocalcemic tetany, strychnine poisoning, and rabies. In rabies, CNS involvement with altered mental status occurs early in disease, and there is prominent early development of respiratory embarrassment and dysphagia; in strychnine poisoning, symptoms advance rapidly, trismus occurs late, and hypertonia alternates with hypotonia. Many patients may be misdiagnosed on initial visit to a physician (Table 20.2).

Complications

Respiratory System

Respiratory insufficiency may result from spasm of the inspiratory muscles or from acute laryngospasm. Early intervention with muscle relaxation, airway control with an endotracheal tube, and assisted ventilation with induction of total or partial neuromuscular blockade has become the mainstay of tetanus therapy in the intensive care unit (ICU) and is responsible for diminution of the death rate.

Table 20.2
Alternative Diagnosis of 47 Patients with Tetanus at the First Visit to a Doctor[a]

Diagnosis	Number of patients
Pharyngitis, common cold	7
Undefined neurologic disease	6
Side effect of phenothiazine	4
Disease of the esophagus	4
Epilepsy	3
Psychogenic symptoms	3
Stomatitis	2
Disease of the temporomandibular joint	2
Encephalitis	2
Facial paresis	2
Other	12
Total	47

[a]Modified with permission from Luisto M. Tetanus in Finland: diagnostic problems and complications. Ann Med 1990;22:15–19.

Autonomic Nervous and Cardiovascular Systems

The cardiovascular complications of tetanus carry the greatest risk of death in today's ICU environment. Involvement of the autonomic nervous system occurs primarily in patients with severe disease who require mechanical ventilation, most of whom are receiving many sedative drugs, muscle relaxants, and usually pharmacologic paralysis. Sympathetic and parasympathetic disinhibition occur.

Sympathetic Overactivity

Symptoms generally occur by the second to third week of illness. The syndrome is heralded by elevation of heart rate and blood pressure, which vary in a hectic fashion, unrelated to generation of spasms (Fig. 20.5). The changes are associated with increased cardiac output, elevation of peripheral vasomotor tone, and elevated venous pressure.

Clinical signs include the following:

- Peripheral vasoconstriction, which may cause actual ischemia and pallor in a stocking-glove distribution
- Profuse sweating of the face and thorax, even with peripheral constriction and the absence of hyperpyrexia
- High fevers
- Electrocardiographic evidence of sinus tachycardia, supraventricular tachycardia, multifocal premature atrial contractions, and premature ventricular contractions

24-HOUR OBSERVATION

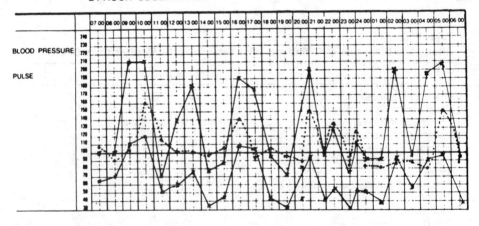

Figure 20.5. Graphic representation of marked cardiovascular disturbances in a patient with severe tetanus, on Day 7 of hospitalization, before treatment with MgSO$_4$. × ——— ×, blood pressure; •••, pulse rate. (From James MFM, Manson EDM. The use of magnesium sulfate infusions in the management of severe tetanus. Intensive Care Med 1985;11:5. With permission.)

The constellation of symptoms may occur spontaneously or in response to even minor stimuli, as is the case with tetanic spasms. It cannot be alleviated through pain control or sedation. Epinephrine and norepinephrine levels are elevated, the significance of which goes beyond symptomatic sympathetic overdrive and may cause direct myocardial damage. Sympathetic overactivity may end with profound and untreatable hypotension and bradycardia, with evolving and progressive myocardial failure and associated alterations in ST segments and T waves, suggesting cardiac ischemia.

Parasympathetic Overactivity

Parasympathetic overactivity may lead to severe bradycardia, sinus arrest, and increased bronchial and salivary secretions. Patients may respond to endotracheal suctioning with marked bradycardia. Direct damage to the vagal nucleus has been implicated, in addition to potential local damage to the sinus node, and to reflex excessive vagal tone.   .

Treatment of Autonomic Dysfunction

Management Approach It is prudent to achieve full control of the respiratory system first, thereby also achieving control of painful muscle spasms. If wide swings in blood pressure or heart rate are occurring with any degree of frequency, the clinician should seek to reduce further stimulation of the patient, if possible, and should provide additional pain relief with a narcotic agent. Additional therapy should aim to further depress the CNS, if tolerated (e.g., through the use of high-dose barbiturate).

Magnesium Therapy Administration of $MgSO_4$ has been successful and without major adverse effects on cardiac function (Fig. 20.6).

Beta Blockade Attempts to control heart rate and blood pressure through β-blockade may risk sudden death because of increased α-activity in the face of diminished cardiac function from β-blockade. Successful therapy with labetalol has been reported. If pure β-antagonist agents are used, they should be given in small doses intravenously and titrated for effect. The use of enterally administered propranolol is contraindicated.

Death Respiratory failure continues to lead the list of causes of death, followed by hemodynamic instability, hemorrhage, and sepsis caused by superinfection of the lung or urinary tract. Although the death rate directly attributable to tetanus has dropped dramatically with the advent of intensive care, deaths caused by iatrogenic and other complications have become more frequent.

Therapy

The goals of acute therapy of tetanus are to support the vital functions and provide pain relief and muscle relaxation.

24-HOUR OBSERVATION

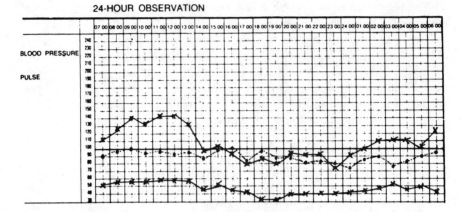

Figure 20.6. Twenty-four hour record of the same patient as in Figure 18.5, 2 days after commencement of magnesium therapy. X ——— X, blood pressure; •••, pulse rate. (From James MFM, Manson EDM. The use of magnesium sulfate infusions in the management of severe tetanus. Intensive Care Med 1985;11:5. With permission.)

Table 20.3
Medical Therapy for Tetanus

Therapeutic Effect	Therapeutic Measure
Muscle relaxation	Diazepam
	Morphine
	Chlorpromazine
	Dantrolene
	Propofol
Stop convulsions, achieve adequate ventilation	Pancuronium bromide
	Atracurium
Airway control	Tracheostomy
	Nasotracheal intubation (preferred in neonates)
Inhibit growth of *C. tetani*[a]	Penicillin
	Chloramphenicol

[a]Prevents generation of more toxin but will not change the natural history of the disease.

Medical Therapy

Treatment options are outlined in Table 20.3.

Surgical Intervention

When the injury is still apparent, especially if there is any chance of a retained foreign body, the wound should be explored and debrided. Tetanus hyperimmune globulin should be administered immediately; if possible, an hour or so before surgical debridement. The value of antitoxin is limited, because it is without effect on toxin that has already bound to nervous tissue and can only inactivate free toxin in the bloodstream.

Immunization

Because natural immunity to tetanus does not occur, the patient with tetanus must receive active immunization to prevent recurrence of disease. Immunization should begin during the acute hospital course. The primary immunization series should be provided over a 6-month period. Patient education is exceedingly important in this regard.

BOTULISM

This disease is caused by a deadly neurotoxin elaborated by the bacterium Clostridium botulinum, an anaerobic Gram-positive bacillus that is distributed widely in nature.

Action of the Toxin

The most deadly substance known to man, botulin toxin is capable of causing death in extremely small doses. This heat-labile toxin blocks release of acetylcholine from nerve endings at four different levels of the peripheral nervous system: the neuromuscular junction, parasympathetic nerve endings, autonomic ganglia, and acetylcholine-releasing sympathetic nerve endings. The effects on the neuromuscular junction are considered the most important.

Clinical Syndromes

Three specific forms of disease are infant, foodborne, and wound botulism. An unclassified disease category includes victims older than 1 year of age in whom a vehicle of infection cannot be identified.

Infant Botulism

Epidemiology This rare disease is caused by the *C. botulinum* toxin, which is produced within the gastrointestinal tract of the victim. Infant botulism is limited to patients 1 to 12 months of age. There is no racial or sexual prevalence. More cases have been identified in California than anywhere else.

Honey has been implicated in approximately 35% of cases. *C. botulinum* spores, but not toxin, have been found in the honey that has been fed to some of these patients. It is therefore recommended that children younger than 1 year of age not be fed honey.

Clinical Features The clinical spectrum of infant botulism ranges from asymptomatic "carriage" of *C. botulinum* to a hyperacute form of disease that may mimic sudden infant death syndrome (SIDS). Most infants suffer from disease of moderate to severe intensity and require hospitalization.

General Signs and Symptoms Common signs and symptoms of infant botulism appear in Table 20.4. The order of progression of some of these symptoms is included in Table 20.5.

Physical Findings Some physical findings that may be helpful in the early diagnosis of infant botulism are listed in Table 20.6. There may be associated findings consistent with pneumonia and metabolic abnormalities accompanying dehydration, which may confuse the clinical picture.

Disease Progression General muscle weakness and hypotonia usually precede the onset of respiratory insufficiency (Fig. 20.7). Not all babies, however, progress to develop respiratory muscle paralysis. Administration of aminoglycosides may worsen the progression of the paralysis because these antibiotics decrease the release of acetylcholine from the nerves innervating the diaphragm. As depicted in Table 20.5, the progression of symptoms in infant botulism is comparable to those elicited in awake adults receiving small sequential doses of competitive muscle relaxants. As in patients who are partially paralyzed by nondepolarizing agents, flexion of the neck may result in acute airway obstruction and apnea.

Once weakness becomes apparent, it generally progresses over a period of several days to a maximal point, remains at a relatively constant state for at least 2 weeks, then gradually improves. Infants who progress to respiratory failure may require assisted ventilation for several months, and tracheostomy may be necessary.

Diagnosis Presumptive diagnosis can be made on the basis of the signs and symptoms and progression of illness. Definitive diagnosis requires demonstration of toxin in the blood or of the organism, toxin, or spores in the stool. Supportive evidence is provided in many cases by electrodiagnostic studies (Fig. 20.8).

Differential Diagnosis The most commonly entertained diagnosis in babies with early infant botulism is sepsis. Other entities to be considered are listed in Table 20.7.

Therapy

Assessment and Critical Care Management Babies with suspected infant botulism who show any signs of muscle weakness should be carefully observed and monitored for apnea and bradycardia, preferably in an ICU or intermediate care unit. If gag and cough reflexes are suppressed, no attempts should be made to feed the patient by mouth. The clinician should assess respiratory mechanics and reserve, and if respiratory insufficiency seems imminent, intubation of the trachea or tracheostomy should be performed and assisted ventilation should be provided as needed.

Antitoxin and Antibiotics Affected infants do not require treatment with antitoxin, nor have antibiotics (i.e., parenteral, oral) been proven to be ef-

Table 20.4
Signs and Symptoms in Hospitalized Patients with Infant Botulism[a]

Autonomic dysfunction
Constipation
Neurogenic bladder
Hypertension

Hypotonia and weakness
Decreased resistance to passive motion
Lack of spontaneous motor activity
Motor response to noxious stimuli diminished
Poor head control

Cranial nerve dysfunction
Decreased suck and swallow ability
Weak cry
Facial diplegia
External ophthalmoplegia
Sluggishly reactive pupils

Absent or diminished deep tendon reflexes

Respiratory insufficiency
Associated with progressive weakness and cranial nerve dysfunction
Provoked by postural manipulation for procedures

[a]From Brown LW. Infant botulism. Adv Pediatr 1981;28:141. With permission.

Table 20.5
Comparison of Symptom Progression in Patients with Infant Botulism and Those Undergoing Competitive Neuromuscular Blockade[a]

Infant botulism	Competitive blockade
Constipation, tachycardia	Blurred vision, tachycardia
↓	↓
Loss of head control[b]	Loss of head lift[b]
Difficulty feeding[b]	Weakness in jaw muscles
Weak cry[b]	Decreased hand grip (sustained)[b]
Depressed gas reflex[b]	Bulbar weakness
↓	↓
Peripheral motor weakness	Peripheral motor weakness
↓	↓
Diaphragmatic weakness	Diaphragmatic weakness

[a]From L'Hommedieu C, Polin RA. Progression of clinical signs in severe botulism: therapeutic implications. Clin Pediatr 1981;20:90.

[b]Repetitive muscle activity.

Table 20.6
Physical Findings that May Be Helpful in the Diagnosis of Infant Botulism[a]

Test	Findings	Interpretation
1. Shine a bright light in the eye and observe the briskness of the pupillary light reflex. Once the iris constricts, remove the light. As soon as the iris dilates, again shine the light in the eye. Continue for 1–3 min without interruption.	Pupillary constriction, which may initially be brisk, eventually becomes sluggish. An initially midposition pupil may become dilated at rest as the test continues.	Fatigability when repetitive muscle contraction is required is one hallmark of botulism. Infection—a most important consideration in the differential diagnosis at presentation—does not impair the pupillary light reflex (unless the infection is of the central nervous system).
2. Shine the light along the optical axis so that it falls directly on the fovea. Keep the light continuously on the fovea for 1–3 min, even if the infant tries to deviate his eyes. Observe the infant's efforts and ability to deviate the eyes. Observe the vigor and purpose-fulness of the infant's efforts to avoid the light.	Latent ophthalmoplegia may be elicited. Efforts to push away the examiner's hand or to squirm away from the light may be feeble or not purposefully continued.	A sustained bright light on the fovea is most uncomfortable, and an infant with normal motor ability will use it to avoid sensation.
3. Place a clean fifth finger in the infant's mouth (but be certain that doing so will not compromise adequate air flow). Note the strength and especially the duration of the reflex sucking efforts. If the infant has an empty stomach, advance the finger and manually gauge the briskness and strength of the gag reflex. (Feeling the gag reflex regularly is also a useful way to follow the infant's recovery.)	The suck is weak and of short duration. The gag reflex is diminished.	Fatigability, as in 1 above.

[a]From Arnon SS: Infant botulism. Annu Rev Med 1980;31:541.

fective, except for therapy of associated infectious complications. If amino-glycoside antibiotics must be used, they should be given in the ICU under the supervision of a physician trained in the care of the infant airway.

Purgatives The use of purgatives and emetics has not been proven effective and is potentially dangerous in the impaired child.

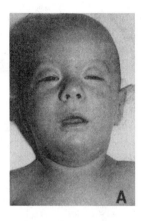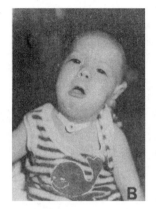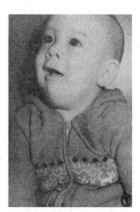

Figure 20.7. Typical case of infant botulism. A. On day of admission, baby had bilateral ptosis and facial diparesis. B. Same infant 4 weeks later with tracheostomy in place because of persistent inadequate protective airway reflexes, multiple cranial nerve involvement, and poor head control. C. Nine weeks after admission; complete recovery. (From Brown LW. Infant botulism. Pediatr Ann 1984;13:135. With permission.)

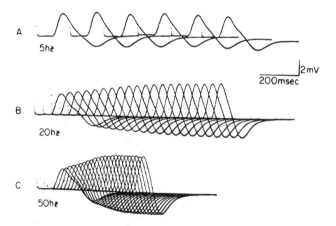

Figure 20.8. Repetitive nerve stimulation of patient with infant botulism at different rates. A. No augmentation at 5 Hz. B. 48% incremental response of staircase phenomenon at 20 Hz. C. Maximal supratetanic rate of stimulation (50 Hz) producing 60% incremental response. (From Brown LW. Infant botulism. Pediatr Ann 1984;13:135. With permission.)

Prophylaxis Because organisms and, more importantly, toxin are excreted in the stool for as long as several months after onset of the infection, caretakers must be instructed in methods for avoiding exposure. Likewise, all specimens sent to the laboratory should be labeled with the possible diagnosis and transported in biohazard containers.

Table 20.7
Differential Diagnosis of Infant Botulism[a]

Systemic
Sepsis/meningitis
Electrolyte/mineral imbalance
Metabolic encephalopathy
Reye syndrome
Intoxication—organophosphates, heavy metals
Hypothyroidism
Substance necrotizing encephalomyelitis
Organic acidurias

Neuromuscular
Poliomyelitis
Infantile spinal muscular atrophy
Acute polyneuropathy—Guillain-Barré syndrome, diphtheria
Tick paralysis
Congenital myasthenia gravis
Muscular dystrophy—"congenital," myotonic dystrophy
Congenital myopathy

[a]From Brown LW, Infant botulism. Adv Pediatr 1981;28:141. With permission.

Foodborne Botulism

Botulism that occurs after ingestion of preformed toxin in contaminated food is the most common of all forms of the disease. Food products most often associated with disease are home-canned vegetables, fruits, meat products, and seafood. An incubation period of several hours to 8 days follows ingestion of the toxin-containing food. In general, the shorter the incubation period, the more severe and protracted the disease.

Diagnostic Signs Symptoms of foodborne botulism include:

- Cranial nerve dysfunction
- Diplopia
- Dysarthria
- Dysphagia
- Gastrointestinal distress (nausea, vomiting, diarrhea, and abdominal pain; constipation later)
- Descending muscle weakness (may be more pronounced in proximal limbs)
- Dry mucous membranes
- Urinary retention
- Normal or fixed and dilated pupils
- Depressed but symmetric reflexes

The cardinal features of botulism are listed in Table 20.8. Tachycardia is not a prominent finding in this form of botulism.

Differential Diagnosis The differential diagnosis includes numerous diseases, mostly noninfectious (Table 20.9). As in infant botulism, definitive diagnosis depends on demonstration of the toxin in the patient's stool or serum, although this is not always possible. Suspect food should also be examined, if available. Electromyography is helpful in foodborne botulism, with findings similar to those in infant botulism.

Therapy

General Approach Treatment consists of induced vomiting and catharsis and careful observation of the patient. Emesis should not be induced if the airway reflexes are impaired or if consciousness is severely depressed. In this case, controlled intubation of the trachea with a cuffed endotracheal tube followed by gastric lavage may be an alternative. Supportive care, including assisted ventilation, is lifesaving.

Use of Antitoxin Administration of antitoxin is effective only if provided early in the course of the disease. Botulinal toxin is irreversibly bound to nerve endings, so antitoxin has no effect once binding has occurred. Toxin may circulate in serum up to 30 days after the onset of disease. The decision to use antitoxin is not a simple one, as great risks such as anaphylaxis and serum sickness are associated with administration of the drug, which is a horse serum product. Nevertheless, the Centers for Disease Control and Prevention (CDC) recommends immediate administration of trivalent (ABE) antitoxin to patients diagnosed as having botulism. It may be obtained from the CDC by calling the Drug Service at (404) 639-3670 during business hours, and at (404) 639-2888 at all other times.

Adjunctive Measures Treatment may include administration of drugs, such as guanidine, that increase the amount of acetylcholine released at the nerve terminals. These agents have not been proven definitely effective and have a long list of potential adverse effects.

Wound Botulism

Wound botulism is rare and consists of signs and symptoms of botulism after an injury in the absence of an identifiable food source and without evi-

Table 20.8
Botulism: Five Cardinal Features as Defined by CDC[a]

Absence of fever except in presence of complicating infection
Normal mental status
Pulse rate normal or slow
Absence of numbness, paresthesias, and sensory deficit
Neurologic manifestations usually symmetrical

[a]Data from Centers for Disease Control. Botulism in the United States, 1899–1977. In: Handbook for epidemiologists, clinicians, and laboratory workers. May 1979.

Table 20.9
Differential Diagnosis of Foodborne Botulism

Other types of food poisoning: *Staphylococcus, Salmonella, Shigella,* chemical
Guillain-Barré syndrome
Carbon monoxide poisoning
Cerebrovascular accident
Viral encephalitis
Neuropsychiatric disorders
Phenothiazine drug reaction
Myasthenia gravis
Alcohol or other chemical intoxication
Diphtheria
Tick paralysis

dence of gastrointestinal disease. Diagnostic and therapeutic considerations are described previously.

TOXIC SHOCK SYNDROME

Toxic shock syndrome is caused by coagulase-positive staphylococci that liberate an exoprotein now known as toxic shock syndrome toxin-1 (TSST-1). Although some patients have evidence of *Staphylococcus aureus* bacteremia or deep tissue infection, simple colonization of a wound or mucous membrane with a TSST-1 liberating strain is enough to cause severe disease. In addition to menstruating women, the syndrome also occurs in burned or scalded children.

Diagnosis

There is no rapid diagnostic test. Diagnosis is based on meeting CDC clinical and laboratory criteria (Table 20.10). The criteria subsequently have been amended to allow blood cultures positive for *S. aureus*. An alternative diagnostic scheme proposed for children is listed in Table 20.11. This scheme has not been adopted by CDC.

Differential Diagnosis

The spectrum of differential diagnoses is presented in Table 20.12.

Clinical Manifestations

Toxic shock syndrome is a multisystem disease (Fig. 20.9). Massive vasodilation with extravasation of fluid and serum proteins result in:

Table 20.10
Toxic Shock Syndrome Case Definition[a]

Criteria A

Fever—Temperature ≥ 38.9° C (102° F)

Rash—Diffuse or palmar erythrodema progressing to subsequent peripheral desquamation (hands and feet)

Mucous membrane—Nonpurulent conjunctival hyperemia, or oropharyngeal hyperemia, or vaginal hyperemia, or discharge

Hypotension—Systolic blood pressure <90 mm Hg for an adult (>16 years) or <5th percentile for age for a child; or orthostatic hypotension as shown by a drop in diastolic blood pressure ≥15 mm Hg from recumbent to sitting; or history of orthostatic dizziness

Multisystem involvement (≥4 of the following):

Gastrointestinal—History of vomiting or diarrhea at onset of illness

Muscular—CPK, ≥2 × ULN 4–20 days after onset

CNS—Disorientation or alteration in consciousness without focal signs at a time when patient is not in shock or hyperpyrexic

Renal—BUN or serum creatinine clearance, ≥2 × ULN, and abnormal findings on urinalysis (≥5 WBCs per high power field; ≥1 RBC per high power field; protein, ≥1 +); or oliguria defined as urine output <1 mL/kg/h for 24 h

Hepatis—Total serum bilirubin level ≥1.5 × ULN; or SGPT ≥2 × ULN.

Hematologic—Thrombocytopenia (platelets <100,000/mm³)

Cardiopulmonary—Adult respiratory distress syndrome; or pulmonary edema; or new onset 2° or 3° heart block; or ECG criteria for myocarditis decreased voltage and ST-T wave changes; or heart failure shown by new onset of gallop rhythm, or by increase in size of cardiac silhouette from one chest roentgenogram to another during the course of the illness, or diagnosed by cardiologist

Metabolic—Serum calcium level, ≤7.0 mg/dL with serum phosphate level, ≤2.5 mg/dL, and total serum protein level, ≤5.0 mg/dL

Evidence for absence of other causes:

When obtained; negative blood, throat, urine, or CSF culture results[b]

When obtained; absence of serologic evidence of leptospirosis, rickettsial disease, or rubeola

Evidence for absence of Kawasaki syndrome; no unilateral lymphadenopathy or fever lasting >10 days

Criterion B

At least two episodes meeting criteria for fever, rash, mucous membrane, hypotension, and one of the situations under multisystem involvement

---

[a]From Chesney PJ, Davis JP, Purdy WK, et al. Clinical manifestations of toxic shock syndrome. JAMA 1981; 246:741.

[b]Blood cultures positive for *S. aureus* are accepted.

CPK, creatinine phosphokinase; ULN, upper limits of normal for the laboratory; BUN, blood uear nitrogen; WBCs, white blood cells; RBC, red blood cell; SGPT, serum glutamic pyruvic transaminase; ECG, electrocardiogram; CSF, cerebrospinal fluid.

- Hypotension
- Oliguria with acute tubular necrosis
- Low central venous pressures
- Pulmonary and peripheral edema
- Low serum albumin levels with hypocalcemia

Table 20.11
Proposed Simplified Diagnostic Criteria for Toxic Shock Syndrome in Children[a]

Pyrexia ≥39° C
Lymphopenia
Rash
Shock
Diarrhea and/or vomiting
Irritability

[a]Modified with permission from Cole RP, Shakespeare PG. Toxic shock syndrome in scalded children. Burns 1990;16:221–224.

Table 20.12
Differential Diagnosis of Toxic Shock Syndrome

Infections
Rash-associated viral syndromes
Rocky Mountain spotted fever
Kawasaki disease
Scaled skin syndrome
Streptococcal scarlet fever
Overwhelming sepsis
Leptospirosis
Tick typhus
Legionnaires' disease
Gastroenteritis
Pelvic inflammatory disease

Noninfectious (or postinfectious)
Acute rheumatic fever
Hemolytic uremic syndrome
Lupus
Adverse drug reactions

Complications

Toxic shock syndrome is associated with:

- Rhabdomyolysis (i.e., increased urine and serum myoglobin values)
- Hypophosphatemia
- Metabolic acidosis
- Hypoventilation secondary to severe muscle weakness
- Acute respiratory distress syndrome requiring mechanical ventilation (more common in children than in adults)
- Tachydysrhythmias potentially requiring drug or countershock therapy

Death occurs as a result of end organ failure: irreversible shock, respiratory failure, cardiac dysrhythmias, untreatable coagulopathy, or severe cerebral ischemia.

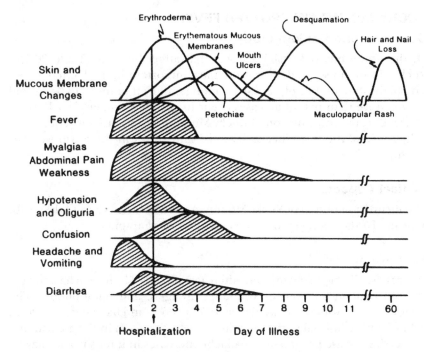

Figure 20.9. Composite drawing of major systemic, skin, and mucous membrane manifestations of toxic shock syndrome. (From Chesney PJ, Davis JP, Purdy WK, et al. Clinical manifestations of toxic shock syndrome. JAMA 1981;246:741–748. © 1981, American Medical Association, with permission.)

Therapy

Therapy consists of supportive care, aimed at preservation of vital organ function, and antibiotic administration. Systemic administration of a β-lactamase-resistant antistaphylococcal antibiotic is recommended. Although such treatment may not have a profound effect on the patient's short-term outcome, antibiotic therapy appears to reduce the incidence of recurrence.

An effort should be made to remove any potentially infected material, such as retained tampons, and to irrigate the vagina or any suspicious wounds to reduce further production and release of toxin. Diseases that might be mistaken for toxic shock syndrome (see Table 20.12) should be ruled out.

Long-term sequelae of toxic shock syndrome include the following:

- Prolonged muscle weakness and fatigue
- Loss of fingers or toes
- Abnormal renal function
- Behavioral changes or memory impairment
- Reversible hair and nail loss

ROCKY MOUNTAIN SPOTTED FEVER

Overview and Epidemiology

Of the numerous rickettsial diseases that affect humans (Table 20.13), Rocky Mountain spotted fever is the most important in the United States. The highest incidence of disease is among children in the 5- to 9-year-old range. More than half of all cases occur in people younger than 19 years of age. Because transmission of Rocky Mountain spotted fever requires activity of ticks, the incidence is seasonal and peaks in the warm weather months.

Clinical Aspects

The incubation period of Rocky Mountain spotted fever is 2 to 14 days, with a mean of 7 days between tick bite and onset of symptoms.

Early Symptoms

Fever is usually the first symptom, often accompanied by headache and generalized malaise followed by vomiting, myalgias, and photophobia. The fever increases, with spikes as high as 105 to 106°F, and has a hectic pattern, falling to near normal in the morning only to rise again in the afternoon.

As the disease progresses, headache increases in intensity and may be

Table 20.13
Rickettsial Diseases that Affect Humans

Organism	Disease	Geographic location	Vector
R. ricketsii	Rocky Mountain spotted fever	Western hemisphere	Ticks
R. conorii	Boutonneuse fever, African and Indian tick fevers	Africa, Europe, India, Middle East	Ticks
R. australis	Queensland tick typhus	Australia	Ticks
R. sibirica	North Asia tickborne rickettsiosis	Siberia, Mongolia	Ticks
R. akari	Rickettsial pox	North America, Europe	Mites
R. prowazeki	Epidemic typhus	Worldwide	Body lice
R. mooseri	Endemic typhus	Worldwide	Fleas
R. tsutsugamushi	Scrub typhus	Asia, Australia, Pacific Islands, Malaysia	Thrombiculid mites
Coxiella burnetti	Q fever	Worldwide	Ticks
Rochalimaea quintana	Trench fever	Worldwide	Body lice

associated with stiffness of the neck. Some children have shaking chills, abdominal pain, or diarrhea. The mental status eventually becomes clouded, and the youngster may be listless, lethargic, apathetic, or frankly comatose.

Rash

Distribution From 2 to 4 days after the onset of fever, a rash begins as discrete erythematous macules on the ankles and feet, progressing to the wrists and hands, the limbs, and, finally, the abdomen. In some children, it may start on the trunk and move outward to involve the extremities. The rash involves the palms and soles and is most pronounced over the extremities.

Appearance A rash of discrete blanching macules of several millimeters in diameter becomes morbilliform, then papular, then darkens in hue; it gradually becomes petechial and, sometimes, frankly purpuric. The purpura is related to the underlying coagulopathy, which is discussed below, and may become severe enough to result in overt gangrene of the ear lobes, scrotum, and digits. In some children, petechiae and purpura do not develop and the rash remains maculopapular or morbilliform, making the etiologic diagnosis less apparent.

Associated Findings

Patients may also manifest the following

- Involvement of mucous membranes (conjunctivitis is frequently present)
- Nonpitting edema of the limbs and periorbital areas
- Isolated splenomegaly or hepatosplenomegaly, associated with mild transient elevation of serum transaminase
- Acute tubular necrosis, because of hypovolemia
- Renal vasculitis
- Interstitial nephritis
- Interstitial pneumonitis and myocarditis
- Hemodynamic collapse, often related to inadequate intravascular volume
- Neurologic abnormalities (course may resemble that of acute encephalitis or meningitis)

When hypotension does not respond to fluid administration, the intensivist must suspect myocardial failure secondary to myocarditis.

Diagnosis

Entertaining and making a presumptive etiologic diagnosis is essential. Specific antibiotic therapy initiated early in the course of disease may be lifesaving.

Laboratory Evidence

Laboratory evaluation generally reveals the following:

- Leukocytosis with increased number of band forms
- Mild anemia
- Thrombocytopenia with hypofibrinogenemia
- Elevation of fibrin degradation products
- Hyponatremia
- Hypochloremia
- Low serum albumin level
- Elevated values of blood urea nitrogen, creatinine, and hepatic enzymes

Examination of the CSF may be normal or may reveal a lymphocytic pleocytosis with elevated protein but normal glucose concentration and absence of organisms on Gram stain.

Antibody Titers

The disease is confirmed when results show a complement fixation titer of at least 16, an indirect fluorescent antibody titer of 64 or greater, or a fourfold rise in either titer. Antibody titers peak 2 to 4 weeks into the illness.

Muscle Biopsy

Muscle biopsy may be useful and would be expected to show perivascular lymphocyte infiltration. Testing of the specimen by direct immunofluorescence may be positive. The tissue should be Giemsa-stained, which may reveal the presence of coccobacillary forms not observed on Gram's stain or hematoxylin and eosin stain.

Differential Diagnosis

The differential diagnosis includes the diseases listed in Table 20.14.

Therapy

Antimicrobial Agents

When the disease is recognized early and appropriate antibiotics are administered, most children will not require the services of the ICU. Antibiotics of choice are chloramphenicol for children or tetracycline for adolescents and adults, each at a dose of 100 mg/kg/day.

Supportive Care

Critical care support of advanced disease may include:

- Assisted ventilation necessitated by pulmonary edema that results from the vasculitis and hypoalbuminemia treatment of pleural effusions or empyema

Table 20.14
Differential Diagnosis of Rocky Mountain Spotted Fever

Other rickettsial diseases
Murine typhus
Typhoid fever
Colorado tick fever

Bacterial and spirochetal diseases
Meningococcemia
Disseminated streptococcal sepsis
Tularemia
Leptospirosis
Rat-bite fever

Viral diseases
Atypical measles
Enteroviruses
Epstein-Barr virus

Others
Juvenile arthritis
Systemic lupus erythematosis
Henoch-Schönlein purpura
Thrombotic thrombocytopenic purpura
Hemolytic uremic syndrome
Kawasaki disease

- Invasive hemodynamic monitoring and support, especially when the hypotensive patient is also in renal failure
- Hemodialysis or peritoneal dialysis for acute renal failure
- Replacement of plasma, platelets, blood, and clotting factors
- Possible heparinization if thrombotic complications are overwhelming
- Neurologic, nutritional, and physical therapy support of the comatose child

Precautions

As in any disorder involving thrombocytopenia and disseminated intravascular coagulation, any procedure such as central line insertion, lumbar puncture, and endotracheal intubation should be performed with great care. Nasotracheal intubation should be avoided. There does not appear to be a role for steroids in any phase of the infection.

21.

Gastrointestinal and Hepatic Failure in the Pediatric Intensive Care Unit

Elizabeth L. Rogers and Jay A. Perman

The gastrointestinal tract may complicate care of any child in the pediatric intensive care unit (PICU). Some gastrointestinal (GI) complications are avoidable, most are treatable if recognized early, and all are potentially lethal. Complications that need to be watched for in all children admitted to PICUs, almost regardless of their primary illness, include:

- Bleeding
- Ileus
- Diarrhea
- Pancreatitis
- Malnutrition

The GI tract also can be an early marker for shock states, using mucosal pH monitoring by tonometry.

EROSIVE GASTRITIS AND STRESS BLEEDING

Bleeding from diffuse, erosive stress gastritis is common in children admitted to the PICU. The potential becomes even greater if the reason for their admission includes:

- Head trauma
- Surgery
- Burns
- Cancer chemotherapy
- Renal failure
- Connective tissue disorders
- Reye syndrome
- Liver disease

Stress bleeding may occur in up to 80% of children with these problems and is usually from multiple locations.

Pathophysiology

Stress gastritis occurs when the normal mucosal defense mechanisms of the gastric mucosa become overwhelmed. The integrity of the mucosal cell membrane itself and the adjacent tight junctions are of prime importance in preventing stress gastritis; decreased cell turnover, hypoxia, the stress of being restrained, and decreased mucosal blood flow impair that integrity. As a result, the gastric mucosa loses its ability to produce sufficient amounts of mucus and, therefore, its protection from damage caused by bile salts, fasting and high concentrations of salt, alcohol, aspirin, and anti-inflammatory agents (e.g., indomethacin, phenylbutazone, naproxen).

Prostaglandin E1 (i.e., misoprostol) has been used to protect the gastric mucosa from the ulcerogenic effects of these nonsteroidal anti-inflammatory drugs; this leads to seepage of hydrogen ion from the lumen through or between mucosal lining cells to the submucosa. Measurement of intramural pH confirms that stress ulceration occurs in those patients whose intramural pH has fallen below the lower limit of normal levels. If the process is allowed to continue, local mucosal damage progresses to deeper ulceration into the mucosa and submucosa.

PRESENTATION

Stress gastritis after thermal injury develops within 72 hours in 74% of patients, and gastric ulceration occurs in 22% and duodenal ulceration occurs in 28% of patients. Life-threatening hemorrhage or perforation occurs mainly in patients with acute duodenal ulcers. Stress lesions can present as hematemesis, melena, hematochezia, or a slow decrease of the hematocrit. Abdominal pain or findings of tenderness on physical examination rarely occur. Nasogastric aspirate reveals coffee-ground material or bright red blood. The rate of bleeding is variable but may be rapid enough to result in exsanguination.

PREVENTION

There are compelling reasons to treat patients at risk for development of mucosal lesions, such as those with:

- Extensive burns
- Central nervous system (CNS) injury
- Prolonged hypotension
- Sepsis
- Acute respiratory failure
- Acute hepatic failure

The degree of mucosal damage and subsequent risk of bleeding correlates with the severity of the underlying illness. This damage will lead to overt bleeding in 15% of untreated patients, with upper intestinal bleeding accounting for as many as 30% of deaths.

The frequency of stress gastritis complicating the progress of intensely ill children and adults decreases when gastric intraluminal pH is carefully controlled.

- Maintain pH at 4.0 to 4.5
- Hourly antacids
- H_2 receptor agonists given by continuous infusion rather than through intermittent dosing
- Sucralfate, given in a dosage of 6 to 9 g daily
- Omeprazole (20 mg daily in adults) as a useful alternative to H_2 receptor agonists
- Lower body temperature
- Early attention to enteral feeding of an elemental diet

There are several mechanisms by which enteral feeding may be useful. The normal turnover of the gastric mucosal lining cells is quite rapid, with a half-life of 12 to 14 hours. When stress has damaged the mucosa, rapid cell renewal becomes most important in avoiding back diffusion of acid. Enteral administration of protein has been shown to release gastrin, a potent stimulator of cell turnover. Additionally, elemental diets act to buffer gastric acid and have been shown to maintain gastric pH above 4 during infusion.

Therapy

Treatment of stress bleeding in patients in the PICU involves the following measures:

- Hemodynamic resuscitation
- Convene treatment team
- Nasogastric lavage, saline
- Endoscopy to determine etiology and treatment
- Treatment specific to etiology

HEMODYNAMIC STABILIZATION

Intravenous fluids, colloid, packed red blood cells, and fresh frozen plasma, if needed, should be given until tachycardia and orthostasis are abolished. A nasogastric tube is useful both to monitor the severity of the bleeding and to apply saline lavage. Room temperature saline is adequate for lavage; chilling is unnecessary. Norepinephrine in a dosage of 8 mg mixed with saline 100 mL and instilled into the stomach, followed by clamping of the lavage tube for 30 minutes, occasionally has been helpful in reducing the rate of bleeding.

Team Approach

At a minimum, this GI and hepatic team should consist of the physician primarily responsible for the child, a gastroenterologist, a surgeon, and frequently, an interventional radiologist.

Locate and Treat Source of Bleeding

Endoscopy should be performed quickly to identify the site of the bleeding. If a discrete ulcer or bleeding site is found, endoscopic therapy is possible—especially in older children—with electrical cautery, laser cautery, or application of topical coagulants.

When endoscopy is unsuccessful in locating the site of the upper intestinal hemorrhage, the clinician should undertake arteriography. An upper GI series are not indicated in this situation because the yield is low and the presence of barium in the GI tract will prevent arteriography from being performed effectively later.

Suppression of Further Bleeding

Intravenous H_2-receptor antagonists frequently are administered to help suppress bleeding, although no data indicate that intravenous H_2-receptor antagonists or enteral antacids stop bleeding faster than does lavage alone.

Sometimes bleeding is brisk and persists despite lavage, in which case, the patient should undergo arteriography. The ability to suppress bleeding with intra-arterial vasopressors or thromboembolic agents is especially useful in patients with acute processes. Rarely, patients with stress gastritis will bleed so quickly and continuously that hemodynamic stability cannot be maintained and blood transfusions become overwhelming. At this time, surgical intervention with vagotomy (not always permanently successful) or total gastrectomy (successful but with a high mortality and morbidity rate) should be considered.

PARALYTIC ILEUS AND PSEUDO-OBSTRUCTION

Definition and Causative Factors

Postoperative Ileus

The functional inhibition of propulsive bowel activity, regardless of pathogenetic mechanism, is common after abdominal laparotomy, with severity inversely related to the child's age. Two kinds of postoperative ileus have been identified: (1) uncomplicated ileus after surgery that resolves spontaneously within 2 to 3 days, and (2) postoperative paralytic ileus that lasts for more than 3 days after surgery. Postoperative ileus is thought to result from temporary inhibition of extrinsic motility regulation. Alteration of sympathetic neuronal hyperactivity in patients who have undergone surgical procedures distant from the intestines results in decreased motility that is more profound and more persistent in the colon, less so in the small intestine, and least in the stomach.

Hypokalemia, hyponatremia, hypomagnesemia, and decreased osmolarity are among the many causes of acute pseudo-obstruction (Table 21.1). Hypokalemia is thought to exert its effects by interfering with acetylcholine release when the serum potassium level is below 2.5 mg/dL. Anoxic damage affects the especially sensitive intramural intestinal ganglia. Regional hypoxia can cause regional paralysis. In shock, blood is shunted away from the GI tract to the brain, heart, and kidneys. Localized areas of hypoxia in the small bowel can develop, associated with dilation of the bowel, loss of peristalsis, and functional obstruction. If the anoxic event persists for a prolonged time, permanent destruction of the mesenteric ganglia can be seen.

Although morphine inhibits small bowel propulsion and endogenous opiates have been proposed as one of the causes of postoperative ileus, reversal with naloxone has not been successful.

Experimental chemical sympathectomy reverses postoperative ileus after laparotomy in rats, and α-adrenergic blockade combined with cholinergic stimulation has been shown to hasten the restoration of colonic function.

Localized Ileus

Localized ileus, or pseudo-obstruction, can be seen with intraperitoneal inflammation, such as cholecystitis or pancreatitis, localized infections and abscesses, and lower lobe pneumonias.

Table 21.1
Factors Associated with Acute Pseudo-obstruction

Metabolic	16
Infections	16
Cardiac failure	15
Postoperative extraabdominal	14
Postoperative intraabdominal	13
Parkinsonism	11
Fractures	11
Acute cardiovascular catastrophe	15
Alcoholism	9
Pancreatitis/cholecystitis	9
Urinary tract disease	7
Malignancy	5
Miscellaneous	9
Total	140

Paralytic Ileus

Paralytic ileus seen after pelvic surgery is attributed to disruption of the sacral parasympathetics. Likewise, certain drugs cause functional obstruction by altering the parasympathetic to sympathetic ratio. These agents include:

- Phenothiazine-like antidepressants, such as chlorpromazine and amitriptyline
- Ganglionic blockers
- Cogentin
- Pro-Banthine
- Morphine
- Meperidine
- Methadone
- Other opioids

A good drug history, therefore, is mandatory for patients without obvious reason for the ileus.

Diagnosis

Signs and Symptoms

Most patients with postoperative ileus have the following:

- Abdominal distention
- Dilation of the intestine
- Nausea
- Vomiting
- Delayed defecation
- Decreased bowel sounds

Patients with localized functional obstruction, however, may have:

- Abdominal pain
- Nausea
- Vomiting
- Normal, decreased, or hyperactive bowel sounds

Imaging

A plain film radiograph of the abdomen can be useful in demonstrating diffuse ileus. A dilated cecum and transverse colon with no air in the descending colon or rectum is classic for mechanical obstruction but is also seen in functional obstruction. This picture can be differentiated from mechanical obstruction by Gastrografin or metrizamide enema or colonoscopy. Metrizamide is used in neonates and young children when barium is contraindicated because of suspected perforation and when Gastrografin is of concern because of its hypertonicity. Real-time ultrasonography also has been used in children to diagnose the reasons for mechanical obstruction, such as intussusception.

Postoperative Ileus versus Mechanical Obstruction/Intussusception

Not all postoperative ileus is functional. Prolonged ileus, or ileus that recurs 1 to 3 weeks postoperatively, may in fact be mechanical obstruction secondary to intussusception, or adhesions. Diagnosis of intussusception is difficult because most of the classic symptoms of obstruction are missing or obscured by the nasogastric suction and by pain medicines given postoperatively.

Postoperative intussusceptions are usually ileoileal, appear within 8 days of surgery, and require surgical correction. Intestinal adhesions as a cause of postoperative obstruction, on the other hand, tend to occur more than 2 weeks after surgery.

Therapy

The first line approach to treatment of the patient with ileus includes:

- Nothing per os (NPO)
- Nasogastric/intestinal suction
- Discontinue narcotics, smooth muscle relaxants, if possible
- Colonic decompression
- Rectal tube
- Colonoscopy

Ileus usually resolves with nasogastric decompression, correction of the underlying metabolic, infectious, or inflammatory processes, and intravenous nutritional support. Presence of bowel sounds and the passage of flatus followed by bowel movements usually marks the end of ileus. Partial small bowel mechanical obstruction also can be helped in some cases by nasogastric suction without increasing the risk of surgery should a definitive operation become necessary.

If the cecum has dilated to more than 12 cm in diameter, a definite danger of perforation exists, even though there is no mechanical reason for the obstruction. If the cecal dilation cannot be reduced by nasogastric decompression, decompression by a long double-lumen colonoscope has been performed successfully. If the cecal dilation cannot be decreased quickly, cecostomy is indicated because perforation carries with it a 35 to 75% mortality. When functional obstruction is suspected, narcotics, smooth muscle relaxants, and parasympathomimetic agents should be avoided because they can increase the chance of perforation.

OTHER DISORDERS OF MOTILITY

Other conditions affecting digestive tract motility may cause critical illness in the pediatric patient.

Chronic Idiopathic Intestinal Pseudo-Obstruction

This recurring condition characterized by bowel obstruction without organic mechanical occlusion of the lumen. There is no known underlying pathologic etiology.

The clinical course in children is characterized by intermittent episodes of abdominal distention, vomiting, abdominal pain, diarrhea, constipation, and malnutrition. Radiographic findings are diagnostic of the following:

- Abnormal esophageal motility
- Delayed gastric emptying
- Dilated loops of small intestine
- Disturbed colonic motility

Esophageal manometric studies are an aid to diagnosis.

Because acute attacks may be life-threatening, the patient with chronic idiopathic intestinal pseudo-obstruction (CIIP) may require intensive care:

- Nasogastric suction
- Fluid and electrolyte support
- Colonic lavage

A review by Schuffler et al. of the causes of and therapies for CIIP is useful for those requiring more detailed information.

Toxic Megacolon

The features of this possibly life-threatening complication of chronic ulcerative colitis are superimposed on those of fulminant colitis.

The condition is characterized by:

- Rapid deterioration with abdominal distention
- Disappearance of bowel sounds
- Toxemia

Precipitating factors are thought to be potassium deficiency, opiate treatment, preparation for and performance of barium enema, and mechanical obstruction.

Plain film radiographs of the abdomen show colonic distention. Because there is a high mortality, the condition demands:

- Intensive medical therapy
- Decompression of the small intestine by intubation
- Consultation with surgical team
- Consideration of steroid administration

Hirschsprung's Disease

This disorder of motility also may be life-threatening. Hirschsprung's disease in infants may be associated with an enterocolitis, either before or after colostomy, that is associated with sudden circulatory collapse and severe mucosal necrosis and ulceration. No specific therapy has been identified. The patient must be sustained with fluid and electrolyte support.

DIARRHEA

Diarrhea is defined as increased frequency of bowel movements to more than three times daily with increased fluidity and volume. Diarrhea in the postoperative or critically ill child occurs principally because of malabsorption, infection, or drugs (Table 21.2). It may also ensue if lymphatic flow from the mesentery is impeded by the surgical procedure. In addition to

Table 21.2
Common Causes of Diarrhea

Malabsorption
Intraluminal problems
    Pancreatic insufficiency
    Severe liver failure—biliary atresia
    Bacterial overgrowth secondary to dysmotility
Enterocyte damage or brush border enzyme depletion
    Postinfection
    Hypoxia
    Necrotizing enterocolitis
    Surgical resection
    Inflammatory bowel disease
    Lymphatic obstruction
Infection
Antibiotic-associated colitis—*Clostridium difficile*
Viral infections—frequently nosocomial
Bacterial infections
    Nonbloody—*Salmonella* and *Escherichia coli*
    Bloody—*Shigella, Yersinia,* and *Campylobacter*
Drugs that Cause Diarrhea
Antibiotics
Antacids
Chemotherapeutic agents
Colchicine
Digitalis preparations
Formula feeding
Lactulose
Potassium supplements
Propranolol
Quinidine

steatorrhea, obstruction of lymphatic flow from the intestine causes protein-losing enteropathy, hypoalbuminemia, and lymphopenia.

Necrotizing Enterocolitis

Necrotizing enterocolitis (NEC), a frequent GI emergency in the neonatal intensive care unit, predominantly affects premature infants, and its etiology may be multifactorial. Mortality appears to be associated with low birth weight and perinatal complications; however, hypoxic injury to the intestinal mucosa is critical to most hypotheses. Under these conditions, sugar malabsorption occurs. Malabsorption of carbohydrates is so typical of NEC that it has become a screening test in many nurseries for the development of NEC.

Infectious Causes of Diarrhea

Young children are at great risk for infectious diarrhea and ensuing dehydration.

Common Causes

Of the infectious causes of diarrhea in the intensive care patient, the following are the most common:

- Salmonella is the most common cause of bacterial diarrhea in children, with the highest attack rate in infants younger than 6 months of age
- *Escherichia coli* with serotype 0157:H7 causes hemorrhagic colitis
- *Giardia lamblia* is the most common cause of parasitic diarrheal disease in children in the United States
- Cryptosporidium is responsible for prolonged diarrheal disease in children with immunodeficiency
- *Clostridium difficile*

Bacterial infections, including *Salmonella* and *E. coli,* may cause fever, crampy abdominal pain, watery diarrhea, and associated hypovolemia and electrolyte problems.

Common antibiotics that cause pseudomembranous enterocolitis, the most severe form of *C.difficile*-induced diarrhea, are:

- Penicillins
- Clindamycin
- Ampicillins
- Cephalosporins

Bloody diarrhea associated with pseudomembranous colitis is rare, and abdominal tenderness may not be marked until the terminal events ensue.

Nosocomial infection is a likely cause of diarrhea in the PICU. Rotavirus androtavirus-like infection are particularly incriminated.

Human Immunodeficiency Virus-Infected Patients

The GI tract is a common target in patients infected with human immunodeficiency virus (HIV), and diarrhea and weight loss are found in more than 50% of patients with acquired immunodeficiency syndrome (AIDS). Cryptosporidium is the most common pathogen isolated from AIDS patients with diarrhea. Infectious causes of diarrhea and malabsorption in AIDS patients are listed in Table 21.3. Up to six stool samples, rectal biopsy, and duodenal biopsy may be required to make a diagnosis. Pathogen-negative diarrhea is also frequently reported and often is attributable to carbohydrate malabsorption.

Diagnosis

Evaluation of the patient with diarrhea includes:

- Document increased stool frequency and volume
- Gross stool examination
- Examination for infectious or inflammatory cause
- Fecal: blood, leukocytes, ova and parasites, culture for enteric pathogens, *C. difficile* toxin
- Blood: enzyme-linked immunosorbent assay (ELISA) for viral pathogens, TORCH for parasitic pathogens
- Sigmoidoscopy
- Evaluation for malabsorption
- Stool pH
- Breath hydrogen test
- D-Xylose test
- Small bowel series
- Small bowel biopsy

The first step in the clinical evaluation of diarrhea is to document the presence of diarrhea and other clinical signs:

Table 21.3
Infectious Etiologies for Diarrhea in Acquired Immunodeficiency Syndrome

Bacteria	Protozoan	Viruses
Salmonella	*Cryptosporidium*	Human immunodeficiency virus
Shigella	*I. belli*	Cytomegalovirus
Campylobacter	*Giardia*	Herpes simplex
M. avium intracellulare	*E. histolytica*	

- Vomiting frequently accompanies diarrhea in viral gastroenteritis
- Fever suggests a bacterial or viral etiology
- *Shigella* dysentery, for example, is frequently associated with a high temperature and febrile convulsions
- Abdominal pain and tenesmus are seen with *Yersinia enterocolitica, C. jejuni, Shigella,* and enteropathogenic *E. coli* infection in the colon
- Infections involving the small bowel usually result in a watery diarrhea
- Infectious colitis usually is associated with stool that contains blood, with or without mucus

Stool examination can prove to be useful.

Blood

The presence of visible blood in diarrheal stools should trigger further investigation for:

- Enteric pathogens such as *Shigella, Yersinia,* and *Campylobacter*
- Idiopathic inflammatory bowel disease
- Allergic colitism which may be induced by intolerance to dietary proteins, especially in the infant
- Ischemic injury
- NEC

Stools containing no visible blood should be tested for occult blood. A variety of methods, including guaiac-impregnated filter paper (i.e., Hemoccult), are available for this purpose.

Fecal Leukocytes

Examination of the diarrheal stool for white cells is useful in identifying infectious or inflammatory causes of diarrhea. A stool sample should be smeared on a glass slide and stained with methylene blue or Wright stain. The presence of neutrophils in the stool suggests *Shigella, Yersinia, Campylobacter,* or invasive *E. coli* as a possible cause. The presence of leukocytes generally eliminates viral or toxigenic bacterial causes of diarrhea.

CULTURE

If a bacterial cause for the patient's diarrhea is suspected, stool culture for enteric pathogens is appropriate. The presence of *C. difficile* can be detected by culture or by assay for *C. difficile* toxin.

Virus Identification

Diarrhea induced by virus can be detected by ELISA for viral antigens. The ELISA test for rotavirus has been shown to be extremely sensitive. ELISA may also be available for other enteroviruses, such as adenovirus.

Screening Tests for Carbohydrate Malabsorption

The screening tests for carbohydrate malabsorption using freshly passed feces are meaningful only if the child being tested is currently being fed a potentially offending carbohydrate. These tests include the measurement of pH (i.e., fecal pH) and reducing substances in the stool. Release of organic acids by bacterial fermentation of malabsorbed sugar forms the basis for utilizing fecal pH as a screening test for carbohydrate malabsorption.

The clinician dips nitrazine paper into the most liquid part of a fresh stool. The resulting color on the paper is compared with a provided chart. A fecal pH equal to or below 5.5 is abnormal. Reducing sugars that escape small bowel absorption and are excreted in the stool may be detected by placing a small amount of fecal material in a test tube and diluting it with twice its volume of water. Fifteen drops of the resulting suspension are then placed in a second test tube with a Clinitest tablet. The color of the reaction is compared with a chart provided in the Clinitest kit used for urine testing. Positive results are considered to be 0.5% or above; 0.25% is considered equivocal. Because sucrose is not a reducing sugar, an accurate test for sucrose malabsorption requires the use of 1 NHCl instead of water.

Breath Hydrogen Test

Hydrogen in breath results when carbohydrate that escapes small bowel absorption is fermented by colonic bacteria. A fixed portion of the H_2 produced is absorbed into the portal circulation and excreted in breath. The choice of sugar substrate for testing depends on the nature of the carbohydrate malabsorption suspected. For example, lactose is used when lactose malabsorption is suspected. The test is commonly performed after an overnight fast, but fasting may be shortened in the smaller infant.

Sigmoidoscopy

Sigmoidoscopic examination is valuable if inflammatory bowel disease or pseudomembranous colitis is suspected. Flexible sigmoidoscopy can be performed conveniently even in small children, and biopsies can easily be obtained. Pseudomembranous colitis is characterized by excrescences and raised yellow pseudomembranes with areas of ulceration. Pseudomembranous colitis induced by *C. difficile* is only one end of the spectrum of *C. difficile*-induced diarrhea; that is, the most common clinical presentation of this infection is self-limited diarrhea.

Therapy

Acute Self-Limited Diarrhea

Acute self-limited diarrhea, such as that attributable to viral agents, requires a short period on a clear liquid diet followed by gradual advancement in feedings. More intensive supportive care may be necessary to correct fluid and electrolyte disturbances. Infants are at higher risk than adults for development of dehydration and malnutrition with diarrhea.

Dehydration

Assessment of hydration state can be made clinically as well as by monitoring urine volume and central venous pressure. Fluid replacement should take into consideration the child's normal daily fluid requirement, electrolyte deficit, and ongoing fluid and electrolyte losses, estimated by measuring losses of stool, vomitus, and urine. Vomiting is not a contraindication to oral rehydration therapy unless ileus or an acute abdomen is present.

In the severely dehydrated child, rapid restitution with intravenous administration of 20 to 30 mL/kg isotonic saline containing 5% dextrose in water should be performed. Children with hypernatremic dehydration should have their electrolyte levels normalized over 2 to 3 days to avoid cerebral edema.

Malabsorptive Conditions

These conditions require modification of the child's enteral feeding. Whenever possible, feeding changes should be based on identification of the nutrients malabsorbed by the patient. Therapy of severe intestinal injury and short bowel syndrome frequently requires intravenous hyperalimentation. Total parenteral nutrition (TPN) has improved survival dramatically after massive small bowel resection and may permit normal infant growth and development. Short bowel syndrome may gradually improve as the bowel adapts by hypertrophy of the bowel lumen, lengthening of villi, and slowing of motility. During this adaptive time, tube feeding of defined constituent or modular formulae should be administered to the degree tolerated. Enteral administration of specialized formulae may increase enterocyte hyperplasia while improving the negative nitrogen balance of the patient and repleting missing nutrients.

Infectious Diarrhea

Therapy depends on identifying the offending agent. Specific therapy is available for children with amebiasis, cholera, giardiasis, and infection with *Salmonella, E. coli, Shigella,* and *Strongyloides.*

- Treatment of choice for *Salmonella* is chloramphenicol, when there is evidence of invasion of the organism with septicemia
- Enterotoxic *E. coli* rarely needs to be treated with antibiotics, but usually responds to trimethaprim-sulfa if necessary
- *Campylobacter jejuni* may respond to erythromycin if needed

Compounds such as the fluoroquinolones, which are effective in adults, are not approved for use in children because of their potential side effects. Such "antidiarrheal" agents as Lomotilor Kaopectate may prolong and worsen the severity of disease, especially in *Shigellosis,* but also in *C. jejuni* infections. These compounds also interfere with identification of enteropathogens in stool specimens and have a high overdose potential in children.

Necrotizing Enterocolitis

In NEC, treatment includes antibiotics, fluids and colloid, nasogastric decompression, and frequent radiographic examinations to rule out perforation. Because disseminated intravascular coagulation is common in this process, fresh frozen plasma frequently is necessary. Feedings should be withheld for 7 to 14 days and then provided by continuous feeding through the nasogastric tube.

Bacterial Infections

Guidelines for therapy of specific bacterial infections may be obtained from a variety of sources. Nonspecific methods for treating *C. difficile* colitis include:

- Discontinuation of the suspected antimicrobial agent
- Avoidance of antiperistaltic drugs
- Supportive care to correct dehydration and electrolyte disturbances
- Metronidazole for initial treatment of the moderately ill patient
- Vancomycin is reserved for the patient who is severely affected by *C. difficile*

HIV and AIDS

Antimicrobial treatment of diagnosed enteric pathogens in HIV-infected patients is indicated. Parenteral therapy usually is necessary for the initial management of bacteremic patients. Although response to antibiotics is generally good, relapses and recurrences are frequent.

PANCREATITIS

In children, the most common causes of obstructive relapsing pancreatitis due to congenital anomalies are:

- Choledochal cysts
- Stricture of the common duct
- Congenital stenosis of the ampulla of vater
- Anomalous insertion of the common bile duct
- Intrapancreatic ductal duplications
- Periampullary duodenal duplication
- Duodenal diverticulum

In addition to the usual reasons for pancreatitis in children (e.g., cystic fibrosis, amino acid dyscrasias, hyperlipoproteinemias), it can also be seen in the PICU setting as a complication of hepatitis and drug therapy.

Presentation

Clinical Features

Physical findings that are diagnostic include:

- Bandlike epigastric pain
- Radiation of pain through to back or left shoulder
- Nausea, vomiting
- Low-grade fever (100 to 103°F)
- Tachycardia, tachypnea
- Blood pressure is normal, although profound orthostatic hypotension may be seen
- Mildly to moderately tender abdomen, rarely with board-like stiffness or rebound
- Bowel sounds are decreased but present in all but the most severe cases
- Localized ileus on plain film

Laboratory Findings

Moderate leukocytosis (12,000 to 18,000) and hemoconcentration of the hematocrit are seen.

Although the serum amylase value usually is elevated, the height of elevation does not correlate with the severity of the clinical disease process. When the elevation is mild, urinary clearance of amylase may be helpful to demonstrate increased renal clearance of amylase compared with that of creatinine, if the patient does not have renal failure or severe burns. Other processes associated with hyperamylasemia include parotitis, esophageal perforation, acute renal failure, pregnancy, and bowel infarction. Serum lipase is also elevated in most cases of pancreatitis and can be obtained when there are other reasons to expect hyperamylasemia.

Laboratory findings that suggest a poor prognosis include:

- Serum calcium level below 7.5 mg/dL
- Leukocytosis above 20,000
- PO_2 below 60
- Azotemia

The hypocalcemia of fatal pancreatitis probably has multiple causes, including extraskeletal calcium sequestration, hypersecretion of glucagon, hypomagnesemia, and saponification of fatty acids.

Other useful laboratory parameters for staging the severity of pancreatitis include the levels of serum cyclic adenosinemonophosphate, albumin, methemalbumin, serum ribonuclease, and C-reactive protein. These levels, in general, have not been found to be of universal value in the clinical management of the patient with acute pancreatitis.

Effects on Other Organ Systems

During pancreatitis, any organs that come in direct contact with the pancreas may exhibit dysfunction secondary to localized inflammation; therefore, one frequently sees localized areas of ileus in those loops of bowel that happen to come in contact with the pancreas. This contact leads to such radiographic findings as "sentinel loop" if the small bowel is involved, and "colon cut-off" if the transverse colon and descending colon are affected.

Through a similar mechanism, one may see red blood cells and white blood cells on urinalysis if the tail of the pancreas involves the left kidney. When the head of the pancreas is swollen and edematous and there is inflammation of the common bile duct, the clinician may see mild cholestasis. At these times, the alkaline phosphatase or 5-nucleotidase may be two to four times normal, and the serum bilirubin will be in the 2 to 5 mg/dL range.

Therapy

Pancreatic Rest

The most effective treatment entails keeping the patient NPO. Particularly important is the need to keep fat and protein out of the proximal bowel, because these food products cause the release of cholecystokinin, which in turn leads to pancreatic enzyme release. This is more destructive to an already inflamed pancreas than is any other single manipulation.

While the child is NPO, nutritional status can be maintained by peripheral parenteral nutrition as long as the child was not malnourished to begin with and the pancreatitis appears to be resolving quickly. The malnourished child should begin central venous parenteral nutrition on the first day of hospitalization to correct nitrogen balance more quickly, to fight infection, and to speed recovery.

Fluid Balance

Intravenous fluids can be lifesaving, because third spacing of fluid becomes a major problem in pancreatitis. Fluid and colloid should be given quickly enough to decrease tachycardia and to correct orthostasis. Central venous pressure or pulmonary artery monitoring may be necessary because of the combined hypovolemia and pulmonary complications. Careful restitution of serum calcium, magnesium, and potassium is necessary in severe cases.

Endoctracheal Intubation and Positive End-Expiratory Pressure

Pulmonary problems occur in as many as 40% of patients with pancreatitis, although this complication is frequently underappreciated. Pulmonary effusion is usually on the left side, although bilateral sympathetic effusions can be seen. Endotracheal intubation and the use of positive end-expiratory pressure (PEEP) are indicated when atelectasis is severe.

Analgesia

Abdominal pain can be severe, requiring narcotic analgesics for relief. This needs to be remembered, especially in the older child who may have taken illicit drugs previously and who may be viewed with skepticism when complaining of pain.

Nasogastric Decompression

For those patients with gastric atony secondary to localized inflammatory response, large volumes of gastric secretion accumulate. These patients feel more comfortable with nasogastric decompression.

Antacids

Although the presence of gastric acid in the duodenum is associated with hormonal release of secretin and thus the stimulation of pancreatic secretion of water and bicarbonate, there is no evidence that this worsens or prolongs the pancreatitis. On the contrary, the addition of antacids or cimetidine to the treatment regimen will not be helpful and may be associated with prolonged pain, fever, or hyperamylasemia.

Trasylol and Glucagon

There are theoretical reasons why Trasylol, a chemotrypsin activation inhibitor, might be useful. Double-blind studies, however, have varied in their ability to demonstrate this usefulness conclusively. Likewise, glucagon has been suggested as a method of suppressing pancreatitis, but controlled studies have thus far been inconclusive.

Refeeding

Patients with pancreatitis should be continued NPO for 3 to 4 days after abdominal discomfort, fever, leukocytosis, and hyperamylasemia disappear. Careful refeeding involves a trial of carbohydrate solids, such as fruit. If tolerated, the diet can be advanced slowly by adding protein, then low fat, and finally regular food. In the more protracted cases, elemental feeding has been used. Intake should be stopped immediately if abdominal discomfort, fever, or leukocytosis recurs.

Complications

Usually, pancreatitis is a mild disease with a low incidence of significant morbidity or mortality. In 10 to 20% of cases, potentially serious complications of pancreatitis can occur, including:

- Pseudocyst
- Pancreatic effusions: ascites, pleural, pericardial
- Pancreatic abscess
- Respiratory distress syndrome
- Shock

Fluid can collect as pancreatic ascites, discrete fluid collections around the pancreas, pleural effusion, and pericardial effusion.

Pseudocysts

From 40 to 60% of patients with acute pancreatitis will develop small pseudocysts. These are the result of pancreatic duct rupture with extravasation of pancreatic juices. Pseudocysts are usually asymptomatic and will disappear with the resolution of the pancreatitis. Prolonged hyperamylasemia, recurrent pain with refeeding, and persistent ileus should raise the suspicion of a larger than usual pseudocyst.

A pseudocyst is a collection of pancreatic enzymes beyond the usual confines of the pancreas. The "walls" of this collection may be any structure or mesentery contiguous to the collection. When the enzymatic proteins in this collection are activated, digestion of the walls begins and can lead to perforation of a viscus, severe cholangitis, thrombosis of a major vein, such as the splenic vein, or perforation into a major artery with exsanguination.

For this reason, large pseudocysts or rapidly expanding pseudocysts are considered ominous in the face of acute pancreatitis. Although each patient must be considered individually, surgical intervention should be considered for patients with acute pancreatitis who are receiving appropriate therapy and develop an acutely expanding or large pseudocyst that appears to be compromising the vascular or biliary systems. Large asymptomatic pseudocysts that are found by serendipity after a bout of acute pancreatitis can be followed for 6 to 12 weeks. If they do not resolve spontaneously, they can be drained surgically. Percutaneous drainage of pancreatic fluid collections is effective in most patients, making the need for laparotomy less frequent.

Pancreatic Abscess

Infected pancreatitis may be suspected when there is higher than usual fever, leukocytosis, or involuntary abdominal guarding or rigidity. Pancreatic abscess is a fairly uncommon complication, but if untreated, there is a 50 to 90% mortality rate.

Contrast-enhanced computed tomography (CT) is the method of choice for anatomic evaluation. Indications for CT include:

- Acute pancreatitis that does not respond within a few days
- Pancreatitis with large and enlarging pleural effusions
- Clinical deterioration after initial improvement

Although prophylactic antibiotics have not been shown to be cost beneficial, antibiotics effective against gut flora should be started as soon as infected pancreatitis or pancreatic abscess is suspected. Additionally, emergency percutaneous or surgical drainage should be considered. With multiple percutaneous catheters, cure rates from 60 to 90% have been reported.

Management of the patient with pancreatic abscess includes the following steps:

- Rapid assessment of physiologic derangement
- Prompt enhanced CT for anatomic evaluation
- Early institution of hemodynamic monitoring
- Adequate fluid resuscitation
- Percutaneous aspiration to identify septic foci
- Aggressive surgical debridement

MALNUTRITION

Critically ill children have intestinal, emotional, and iatrogenic reasons for failing to consume sufficient intake to remain in nitrogen balance.

Hypermetabolic State

Conditions such as stress and infection make attention to nutrition critical. Response to stress includes such hormonally mediated effects as:

- Increased metabolic rate
- Increased sodium levels
- Water retention
- Need for blood pressure maintenance
- Hyperglycemia
- Breakdown of skeletal muscle

Therapy

Initiation of nutritional support for a malnourished child undergoing stress requires monitoring of weight, fluid balance, and serum electrolyte values. Nutritional support should consist of the least invasive effective method of maintaining the child in positive nitrogen balance. Enteral alimentation prevents the decrease in function and structure of the GI tract associated with pure parenteral nutrition.

Tube Feeding

Tube feeding should be administered in small continuous volumes of dilute concentrations in the beginning, with gradual increases in volume and strength as they are tolerated by the patient. Use of a delivery system that pumps the tube feeding at a constant slow rate is associated with less reflux and diarrhea than one that feeds by bolus. Tube feeding directly to the jejunum is associated with a somewhat higher incidence of diarrhea but with less risk of aspiration pneumonia.

Total Parenteral Nutrition

When insufficient nutrition can be provided orally or through tube feeding, nutritional intake can be supplemented with peripheral parenteral alimentation. Such techniques allow for glucose, saline, and volume. Protein-sparing therapy is achieved by administering intravenous amino acids. Daily addition of fatty acids act as an easy source of calories as well as preventing fatty acid deficiency.

If the child will likely require prolonged parenteral alimentation or was malnourished before entering the PICU, that child should be started immediately on TPN. When the child can tolerate enteral alimentation, TPN can be discontinued.

FULMINANT HEPATIC FAILURE

Etiology

Liver failure in the PICU is most frequently associated with toxins or drugs, viral hepatitis, or Reye syndrome.

Toxic Hepatitis

Accidental ingestion of toxic amounts of iron, acetaminophen, and vitamin A, as well as idiosyncratic hypersensitivity to isoniazid, α-methyldopa, nonsteroidal anti-inflammatory drugs, and some antibiotics and anticonvulsants can cause acute hepatic failure. If the child does not die of the liver failure itself or of the associated complications, recovery can be complete, as there is rapid regeneration of the injured hepatic tissue after toxic damage.

Hepatitis Non-A, Non-B

Although hepatitis A most frequently affects children, hepatitis non-A, non-B is the one most likely to cause fulminant hepatic failure (75% of some series). If the child can be maintained throughout the hepatic failure, recovery can be complete, without chronic liver scarring or damage. Recovery, however, is slower after viral hepatitis than after toxic hepatitis because of suppressed regeneration associated with viral exposure.

Reye Syndrome

This disease process (see Chapter 13) affects the mitochondrial system of the body (Fig. 21.1). Reye syndrome most frequently affects children 6 to 12 years old, usually appearing shortly after an acute viral syndrome. Fre-

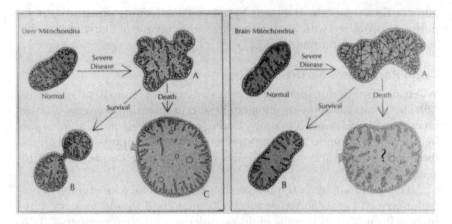

Figure 21.1. Liver Mitochondria in Severe Disease (left, A) Often Assume a Pleomorphic Form and Show Less of Dense Bodies and Expanded Matrix Space. In survivors **(left, B)**, most mitochondria appear quite normal except for increased fission. Nonsurvivors **(left, C)** present expanded matrix, protein disorganization, and membrane rupture. In the brain, mitochondrial changes are less well studied, but it is thought that substantial matrix expansion occurs in severe disease **(right, A)**, although "web-work" may remain intact. In one patient who survived **(right, B),** expanded matrix, "broken" protein, and membrane ruptures were demonstrated. Changes in fatal cases are unknown. (From Haller JS. The enigmatic encephalopathy of Reye's syndrome. Hosp Pract 1975;10:93.)

quently, the child has been treated with aspirin. Since this association has been made, efforts have been undertaken to limit the use of aspirin, especially during varicella and influenza infection. As a result, the incidence of Reye syndrome has decreased.

Pronounced nausea usually is followed by protracted vomiting, confusion, and coma. Unlike hepatic failure from other causes, jaundice is conspicuously absent in Reye syndrome. Although liver failure itself can be profound, the most frequent cause of death in children with Reye syndrome is cerebral edema.

Clinical Features

Patients with Reye syndrome may demonstrate the following:

- Mild to moderate nausea
- Anorexia
- Fatigue
- Protracted vomiting
- Altered behavior
- Increased tendency to bruise
- Ascites

Changes in behavior range from euphoria to belligerence and the unexpected use of foul language. Sleep patterns may be altered, with the child sleeping all day and being up all night. Confusion may range from altered spatial orientation to slurred speech and complete disorientation. Asterixis may be present. Hyperventilation, hyperthermia, and hyperreflexia reflect significant CNS involvement. The child may be lethargic, difficult to rouse, unarousable, or may demonstrate decerebrate posture.

Throughout its course, the depth of hepatic encephalopathy is one of the most reliable means of assessing and studying the severity of the hepatic failure. Although the more severe grades of encephalopathy are associated with more severe fulminant hepatic failure (FHF) and poorer prognosis, recovery from FHF can be complete and frequently without permanent neurologic sequelae. Mortality in patients with FHF when encephalopathy occurs within 8 weeks of the onset of jaundice ranges from 60 to 90%.

Laboratory Findings

The absolute height of transaminase elevation does not correlate with the severity of the disease; however, it is usually elevated 10- to 100-fold in FHF. As alkaline phosphatase is expected to be high in children because of bone growth, 5-nucleotidase may be useful to differentiate bone from liver alkaline phosphatase and is better than heat fractionation for this purpose.

Neither transaminases nor alkaline phosphatase defines liver function, however. This can best be appreciated by carefully monitoring serum bilirubin, albumin, and prothrombin time, all of which require active hepatocyte metabolism and thus reflect "function." With severe deterioration of liver function, there will be a mixed hyperbilirubinemia in the range of 15 to 40 mg/dL, the albumin will decrease to less than 3.0 mg/dL, and the prothrombin time will become more than 3 seconds beyond control.

Mortality Rates

Mortality rates are high for FHF, being almost 60% in the Fulminant Hepatic Failure Surveillance Study and rising to 80% when grade IV encephalopathy is present.

Therapeutic Guidelines

The essential elements of management of the child with FHF are:

- Admit to a PICU, preferably a liver failure unit
- Develop a team approach for the patient's projected needs
- Distinguish between FHF and exacerbation of chronic liver disease
- Establish a cause: draw blood for diagnostic serologic and drug testing
- Carefully control fluid and electrolyte status

- Give prophylaxis against stress bleeding and encephalopathy, treat aggressively
- Monitor for infection and encephalopathy
- Consider transplantation if rapid deterioration ensues

Monitoring

Basic monitoring should consist of the following:

- Hourly observations of blood pressure, pulse, respiration, mental status, urine output, and central venous pressure
- Check arterial blood gases routinely
- Single toxic screen should be run on admission, to rule out other treatable causes of coma
- Serum ammonia levels (preferably arterial) to confirm a hepatic origin to coma and in monitoring progress
- Serial electroencephalograms
- Intracranial pressure monitoring, when grade III encephalopathy ensues

Fluids and Electrolytes

The mainstays of therapy are to keep the child normovolemic with normal electrolytes. Profound hypoglycemia, found in as many as 40% of children with acute hepatic failure, must be treated vigorously. Large doses of intravenous potassium may be required to maintain a normal serum level because of the kaliuresis associated with secondary hyperaldosteronism. Decreased serum sodium, because of an antidiuretic-like activity, is combined with increased total body sodium and fluid retention caused by a hyperaldosterone-like activity.

Encephalopathy

Because most children with acute hepatic failure have severe hepatic encephalopathy, TPN should be started at once if oral nutrition cannot safely be maintained. Attention must be given, however, to adding those amino acids most needed by the body and avoiding those that tend to make encephalopathy worse (see subsequent discussion of hepatic encephalopathy).

Steroid Therapy

Figure 21.2 represents the relative 16-week survival of patients treated with the steroid methylprednisolone versus those receiving a placebo.

A randomized, controlled therapeutic trial in 38 patients with FHF failed to show that the combination of insulin and glucagon demonstrated any benefit related to morbidity or mortality.

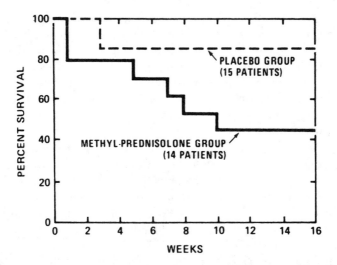

Figure 21.2. Survival Curves for Two Treatment Groups during the 16-Week Study Period. (From Gregory PB, Knaver CM, Kempson RL, Miller R. Steroid therapy in severe viral hepatitis: A double-blind randomized trial of methylprednisolone vs. placebo, N Engl J Med 1976;294:683. Reprinted by permission of the New England Journal of Medicine.)

GASTROINTESTINAL BLEEDING

As many as 70% of patients with acute hepatic failure may experience GI bleeding, and as many as 30% will die from this complication. Bleeding occurs for a number of reasons, including stress gastritis and portal hypertension. Both of these problems are exacerbated by the coagulopathy of liver disease.

Coagulopathy

Coagulopathy occurs from inadequate synthesis of factors V, VII, and X. Vitamin K should be administered, but the coagulopathy frequently does not respond. In chronic liver disease, hypersplenic sequestration of platelets also may occur. Diffuse intravascular coagulopathy also exists in most patients with acute or chronic liver disease, with exacerbation during stress induced by bleeding or infection. Trasylol, heparin, and ε-aminocaproic acid are not recommended for prophylactic use but have been used when bleeding from disseminated intravascular coagulation develops.

Stress Gastritis

The incidence of stress gastritis in patients with hepatic failure can be reduced, although the risk of nosocomial pneumonia may be increased by maintaining the pH of the gastric contents at 4.5 or greater. Use of H_2-receptor antagonists or antacids and gentle nasogastric suction has been associated with a decrease in severe bleeding from 54 to 4% and a decrease in mortality. Care must be taken that high vacuum pressures are not used through the nasogastric tube, to prevent mucosal denuding through the suction holes and by a whip-like action of the tube under pressure.

Portal Hypertension

Bleeding from esophageal varices caused by portal hypertension occurs commonly in childhood, and extrahepatic portal vein obstruction is a common reason for those varices. Of these patients, 73% are under the age of 10 years.

Frequently, the initial presentation responds acutely to supportive measures of blood volume restoration and vasopressin, followed by propranolol prophylaxis. Rebleeding or failure of bleeding to stop are indications for more invasive therapy.

Shunt surgery often is effective but is associated with a high rate of shunt thrombosis in this age group. Endoscopic sclerotherapy has been used for several decades in adults, with promising results. Complications of sclerotherapy include:

- Retrosternal discomfort
- Transient pyrexia
- Esophageal ulceration
- Esophageal stricture

Rebleeding after supposedly successful sclerotherapy can occur in one-third of patients, presumably because of reformation of esophageal varices or presence of gastric varices.

ASCITES

A common complication of acute and chronic liver disease is ascites, which can be a cosmetic problem, be responsible for exacerbating respiratory or renal failure, or can serve as a medium for the development of spontaneous bacterial peritonitis. Ascites develops in association with portal hypertension and is related to weepage from obstructed lymphatics, altered aldosterone status with sodium retention, and decreased tissue oncotic pressure due to low serum albumin. With new-onset ascites, diagnostic paracentesis is indicated to assure that the fluid is a transudate and not infected.

Treatment of ascites focuses on:

- Restricting sodium intake to less than the amount put out in the urine
- Administering spironolactone
- Slow diuresis
- Therapeutic paracentesis associated with albumin infusion and close monitoring of intravascular status.

This safer form of therapeutic paracentesis is indicated in situations of respiratory embarrassment or umbilical necrosis. For patients without frank pedal edema, diuretics remains the best treatment.

RESPIRATORY FAILURE

Hypoxia seen in 40 to 60% of patients with hepatic failure is attributable to:

- Neurogenic pulmonary edema
- Fluid overload from antidiuretic-like activity seen in patients with liver failure
- Intrapulmonary shunting due to the release of vasoactive products in liver failure

Increasing the concentration of inspired oxygen may be all that is necessary in some patients to correct the hypoxia. Others may benefit from PEEP.

Although intubation may help correct hypoxia and improve hepatic function theoretically, the use of increased pressure to open the alveoli leads to increased pressure in the inferior vena cava, which is transmitted to the hepatic veins. Increased pressure and decreased flow from the hepatic veins result in increased ischemia of the hepatocytes surrounding the central veins. In addition, increasing the tidal volume may be associated with increased splanchnic resistance and decreased flow through the splanchnic circulation. This may result in decreased portal blood flow, with potential ischemic liver damage.

HEPATORENAL SYNDROME

Although most patients with liver disease seem to be volume overloaded and have both inappropriate aldosterone-like activity and inappropriate antidiuretic hormone-like activity, much of the volume load does not recirculate because of the portal hypertension. The effective intravascular volume seems to be decreased in patients with hepatorenal syndrome; their urine volume may decrease, and the urine sodium level may drop to less than 10 mg/dL.

Evidence of renal failure occurs in as many as 70% of patients with acute hepatic failure. The term hepatorenal syndrome connotes previously normal kidneys that decompensate in the presence of severe liver disease (Fig. 21.3).

Diagnosis

The diagnosis of hepatorenal syndrome should be suspected in a patient with significant liver disease with:

- Oliguria
- Elevated serum urea nitrogen (i.e., BUN)
- Normal urinary sediment
- Low urine sodium level

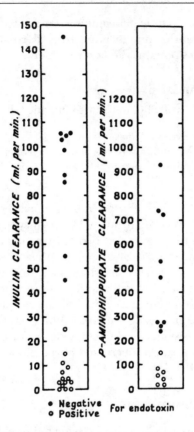

Figure 21.3. Relationship between Endotoxemia and Glomerular Filtration Rate and Renal Plasma Flow. (From Wilkinson SP, Gazzard BG, Arroyo V, et al. Relation of renal impairment and hemorrhagic diathesis to endotoxemia in fulminant hepatic failure. Lancet 1974;1:523. © The Lancet Ltd., with permission.)

Management

A central venous pressure of 3 to 8 mm Hg will allow sufficient volume to perfuse the kidneys adequately without impeding hepatic vein overflow. If hepatorenal syndrome is suspected, a rapid fluid load should be given to raise the central venous pressure to 10 mm Hg quickly, using salt-poor albumin and fluid. Additional volume or an increase of central pressure greater than 10 mm Hg may lead to decreased portal flow and greater hepatic damage. For patients who require exquisitely sensitive fluid management, particularly those with pulmonary edema, a pulmonary artery catheter may be used instead of a central venous catheter.

In the absence of pulmonary edema, therefore, addition of a plasma expander such as mannitol plus concomitant furosemide may increase diuresis and can be tried as long as the central venous pressure is maintained by minute-to-minute observation in a range of 3 to 10 mm Hg. Excessive diuresis with a drop of central venous pressure may result in irreversible renal shutdown; an increase in the central venous pressure may result in either pericentral hepatic ischemia or variceal bleeding or both.

INFECTIONS

Four types of infection in children with liver disease are: (1) bacteremia by gut organisms, because of poor hepatic clearing of organisms seeded from the edematous bowel of portal hypertension; (2) spontaneous bacterial peritonitis; (3) urinary tract infections; and (4) aspiration pneumonias. There is ample evidence that prophylactic antibiotics are not of value. Clues to the possibility of infection, however, include:

- Worsening of encephalopathy
- Sudden development of hepatorenal syndrome
- New onset of leukocytosis or fever

HEPATIC ENCEPHALOPATHY

As liver failure increases, the stage of hepatic encephalopathy increases. Other factors that make encephalopathy worse include:

- Excessive protein load
- Respiratory alkalosis
- Hyponatremia
- Hypokalemia
- Hypoglycemia
- Infection
- Upper intestinal bleeding
- Azotemia
- Hypoxia
- Administration of medications that suppress the sensorium

Ammonia Level

The ammonia level per se does not correlate with the grade of encephalopathy. If the ammonia level is elevated in an individual with encephalopathy, however, this level will tend to rise as the encephalopathy worsens and decrease as the encephalopathy improves.

Likewise, interventions that increase ammonia levels, such as increased ingestion of nitrogen-containing products, are associated with worsening encephalopathy. Therapeutic interventions that decrease ammonia levels, such as trapping ammonia in the gut (lactulose) or decreasing the urea-producing gut organisms (antibiotics and lactulose), are associated with concomitant improvement in encephalopathy.

Arterial ammonia correlates better with the degree of encephalopathy than does venous ammonia; however, venous ammonia levels are generally used for sequential monitoring. When the ammonia level is not elevated, the serum or cerebrospinal fluid glutamine level elevation may be diagnostic.

Altered Neurotransmission

Branched-chain amino acid solutions are better tolerated than are nonselective protein solutions, so more nitrogen can be given to malnourished patients, improving their nitrogen balance (Table 21.4). The neuroinhibitory actions of benzodiazepines and barbiturates are mediated by the γ-aminobutyric acid (GABA) neurotransmitter receptor system. Preliminary studies in humans with hepatic encephalopathy indicate that GABA plasma levels are elevated, perhaps suggesting increased formation or increased release from neurons.

Staging System

The patient with hepatic encephalopathy is best monitored by the crude clinical criteria for grade scoring of encephalopathy:

Grade O: Normal
Grade I: Altered spatial orientation, sleep patterns, and affect
Grade II: Drowsy but arousable, slurred speech, confusion, and
            asterixis

Table 21.4
Controlled Trials of Branched-Chain Amino Acid Therapy in Hepatic Coma

Investigator	Number of patients	Test solution	Control	Results
Mendenhall	57	Oral BCAA	Hospital diet	Improved nutrition in BCAA group; no difference in coma
Egberts	22	Oral BCAA	Casein	Improved psychometric tests, but no difference in "ability to drive" for BCAA group
Michel	70	IV BCAA	Amino acids	No difference between groups
Cerra	70	IV FO80	Neomycin/ dextrose	BCAA superior; only 13 of 35 survived control therapy
Wahren	50	IV BCAA	Glucose	No difference in encephalopathy; more deaths in BCAA group

BCAA, branched-chain amino acid.

Grade III: Stuporous but responsive to painful stimuli
Grade IV: Unresponsive, with decorticate or decerebrate
             posturing possible

Treatment

The focus of treatment is on:

- Prevention and therapy of processes known to precipitate encephalopathy
- Reduction in protein intake (especially aromatic and straight-chained amino acids)
- Reduction of serum ammonia levels by the addition of neomycin plus a laxative or lactulose

Neomycin, an antibiotic that is poorly absorbable (<1%) and effective at least acutely against urea-splitting gut flora, has become less popular because of toxicity and GI side effects. Lactulose, a nonabsorbable synthetic disaccharide, causes a watery osmotic diarrhea of low pH, which results in loss of the normal urea-splitting colonic flora and overgrowth of lactobacillic organisms. The low pH may also prevent the absorption of ammonia and aromatic amino acids. Although lactulose is more expensive than neomycin, it has become the standard therapy of hepatic encephalopathy because of its low toxicity. Lactulose or lactose enemas also reduce encephalopathy.

   Addition of branched-chain amino acids to hypertonic (20%) glucose may help improve nutritional status and reduce the concentration of aromatic amino acids (see Table 21.4). GABA antagonists have also been administered, albeit in an uncontrolled fashion (Table 21.5).

CEREBRAL EDEMA

Cerebral edema is the cause of death in as many as 40 to 70% of patients with hepatic failure.

Etiology

The causes of cerebral edema are as poorly understood as those of encephalopathy, but they appear to be related to each other. Patients who develop progressively deeper levels of encephalopathy eventuate into cerebral edema if the process is not stopped. It has been postulated that one mechanism may include altered permeability of the blood-brain barrier. Many toxic substances that accumulate during FHF are known to inhibit membrane Na+K+-APTase. Any reduction in brain Na+K+-ATPase activity is likely to impair neurotransmission and potentially cause glial cell swelling. The degree of enzyme activity reduction, however, correlates more closely with the degree of encephalopathy than with the development of cerebral edema. Inappro-

Table 21.5
Flumazenil-Induced Improvements in the Degree of Hepatic Encephalopathy in Humans[a]

Study	Clinical setting	Cases (n)	Responses[b]
Bansky et al.	Cirrhosis	14	10
Grimm et al.	Cirrhosis	8	5
Meier and Gyr	Cirrhosis	3	3
Burke et al.	Alcoholic liver disease	1	1
Scollo-Lavizzari and Steinmann	Fulminant hepatic failure	2	2
Grimm et al.	Fulminant hepatic failure	4	5
Sutherland and Minuk	Fulminant hepatic failure	1	0
Olf[c]	Fulminant hepatic failure	2	2
Ferenci et al.	Chronic portal-systemic encephalopathy	1	1

[a]Fulmazenil is an investigational drug Ro 15-1788 from Hoffman La Roche, Basel, Switzerland.

[b]Responses were achieved in 29 of 41 cases (71%).

[c]Olf J. Personal communication.

priate pathologic cerebral vasodilation may also be an important cause of increased intracranial pressure in the brains of patients with hepatic encephalopathy that are suffering a number of generalized insults.

Elevated Intracranial Pressure

Clinical Signs

The neurologic signs associated with high intracranial pressure (ICP) are:

- Increased muscle tone
- Increased deep tendon reflexes
- Abnormal pupillary reflexes
- Hyperventilation

Treatment

When ICP has reached a persistent level of 30 mm Hg, the first-step approach includes:

- Elevation of head of bed 45°
- Avoid turning the head, which increases resistance to venous flow in neck
- Hyperventilate mechanically
- Mannitol plus furosemide if possible
- Maintain cerebral perfusion pressure below 30 mm Hg

Maintaining Carbon Dioxide Level

Because the level of consciousness correlates with the degree of respiratory alkalosis, some researchers recommend initiating ICP monitoring when

PCO_2 exceeds 25 torr, because this is the level associated with cerebral vasodilation. ICP monitoring may also be indicated when PCO_2 is below 20 torr, which has been correlated with inadequate cerebral blood flow. To maintain CO_2 in a fixed narrow range, elective intubation with mechanical ventilation and immobilization of the child with pancuronium have been recommended (Table 21.6).

Decreasing Fluid Level

Mannitol has been used, at least in part, to induce an osmolar gradient between brain cells and the intravascular system, so that fluid can be drawn out of the brain. Achieving an intravascular osmolarity of 300 to 350 mOsm reduces the water volume in the brain, and the ICP can be reduced. Appropriate rapid infusion of mannitol at 0.5 mg/kg may decrease ICP a mean of 22 mm Hg and reverse early clinical signs of cerebral edema. Glycerol has also been used to induce an osmotic gradient. After glycerol is metabolized to glucose, however, it equilibrates with brain tissue and, therefore, no longer acts as an osmolar sump pump.

Hypothermia and Barbiturates

"Brain resuscitation" associated with decreasing the metabolic demands of the brain have been accomplished by using hypothermia and barbiturates. Both techniques may also reduce blood flow and blood volume in the brain, thereby reducing ICP.

Steroid Therapy

Although steroids are of use in patients with increased ICP from tumors, they do not prevent cerebral edema or increase survival in patients with FHF. A comparison of the use of mannitol and dexamethasone is shown in Table 21.7.

Table 21.6
Frequency of Development of Cerebral Edema and Mannitol Requirement in Electively Hyperventilated Patients (Group A) and Nonelectively Ventilated Patients (Group B)

	Group A	Group B
No. of patients	20	35
Increased intracranial pressure	17 (85%)	30 (85)
Total volume of mannitol (mean)	1689 ± 246 mL	1294 ± 250 mL
Total no. of episodes of cerebral edema	12	8.8
Volume of mannitol per episode	141 mL	146 mL
Duration of mannitol treatment (h)	60.0 ± 11.0	40.0 ± 7.7
No. of episodes of cerebral edema per 24 h	4.8	5.3

Table 21.7
Comparison of Mannitol and Dexamethasone in the Treatment of Patients with FHF

Treatment Group	Total	No. with Increased ICP	Survivors No.	%
Mannitol	10	10	5	50
Mannitol and dexamethasone	10	7	3	43
Dexamethasone	11	9	1	11
Neither drug	13	8	0	0

OTHER TECHNIQUES

Charcoal hemoperfusion, peritoneal dialysis, polyacylonitrile membrane hemodialysis, and exchange transfusion procedures have been tried to support the patient until hepatic regeneration occurs. Each of these techniques has been associated with temporary arousal of children or adults from deep stages of encephalopathy. Despite initial enthusiasm, however, increased survival has not been found with these techniques.

Liver transplantation should be considered early for patients with poor prognosis from FHF to allow as much time as possible for a donor organ to become available. The indications and contraindications for liver transplantation are delineated in Chapter 22 (Table 22.1).

22.

Liver Transplantation

Charles L. Schleien, G. Patricia Cantwell, and Andreas G. Tzakis

INDICATIONS

With continuing improvement in patient survival rate after orthotopic liver transplant (OLT), the scope of indications also continues to broaden. With wide application of OLT, the principal problem is limited donor availability. This problem has been alleviated somewhat by the use of reduced-size livers and split-liver grafting.

Patients who require OLT are summarized in Table 22.1. The most common indication for liver transplantation in children is biliary atresia.

CONTRAINDICATIONS

The list of contraindications for OLT in children and infants has decreased with better survival rates and greater understanding of perioperative principles, including immunosuppression, nutrition, and management of other organ systems. Relative contraindications for OLT are:

- Acceptable alternative medical therapy
- Expected suboptimal outcome
- Impairment of other organ systems that would compromise function of the graft
- Major systemic infection
- Cancer with a high postsurgical recurrence rate

Absolute contraindications for OLT are:

- Uncontrollable extrahepatic sepsis
- Unresectable hepatic malignant tumor

PREOPERATIVE MANAGEMENT OF THE DONOR

After declaration of brain death, meticulous management of the donor's physiologic parameters is imperative to avoid unnecessary loss of donor organs (Table 22.2). The basic principles of intensive care should be followed, with close monitoring of vital functions (i.e., blood pressure, heart rate, body temperature, urine volume, arterial blood gas determination, electrocardiographic data).

DONOR ORGAN
Size of Graft

The liver graft to be implanted must be similar in size to the diseased liver being removed. The shortage of pediatric donors and the great variability in the liver size needed has led to the use of reduced-size grafts. Liver fragments formed from hepatectomies include the results of a right hepatectomy, right trisegmentectomy, and left lateral segmentectomy.

Disadvantages to using a liver segment include hemorrhage, biliary fis-

Table 22.1
Indications

Conditions likely to progress to hepatic failure
    Biliary atresia
    Fulminant hepatic failure: infection, toxin, drug
    Chronic active hepatitis—hepatitis B or C
    Metabolic diseases (e.g., Wilson's disease)
    Cryptogenic cirrhosis
    Progressive cholestasis
    Byler disease
    Sclerosing cholangitis
Nonprogressive liver disease
    Intrahepatic cholestasis
    Alagille's syndrome
    Neonatal hepatitis
Systemic disease with hepatic involvement
    Cystic fibrosis
    α_1-Antitrypsin deficiency
    Tyrosinemia
    Crigler-Najjar syndrome
    Over-the-counter deficiency
    Wilson's disease
    Familial hypercholesterolemia
    Glycogen Storage disease types III and IV
    Perinatal Hemochromatosis-iron storage disease
Hepatic malignancy
    Primary malignancy
    Disease with secondary hepatic malignancy
        Tyrosinemia
    α_1-Antitrypsin deficiency
        Glycogen storage disease type I
        Biliary tract trauma

tula, and infections of the raw surface; however, the larger size of the donor artery decreases the incidence of hepatic artery thrombosis.

Suitability

The donor's surgeon evaluates the donor organ and determines its acceptability. Even perfect donors with hemodynamic stability and normal blood biochemistry values do not ensure a great advantage in graft survival. Insistence on these ideal donor conditions results in a waste of an already scarce resource.

Harvest

The liver is harvested as part of a multiple organ procurement, which usually involves liver, renal, and thoracic teams working in harmony. When the

Table 22.2
Donor—Preoperative Management

Respiratory
   Optimize arterial blood gases
   Maintain pulmonary physiotherapy
   Avoid respiratory alkalosis
   Anticipate pulmonary edema (neurogenic, fluid overload, cardiogenic, aspiration)
Cardiovascular
   Monitor blood pressure, heart rate, electrocardiogram
   Monitor central venous pressure and pulmonary artery pressure as indicated
   Maintain urine output ($\geq$ 1 mL/kg/h)
Renal
   Avoid consequences of excessive diuresis
      Hyperosmolality
      Hypokalemia
      Hypernatremia
Endocrine
   Treat diabetes insipidus
      Free water replacement
      Exogenous vasopression
   Treat hyperglycemia
   Avoid effects of hypothermia
      Electroencephalogram changes
      Electrocardiogram abnormalities
      Arrhythmias
      ↓ Cardiac contractility
      ↓ Glomerular filtration rate
      Coagulopathy
      Altered cellular metabolism
Infection
   Appropriate antibiotics
Central nervous system
   Treat autonomic instability (blood pressure ↑ or ↓, heart rate ↑ or ↓)
   Often secondary dehydration → liberalize fluids

donor's condition is stable, the surgeon performs a preliminary dissection of all the organs to be removed and the anatomy is defined. The organs are then cooled in situ by the rapid infusion of a chilled solution into the aorta. Additional perfusion is provided for the liver through a separate cannula, which is inserted through the splenic vein or other major side branch of the portal vein. When the donor is unstable, cooling through the aorta is performed on an urgent basis before careful dissection is performed.

Organ Preservation

The liver is preserved in special solutions. The solution developed by University of Wisconsin provides safe preservation of the liver for at least 12 to 16 hours, compared with 6 to 8 hours for previously used solutions. Advantages of increased length of preservation include:

- Longer distances between donor and recipient are allowed
- The procedure need not be performed as urgently
- Better surgical preparation of the operative field and back table procedures is facilitated, especially for reduced-size liver transplants

PREOPERATIVE MANAGEMENT OF THE RECIPIENT

Issues that must be resolved by the time the patient presents for preoperative management include:

- Confirmation of the diagnosis, consisting of full anatomic definition of the portal circulation and biliary tree
- Staging of the patient's condition
- Determination of possible contraindications to OLT
- Evaluation of other organ system dysfunction that may complicate the perioperative period
- Financial and social arrangements (Table 22.3)

INTRAOPERATIVE MANAGEMENT

Most patients undergoing hepatic replacement therapy receive an orthotopic transplant, with the native liver removed entirely and a whole or partial organ surgically implanted in another (i.e., orthoptic) position. In some centers, segmental auxiliary transplantation is performed in patients having metabolic deficiencies without removing the native liver. The following discussion of surgical technique and complications after OLT is confined to orthotopic transplants.

Surgical Technique

The surgery itself involves three phases (Table 22.4), each with its inherent problems and complications that must be anticipated.

The recipient hepatectomy phase may be lengthy, depending on the number of complicating factors (see Table 22.4). Patients with coagulopathy may require factor replacement during the hepatectomy stage to avoid an exsanguinating hemorrhage.

The anhepatic phase begins after placement of vascular clamps on the hepatic artery, portal vein, and suprahepatic and intrahepatic inferior vena cava (IVC) and subsequent removal of the liver.

The reperfusion phase begins on release of the vascular clamps. As the liver fills with blood, washout of small amounts of potassium-containing residual perfusion solution and release of congested blood from within the portal system and IVC may result in transient hypotension and bradycardia. This condition necessitates administration of vasopressors such as phenylephrine and ephedrine, atropine, and agents to buffer the increased acid and potassium load.

Table 22.3
Preoperative Evaluation of Potential Liver Transplant Recipient

History and physical examination
  Previous medical/surgical history
  Body weight and height
  Nutritional status
Laboratory evaluation:
  Complete blood cell count, platelets
  Electrolytes, serum urea nitrogen, creatinine, glucose, calcium (total & ionized),
    magnesium, phosphorus, uric acid
  Protein electrophoresis
  Bilirubin, γ-glutamyl transpeptidase (GGTP), amylase, ammonia
  Prothrombin time, partial thrombo-plastin time
  Arterial blood gas/pH
  Hepatitis A and B screen
Blood, urine, sputum, ascitic fluid cultures as needed
Blood typing, HLA type, cytotoxic antibody screen
Other evaluation
  Ceruloplasmin
  α_1-Antitrypsin level and phenotype
  Antimitochondrial, antithyroid, and antinuclear antibodies
  Iron, iron binding capacity, ferritin
  Quantitative immunoglobulins
Radiologic imaging
  Chest
  Abdominal ultrasound
  Abdominal computed tomography
  Cholangiography (if indicated)
  Arteriography (if indicated)
Ancillary evaluation
  Upper gastrointestinal panendoscopy
  Colonoscopy (as indicated)
  Endoscopic retrograde cholangiopancreatography (as indicated)
  Ophthalmologic evaluation
  Neuropsychiatric evaluation
  Electroencephalogram
  Psychosocial services

Intraoperative Complications

Complications that may occur during the surgical procedure include the following:

- Hemodynamic instability, usually a result of hypovolemia secondary to bleeding, may also result from myocardial depression associated with hypocalcemia, acidosis, or other factors released after reperfusion of the liver.
- Metabolic disturbances include hypoglycemia, hypocalcemia, and citrate intoxication from transfused blood; hyperkalemia; metabolic acidosis; and late metabolic alkalosis

Table 22.4
Surgery

Before incision
  Vascular access—large bore catheters
  Arterial access
  Correct dehydration
  Optimize cardiovascular and coagulation status
  Proper positioning
First phase: recipient hepatectomy
  Dissect liver
  Complications:
    Adhesions
  Portal hypertension/bleeding
  Anatomic abnormalities
  Pneumothorax
Second phase: anhepatic stage
  Clamps placed
  Established veno-veno bypass (>25 kg)
  Remove liver
  Superior vena cava anastomosis
  Inferior vena cava anastomosis
  Portal vein anastomosis
  Complications:
    Air embolus
Third phase: reperfusion stage
  Remove clamps
  Hemostasis established
  Hepatic artery anastomosis
  Biliary reconstruction
  Complications:
  Hypotension/bradycardia
  Surgical bleeding

- Air embolism may occur during venovenous bypass or because of inadequate flushing of the liver during implantation
- Pulmonary complications include pneumothorax, pleural effusion, and atelectasis
- Difficult abdominal closure, resulting in increased intra-abdominal pressure

Increased intra-abdominal pressure causes hypotension and high venous mesenteric and renal pressures, which cause intestinal and renal ischemia. This situation occurs most often in smaller patients with a donor liver that is too large. Infrequently, a silo or fascial patch is necessary to close the abdomen.

POSTOPERATIVE MANAGEMENT

The success of OLT hinges on the management of the patient in the operating room and during the first few postoperative days. Rapid changes in liver function and extrahepatic dysfunction require the skills of the many subspecialty services forming the multidisciplinary critical care team.

Patient Care and Monitoring

Children undergoing liver transplantation require extensive postoperative monitoring:

- Arterial blood pressure
- Central venous pressure
- Heart rate
- Electrocardiogram (ECG) tracings
- Respiratory rate
- Oxygen saturation
- Body temperature
- Urinary output
- Abdominal drain output
- Bile output
- Abdominal girth and body weight (twice daily)
- Hourly neurologic checks

A pulmonary artery catheter is useful in patients with congestive heart failure, cardiac dysfunction, or pulmonary hypertension.

On arrival at the pediatric intensive care unit (PICU), the patient may be hypothermic. Active warming should be undertaken, using warmed and humidified inspired ventilator gases, warmed fluid and blood products, and warming blankets.

Routine intensive care should include all methods available in PICUs, including respiratory and ventilator management and attention to fluid, electrolytes, and nutrition.

Hepatic Complications

Some primary hepatic complications that occur after liver transplantation result in loss of graft function and ultimately may necessitate retransplantation (Table 22.5). Retransplantation rates vary from 5 to 30% of first-time recipients, depending on the institution and characteristics of the donor graft.

Hemorrhage

Early postoperative bleeding is relatively common, requiring a second surgery in 5 to 10% of patients. Coagulopathy occurring after reperfusion of the donor liver is associated with multiple vascular anastomoses; the cut edge of segmental grafts provides the setting for postoperative bleeding. When bleeding from surgical drains increases and persists in spite of normalization of clotting factors, the patient should undergo an exploratory laparotomy to achieve hemostasis.

Table 22.5
Evaluation of Liver Dysfunction—Posttransplant

	Primary Nonfunction	Acute Rejection	Hepatic Artery Thrombosis	Portal Vein Thrombosis	Biliary Leak/Obstruction	Infection
Clinical symptoms	Hypoglycemia Coma Renal Failure Metabolic acidosis Cardiogenic shock Hyperammonemia	Fever Encephalopathy	Fever	Fever Intestinal swelling Ascites GI bleeding	Fever Peritonitis	Fever Malaise Anorexia
Lab						
Aspartate aminotransferase/ Alanine aminotransferase	+/+++	+/+++ (3–7 days)	+/+++ (3–7 days)	+/+++ (3–7 days)	0/+	+/++
GGT	+	+	+	+	+++	+
Bilirubin	+/+++	+/+++	+/+++	+/+++	+/+++	0/++
Coagulation profile	+/+++	+/+++	+/+++	+/+++	0/+	0/+
White blood cells	0/+	+/+++	+/+++	+/+++	0/+	+/+++
Cultures	Negative	Negative	+/–	+/–	+/–	+
Ancillary tests						
Ultrasonography	Normal blood flow	Echogenicity	Absent flow/ infarction Intrahepatic air	Absent flow/ infarction	Dilated bile ducts	Abscess
KUB						
CT			Occluded vessel Infarction Bowel/biliary disruption, extrinsic compression (hematoma, biloma, intrahepatic abscess)	Occluded vessel Infarction Bowel/biliary disruption	Dilated bile ducts Biloma Extrinsic compression of common duct	Abscess ileus Abscess

continued

Table 22.5
Evaluation of Liver Dysfunction—Posttransplant

	Primary Nonfunction	Acute Rejection	Hepatic Artery Thrombosis	Portal Vein Thrombosis	Biliary Leak/Obstruction	Infection
Angiography			↓/Absent flow	↓/Absent flow		Parenchymal defect
Radionuclide scan	Delayed ejection	↓Uptake Delayed excretion	Delayed excretion	Delayed excretion	Abnormal T-tube cholangiogram	
Biopsy		Portal inflammatory infiltrate Portal/central vein Endothelialitis Bile duct damage	Severe necrosis	Severe necrosis	Dilated ducts	Inflammatory infiltrates Inclusion bodies +Cultures Viral stains

A large hematoma often is found in the perihepatic area without a discrete bleeding site. Hematoma removal results in decreased consumption of clotting factors and often suffices to control the hemorrhage.

Graft versus Host Disease

The liver graft is capable of mounting an immunologic reaction against the host. Graft versus host disease (GVHD) may arise from a humoral cause, in which the donor is of a compatible but unidentified major blood group (e.g., O to A). Rarely, cellular GVHD is seen, including involvement of skin, gastrointestinal (GI) tract, lungs, and hematopoietic elements.

Diagnosis and Evaluation

Liver Function Tests Frequent assessment of liver function is routine, including measurement of total and direct bilirubin levels and transaminase levels (i.e., aspartase transaminase (AST), alanine transaminase (ALT), gamma-glutamyl transferase (GGT); alkaline phosphatase). When postoperative complications do not occur, liver enzymes typically reach peak levels within 72 hours and rapidly fall to normal levels thereafter.

Abnormal findings warrant further investigation.

- Persistent or increasing elevation of liver enzymes may indicate primary non-function
- Rising levels of liver enzymes between postoperative days 3 and 7 may indicate vascular occlusion or acute rejection
- Elevation of bilirubin and alkaline phosphatase levels may indicate cholestasis from liver injury, biliary leak, or infection of the biliary tree
- AGGT level greater than 500 IU/L is usually a sign of acute rejection or biliary tract obstruction

Synthetic and Metabolic Function Further discrimination among the causes of liver dysfunction requires assessment of synthetic and metabolic function. Prothrombin time (PT), partial thromboplastin time (PTT), and fibrinogen level are measured daily and should normalize over the first 72 hours after surgery. A sudden change in clotting function level signifies graft dysfunction caused by vascular occlusion or acute rejection. The serum ammonia level also may rise in the first week after surgery, indicating severe graft dysfunction.

Doppler Ultrasound Color Doppler ultrasonography assesses blood flow through the hepatic artery, portal vein, hepatic veins, and vena cava as well as fluid collections in the perihepatic area. This test usually is performed within 36 hours after surgery to gather baseline information and, later in the course when any complication ensues. Diagnosis of a vascular thrombosis by ultrasonography may be confirmed by selective arteriography.

Biliary Tract The biliary tract is assessed on the fifth to seventh day after surgery. T tube cholangiography is performed to assess healing of the biliary tract and provide evidence of obstruction or leak in the older patient who has a duct-to-duct anastomosis with a T tube.

Patients with a Roux-en-Y choledochojejunostomy routinely receive a 99mTc-diisopropyliminodiacetic acid (i.e., DISIDA) scan in the first postoperative week to assess uptake and excretion of radioactive tracer into the intestinal tract. Delayed uptake of tracer is associated with an improperly preserved donor liver, vascular compromise, or rejection. Delayed excretion into the biliary system may indicate hepatocellular damage from rejection, ischemia, or viral infection.

Liver Biopsy When liver function test results are normal, a liver biopsy is useful to test for early rejection. A biopsy is performed routinely after reperfusion of the liver and on posttransplant days 7 and 30. Results are used to refine immunosuppressive management.

Computed Tomography Scanning An abdominal computed tomography (CT) scan is useful in searching for the presence of an intra-abdominal fluid collection, which may be a source of infection and should be drained percutaneously or by laparotomy.

IMMUNOSUPPRESSION

Types of Rejection

Humoral or Hyperacute Rejection

This type of rejection typically occurs only hours or days after transplantation; hence, hyperacute refers to rejection of the donor organ by preformed antibodies. These antigraft antibodies are isoagglutinins of both IgG and IgM classes, which can cause clots that plug the liver microvasculature. Other cytotoxic antibodies, although less of a problem with liver transplants compared with heart or kidney grafts, may cause hyperacute rejection.

Cellular or Acute Rejection

This type of rejection occurs acutely usually days or weeks after transplantation. Mononuclear-cell infiltration of the liver is concentrated in the portal triads. The intrahepatic bile ducts are most affected, and there is some inflammatory attack of arteries and central and portal veins. These changes account for the following clinical effects:

- Decreased total liver blood flow
- Obliterative endophlebitis and subsequent outflow block, as in the Budd-Chiari syndrome
- Graft edema
- Intrahepatic cholestasis
- Parenchymal damage with biochemical changes

Successful treatment may resolve all of these problems if instituted before graft destruction occurs or chronic rejection ensues.

Chronic Rejection

Chronic rejection, usually seen months or years after transplant, also has been observed as soon as 3 or 4 weeks after transplant. It is heralded by:

- Occlusive arterial disease
- Disappearance of intrahepatic bile ducts
- Parenchymal fibrosis
- A sparse cellular infiltrate in the portal tracts

Clinically, chronic rejection is manifested by obstructive jaundice progressing over time to liver failure. Preservation of synthetic and other parenchymal function are early findings.

Pharmacology

Corticosteroids

High-dose corticosteroids, used in the initial management and treatment of rejection in combination with other immunosuppressant agents, work via a direct lymphocytotoxic effect. In moderate doses, these agents affect lymphocyte and macrophage activation and proliferation as well as cytokine production.

Complications of corticosteroid therapy include:

- Salt and water retention
- Hypertension
- GI hemorrhage
- Stunting of growth
- Cosmetic deformation, including moon facies, buffalo hump, striae, and bone abnormalities

Azathioprine

Azathioprine has a direct effect on all lymphocyte subsets and suppresses the bone marrow production of all cell lines. It also is used in combination with other immunosuppressant drugs for the prevention, but not the reversal, of rejection.

Side effects of azathioprine therapy are related to bone marrow suppression with decreased white blood cell count, red cell mass, or platelet count. Dosage adjustment is required for significant leukopenia or other evidence of bone marrow suppression.

Cyclosporine

The clinical availability of the fungal peptide cyclosporine has had a significant impact on the success of liver and all other organ transplantation. At immunosuppressive doses, cyclosporine selectively inhibits T-helper lymphocytes, sparing B lymphocyte, macrophage, and bone marrow function. At the cellular level, cyclosporine inhibits T- helper cell production of cytokines, particularly interleukin-2 (IL-2), as well as the elaboration of the high affinity IL-2 receptor by the cytotoxic T cell. The suppressor T cell is spared by cyclosporine, which may result in tolerance to the drug.

Use of cyclosporine requires the clinician be aware of many potential drug interactions (Table 22.6). Complications of cyclosporine therapy are summarized in Table 22.7. Significant renal dysfunction requires a dosage reduction.

FK 506

The major advantage of the macrolide FK 506 compared with cyclosporine is the ability to use it as a single agent, thus avoiding the toxicity of drugs such as corticosteroids and azathioprine. Typically, it is used as a sole agent for up to 3 months after transplant.

Complications attributed to FK 506 include toxicities also associated with cyclosporine:

- Nephrotoxicity with hypertension, hyperglycemia, and neurotoxicity
- Hyperglycemia, which may require the chronic use of insulin
- Neurologic toxicity, manifested by agitation, tremors, insomnia, and seizures

The incidence of nephrotoxicity is similar to that with cyclosporine, but usually is accompanied by less severe hypertension. The hirsutism and coarsening of facial features seen with cyclosporine are not observed with FK 506.

Another devastating complication secondary to both FK 506 and cyclosporine is lymphoproliferative disease, usually of the B-cell type associated with Epstein-Barr virus and epithelial or hematopoietic malignant tumors. When a pathologic diagnosis is made, immunosuppressive drugs usually are stopped in order to treat the cancer. Chemotherapy may be instituted in these instances.

Antilymphocyte Globulins (ALG)

Antilymphocyte globulins (ALG) are polyclonal or monoclonal antilymphocyte antibodies designed to eliminate lymphocytes from the circulation and lymphoid depots of the transplant recipient. ALGs are used either to treat rejection or as prophylaxis. Polyclonal antibodies may be used several times without creating resistance.

Table 22.6
Cyclosporine Drug Interactions

Drugs that ↑ cyclosporine levels
  Cimetidine
  Erythromycin
  Ketoconazole
  High-dose methylprednisolone
  Nonsteroidal anti-inflammatory agents
Drugs that ↓ cyclosporine levels
  Phenobarbital
  Phenytoin
  Rifampin
  Isoniazid
  Trimethoprim (intravenous)
Drugs that potentiate nephrotoxicity
  Aminoglycosides
  Amphotericin B
  Acyclovir

Antithymocyte Globulin (ATG) Antithymocyte globulin (ATG) is a polyclonal sheep or horse immunoglobulin active against human T lymphocytes. It specifically binds to mature T lymphocytes and inactivates or destroys them in association with macrophages. Although ATG is highly purified, serious systemic reactions occur, including fever, chills, skin rash, and serum sickness secondary to antibody complexes in the transplant recipient.

OKT3 A more sophisticated ALG, OKT3 is a murine antihuman T-lymphocyte monoclonal antibody. Binding of OKT3 to mature T-lymphocytes may eliminate them from their role in rejection by blocking the T-cell receptor or by specifically killing the T lymphocyte. OKT3 is highly effective in stopping established rejection episodes and has been used to prevent rejection in the early transplant period. The effectiveness of the monoclonal antibody may be eliminated by formation of blocking antimurine antibodies.

Complications associated with OKT3 therapy include a capillary leak syndrome, which causes pulmonary edema, and result in hypoxemia, fever, and occasionally, neurologic symptoms characterized by headache and meningismus.

Drug Regimens

Immunosuppressive regimens vary widely among institutions. A comprehensive understanding of the possible side effects of different immunosuppressive agents is essential (see Table 22.7).

The recent trend in therapy has been toward the use of methylprednisolone and FK 506 in the early postoperative period.

Table 22.7
Immunosuppressive Drugs—Side Effects

Corticosteroids
  Hypertension
  Na/H_2O retention
  Hyperglycemia
  Gastrointestinal bleeding
  Muscle weakness
  Personality changes
  Infection
Azathioprine
  Bone marrow suppression
  Infection
  Nausea, vomiting
  Mucosal ulceration
Cyclosporine
  Hypertension
  Renal dysfunction
  Hirsutism
  Hyperuricemia
  Neurologic dysfunction—tremors, seizures
  Hyperglycemia
  Muscle weakness
  Personality changes
  Infection
  Na/H_2O retention
FK506
  Renal dysfunction
  Hyperglycemia
  Hyperuricemia
  Neurotoxicity—tremors, agitation, insomnia, seizures
  Hypertension
OKT-3
  Fever
  Headache
  Pulmonary edema
  Meningismus/headache
Antithymocyte globulin (ATG)
  Anaphylaxis
  Serum sickness
  Infection
  Lymphopenia
Antihuman lymphoblast globulin (ALG)
  Thrombocytopenia
  Lymphopenia
  ↑ BUN, creatinine
  Anaphylaxis
  Serum sickness
  Chills, rashes, dyspnea

- FK 506 typically is begun at a dose of 0.15 mg/kg/day as a single, slow intravenous infusion
- When oral doses are tolerated, 0.15 mg/kg is administered twice per day
- Methylprednisolone or prednisone are started immediately postoperatively and discontinued when graft function is stable

The dose usually is increased in cases of rejection if the trough level is less than 2 ng/mL and there is no nephrotoxicity. The dose is decreased in the absence of rejection if the trough level is more than 3 ng/mL or if there are signs of nephrotoxicity.

In cases of rejection, FK 506 doses are in the high therapeutic range, and corticosteroids are pulsed intravenously. OKT3 typically is used in steroid-resistant rejection episodes.

NONHEPATIC MANAGEMENT

Fluids, Electrolytes, Nutrition, Gastrointestinal Tract

Fluid status, electrolyte balance, coagulation status, and liver and kidney function are assessed as outlined in Table 22.8, unless the clinical course mandates tighter monitoring.

Table 22.8
Laboratory Assessment After Liver Transplantation

Frequent (every 6–8 h)
   Hematocrit, platelets
   Prothrombin time, partial thromboplastin time
   Electrolytes
   Arterial blood gas/pH
   Ionized calcium
Daily
   Complete blood cell count
   Serum urea nitrogen
   Creatinine
   Total and ionized calcium
   Phosphorus
   Total and direct bilirubin
   Aspartate aminotransferase
   Alanine aminotransferase
   Alkaline phosphatase
   Gamma-glutanyl-transferase (GGT)
   Ammonia
   Amylase
   Total protein/albumin
   Immunosuppressive drug level (e.g., cyclosporine/FK 506)
   Chest radiograph

Fluid Management

Frequent alterations are required to balance fluid status after liver transplantation. Generally, the postoperative patient is fluid overloaded; fluids are given initially at 80% of maintenance requirements. Nasogastric and abdominal drain outputs are replaced by an isotonic crystalloid or colloid solution. Other physiologic parameters should be followed closely to maintain:

- High-normal central venous pressure (7 to 10 mm Hg)
- Urine output of 1 to 2 mL/kg/hour
- Normal mean arterial blood pressure

Low-dose dopamine, 0.5 to 3.0 μg/kg/minute, may be administered to enhance kidney and mesenteric perfusion. At all times, however, hypovolemia must be avoided because of its catastrophic effect on graft function.

Electrolytes

Electrolyte imbalances are common and should be corrected (see Chapters 8 and 23).

Nutrition

Careful assessment of the patient's nutritional status is imperative. Nutritional markers include:

- Total protein
- Albumin
- Prealbumin
- Cholesterol
- Triglyceride
- Retinal-binding protein
- Transferrin

Patients with preexisting cirrhosis, biliary atresia, or cancer are typically profoundly deficient in protein calories in the postoperative period.

Supplying Nutrients Intravenous hyperalimentation usually is instituted on the second postoperative day. Postoperative ileus generally resolves by the third to fourth postoperative day; therefore, enteral feedings may be initiated at that time. A silastic feeding tube may be placed beyond the pylorus if the patient is unable to take adequate oral feedings. Refeeding bile into the GI tract increases the capacity to absorb fat and also may protect against endotoxemia and renal failure.

Hyperglycemia Glucose intolerance, manifested by hyperglycemia and glucosuria, is commonly associated with high doses of corticosteroids, along with FK 506 and cyclosporine; release of glucose from dead donor-hepatocytes; or an elevated glucagon level. Insulin infusion allows adequate caloric intake until glucose tolerance improves. Intravenous lipids should not be administered until the triglyceride level falls below 200 mg/dL.

Hypoglycemia Severe hypoglycemia is associated with primary graft failure and should be treated with a glucose infusion until retransplantation.

Gastrointestinal Tract

Nasogastric Suction A nasogastric tube, usually placed during surgery, is maintained at low continuous suction. An antacid at a dose of 0.5 to 1.0 mL/kg is administered via the nasogastric tube every 2 to 4 hours to maintain the gastric pH level at more than 5.0. When normal bowel function returns during the first postoperative week, nasogastric suction can be discontinued.

H$_2$-Receptor Antagonists Elevated aminotransferase levels generally occur in patients receiving large doses of intravenous H$_2$-blockers. Cimetidine (30 mg/kg/day in four divided doses) and ranitidine (1 to 2 mg/kg/day in divided doses every 8 hours) have been implicated in causing hepatitis (cholestatic, mixed cholestatic-hepatocellular or pure hepatocellular pattern), although this complication is rare. Hepatic blood flow is probably not markedly altered by the use of H$_2$-blockers. Ranitidine has less of an effect on the metabolism of other drugs compared with cimetidine.

During the postoperative period, it remains imperative to maintain an index of suspicion for surgical complications including GI perforation.

Pulmonary Management

Extubation

Ventilator weaning and tracheal extubation usually are accomplished within 36 hours of the operation. Routine criteria for weaning from mechanical ventilation are used.

Some patients, however, require extended periods of ventilatory support. Extubation is delayed because of:

- Generalized weakness or abnormal chest wall mechanics in malnourished and very young infants
- Depressed respiratory drive secondary to oversedation
- Prolonged paralysis
- Impaired hepatic recovery
- Pain

Other pulmonary complications after transplantation are outlined in Table 22.9. Daily chest radiographs allow diagnosis of these complications in addition to observation of the position of indwelling tubes and intravascular catheters.

Table 22.9
Respiratory Complications

Depressed respiratory drive
　Oversedation
　Prolonged paralysis
　Impaired hepatic recovery: hyperammonemia
　Pain
Pulmonary edema
Atelectasis
Restrictive effect of large donor liver
Pneumonia
Pleural effusion, commonly right-sided
Diaphragmatic paralysis—phrenic nerve injury
Absent gag reflex
Inability to handle secretions—associated with hepatic encephalopathy
Metabolic alkalosis
Electrolyte disorder (hypophosphatemia, hypocalcemia, hypokalemia)
Adult respiratory distress syndrome
Abdominal distention

Pulmonary Edema

Pulmonary edema occurs secondary to fluid overload, but generally is controlled with:

- Diuretics
- Fluid restriction
- Positive end-expiratory pressure (PEEP) maintained at 5 cm H_2O (unless higher levels are required to maintain the PaO_2 at more than 70 mm Hg despite a fraction of inspired oxygen [FIO_2] of 0.5)
- Aggressive chest physiotherapy, including frequent suctioning, turning, clapping, postural drainage, incentive spirometry, and early mobilization

Atelectasis

Symptoms include:

- Pain
- General anesthesia
- Decreased movement
- Abdominal distention
- Pneumonia

Bronchoscopy is a useful therapeutic tool with persistent atelectasis.

Sepsis or Pneumonia

These conditions should be treated in the presence of acute respiratory distress syndrome. After transplantation, pneumonia or sepsis is associated with cytomegalovirus (CMV), *Pneumocystis carinii*, *Streptococcus faecalis*, *Pseudomonas aeruginosa*, *Aspergillus fumigatus*, and streptococcal pneumonia.

Pleural Effusions

Pleural effusions are usually right-sided and are often associated with ascites or fluid overload. They result from trauma induced by inadvertent clamping of a small section of the right hemidiaphragm as the suprahepatic vena cava is clamped. A coexisting phrenic nerve palsy with temporary paralysis of the right hemidiaphragm may also be seen.

Diuretics may be used to lessen the ascites and pleural effusion. Pleural drainage is indicated when respiratory compromise is present. This procedure should be undertaken with caution in the presence of coagulopathy and because of the numerous collateral vessels that are present secondary to the preexisting liver disease.

Restricted Movement

Normal respiratory movements may be hindered by high intra-abdominal pressures caused by a large donor liver or by ascites. If the pressure is secondary to ascites, drainage by peritoneal dialysis catheter may be done.

A donor liver that is larger than the recipient's native liver may cause pulmonary compromise by decreasing total lung volume, restricting diaphragmatic movement, and causing ventilation/perfusion ($\dot{V}/\dot{Q}$) mismatching from atelectasis.

Cardiovascular Management

Preoperatively, hepatic failure is associated with increased cardiac output, left ventricular dilation and hypertrophy, low systemic and pulmonary vascular resistance, and systemic and pulmonary shunting because of arteriovenous malformations.

After transplantation, the systemic vascular resistance normalizes and the cardiac output decreases. The low diastolic pressure in the pretransplant patient, owing to decreased systemic and pulmonary vascular resistance, is usually not a problem after surgery.

Myocardial Dysfunction

Postoperatively, fluid overload may result in decreased left ventricular compliance and decreased contractility. When myocardial dysfunction exists, the clinician should managed it with inotropic agents or afterload reducing agents, such as nitroprusside or nitroglycerin. Many patients are selenium-deficient or have an occult cardiomyopathy.

Hypertension

Hypertension encountered in the immediate postoperative period usually is attributed to pain. Morphine, 0.1 mg/kg, or fentanyl, 1 to 2 μg/kg may be effective in achieving postoperative analgesia, or patient-controlled analgesia may be used.

If there is no response to appropriate doses of analgesics, other causes of hypertension should be considered:

- Intravascular volume overload
- Elevated renin and catecholamine levels
- Renal toxicity caused by corticosteroids, FK 506, cyclosporine, or other drugs.

When systemic hypertension does not respond to pain control or diuresis, medications such as nitroprusside, a calcium channel blocker (e.g., nifedipine), or hydralazine should be used. The hypertension is generally transient and usually does not require treatment beyond the first month after transplant.

Hematologic Management

Hemolytic anemia may occur in ABO-compatible, nonidentical recipients, producing a graft-versus-host response that is seen within the first month after transplantation, is typically self-limited, and lasts approximately 2 to 4 weeks.

Signs of a graft versus host response encompass:

- Hemoglobinuria
- Sudden increase in total bilirubin level
- Minimal hepatic parenchymal enzyme changes
- Decreased serum hemoglobin level
- Increased reticulocyte count
- Sonographic evidence of an unobstructed biliary tract

Serial reticulocyte counts are the most useful tool in studying the progression of hemolysis. When evidence of hemolysis persists, the patient should receive type O blood.

Coagulation Disorders

Typically, after transplantation, PTT decreases to control levels within 2 days, and PT normalizes by 5 to 7 days. Postoperative coagulopathy, manifested by prolonged PT and PTT and thrombocytopenia, usually is responsive to appropriate component therapy. It should be corrected only if active bleeding is present or if the coagulation tests are more than twice their control level.

Graft dysfunction is associated with a lack of response to therapy with fresh frozen plasma or platelets. The degree of ongoing liver dysfunction, preoperative aspirin use, and large amounts of blood transfusion contribute to a clinically apparent coagulopathy. When repeated packed red blood cell transfusions are needed to maintain the hematocrit above 25 to 30%, surgical reexploration may be necessary to establish hemostasis.

Renal Management

Impaired Renal Function

The combination of FK 506, cyclosporine, corticosteroids, and an increase in serum renin level prevents the kidneys from responding appropriately to salt and volume overload with adequate diuresis and natriuresis. Appropriate postoperative therapy should include:

- Salt restriction
- Liberal use of diuretics
- Angiotensin-converting enzyme inhibitors for patients with a low creatinine excretion index

Acute Renal Failure

Acute renal failure most often occurs in patients with:

- Preexisting renal disease, including hepatorenal syndrome
- FK 506 or cyclosporine toxicity
- Other drug toxicity
- Acute tubular necrosis

Good graft function usually results in prompt resolution of preexisting hepatorenal syndrome. Refractory postoperative renal failure, even in patients with preexisting hepatorenal syndrome, is suggestive of systemic infection or graft dysfunction.

Venovenous bypass, which significantly reduces the incidence of acute renal failure after liver transplantation in adults, is generally not used in children who weigh less than 15 kg. In these patients, the suprarenal vena cava is occluded during the implantation of the new liver, resulting in a decrease in urine output. Mannitol may be administered in an effort to increase urine output and to minimize renal injury resulting from caval cross-clamping.

Acute Tubular Necrosis

Acute tubular necrosis generally is attributed to perioperative hypotension and massive intraoperative transfusions. FK 506 or cyclosporine levels must be monitored meticulously because of their propensity to cause acute tubular necrosis. The combination of hypovolemia and FK 506 administration increases the incidence of postoperative renal failure.

Metabolic Acidosis

When metabolic acidosis occurs in the immediate postoperative period, it is secondary to hepatic or renal failure. When severe, it may be controlled with continuous arteriovenous hemofiltration and predilution with sodium bicarbonate.

Infection Management

Infection is a common cause of death in the postoperative phase. Distinguishing between infection and rejection is necessary, because infection requires a decreased dose of immunosuppressive drugs whereas rejection usually necessitates an increased dosage.

Identifying the Cause of Infection

Surveillance cultures should be obtained from the throat, endotracheal tube, urine, blood, stool, and bile. A lumbar puncture should also be done to rule out central nervous system (CNS) infection, if warranted by the clinical examination. Samples must be cultured for aerobes, anaerobes, viruses, and fungi. An index of suspicion should also be maintained for reactivation of tuberculosis, Legionella species, and hepatitis B virus (HBV). The prevalence of hepatitis C infections in infants and children is substantially less than that in adults.

Children who have an enterostomy in place from a previous Kasai procedure are at increased risk for wound infections and, for this reason, the enterostomy should be closed before the transplant.

Protective isolation is not mandatory in the postoperative period; however, strict hand washing should be enforced to limit the spread of infection by hospital personnel. The patient's own GI flora is the greatest threat of infection. Various posttransplant infectious agents have been reported.

Antibiotic Therapy

Antibiotics effective against biliary pathogens (Klebsiella species, *Escherichia coli,* and enterococcus) should be continued postoperatively. The combination of ampicillin and cefotaxime is an effective regimen.

Mycostatin oral suspension given four times a day via nasogastric tube and mycostatin vaginal suppositories (for adolescent girls) given three times a day help minimize the incidence of oral and vaginal candidiasis.

Selective bowel decontamination may be used to eliminate an endogenous source of gram-negative and fungal organisms from the GI tract. Treatment consists of a solution of gentamicin (80 mg), polymyxin E (100 mg), and nystatin (2,000,000 U) administered through a nasogastric tube or orally as tolerated. The solution can also be applied to the oral cavity while the patient is still tracheally intubated.

Bacterial Infection

Bacterial pneumonia is relatively uncommon as a cause of infection after surgery. It is most often seen in immunosuppressed children with an underlying disease such as cystic fibrosis, α_1-antitrypsin deficiency, or chronic bronchitis. The antibiotic regimen may be altered in accordance with results of surveillance cultures. Fiberoptic bronchoscopy with bronchoalveolar lavage may be helpful in specific cases of pneumonia. In the event of a new pulmonary infiltrate, erythromycin and trimethoprim-sulfamethoxazole (TMP-SMX) provide adequate coverage for Legionella and *P. carinii* infection before culture results are available.

Other bacterial infections include cholangitis and intra-abdominal abscesses. Cholangitis may be associated with mechanical obstruction of the biliary tree; therefore, biliary obstruction must be excluded.

Viral Infections

Cytomegalovirus, herpes simplex virus (HSV), and Epstein-Barr virus (EBV) are the most common viral infections seen after transplantation. Adenovirus has been associated with overwhelming pneumonitis and hepatitis.

Cytomegalovirus

CMV titers may be elevated because of a new infection or reactivation of a previous infection. Asymptomatic shedding of CMV is detected by isolation of the virus in the urine or pharynx in the absence of clinical illness or an increase in the anti-CMV–IgM titer. When symptoms of active infection are not present, the patient should be treated for rejection. Whenever possible, CMV-positive donors are used in CMV-positive recipients. Prophylaxis with intravenous CMV immune globulin has not triggered a decreased incidence of posttransplant infections.

Clinical Signs Manifestations of CMV infection include:

- Fever
- Malaise
- Anorexia
- Abnormal results on liver function tests (levels of bilirubin and transaminases)
- Leukopenia
- Pneumonitis (interstitial pulmonary infiltrates and positive results on culture of bronchoalveolar lavage)
- Enteritis (abdominal pain, nausea, vomiting, GI hemorrhage, diarrhea, and mucosal ulcerations that are positive for CMV seen at endoscopy)
- Hepatitis
- Pneumonitis
- Colitis

- Sepsis
- Cerebritis

Evidence of viral infection is occasionally found on liver biopsy, usually with evidence of concomitant rejection. Primary infection is associated with a more severe clinical course than does a reactivation-associated infection.

Treatment When CMV infection is severe, the dose of immunosuppressive agents is decreased and gancyclovir is added to the patient's regimen. In severe cases of hepatitis, pneumonitis, duodenitis, gastritis, or colitis, immunosuppressive agents may have to be discontinued. Patients with severe CMV infection and concomitant rejection have been successfully treated with a combination of OKT3 and gancyclovir.

Herpes Simplex Virus

Acyclovir is used to treat any sign of HSV infection. Topical therapy is used for cutaneous lesions; invasive infection requires systemic therapy. Herpes encephalitis is usually fatal despite prompt institution of acyclovir therapy and withdrawal of immunosuppressive drugs.

Epstein-Barr Virus

Epstein-Barr Virus (EBV) infections range from an asymptomatic, isolated rise in viral titers to mononucleosis or lymphoma. Acyclovir is used to treat EBV infections. Lymphoma is secondary to immunosuppressive drug use; therefore, it is managed by withdrawal of immunosuppressive drugs rather than with chemotherapy. Breinig and coworkers reported a 57% incidence of EBV infection by means of serologic testing with only 12% of cases being symptomatic. Of the patients with primary EBV infections, 14% contracted an EBV-associated lymphoproliferative syndrome between 2 months and 2 years after the infection.

Fungal Infections

Candida albicans is often encountered in the immunocompromised host. Aspergillus species cause the next most frequent fungal infection, which is usually fatal. Other risk factors for fungal infections include prolonged surgical time and the use of relatively high doses of antibiotics and immunosuppressive agents.

Positive results on blood cultures should not be merely attributed to central line colonization. Specimens from indwelling venous and arterial catheters must be cultured often.

Amphotericin B should be strongly considered if fungemia is suspected, but the dose should be adjusted cautiously in the presence of altered renal function. Ketoconazole is not recommended for use in transplant recipients.

Pneumocystis carinii Infection

When this life-threatening nonviral infection is suspected, prompt institution of TMP-SMX therapy is warranted. The diagnosis may be facilitated by examination of samples from bronchoalveolar lavage. In the event of a resistant infection or an allergy to sulfa drugs, pentamidine isethionate may be used. The incidence of *P. carinii* infection in the immunocompromised patient may be reduced by using TMP-SMX prophylaxis.

Neurologic Management

Neurologic function may be depressed after liver transplantation because of the lingering effects of anesthetics, narcotics, and neuromuscular blocking agents. Compromised liver or kidney function may prolong the excretion of many of these drugs and lengthen the period of neurologic derangement. Most patients become responsive within the first postoperative day. Patients who had preoperative encephalopathy may take many days to recover normal CNS function.

Central nervous system complications include seizures, strokes, peripheral neuropathy, and "dulled mentation."

Seizures

Seizures are usually grand mal. Although CT scanning and lumbar puncture generally reveal negative results, the possibility of an intracranial hemorrhage, infarct due to clot or air embolism, or metabolic disorder, such as hyponatremia, hypoglycemia, FK 506 or cyclosporine toxicity, should be ruled out.

Other factors associated with seizures are:

- Fluid retention
- Hypertension
- High-dose corticosteroid therapy
- Hypomagnesemia
- Graft dysfunction
- Demyelination

Reduction of the FK 506 or cyclosporine dosage is advisable in cases of suspected toxicity. Cyclosporine-induced CNS toxicity has also been seen in association with a low serum cholesterol level.

Phenobarbital controls most seizures. When anticonvulsant therapy is instituted, it is important to monitor FK 506 or cyclosporine levels, because both phenobarbital and phenytoin are associated with decreasing plasma levels of these agents.

Cerebral Edema

Cerebral edema, either vasogenic or cytotoxic, may complicate management both before and after transplant. Intracranial pressure monitoring may be prudent, although placement of a monitoring device may be problematic in respect to a coincident profound coagulopathy.

Psychosocial Management

Social and financial management are important aspects of successful transplantation. Social problems encountered are related to finances, chronic disease, interpersonal relationships within the family, age of the patient, and sophistication of caretakers.

23.

Renal Disorders in Pediatric Intensive Care

Matthew M. Hand, Michael L. McManus, and William E. Harmon

INTRODUCTION

Renal failure may be caused by a variety of insults, including ischemia, nephrotoxins, and a range of primary renal diseases. A comprehensive list of conditions that may lead to renal failure is provided in Table 23.1.

FLUID AND ELECTROLYTE MANAGEMENT

Basal Requirements

Fluid, electrolytes, and caloric requirements per kilogram of body weight are much greater in infants than in children and adults. Additionally, patients with increased energy expenditure beyond a basal metabolic state have greater fluid requirements. Fever, for example, increases basal requirements by about 12.5% for every degree of temperature more than 38°C (Tables 23.2 and 23.3).

Replacement

The basis of fluid replacement therapy is to return to the patient the same composition and volume of fluid that has been lost. The composition of replacement fluids for insensible losses is generally free water. The replacement fluids for other losses are variable, yet generally should be isotonic (Table 23.4).

Table 23.1
Causes of Renal Failure in Children

Prerenal/Hypoperfusion
  Hemorrhage
  Dehydration
  Septic shock
  Surgery
  Diabetes mellitus
  Diabetes insipidus
  Burns
  Decreased cardiac function
Anatomic
  Obstruction (posterior urethral valves, tumor, blood clots)
  Congenital renal disease
    Multicystic dysplastic kidneys
    Autosomal recessive polycystic kidney disease
    Renal agenesis/hypoplasia
  Papillary necrosis
Toxins
  Organic solvents (ethylene glycol, methanol)
  Metals (lead, mercury, gold, bismuth)
  Chelating agents
  Radiocontrast dyes
  Myoglobin (rhabdomyolysis, crush injuries, malignant hyperthermia)
  Hemoglobin (transfusion reaction, venomous bites)
  Uric acid
  Oxalate
Immunologic/Vasculitis
  Hemolytic uremic syndrome
  Acute postinfectious glomerulonephritis
  Rapidly progressive glomerulonephritis
  Systemic lupus erythematosus
  Goodpasture's syndrome
  Wegener's granulomatosis/ANCA—positive vasculitis
  Membranoproliferative glomerulonephritis
  Henoch-Schönlein purpura
  Nephrotic syndrome
Infectious
  Bacterial
  Viral
  Mycoplasma
  Bacterial endocarditis
Drugs
  Antibiotics
    Aminoglycosides
    Penicillin
    Amphotericin B
  Angiotension converting enzyme inhibitors
  Acyclovir
  Nonsteroidal antiinflammatory drugs (indomethacin, ibuprofen)
  Anesthetic agents (methoxyflurane)
Vascular
  Bilateral renal artery/vein thrombosis

Table 23.2
Caloric Expenditure/kg of Body Weight

1–10 kg	100 kcal/kg/d
10–20 kg	1000 kcal + 50 kcal/kg over 10 kg/d
>20 kg	1500 kcal + 20 kcal/kg over 20 kg/d

Table 23.3
"Maintenance" Fluid and Electrolyte Requirements[a]

Fluid requirements by body weight:	
1–10 kg	100 mL/kg/d
10–20 kg	1000 mL + 50 mL/kg over 10 kg/d
>20 kg	1500 mL + 20 mL/kg over 20 kg/d
Electrolyte composition of solutions:	
Sodium	3–5 mEq/100 mL
Potassium	2–4 mEq/100 mL
Chloride	2–3 mEq/100 mL

[a]Patients with normal renal function

ACUTE RENAL FAILURE

Renal failure is defined as the cessation of kidney function with or without changes in urine volume. Anuria is arbitrarily defined as urine output of less than 0.5 mL/kg/hour, whereas oliguria is urine output of more than 1 mL/kg/hour.

Nonoliguric versus Oliguric Renal Failure

Maintenance of adequate urine output and prevention of further renal injury is critical. Because of the better outcome in patients with nonoliguric renal failure, many investigators have attempted to "convert" oliguric to nonoliguric renal failure.

Diagnostic Studies

Renal failure often is separated into three major categories: prerenal, renal (intrinsic), and postrenal. Each condition can progress to another, and acute renal failure (ARF) is often multifactorial in nature.

Fractional Excretion of Sodium

In prerenal azotemia, the fractional excretion of sodium is low and the serum urea nitrogen level (i.e., BUN) to creatinine level ratio is more than 20. The fractional excretion of sodium (FE_{Na}) is calculated as follows:

$$U_{Na}/P_{Na} \times P_{cr}/U_{cr} \times 100 = FE_{Na}$$

Table 23.4
Composition of Body Fluids

Fluid	Electrolyte (mEq/L)		
	Na	K	Cl
Gastric	20–80	5–20	100–150
Pancreatic	120–140	5–15	40–80
Biliary	120–140	5–15	80–120
Small intestinal	100–140	5–15	90–130
Ileostomic	45–135	3–15	20–115
Diarrheal	10–90	10–80	10–110

Table 23.5
Urine and Serum Laboratory Values in Prerenal and Intrinsic Renal Failure

	Prerenal	Renal
BUN/Cr	>20	<20
FENa	<1%	>2%
Renal Failure Index	<1%	>1%
U_{Na}	<20 mEq/L	>40 mEq/L
Specific Gravity	>1.020	<1.010
U_{osm}	>500 mOsm/L	<350 mOsm/L
U_{osm}/P_{osm}	>1.3	<1.3

in which the U_{Na} is urinary sodium, P_{cr} is plasma creatinine, P_{Na} is plasma sodium, and U_{cr} is urinary creatinine, all from simultaneously obtained "spot" blood and urine samples. Values in neonates and infants differ slightly from those in older children because of their greater urinary losses of sodium. In the presence of loop diuretics, such as furosemide, the FE_{Na} is artificially high and not particularly useful. In such cases, when diuretics must be given, the fractional excretion of urea (calculated similarly) may be used.

Renal Failure Index

The renal failure index (RFI) is based on similar variables. Like the FE_{Na}, the values are slightly different for neonates. RFI is calculated as follows:

$$RFI = (U_{Na} \times 100)/U_{cr}/S_{cr}$$

in which S_{cr} is the serum creatinine and other variables are as above.

A comparison of the laboratory values and calculated indices in prerenal and intrinsic renal failure is shown in Table 23.5.

Imaging

Ultrasound examinations can be helpful in the diagnosis of ARF. Nuclear medicine scans are available to evaluate renal function and anatomy. Renal scans are not necessary to diagnose ARF, but they may aid in identifying its cause. They are also particularly useful in evaluating renal transplant recipients in the postoperative period.

Specific Prevention Strategies

If specific treatment is undertaken early, hemoglobinuria, myoglobinuria, and uric acid nephropathy may often be predicted and renal damage limited.

Hemoglobinuria

Hemoglobinuria is seen in patients with red blood cell lysis (as in transfusion reaction, hemolytic uremic syndrome, ethanol sclerotherapy, extracorporeal circulation). In massive hemolysis, the stromal component of the red blood cell likely causes mechanical obstruction and has a greater nephrotoxic effect than hemoglobin. Treatment of hemoglobin nephropathy focuses on preventing and inhibiting the toxic mechanisms:

- Increasing urine flow by aggressive hydration decreases tubular obstruction
- Alkalinization of the urine increases hemoglobin solubility and decreases the toxic effect of hemoglobin
- Urine pH level may be raised by bicarbonate infusion and carbonic anhydrase inhibitors
- Mannitol and furosemide increase urine flow and reduce tubular obstruction
- Exchange transfusion or plasmapheresis lowers serum hemoglobin levels in refractory cases

Myoglobinuria

Myoglobin-induced nephrotoxicity occurs in patients with muscle injuries (e.g., electrocution, malignant hyperthermia, crush injuries, other causes of rhabdomyolysis); therefore, myoglobin may pose a greater risk for nephrotoxicity than hemoglobin. Preventing renal damage is the goal in susceptible patients.

Diagnosis The hallmark of myoglobinuria is urine that tests positive for blood without the presence of red blood cells. The diagnosis is confirmed by an elevated serum creatine phosphokinase (CPK) level. Myoglobinuria associated with rhabdomyolysis involves extensive muscle damage and creatinine release. With rhabdomyolysis, the serum creatinine level may increase by more than 2 mg/dL/day early in the course. The BUN:creatinine ratio is typically less than 10. The massive tissue destruction usually involved can lead to significant hyperkalemia.

Treatment Treatment of myoglobin nephropathy is the same as for hemoglobin-induced nephropathy:

- Aggressive hydration
- Diuresis
- Alkalinization (to a urine pH level of more than 7)

Uric Acid Nephropathy

Significant elevation of uric acid may cause ARF. The typical patient at risk has tumor lysis syndrome as a result of the initiation of chemotherapy for solid tumors or acute lymphoproliferative diseases with high cell turnover rates. Uric acid precipitates in acidic urine, intratubular obstruction, and renal failure then occur.

Treatment involves:

- Aggressive hydration to produce high urine flow rates
- Bicarbonate infusion to alkalinize the child's urine
- Administration of xanthine oxidase inhibitors before chemotherapy is started

If renal failure develops, even with aggressive therapy, dialysis is indicated.

Management of Renal Failure

Fluid Therapy

Standard "maintenance fluids" that are appropriate for patients with normal renal function can cause fluid overload, hypertension, and pulmonary edema in patients with ARF. In polyuric states, these fluids may lead to dehydration.

Proper management of the patient in renal failure involves replacing losses. Fluid losses include insensible losses, urine output, and other losses (i.e., surgical drains, nasogastric tubes, diarrhea). Insensible losses are calculated generally at 300 mL/M^2/day. Other losses should be measured.

Electrolyte concentrations of replacement solutions should be guided by the concentration found in lost fluids. Standard concentrations of body fluids are indicated in Table 23.4. Urine replacement is calculated using urine electrolytes.

As long as the patient has ARF, no potassium should be given until normal serum potassium concentration is attained and some potassium is excreted. If the patient has substantial urine output, significant potassium depletion could occur.

Daily measurement of body weight (occasionally twice a day) and frequent assessment of serum electrolyte levels are essential for determining the accurate composition of fluid and electrolyte replacement.

Electrolyte Therapy

Sodium The usual sodium abnormality in ARF is hyponatremia caused by water retention. In patients with hyponatremia and volume overload, restriction of free water intake to less than the volume of output allows for hypotonic fluid loss and leads to correction of hyponatremia. Serum sodium should be viewed as a reflection of total body water, whereas urine sodium is often an indicator of total body sodium.

Calculating Deficit The following formula:

Sodium deficit = (normal serum sodium level − actual serum sodium level) × 0.6 × (body weight in kg)

describes the total cation deficit, but it is safe to assume that the losses are sodium. Normal serum sodium level should be 135 mEq/L.

Treating Hyponatremia Symptomatic hyponatremia (i.e., obtundation and seizures) may be treated with 3% saline infusions. In an emergency, standard (1 mEq/mL) $NaHCO_3$ solution, available with resuscitative medications, may be used. The sodium deficit formula is used for calculation of the amount of sodium that must be replaced. Although hyponatremic seizures are difficult to control using anticonvulsants, they respond well to relatively modest rises in serum sodium level.

Because rapid return to normonatremia may precipitate neurologic injury, it is most prudent to use lower goals (such as 125 mEq/L) for target serum sodium level. Three percent saline contains 513 mEq/L of sodium, is extremely hypertonic, and should be administered with extreme caution.

Potassium

Decreased Excretion Patients with ARF accumulate potassium because the kidney is responsible for elimination of 85 to 90% of daily potassium excretion. The remaining 10 to 15% is removed by the gastrointestinal tract. Patients with chronic renal failure may compensate by increasing their gastrointestinal losses, but similar compensation in patients with ARF is unlikely.

Increased Generation Many patients not only have decreased potassium excretion but also have increased potassium generation. Patients with rhabdomyolysis, hemolysis, tissue necrosis, and other cellular damage experience a large release of intracellular potassium. When a decrease in excretion and an increase in generation are combined with acidosis, commonly occurring in the critically ill child, serum potassium levels can increase dramatically. For each 0.1 unit decline in pH level, K^+ increases by 0.5 mEq/L.

Treating Hyperkalemia Hyperkalemia is life-threatening because of the importance of the intracellular potassium gradient in regulation of cardiac action potential generation and conduction. As a consequence, aggressive therapy is warranted. Treatment should be started when the serum K^+ is more than 6 mEq/L or at lower levels if the serum K^+ is rising rapidly.

Therapy involves:

- Protection of the myocardium by infusion of calcium (10 mg/kg elemental Ca^{++} as CaCl or calcium gluconate) in an effort to increase conductance and contractility
- Shift of K^+ from extracellular to intracellular sites
- Removal of K^+ via the gastrointestinal tract or dialysis

Treatment options for hyperkalemia are outlined in Table 23.6.

Nutrition Therapy

Patients with ARF are initially in a catabolic state. The primary goals in managing the nutritional needs of patients in ARF are:

- Maintaining adequate caloric intake
- Avoiding excessive protein intake to control the rise in BUN
- Minimizing potassium and phosphate intake
- Reducing fluid intake

Renal Replacement Therapy

A number of factors influence the need for renal replacement therapy (Table 23.7). Renal replacement therapy is available through a large number of methods, all of which are based on principles of solute mass transfer and ultrafiltration (i.e., fluid removal). The choice depends on the clinical scenario and the experience at individual centers.

Hemodialysis Hemodialysis results in removal of solutes from a patient's serum.

Ultrafiltration Removal of fluid (ultrafiltrate) can be performed independently of solute transfer with modern dialysis machines, and extremely accurate control of ultrafiltration can be accomplished. Ultrafiltration is controlled independently of blood flow and is regulated by a transmembrane pressure applied by the dialysis machine.

Central Access A continuous circuit from "arterial" to "venous" site is required. Three techniques are used.

1. Separate access lines, one arterial and one venous, may be placed. Rarely, however, is an arterial catheter used for hemodialysis.
2. More commonly, a single catheter with a distal or "venous" port and a proximal "arterial" side port is placed in a large vein. The dialysis pump pulls blood from the "arterial" port and after passing through the dialyzer, returns it to the patient via the "venous" port. Unfortunately, the proximity of the catheter ports permits approximately 15% "recirculation" of blood (i.e., blood returning to the patient is sucked back into the dialyzer without first circulating in the patient). Recirculation decreases clearance but can be offset by increasing the duration of the dialysis treatment.

Table 23.6
Treatment of Hyperkalemia

Drug or Method	Dose and Route	Onset (Duration)	Mode of Action	Comments
Calcium gluconate (100 mg/mL)	10 mg/kg over 5 min; may repeat ×2	Immediate (30–60 minutes)	Counteracts electrophysiologic effects of hyperkalemia	Monitor electrocardiogram for bradycardia; stop infusion if pulse < 100/min
Sodium bicarbonate (1 mEq/mL)	1–2 mEq/kg IV bolus or infusion over 20 min	20 min (1–4 h)	Causes movement of K+ intracellularly	Assure adequate ventilation; do not give simultaneously with calcium
Glucose and Insulin	1–2 g/kg and 0.3 U/kg together over 1–2 h	15–30 min (3–6 h)	Causes movement of K+ intracellulary	Monitor blood sugar
Kayexalate	1 gm/kg in 30% sorbitol PR or in 70% sorbitol PO	15–30 min	Removes K+ from body	Removes 1 mEq K+/g resin; exchanges Na+ equimolarly with K+
Dialysis	Hemodialysis is most rapid	Immediate	Removes K+ from body	Do not ignore first four steps while preparing for dialysis

Table 23.7
Indications for Acute Dialysis or Hemofiltration

Intractable acidosis
Fluid overload, pulmonary edema
Serum urea nitrogen > 150 mg/dL
Symptomatic uremia (encephalopathy, pericarditis)
Hyperkalemia (serum K+ >7 mEq/L)
Hyperammonemia
Ultrafiltration for nutritional support, transfusions
Exogenous toxins (lithium, salicylate, ethanol, methanol, ethylene glycol,
    aminoglycosides, bromide, theophylline, phenobarbital)
Hyponatremia or hypernatremia

Table 23.8
Temporary and Permanent Hemodialysis Catheters for Pediatric Patients

Type	Manufacturer	External Diameter	Length	Indication
Temporary	MedComp	7F	4 in	Newborn-infant subclavian
	MedComp	7F	6 in	Newborn-infant femoral
	MedComp	7F	8 in	Newborn-infant femoral
	MedComp	7F	12 in	Newborn-infant femoral
	MedComp	9F	4 ¾ in	Toddler subclavian
	MedComp	9F	6 in	Toddler femoral
	MedComp	9F	8 in	Toddler femoral
	Quinton	10F	4 ¾ in	Child, small adult
	Quinton	11F	5 in	Child subclavian/femoral
	Quinton	11F	7 in	Adult subclavian
Permanent	MedComp	8F	18 cm	Infant
	MedComp	8F	24 cm	Infant/Child
	Quinton	10F	28 cm	Child
	MedComp	11.5F	28 cm	Adult
	Quinton	12F	36 cm	Adult
	Quinton	12F	40 cm	Adult

3. A single-lumen catheter can be used with special equipment that permits "single-needle" dialysis. This equipment includes special clamps and pumps that alternate pumping blood into the patient and removing it sequentially through the same catheter. Recirculation is extensive with this method, and therefore is not often used.

Catheters and Insertion Sites Large-bore catheters are required for dialysis because the blood flow can be a limiting factor. Catheter size is dictated by patient size. Suitable dual-lumen catheters are available now for infants (Table 23.8). Preferred sites of insertion include

- Left subclavian vein
- Right internal jugular vein
- Femoral veins

For adequate flows through femoral catheters, ports must reside in an inferior vena cava that is free from clots and external compression.

Treatment Schedule To avoid sequelae related to osmotic shifts during treatment, dialysis should be initiated before BUN level exceeds 150 mg/dL. The initial treatment should decrease BUN level by 20 to 30%. Urea clearance can then be increased by 25% per day. Dialysis often is performed on three consecutive days, increasing gradually to a maximum of 75% reduction of BUN level. Treatments then are changed to an alternate day schedule unless urea generation is excessive or daily ultrafiltration is necessary.

Complications Complications of hemodialysis are listed in Table 23.9.

Osmotic Shifts Dialysis disequilibrium syndrome and other symptoms occurring during dialysis are generally related to osmotic shifts. Mannitol can be used to maintain serum osmolarity in patients who are likely to experience difficulty with osmotic shifts, specifically those with cerebral edema.

Hypotension Hypotension usually is associated with rapid ultrafiltration and subsequent intravascular depletion. To avoid large shifts in extracorporeal blood volume, no more than 10% total blood volume should be in the tubing and dialyzer. If the tubing and dialyzer volume requires more than 10% of total blood volume or the patient is hemodynamically compromised, the tubing should be primed with albumin and packed red blood cells (PRBC). The hematocrit of the prime should be 40 to 45%.

Peritoneal Dialysis Placement of a catheter, surgically or percutaneously, into the intraperitoneal space and instillation of dialysate allows mass transfer of solute and ultrafiltration.

Comparison to Hemodialysis When comparing peritoneal dialysis to hemodialysis:

- Urea clearance is not as efficient but is more gradual and steady
- Easier to administer, particularly in infants
- Similar principles pertain to both forms of therapy
- Blood flow or dialysis size cannot be changed in peritoneal dialysis. Dialysate volume and frequency of dialysate exchanges may be increased or decreased to effect solute clearance.

Table 23.9
Complications of Hemodialysis

Hypotension
Bleeding
Muscle cramps
Embolism
Disequilibrium syndrome
Catheter infection
Complement activation

Assessing Efficiency There is no conclusive test of the effectiveness of peritoneal dialysis. In ARF, the need for extensive calculations of peritoneal dialysis kinetics is rare. The dialysis prescription is derived from the patient's clinical status and metabolic status and by the need for ultrafiltration.

Ultrafiltration Ultrafiltration in peritoneal dialysis is obtained through the use of dextrose as an osmotic agent in the dialysate. Increasing the dextrose concentration increases ultrafiltrate removal: The standard concentrations are 1.5%, 2.5%, and 4.25%. The solutions may be combined to produce intermediate concentrations.

Contraindications Relative contraindications to peritoneal dialysis are found in patients with:

- Intraperitoneal drains and bowel rupture
- Diaphragmatic hernia
- Diaphragm surgery
- Communication between the abdominal and the thoracic cavities

Treatment Schedule After the catheter is placed, the proper dialysate volume is critical for adequate dialysis and patient tolerance of the procedure. After three successive, rapid flushes to ensure catheter patency, the clinician begins dialysis with 10 mL/kg of dialysate. Initially, 1.5% dextrose concentration dialysate is used to avoid excessive ultrafiltration. As the patient adapts to the intraperitoneal volume, the dialysate volume is increased by 10 mL/kg/dwell to a maximum of 40 to 50 mL/kg/dwell. Clearance is increased by administering short, frequent dwells. Ultrafiltrate is increased by increasing dextrose concentration and dwell frequency. Dwell times vary from 30 minutes to 6 hours. Peritoneal dialysis cyclers can be used to instill and drain dialysate and are particularly useful for treatment of infants.

Complications Complications of peritoneal dialysis include:

- Peritonitis
- Dialysate leakage
- Catheter blockage
- Hyperglycemia
- Decreased vital capacity
- Pleural effusions
- Hypotension
- Protein loss
- Visceral rupture

Meticulous care and sterile technique are required when handling the catheter and the catheter site. To prevent leakage, surgical placement with tunneling of a cuffed catheter improves closure around the catheter.

Catheter Obstruction Obstruction can limit instillation and draining of the dialysate. Causes include:

- Fibrin deposition
- Infection
- Omentum around the catheter
- Impingement by abdominal organs

If infection or fibrin deposition is suspected, urokinase instillation (from 5,000 to 20,000 U) and removal may clear the obstruction. Positioning of the patient may help relieve some obstructions.

Peritonitis

Causative Factors Typically, the causative bacterial organism is skin flora. Enteric flora, fungus, and other gram-negative rods, such as *Pseudomonas* species, may cause peritonitis, particularly in infants and malnourished patients.

Clinical Findings Clinical findings include:

- Fever
- Abdominal pain
- Vomiting
- Cloudy dialysate
- Catheter obstruction
- Hypotension

Occasionally, urea clearance and ultrafiltration decrease in patients with peritonitis.

Laboratory Evaluation Evaluation of suspected peritonitis includes complete blood count (CBC) and peritoneal fluid cell count and culture. If peritonitis is suspected, the clinician should institute therapy before culture results are available.

Therapy Intraperitoneal antibiotics and aggressive dialysis are the principle therapies for peritonitis. Vancomycin and gentamicin are added to the dialysate and instilled. The initial concentration of vancomycin is 500 mg/L; subsequent dwells contain 20 mg/L vancomycin. Gentamicin is instilled at a concentration of 8 mg/L. Frequent exchanges help clear the infection and maintain urea clearance. Third-generation cephalosporins can be used instead of gentamicin.

Hemofiltration

Continuous venovenous hemofiltration (CVVH) and continuous arteriovenous hemofiltration (CAVH) are alternative methods of renal replacement therapy. CVVH and CAVH are used primarily for ultrafiltration, (i.e., fluid removal).

Continuous Venovenous Hemofiltration CVVH requires:

- Central venous access
- A blood pump

- An ultrafiltrate pump
- A suitable hemofilter

The central venous access is the same as for hemodialysis. A single catheter with dual lumens or two separate venous sites may be used. In the single catheter technique, the distal port is the "venous" port and the proximal port is the "arterial" port. Blood flow is controlled by the blood pump. Blood flows from the "arterial" side through the hemofilter and returns to the body via the venous side. Ultrafiltrate flow rate can be controlled by an intravenous pump. CVVH does not rely on the patient's blood flow or cardiac output to maintain hemofiltration. CVVH is pump-driven and, therefore, is suitable for patients with marginal perfusion pressure. Modern CVVH machines can control all aspects of the treatment.

Complications Complications of CVVH include:

- Bleeding
- Hypotension
- Catheter infections
- Decreased intravascular volume

In the patient with marginal renal functions (i.e., glomerular filtration rate [GFR] less than 50 to 75%), removal of intravascular volume may result in decreased renal perfusion and worsened renal insufficiency. This situation is particularly difficult in the patient with total body fluid overload and intravascular depletion.

Anticoagulation Heparin is required to avoid clotting of the filter and tubing. The goal of heparinization is an activated clotting time of 120 to 150 seconds. Patients who cannot tolerate systemic anticoagulation may not be suitable for undergoing hemofiltration. Also, small patients may be "chilled" by the procedure unless some type of blood warmer is used.

Continuous Arteriovenous Hemofiltration With this form of hemofiltration, blood flow through the filter is not driven by a mechanical pump but rather depends on the patient's perfusion pressure. Therefore, CAVH is difficult to perform in the hypotensive patient.

Comparison to CVVH The blood flow circuit is similar to CVVH, but there are significant differences. Two access sites are required in CAVH: an arterial site to generate blood flow and a venous site for blood return. Ultrafiltrate generation is dependent on blood flow. The ultrafiltrate flow may be controlled by intravenous pumps as in CVVH. If a patient has poor perfusion pressure, blood flow is slow and therefore ultrafiltrate generation is low. To some extent, this safeguards against excessive ultrafiltration but may be the rate-limiting factor in patients who need fluid removal.

Priming As in hemodialysis, the extracorporeal blood volume required to prime the tubing should not be more than 10% of the patient's total blood volume, particularly for pediatric patients. To avoid hemodynamic compromise or worsening of hemodynamic instability, the tubing is primed with PRBC and albumin. The priming hematocrit should be 40 to 45%. The patient who requires dopamine, epinephrine, or norepinephrine often needs the dosage increased when initiating hemofiltration or hemodialysis, which may result from either dilution from the tubing prime or clearance from the filter.

Hemofiltration with Dialysis

Equipment and Technique Continuous venovenous hemofiltration dialysis (CVVHD) combines CVVH with continuous dialysis. The blood flow circuit is the same as for CVVH. There are two dialysate ports on the Amicon filter. Peritoneal dialysate is pumped countercurrently to the blood flow through the filter. The dialysate generally has a 1.5% glucose concentration and uses lactate as a buffer, which may restrict the use of this method in patients who cannot convert lactate. The dialysate removed from the filter is controlled by a pump, which controls not only the dialysate flow but also the ultrafiltrate volume. Urea clearance is dependent on dialysate flow rate.

Ultrafiltrate A particularly important aspect of hemofiltration, hemodialysis, and peritoneal dialysis is the ultrafiltrate composition. Ultrafiltrate is isotonic. The electrolyte urea and creatinine concentrations are isotonic to serum. As ultrafiltrate volume increases, particularly in small patients, large sodium losses may occur; therefore, appropriate fluid and electrolyte replacement is required.

HEMOLYTIC UREMIC SYNDROME

Hemolytic uremic syndrome (HUS) is a multisystem disease of the microcirculation and is a common cause of renal failure. Although many noninfectious causes are recognized, the syndrome most commonly accompanies enteric infection with *E. coli.*

Clinical Findings

Signs and symptoms of HUS include:

- Pallor
- Anuria or oliguria
- Tachycardia
- Irritability
- Ataxia
- Tremors
- Behavioral changes

Central nervous system (CNS) involvement is sometimes the presenting complaint of HUS.

Laboratory evaluation reveals:

- Anemia
- Uremia
- Thrombocytopenia
- Blood smear evidence of microangiopathic hemolysis

Complications

With initiation of short-term dialysis, the mortality rate from HUS is generally less than 5%. Early mortality is most often the result of neurologic involvement, and such involvement remains the primary indication for admission to our pediatric intensive care unit (PICU).

Other serious complications of HUS include:

- Hemorrhagic colitis
- Sepsis
- Myocarditis/pericarditis
- Pericardial effusion with tamponade
- Ventricular dysfunction

Treatment

Plasma infusion and plasmapheresis have been instituted with some success. Administration of immunoglobulin preparations to children with HUS has met with mixed results.

HYPERTENSION

Definition and Classification

Hypertension in children is defined as an average blood pressure greater than the 95th percentile for age and gender; normal blood pressure is less than the 90th percentile for age and gender. Blood pressures between the 90th and 95th percentile are borderline hypertension. Normal blood pressures are shown in Table 23.10.

Hypertension is either essential or secondary.

- Essential hypertension is hypertension for which no obvious source is found.
- Secondary hypertension is caused by underlying organ damage or disease process.

The rule of thumb for pediatric hypertension is the younger the patient and the higher the blood pressure, the greater probability of secondary hypertension.

Table 23.10
Range of Blood Pressure in Children

Age Group	95th Percentile		99th Percentile	
	Systolic	Diastolic	Systolic	Diastolic
≤ 7 days	96		106	
8–30 days	104		110	
1–24 months	112	74	118	82
3–5 years	116	76	124	84
6–9 years	122	78	130	86
10–12 years	126	82	134	90
13–15 years	136	86	144	92
16–18 years	142	92	150	98

Table 23.11
Physical Findings as Clues to Causes of Hypertension

Causes	Physical Clues
Renovascular disease or cystic renal disease	Cafe au lait spots
	Abdominal bruits (30% of patients)
	Abdominal masses
	Diminished femoral pulses
	Elfin facies
Corticosteroid excess	Cushingoid appearance
Severe hypertension or increased central nervous system pressure	Papilledema
Volume overload	Fluid intake greater than output
	Weight gain
	Edema
Pheochromocytoma	Hypertension associated with anesthesia
	Sweating
	Flushing

Evaluation and Causes

History and Physical Examination

Clinical history and physical examination are critical in determining the cause of hypertension. Review of the patient's history reveals:

- History of hypertension
- Family history of hypertension or renal disease
- Medications or illicit drug use

Findings from the physical examination may give clues to the underlying cause of hypertension (Table 23.11).

Laboratory Findings

Laboratory investigation of hypertension focuses on the kidneys.

- Urinalysis for hematuria, red blood cell casts, and proteinuria
- Serum electrolytes
- BUN
- Creatinine levels

If the diagnosis is not apparent from the previous evaluation, the clinician obtains a plasma renin activity and aldosterone level. If the clinical setting suggests mineralocorticoid excess, measurement of aldosterone level may be indicated. Pheochromocytomas are rare, but if suggested by the clinical picture, urinary and serum catecholamine levels may be measured.

Imaging

Renal ultrasonography is necessary to visualize:

- Renal parenchyma
- Collecting system
- Blood flow through the renal arteries (evaluated for renal artery stenosis or thrombus)

Ultrasound is specific but not sensitive for renal artery stenosis; a definitive diagnosis is made by arteriography.

Magnetic resonance angiography and angiotensin-converting enzyme inhibitor renal scans have been used, but arteriography is still the gold standard.

The clinician should order computed tomography and ^{131}I metaiodobenzylguanidine (i.e., MBIG) scanning when he or she suspects pheochromocytoma, because there is a possibility of multiple tumors. Renal scans are not usually necessary in the PICU unless the patient has a history of frequent urinary tract infections or vesicoureteral reflux. In this situation, a renal scan may show areas of scarring that may be the cause of hypertension.

Treatment in the Pediatric Intensive Care Unit

Indications

After the clinician makes the diagnosis of hypertension and determines it, therapy may be initiated. Immediate intervention is necessary:

- In a hypertensive crisis or emergency
- When blood pressure is greater than the 95th percentile for age

Patients with borderline hypertension generally do not require immediate therapy.

Medications

A list of antihypertensive agents is provided in Table 23.12.

Diuretics The patient with hypertension and volume overload who still can generate adequate urine output may benefit from diuretic use. Diuretics also are helpful in decreasing the fluid retention that occurs with vasodilators.

Loop Diuretics Loop diuretics, such as furosemide, work at the level of the loop of Henle. These agents typically produce a brisk diuresis and, in doing so, may have a number of adverse effects, which include:

- Hypokalemia
- Dehydration
- Metabolic alkalosis
- Nephrocalcinosis
- Ototoxicity

Furosemide can be administered orally or intravenously as a bolus or continuous drip.

Thiazide Diuretics These agents block sodium reabsorption in the distal tubule. When combined with loop diuretics, thiazides can cause significant sodium loss and hyponatremia. Thiazides have little use in acute hypertension but, like loop diuretics, may help to decrease fluid retention associated with vasodilators.

Carbonic Anhydrase Inhibitors Carbonic anhydrase inhibitors have little use in the treatment of acute hypertension in the PICU.

Aldosterone Antagonists These agents (e.g., spironolactone) inhibit aldosterone in the cortical collecting duct. Although their use is limited in acute hypertension, they often are used in patients with elevated aldosterone levels (e.g., those with liver failure or primary hyperaldosteronism-induced hypertension). These patients typically present with hypokalemia and metabolic alkalosis. Elevated serum aldosterone levels and low plasma renin activity help confirm the diagnosis.

Hypertensive Emergency

Hypertensive emergencies require blood pressure management within hours. They include:

- Hypertension-induced cardiac failure or pulmonary edema
- Hypertensive encephalopathy
- Hypertension from pheochromocytoma
- Hypertension with intracranial hemorrhage
- Hypertension-induced blindness.

Hypertensive encephalopathy can occur when the mean arterial pres-

Table 23.12
Treatment of Hypertension in Children

Agent	Dose	Onset (Duration)	Comments
Parenteral Agents			
α-Blocker			
Phentolamine (Regitine) (5 mg powder supplied with 1 mL diluent—further dilute to 10 mL for 0.5 mg/mL)	0.05–0.2 mg/kg IV	<30 sec (15–30 min)	For diagnosis of pheochromocytoma; may cause marked tachycardia, hypotension, arrhythmias from unopposed β effect
β-Blockers			
Propranolol (Inderal) (1 mg/mL vial—dilute to 10 mL with saline 0.1 mg/mL)	Test dose of 0.005 mg/kg IV then 0.01 mg/kg IV may repeat every 10 min to effect	2–4 min (3–6 h)	Contraindication: myocardial disease, asthma; useful adjunct to vasodilator therapy to control tachycardia; may cause atrioventricular block, bradycardia, hypoglycemia; infants may be relatively resistant to blockade; do not give if heart rate <90, if age <3, if cardiac output is heart rate dependent.
Labetalol (Normodyne, Trandate) (5 mg/mL vial)	0.25 mg/kg repeated incrementally to 1–3 mg/kg/h	Within minutes	β and α blocker, rare cases of hepatocellular injury
Direct vasodilators			
Diazoxide (Hyperstat) (15 mg/mL–20 mg vial)	1 mg/kg IV bolus (5 mg/kg maximum) may repeat in 5 min	1–5 min (up to 12 h)	Hyperglycemia, sodium + water retention—may need concomitant diuretic therapy; contraindications: diabetes, marked tachycardia, thiazide sensitivity
Hydralazine (Apresoline) (20 mg/mL vial)	0.1–0.2 mg/kg every 1–2 h IV 0.2–0.5 mg/kg IM every 3–4 h	10–20 min/3–4 h	Lupus-like syndrome
Nitroprusside (Nipride) (50 mg lyophilized powder):	0.5–8 µg/kg/min titrated to blood pressure	Immediate (diseases on termination of	a. Monitor with arterial line b. Administer with controlled infusion pump

continued

Table 23.12
Treatment of Hypertension in Children

Agent	Dose	Onset (Duration)	Comments
dilute [3 × body weight (kg)] = mg in 100 mL for 1 mL/h = 0.5 µg/kg/min; protect from light-photodegradation (wrap in foil)—change solution every 24 h		infusion	c. Administer through central line if possible d. Positioning with head up may potentiate hypotensive effect e. Monitor blood thiocyanate if: 1. used > 24 h 2. rate > 10 µg/kg/min for > 6 h 3. discontinue if thiocyanate level > 10 mg/dL Thiosulfate is antidote Monitor arterial blood gases for: 1. Metabolic acidosis-cyanide toxicity 2. ↓PO_2 caused by intrapulmonary shunting: May increase intracranial pressure
Calcium channel blocker			
Verapamil (Calan/Isoptin) (5 mg/2-mL vial)	Test dose of 0.01 mg/kg IV then 0.05–0.2 mg/kg	2–4 min (1–2 h)	May cause high-grade AV block if given along with propranolol; not used widely in children
ACE inhibitor			
Enalaprilat	5–28 µg/kg/d divided every 8–24 h	5–15 min (6 h)	May cause oliguria, hyperkalemia, acute renal failure
Enteral agents			
α-Blockers			
Prazosin (Minipress) capsules: 1, 2, 5 mg	1 mg first dose 0.05–0.1 mg/kg every 8–12 h, maximum 0.4 mg/kg/24 h		Hypotension frequent after first dose
β-Blockers			
Propranolol (Inderal) Tablets: 10, 20, 40, 60, 80 mg	0.5 mg/kg every 6–12 h; may increase every 3–6 d		Contraindications; heart failure, asthma, atrioventricular block, pheochromocytoma before blockade, liver disease; may mask sympathetic response to shock, hemorrhage;

Metoprolol (Lopressor) tablets: 50, 100 mg	1 mg/kg every 12 h; may increase every 7 d	may cause bradycardia, atrioventricular block, central nervous system depression β_1-selective (less bronchospasm, otherwise same as propranolol); tablet size limits use in young children
Aetnolol (Tenormin) tablets: 50, 100 mg	1 mg/kg every 24 h	Same as metoprolol; renal elimination ($T_{1/2}$ 6–9 h if CrCl normal), if CrCl 15–35 mL/min/1.73 m², $T_{1/2} = 16$–27 h; if CrCl <15, $T_{1/2} > 27$ h
Labetalol (Trandate) tablets: 100, 200 mg	0.25 mg/kg repeated incrementally to 1 mg/kg every 8 h	β and α_1 blocker, not studied in children
Calcium channel blocker		
Nifedipine (Procardia) 10/20 mg capsules	Capsule 5–20 min Acute: 0.25–0.5 mg/kg S.L./P.O.	Side effects: Flushing, headache, hypotension, edema, tachycardia, constipation
Sustained release tablets: 30, 60, 90 mg	(4–12 h) Repeat q 30–60 min Sustained release (12–24 h) Chronic: 1 mg/kg/d divided every 6–24 h	
Vasodilators		
Hydralazine (Apresoline) tablets: 10, 25, 50, 100 mg	1–2 mg/kg every 4–6 h, maximum 8 mg/kg/24 h, increase every 3–4 days	Lupus-like syndrome is side effect
Minoxidil (Loniten)	0.1–0.2 mg/kg/d (duration 12–14 h), maximum 1 mg/kg/24 h, increase every 3 d	Sodium retention; use with diuretic, hypertrichosis, fluid retention; discontinue gradually; may cause pericardial effusion
Central α-agonist α-Methyldopa (Aldomet) tablets:	25–50 mg/kg every 6–8 h,	Can cause liver function abnormalities;

continued

Table 23.12
Treatment of Hypertension in Children

Agent	Dose	Onset (Duration)	Comments
125, 250, 500 mg; suspension: 250 mg/5 mL	increase every 2 d		contraindication in liver disease—follow liver function tests; Coombs-positive hemolytic anemia, sedation
Clonidine (Catapres) tablets: 0.1, 0.2, 0.3 mg	0.01–0.03 mg/kg b.i.d., maximum 0.06 mg/kg/24 h, increase every 2–4 d		Discontinue gradually to avoid rebound hypertension, dry mouth/sedation; follow fundus examination for retinal degeneration, used infrequently in children.
Angiotension converting enzyme (ACE) inhibitors			
Captopril (Capoten) tablets: 25, 50, 100 mg (scored)	0.5–1 mg/kg t.i.d., maximum dose: CrCl Normal 6 mg/kg/d CrCl 40–80 4 mg/kg/d CrCl 20–40 2 mg/kg/d CrCl 10–20 1 mg/kg/d CrCl <10 0.5 mg/kg/d		Give 1 h before meals—food inhibits absorption 20–40%, can cause decline in renal function: rash, eosinophilia, leukopenia 0.3% (in patients on immunosuppressants or those with autoimmune disease), proteinuria 1%, monitor for hyperkalemia, taste disturbance; renal excretion
Enalopril tablets: 2.5, 5, 10, 20 mg	0.15 mg/kg/d in 1–2 divided doses		Give 1 h before meals—food inhibits absorption 20–40%, can cause decline in renal function: rash, eosinophilia, leukopenia 0.3% (in patients on immunosuppressants or those with autoimmune disease), proteinuria 1%, monitor for hyperkalemia, taste disturbance; renal excretion

sure exceeds autoregulation capability of the cerebral vessels. The differential diagnosis includes:

- Encephalitis
- Intracranial hemorrhage or thrombosis
- Tumor
- Pseudotumor cerebri

Investigation

Evaluation of a hypertensive emergency is similar to evaluating other forms of hypertension. A renal cause needs to be ruled out immediately. The clinician should examine disorders of the CNS. An electrocardiogram or echocardiogram can discern cardiac complications from hypertension.

Therapy

Hypertensive emergency requires immediate treatment and PICU monitoring (see Table 23.12). Frequent automated blood pressures should be available or an arterial line may be necessary. One author recommends decreasing blood pressure by one-third of the planned reduction in the first 6 hours, by one-third over the next 12 to 36 hours, and by the final third over the next 48 hours.

Nitroprusside is one of the first-line drugs for hypertensive crisis. Continuous infusion begins at 0.5 µg/kg/minute to a maximum of 8 to 10 µg/kg/minute. Labetalol is often effective in moderate blood pressure disturbances; its potency is usually insufficient for severe, sustained hypertension. Bradycardia may be reversed by atropine. Diazoxide, administered by rapid intravenous infusion, is usually very effective.

RENAL TRANSPLANTATION
Renal Transplantation in Infants and Children

Renal transplantation is the treatment of choice for children with chronic renal failure. Despite technical improvements in chronic dialysis, children with end-stage renal disease are not afforded a continuous normal metabolic state and generally do not grow and develop normally.

Dialysis generally is regarded as a bridge to transplantation. Most children with chronic renal failure undergo a course of treatment with chronic dialysis before receiving a renal transplant. Nonetheless, virtually all of these children ultimately are considered candidates for renal transplantation.

Adult Donors

The use of living donors provides important advantages in patient and graft survival, particularly for young infants. Living donors typically are the child's parents; therefore, the donor is generally adult. Even if a cadaver donor is used, there are reasons to avoid young donors, particularly for small infants; thus, the usual donor for a young infant is an adult. In addition to difficulty fitting an adult kidney into the abdomen of an infant, mismatches in blood flow to the transplanted graft, compared with what it had received in the donor, produces an opportunity for graft dysfunction, hypertension, and possibly graft thrombosis. Appropriate postoperative care in these patients requires special consideration and experience.

Incidence of Graft Failure

Pediatric recipients of renal transplants are at particular risk for loss of graft function from acute irreversible rejection episodes and from graft thrombosis.

Rejection In older children and adults, the incidence of acute rejection is at least 50%, but most of these episodes are treatable and reversible. In children younger than 2 years of age, between 25 and 50% of acute rejection episodes are irreversible, and in those aged 2 to 5, up to 10% are irreversible. Reasons for poor outcome of acute rejection episodes in children include:

- Immune reactivity of children
- Severity of the rejection episodes
- Delays in diagnosis and treatment

Thrombosis Thrombosis is a unique cause of graft failure in young children. It rarely occurs in adult recipients but may represent up to 15% of graft failures, particularly in young recipients.

Perioperative Treatment

Fluid and Electrolyte Management

Adequate Perfusion Adequate perfusion of the transplanted graft is an essential component of successful posttransplant management of the pediatric recipient, particularly of infants. Because of the substantial risk of thrombosis of the transplanted organ, careful monitoring of blood pressure and central venous pressure are extremely important. Blood pressure should be maintained at least at the upper limits of normal for age. Central venous pressure is typically maintained between 8 to 12 mm Hg.

Replacement Solutions Fluid management generally is provided by separate replacement solutions for different sources of output:

- Calculated insensible losses can be replaced by 5% dextrose solutions
- Urine output is replaced initially by half normal saline, with subsequent changes in concentration guided by frequent assessment of urinary electrolyte concentrations. Generally, a 1:1 replacement of urine volume is maintained for at least the first 2 to 3 days postoperatively.

- Nasogastric output is replaced as usual
- Drainage from other sources, particularly surgical drains, must also be replaced
- Peritoneal losses must be replaced by at least isotonic solutions and perhaps by albumin

Assessment of the patient is achieved by frequent monitoring of serum electrolytes, osmolality, and body weight. Frequently, total body water is expanded by 10% in the first few days postoperatively.

Fluid Removal Subsequent management in patients who have regained good renal function permits slow removal of this excess fluid over several days. Typically, this goal is achieved by replacing only a fraction of the urine output to keep the patient in a negative balance each day. The patient must not be allowed to lose an excessive amount of fluid each day.

Postoperative Dialysis Some patients do not have immediate graft function after surgery. In these cases, postoperative dialysis may be necessary for several days or weeks. The usual indications and techniques of dialysis are applicable, but excessive ultrafiltration must be avoided to reduce the risk of poor perfusion to the graft.

Peritoneal Dialysis If patients have had pretransplant peritoneal dialysis, the peritoneal catheter often is not removed, particularly if there is a high risk of acute tubular necrosis. Peritoneal dialysis may be continued, using the same techniques that had been used before transplant. Complications may arise in small infants because of the large mass of the transplanted kidney and because of pain associated with the surgical incision.

Hemodialysis Hemodialysis is possible in all infants using dual-lumen catheters. It is important to avoid hypotension resulting from either high blood flow rates or excessive ultrafiltration during dialysis. Use of ultrafiltration controlling devices is mandatory in these circumstances.

Continuous Venovenous Hemofiltration CVVH may be used for gentle ultrafiltration but, as indicated previously, the risk of bleeding secondary to continuous heparinization is increased in the postoperative patient. During all of these procedures, infusion of normal saline or albumin may be necessary when hypotension occurs.

Immunosuppression

All transplant patients require substantial immunosuppression to prevent or treat acute rejection episodes. Immunosuppression therapy delivered in the first 1 to 2 weeks after transplant is often referred to as "induction" therapy. Most patients receive high-dose induction therapy and then the medication dosages are gradually reduced to reach "maintenance" levels of immunosuppression several months later. Maintenance immunosuppression for renal transplant patients generally consists of:

- Prednisone
- Azathioprine
- Cyclosporine
- FK506
- Mycophenolate mofietel

Antibody Induction Antibodies directed toward human leukocyte antigens have been used as induction therapy for renal transplantation, although few controlled trials have occurred. Substantial benefits of antibody induction therapy, particularly in young infants, have been suggested from retrospective analysis of pediatric registry data. Although many preparations seem to be highly effective (i.e., horse and rabbit sera), lot-to-lot variation has produced variable results. Complications, such as anemia or thrombocytopenia caused by concurrent presence of antibodies to these elements, also have limited usefulness of these substances.

OKT3 OKT3 is a monoclonal antibody that has been used for both prophylactic and antirejection therapy in organ transplant recipients (see Chapter 22). Because of reported "first use" side effects, it is imperative to monitor respiratory status and to avoid severe fluid overload in patients receiving the first several doses of OKT3. Often, patients who are receiving prophylactic OKT3 receive the first dose intraoperatively while they are still intubated. Careful attention to pretreatment control of respiratory status has lessened the frequency of serious first-dose reaction substantially. Subsequent doses of this agent have few immediate side effects. When antibody induction therapy is provided, concurrent treatment with azathioprine and cyclosporine often is delayed, but prednisone is usually provided concurrently.

Cyclosporine or FK506 Intravenous infusion of these agents often is necessary because oral administration may be unsuccessful as a result of postoperative ileus and poor absorption. Avoidance of a high serum level of these agents is important, because each is nephrotoxic. Concurrent provision of calcium channel blockers, such as nifedipine, seem to ameliorate nephrotoxicity.

Rejection Prophylaxis Although most acute rejection episodes can be treated and reversed successfully, prevention is preferable. Provision of immunosuppression drugs must be consistent, and careful monitoring of their efficacy is important. Lack of sufficient administration of cyclosporine and FK506 may be assessed by frequent monitoring of trough blood levels. Total peripheral lymphocyte counts can be assessed when antilymphocyte preparations are provided. Assessment of circulating T3-positive cells is important if OKT3 preparations are used.

Complications of Use of Immunosuppressants Corticosteroid medications often cause hypertension, sodium retention, and hyperglycemia. Cyclosporine and FK506 administration have been associated with hyperkalemia, decreased GFR, and hypertension. Careful monitoring and treatment of these complications is necessary, but decreasing or eliminating doses of the drugs because of the complications should be avoided.

Rejection Episodes

Clinical Evidence In the immediate posttransplant period, clinical symptoms of rejection include:

- Fever
- Swelling of the graft
- Tenderness over the graft site
- Decreased urine output
- Rising serum creatinine levels

In these circumstances, multiple tests (e.g., renal ultrasound, renal nuclear medicine scan) are obtained to detect causes for these symptoms other than rejection, such as obstruction of the graft, urinary leak, and others. None of these tests, however, produce clear evidence of rejection.

Diagnosis and Confirmation Diagnosis of rejection often is based on the clinical signs and symptoms and sometimes is confirmed by percutaneous graft biopsy. Rejection must always be included in differential diagnosis of posttransplant fever. In the pediatric patient, particularly very small infants who receive an adult kidney, decreases in renal function are often difficult to ascertain in the early stages of rejection; therefore, heightened suspicion must be maintained to avoid having a rejection episode remain untreated for a long period.

Reversibility Rejection episodes are most often reversible if diagnosed quickly and treated with either pulse corticosteroids (Solumedrol, 25 mg/kg daily for 3 days) or antilymphocyte preparations, such as ATGAM or OKT3. Provision of antirejection therapy leads to a rapid decrease in symptoms such as fever and graft tenderness. Depending on the severity of the rejection episode, the graft may suffer acute tubular necrosis, and recovery of renal function is often delayed.

Unfortunately, rejection episodes in young infants are more often irreversible than in older patients. The reasons for this irreversible nature of rejection episodes are not clear but may be related to delays in diagnosis.

Assessment of whether the rejection episode has been reversed is sometimes difficult. Repeated or therapeutically unresponsive rejection episodes are sometimes treated by changes to other immunosuppressant medication, such as FK506.

Graft Thrombosis

Risk Factors For pediatric cadaver donor transplants, the incidence of graft thrombosis is principally related to young donor age. A recent change in the U.S. allocation system has led to a decreased use of young donors, particularly for young recipients. Other factors that place patients at highest risk include:

- Volume depletion or hypotension during or after the transplant procedure
- Acute tubular necrosis and subsequent swelling and increased pressure within the graft
- Compromised perfusion of the graft

Compromised perfusion may place young infants who retain their own native kidneys or those who have high urine output from the kidneys at particular risk. Lack of pretransplant donor nephrectomy has not been associated with increased risk of graft thrombosis, but those who did not have any pretransplant dialysis may be at a higher risk.

Prevention Preventing graft thrombosis involves:

- Avoiding young cadaver donors for infant recipients
- Paying meticulous attention to fluid and electrolyte management
- Maintaining adequate perfusion of the graft
- Avoiding procedures that may compromise perfusion of the graft

Posttransplant Infections

Patients at Risk

The cytomegalovirus (CMV)-negative recipient/CMV-positive donor group is at highest risk for occurrence of posttransplant CMV disease and has the most severe symptoms and the highest mortality. Pediatric recipients, who are more likely to be CMV-negative, may be at much higher risk, particularly if they receive grafts from adult donors.

Prevention

In CMV-negative recipients of CMV-positive grafts:

- High titer CMV gammaglobulin does not prevent disease but ameliorates its severity
- Oral acyclovir prevents disease, but there is significant controversy about its efficacy
- Intravenous ganciclovir, administered at the time of treatment with antilymphocyte antibody preparations, is currently under study

Therapy

Treatment of severe CMV disease with intravenous ganciclovir has been shown to be efficacious in most recipients. This treatment is often given to leukopenic patients who have high fevers, but it is clearly indicated in patients with visceral involvement, including those with pneumonia, hepatitis, or enteritis.

Varicellavirus

Infection is generally mild in normal children but may be severe or even fatal in children receiving immunosuppressant medications. Children who have not had chickenpox before transplantation should receive varicella zoster immune globulin at the time of any exposure if they are receiving immunosuppression. Treatment with intravenous acyclovir is currently warranted if patients have clinical disease.

Unfortunately, even aggressive and early treatment is sometimes insufficient for patients who present with visceral varicella disease. The efficacy of pretransplant varicella vaccine is not yet known, but susceptible patients probably should be appropriately vaccinated before immunosuppression.

Pneumocystis carinii

Pneumocystis carinii pneumonia occurs in approximately 3% of all renal transplant recipients, including children, from 2 to 6 months after transplantation. Patients typically present with fever, tachypnea, and moderately severe hypoxia without cough or dyspnea. Diagnosis often is suspected on the basis of characteristic radiographic findings and can be verified by bronchial washing or even analysis of sputum.

Treatment with intravenous trimethoprim-sulfamethoxazole or pentamidine usually is successful. Most renal transplant recipients receive trimethoprim-sulfamethoxazole prophylaxis in the first several months after transplantation. Prophylaxis can be achieved with aerosolized pentamidine, but this form of prevention is generally not applicable to young infants.

HEPATORENAL SYNDROME

Hepatorenal syndrome (HRS) is renal failure with liver failure when no other source of renal insufficiency can be found, such as in acute tubular necrosis, prerenal azotemia, or obstructive nephropathy. The cause of hepatorenal syndrome remains elusive, but more recent advances have helped identify the pathologic mechanisms.

Pathophysiology

The hallmarks of HRS are:

- Intense, functional vasoconstriction of the renal vasculature
- Decreased renal perfusion with preservation of tubular function

Vasoconstriction in this case is described as functional because, as the liver disease is repaired, renal insufficiency improves. A patient who receives a functioning liver transplant may experience improvement of their renal disease. Also, a kidney transplanted from a patient with HRS may function normally in a patient without HRS.

Clinical Presentation

The typical clinical scenario is a patient with cirrhosis, ascites, and progressive renal insufficiency. Because renal disease is a frequent concomitant to liver disease, distinguishing between HRS and other causes of renal insufficiency may be difficult. Commonly, the patient with HRS sustained a precipitating event resulting in decreased intravascular volume (e.g., gastrointestinal bleeding, aggressive diuresis, paracentesis) or nephrotoxin exposure. HRS can occur without a precipitating event, however.

Diagnostic Findings

Renal Arteriography

Renal vasoconstriction has been revealed with labeled xenon washout and selected renal arteriograms. Postmortem renal arteriogram shows a return of renal vasculature architecture.

Doppler Sonography

Doppler ultrasound typically demonstrates an increased intrarenal-resistive index in patients with HRS.

Laboratory Values

Patients with HRS reabsorb sodium and water avidly; urine is often concentrated. Characteristic findings follow:

- Increased plasma renin and aldosterone levels
- Low urine sodium level
- High urine-specific gravity or osmolarity
- Increased BUN to creatinine ratio

Differential Diagnosis

Distinguishing HRS from acute tubular necrosis (ATN) and prerenal azotemia may be difficult.

Acute Tubular Necrosis

Patients with HRS have the characteristic laboratory findings of volume depletion and renal vasoconstriction just mentioned. In ATN, the urine sodium is elevated (>30 mEq/L); urine osmolality is similar to serum osmolality; and there is a low urine-to-plasma osmolality and low BUN to creatinine ratio (less than 20:1).

Prerenal Azotemia

Unfortunately, prerenal azotemia has the same urinary and serum findings as HRS. Prerenal azotemia usually responds to volume repletion, whereas

HRS may not. Volume repletion may not be accurate in distinguishing HRS from prerenal azotemia because often patients with liver failure and altered Starling forces in their intravascular space require large-volume colloid replacement to adequately improve their volume status.

Treatment

Although attempts to improve outcome in HRS have been dismal and the syndrome is considered universally fatal, the following therapeutic measures may decrease progression to or improve HRS:

- Prevent volume depletion
  - Avoid aggressive diuresis, paracentesis or hemorrhage and use of nephrotoxic agents (e.g., nonsteroidal anti-inflammatory drugs) in patients with cirrhosis
  - Monitor volume status (central venous access)
- Perform orthotopic liver transplantation

Prevention and liver transplantation remain the mainstay of therapy.

24.

Endocrine, Mineral, and Metabolic Disease

Daniel S. Kohane, Joseph R. Tobin, and Isaac S. Kohane

INTRODUCTION

In this review of endocrinologic disease, special considerations relating to airway management, control of circulation, and perioperative care, as well as special implications of intensive care pharmacotherapy to the disease state will be discussed. It is important to recall that in all situations, the airway, breathing, and circulation are the most important issues and should be addressed first and in that order. Everything else is secondary.

DISORDERS OF THE ADRENAL CORTEX

Adrenal Disease

The pathophysiology of adrenal disorders can be categorized into hyperfunction and hypofunction and further classified as primary or secondary (i.e., to hypothalamus or pituitary disease) disorders. Nevertheless, because of the diagnostic approach to these disorders, classification is functional and anatomic for some disorders (e.g., Cushing's syndrome) and biochemical for others (e.g., many congenital adrenal hyperplasias).

Adrenal Hypofunction

Adrenal insufficiency can be primary, secondary, or tertiary. Primary insufficiency can result from one or more defects in production of mineralocorticoids and/or glucocorticoids or from global adrenal failure (Addison's disease). Secondary insufficiency results from disorders of the pituitary (i.e., corticotropin (adrenocorticotropic hormone [ACTH] deficiency) and tertiary insufficiency from disorders of the hypothalamus (CRH deficiency). Presentation and treatment of specific types of adrenal hypofunction depend on the underlying disorder.

Primary Adrenal Insufficiency (Addison's Disease) In primary adrenal insufficiency, all three adrenal cortical layers are destroyed or inactive. Acute adrenal crisis is uncommon in the pediatric intensive care unit (PICU) but can be catastrophic.

Presentation

Autoimmune Adrenalitis The most frequently seen cause (up to 90% of cases in some series) is autoimmune adrenalitis, occurring in isolation or part of polyglandular autoimmune endocrinopathy. Increasingly, opportunistic infections in patients infected with HIV have been found in association with necrotizing adrenalitis or more subtle blunting of the normal adrenal output. Adrenal insufficiency in these patients is worsened by the use of ketoconazole, which inhibits several steroidogenic enzymes, and r fampin, which increases cortisol clearance. Infiltration of the adrenal gland by tumor is far more rare in pediatric patients than in adults.

Adrenoleukodystrophy Increasingly recognized as a potential cause of Addison's disease, adrenoleukodystrophy can present first as Addison's disease before any neurologic findings are seen. Diagnosis is made by urine or serum assays for the presence of very-long-chain fatty acids; therefore, it should be considered in the patient with Addison's disease of unknown cause.

Severe Systemic Illnesses Poor adrenal perfusion due to shock has been associated with reduced corticosteroid output, although data demonstrate that the adrenal medulla is protected during shock and the adrenal cortex and medulla are protected during hypoxia. The Waterhouse-Friderichsen syndrome, which can present at any age, represents acute hemorrhage into the adrenal glands as the result of coagulopathy associated with sepsis (classically meningococcemia).

Congenital Adrenal Hyperplasia In the neonate, several disorders of adrenal enzymes may result in inefficient or absent production of both mineralocorticoid and glucocorticoid. They are classified as types of congenital adrenal hyperplasia (CAH) because cortisol insufficiency leads to stimulation of the adrenal enzymatic machinery, with glandular hypertrophy and hyperplasia.

Congenital adrenal hyperplasia presents typically as a "salt-wasting" crisis between days 5 and 15 of life. Girls with 21-hydroxylase deficiency often are easier to diagnose because of the virilization that results from excessive adrenal androgen production. Less common forms of CAH cause combined deficiency of adrenal steroid synthesis. In 3-beta-hydroxylase deficiency and deficiency of side chain cleavage enzyme, androgen production in the testes and adrenal gland is so compromised that boys have incomplete or even absent virilization (i.e., pseudohermaphroditism).

Clinical Manifestations Clinical presentation of Addison's disease is determined by deficiency of glucocorticoid and mineralocorticoid and a resulting rise in ACTH, CRH, renin, and angiotensin II.

The mineralocorticoid lack is responsible for disordered electrolytes (i.e., hyponatremia, hyperkalemia, hypercalcemia, acidosis) and for loss of extracellular fluid (ECF) volume, presenting as weight loss, dehydration, hypotension, or frank shock. Quadriplegia has been reported in association with hyperkalemia. The shock or preshock state has some unusual features, in that it may be poorly responsive to volume and catecholamine infusions. This is likely due to the glucocorticoid deficit.

The secondary elevations in ACTH, CRH, renin, and angiotensin II in response to the primary deficiency may contribute to the discomfort and nausea experienced by patients with Addison's disease.

Physical Signs and Symptoms Symptoms on presentation invariably include:

- Weakness
- Fatigue
- Anorexia
- Nausea and other gastrointestinal (GI) symptoms
- Salt craving
- Muscle and joint pain
- Hypoglycemia, especially after a prolonged fast
- Increased pigmentation of the skin and mucosa, particularly at skin folds, in sun-exposed areas, and at scars
- Weight loss
- Hypotension

Laboratory Findings Laboratory abnormalities include:

- Hyponatremia
- Hyperkalemia
- Hypercalcemia
- Eosinophilia
- Lymphocytosis
- Mild normocytic, normochromic anemia

Hyperkalemia can be life-threatening and should be treated immediately to prevent fatal dysrhythmias.

TREATMENT

The steps in treating a patient with suspected adrenal crisis are outlined in Table 24.1.

Hydrocortisone Therapy "Stress" hydrocortisone administration in patients in adrenal crisis usually is begun at intravenous daily doses equivalent to 28 to 56 mg/m^2. This recommended dosage is approximately four to eight times the nonstressed physiologic daily dose of 7 mg/m^2.

When the child's condition is stable, the dose can be tapered to the physiologic range within a day. Slower tapering is necessary only if glucocorticoids are being used for an underlying disease (e.g., asthma, cerebral edema) that could worsen with rapid tapering. When converted to oral maintenance therapy, the dose should be 14 mg/m^2 daily (i.e., double the intravenous dose).

Other Specific Therapeutic Measures

- In hyponatremia, salt can be replaced by normal saline infusion or in tablets, depending on the severity of the hyponatremia and the mental status of the patient

Table 24.1
Treatment of the Patient with Suspected Adrenal Crisis

1. Establish a secure intravenous line and withdraw blood for determination of baseline cortisol, electrolytes, blood urea nitrogen, glucose, and Ca^{2+}. Do Chemstrip test.
2. Give 2 mL of 25% dextrose in water per kilogram intravenously unless glucose is known to be normal.
3. Start 5% dextrose in normal saline solution at double the usual maintenance rate. For shock, infuse 20 mL of normal saline or lactated Ringer's solution per kilogram as rapidly and as often as is needed to reverse shock.
4. Give 0.2 mg dexamethasone (or 1 mg methylprednisolone) per kilogram intravenously.
5. Give 250 μg corticotropin intravenously.
6. Repeat the plasma cortisol determination (30 to 60 min) after the administration of corticotropin
7. Begin intravenous hydrocortisone replacement.

- In mineralocorticoid deficiency, cortisol is often sufficient when used in stress doses
- 9-alpha-fluorocortisol typically is only instituted when the patient transfers out of the PICU and is only available as an enteric preparation

Central Adrenal Insufficiency Several disorders of the HPA axis result in insufficient ACTH or ACTH effect. Although ACTH can acutely stimulate mineralocorticoid production, aldosterone is adequately controlled by the renin-angiotensin system in its absence. Only glucocorticoid and androgen production are significantly affected by the absence of ACTH or ACTH effect.

Secondary Adrenal Insufficiency Insufficient ACTH production can be caused by any destructive process in the pituitary:

- Pituitary tumors
- Craniopharyngiomas
- Autoimmune hypophysitis
- Granulomatous disease
- Trauma to the sella

A CRH challenge in a patient with secondary insufficiency results is minimal ACTH response, in contrast to the marked response in tertiary insufficiency. Diagnosis and management of secondary adrenal insufficiency in the PICU is similar to that of tertiary insufficiency.

Tertiary Adrenal Insufficiency This common cause of adrenal insufficiency in the PICU is caused by previous administration of glucocorticoids, which have suppressed the HPA axis.

Glucocorticoid Exposure Although the length of the glucocorticoid exposure required to achieve this suppression is controversial, it appears to be between 1 and 3 weeks and is likely to be dose- and preparation- related. If a patient has received high-dose glucocorticoid for more than 1 week, it is prudent to assume tertiary adrenal insufficiency is present and to administer stress-dose levels of glucocorticoids in a critically ill patient.

The apparent low mortality of this condition may be that anticipation and aggressive treatment are successful in preventing such deaths. Alternatively, it may be that HPA failure is under-recognized because of difficulties in documenting its presence in situations where corrective therapy is readily available.

Other Causes Other causes of tertiary adrenal insufficiency include a tumor or surgery that affects the hypothalamus. Radiation can also cause deficiency, although the central components of the HPA axis appear to be much more resistant to ablation than other hypothalamic and pituitary hormones. Current central nervous system (CNS) radiation doses for malignant tumor rarely lead to HPA insufficiency.

Associated Diuresis Free-water clearance is decreased by decreased levels of glucocorticoid. Consequently, if adrenal insufficiency has been profound and of long duration, transient diuresis may be noted during the initial period of treatment with stress levels of glucocorticoids.

Isolated Mineralocorticoid Deficiency

Any disruption of the renin-angiotensin-aldosterone axis can result in isolated mineralocorticoid deficiency. The typical presentation includes hyperkalemia, hyponatremia, and sometimes hypotension.

Pseudohypoaldosteronism Pseudohypoaldosteronism is characterized by deficient mineralocorticoid effect despite hyperreninemia and hyperaldosteronism. It may be acquired or congenital. The acquired form is found in association with obstructive uropathy and/or urinary tract infections and presents as a salt-wasting crisis with high PRA and aldosterone levels. The salt-wasting state resolves spontaneously, as does the hyperaldosteronemia, often with treatment of the underlying disorder.

Acquired Hypoaldosteronism In hyporeninemic hypoaldosteronism, renin is not secreted in response to the usual stimuli (low systemic arterial pressure, low sodium and high potassium levels); therefore, the mineralocorticoid response is inadequate. The underlying disorder is not known in most cases, although there is a strong association with diabetes mellitus.

Anesthesia, Intubation, and the Perioperative Period Of principal concern to clinicians are acutely hypocortisolemic and inadequately treated patients. The provision of stress-dose steroids is recommended. Further interventions and monitoring needs are determined by the patient's clinical status. Dehydration and electrolyte abnormalities (i.e., hyponatremia, hyperkalemia, hypercalcemia, acidosis) should be corrected. Hyperkalemia is a contraindication to the use of succinylcholine. Patients in shock may require little or no anesthesia. The need for muscle relaxants may be reduced if the patient has muscle weakness.

Cushing's Syndrome

Cushing's syndrome refers to the set of clinical findings that develop as the result of chronic exposure to glucocorticoids. Nevertheless, some causes of Cushing's syndrome also demonstrate androgen and mineralocorticoid excess. Other forms of adrenal hyperfunction that primarily affect mineralocorticoid function are described in the section concerning endocrine hypertension.

Causes Probably the most common cause of hypercortisolism is administration of glucocorticoids, typically to treat chronic inflammatory disease. In this case, the history will be informative, making diagnosis simple.

Endogenous causes of hypercortisolism present diagnostic challenges. These are classified as either ACTH-dependent (secondary adrenal hyperfunction) or ACTH-independent (primary adrenal hyperfunction).

Approximately one third of cases of ACTH-independent Cushing's syndrome are due to adrenal adenoma and two thirds to adrenal carcinoma. Rarely, the patient may have micronodular adrenal disease.

Clinical Presentation In the PICU, the earliest and most suggestive signs of Cushing's syndrome are missed unless a careful history is taken, including a growth curve. Children typically have a decrease in their height centile with acceleration or maintenance of their weight centile.

Diagnosis Making the biochemical diagnosis of Cushing's syndrome is difficult in the PICU. The usual screening studies (8 A.M. serum cortisol level checked after 15 μg/kg of dexamethasone given the previous night or 24-hour urinary free-cortisol excretion) are likely to be positive if only because the stress of critical illness is likely to stimulate the HPA axis. Consequently, diagnosis in the PICU is made on clinical grounds using features of the history and physical examination.

Anesthesia, Intubation, and the Perioperative Period Because children exposed to high doses of endogenous or exogenous steroids are susceptible to pathologic fractures, great care is taken during positioning for procedures and even during seemingly innocuous activities such as physical therapy. There may be coexisting muscle weakness; neuromuscular blocking drugs should be used judiciously. Serum electrolyte and glucose levels may be abnormal (e.g., hyperglycemia, hypokalemia, alkalosis). In general, it is best to return serum levels to normal.

Synthetic Corticosteroids

The preceding general discussion of glucocorticoid and mineralocorticoid effects can be applied to the broad array of synthetic adrenocorticosteroids available to clinicians. To use these adrenocorticosteroids sensibly, however, clinicians must understand the differences between them in terms of potency and proportion of glucocorticoid and mineralocorticoid effects.

Table 24.2
Intravenous Adrenocorticosteroids

Steroid	Glucocorticoid Potency	Mineralocorticoid Potency
Hydrocortisone	1	1
Prednisolone	4	0.8
Methylprednisolone	5	0.5
Dexamethasone	25	0

Adapted from Haynes RJ, Murad F. Adrenocorticotropic hormone; adrenocortical steroids and their synthetic analogs; inhibitors of adrenocortical steroid biosynthesis. In: Gilman A, Goodman L, Rall T, et al, eds. The pharmacologic basis of therapeutics. New York: Macmillan, 1985:1459.

Choice of Agents

In many PICU patients, the intravenous route is the only effective means of administration of drugs. Only four commercially available intravenous corticosteroids are of concern here: hydrocortisone (cortisol), prednisolone, methylprednisolone, and dexamethasone (Table 24.2).

Distinctive Properties

The important differences among the four intravenous steroids pertain to their mineralocorticoid effects. Hydrocortisone (cortisol) has the greatest sodium-retaining properties, dexamethasone has none, and prednisolone and methylprednisolone have intermediate properties. For patients in shock from adrenal insufficiency, the balanced effects of hydrocortisone are appropriate. When glucocorticoid effect (i.e., anti-inflammatory property) and hypovolemia are desired, however, as in patients with intracranial hypertension from a brain tumor, dexamethasone is the appropriate drug.

Duration of Action

The plasma half-lives of intravenous steroids are approximately 80 minutes for cortisol (hydrocortisone), 3.5 hours for prednisolone, and 4.7 hours for dexamethasone. Their biologic half-lives are approximately one and a half to two times as long. Degradation occurs in both hepatic and extrahepatic sites, followed by renal excretion of the metabolites. Liver disease or uremia, therefore, prolong the effects of administered glucocorticoids.

HYPERTENSION

Hypertension in the PICU rarely is caused by primary endocrine disease. More often, hypertension has an iatrogenic cause, such as fluid and/or solute overload, medication administration, or increased intracranial pressure (ICP).

High-PRA Hypertension

When a cause can be found, childhood hypertension (presenting outside the PICU) is most likely to be due to renal, cardiovascular (coarctation), or renovascular factors (which only secondarily result in endocrinopathy). The high renin state associated with these renal diseases results in hypertension.

Other Endocrine Disorders Associated with Hypertension

These disorders include:

- Hypercalcemia
- Hyperparathyroidism
- Acromegaly
- Hyperthyroidism
- Hypothyroidism

DISORDERS OF GLUCOSE METABOLISM

Diabetic Ketoacidosis

Diabetic ketoacidosis (DKA) is certainly among the most frequently discussed, if not the most frequently seen, metabolic disorders in PICUs.

Insulin

Insulin has both facilitative and inhibitory metabolic effects. Insulin:

- Stimulates anabolism and, therefore, storage of glycogen, protein, and fat in muscle, liver, and adipose tissue
- Enhances cell uptake of ketone bodies
- Inhibits glycogenolysis, gluconeogenesis, proteolysis, lipolysis, and ketogenesis

Insulin exerts its effects by rapidly changing the kinetics of key enzymes through phosphorylation and by slowly changing the quantity of these enzymes.

Counterregulatory Hormones

Glucagon and insulin have an intricate metabolic relationship that is central to DKA pathogenesis. The liver is the main target organ for glucagon, where it stimulates glycogenolysis, gluconeogenesis (from glycerol and amino acid precursors), and production of ketone bodies (from fatty acids). These effects follow the induction of several enzymes by an increase in the relative proportion of glucagon to insulin.

Metabolic Derangements

Lipemia and Ketosis Insulin suppresses ketogenesis and lipolysis at lower levels than are required to increase glucose transport. An important hallmark of DKA is acidosis resulting from elevated plasma concentrations of the ketoacids acetoacetate and β-hydroxybutyrate.

Commonly used tests for serum ketones employ nitroprusside reaction, which reflects acetoacetate levels well and acetone less well (approximately 20 moles of acetone react the same as 1 mole of acetoacetate). Hydroxybutyrate does not react at all, which is important for correct interpretation of reported ketone levels because the relative proportions of the three compounds may vary greatly, influenced by acid-base and redox states. Normally, the β-hydroxybutyrate/acetoacetate ratio is approximately 3:1, but it may reach 15:1 in severe DKA, and acetone may represent one and one-half to four times the molar concentration of acetoacetate.

Lactic Acidosis Lactic acid in DKA may arise, in part, from anaerobic glycolysis in hypoperfused tissues during hypovolemia caused by osmotic diuresis. Measuring lactate and acetoacetate gives a crude indication of the relative proportions of ketoacids.

Non-Anion Gap Acidosis

Hyperchloremic acidosis in DKA has been reported by several investigators.

Hyperosmolality

The hyperosmolar state induced by insulin deficiency is as harmful as ketoacidosis. Osmolality can be measured in the laboratory or can be estimated:

$$\text{Osmolality} = [\text{glucose (mg/dL)}/18] + [\text{BUN (mg/dL)}/2.8] + 2[\text{Na (mEq/L)} + \text{K (mEq/L)}]$$

Both hyperglycemia and dehydration, therefore, contribute to hyperosmolality. In fact, the values generally reported suggest that in a typical child with DKA, glucose is elevated by approximately 400 mg/dL, and serum urea nitrogen (i.e., BUN) by approximately 15 mg/dL, therefore contributing approximately 22 and 5 mOsm/L, respectively. The volume of fluid loss for this typical child in DKA represents 15% of body weight.

The fluid loss is due to osmotic diuresis induced by glucose. When fluid loss is severe enough to impair glomerular filtration rate (GFR), excretion of excess glucose is slowed and hyperglycemia accelerates. The combination of rapidly rising glucose and BUN results in extreme hyperosmolality. Hyperosmolality has been noted to correspond with levels of obtundation and with electroencephalogram (EEG) abnormalities better than other laboratory measurements in DKA.

Derangements in Serum Electrolytes and Minerals

Water Loss Loss of water through osmotic diuresis is, arguably, the most dangerous process brought about by DKA. Cardiorespiratory function can remain adequate to sustain life even at the extremes of pH and osmolality seen in DKA, but shock invariably occurs when dehydration is severe.

Sodium Loss Hyponatremia is usually reported in DKA patients, and often the reportedly low value is an artifact. Extreme lipemia can decrease the measured sodium value simply by decreasing the aqueous phase of blood, in which sodium is found. A correction formula has been proposed:

$$\text{True (aqueous phase) serum sodium (mEq/L)} = [\text{reported sodium (mEq/L)}][0.021 \text{ (triglycerides (g/dL)} + 0.994)]$$

Hyperglycemia also causes a shift in sodium measurement, although this is not an artifact in the sense that the measured sodium correctly reflects the dilutional effects of water flowing into the vascular compartment due to the osmotic gradient. The shift in sodium concentration is closer to 1.6 mEq/L for every elevation in glucose concentration of 100 mg/dL, producing the following formula for predicted serum sodium if the patient was rendered euglycemic (corrected):

$$\text{Sodium (mEq/L) predicted} = [\text{reported sodium (mEq/L)} + 0.016 \text{ (glucose [mg/dL])}]$$

In formulas 2 and 3, the sodium concentration that would be measured if hyperglycemia and lipemia were cleared can be approximated:

$$\text{Sodium (mEq/L) predicted if euglycemic and eutriglyceridemic}$$
$$= (\text{reported sodium [mEq/L]})(0.021 \text{ [triglycerides (g/dL)]}$$
$$+ 0.994) + 0.016 \text{ (glucose [mg/dL])}$$

Although some intensivists believe this calculated correction of sodium concentration provides a useful guideline for hydration, the measured serum sodium level is the "real" actual sodium concentration in blood. The corrected sodium level is a theoretic calculation.

Potassium Hyperkalemia found at presentation with DKA is commonly believed to be the result of the elevated extracellular hydrogen ions being exchanged for the major intracellular cation, potassium. According to theory, the protons from the increased amount of ketoacids travel down their concentration gradient into the intracellular fluid (ICF).

Phosphate, Calcium, and Magnesium Profound hypophosphatemia and depressed levels of red blood cell (RBC) 2,3-diphosphoglycerate (2,3-DPG) have been described. During treatment of DKA, exuberant replacement of phosphate can result in depressed serum levels of calcium and magnesium. In spite of this, tetany is rarely seen.

Clinical Presentation

Physical Signs and Symptoms Children with DKA often present with:

- Familiar history (i.e., polyuria, polydipsia, polyphagia, and weight loss)
- Headache
- Abdominal pain
- Vomiting
- Lethargy
- Hyperpnea

The child with DKA who arrives in the emergency department with a clear sensorium and good peripheral circulation may not require admission to the PICU. Indications for PICU admission include:

- Profound shock
- Coma
- Respiratory failure
- Dysrhythmias
- Suspicion that the child is at risk for any of the above

As in all situations, treatment priorities follow the "ABCs"; first the airway, then breathing, then circulation.

Evaluation of Patients with Diabetic Ketoacidosis

Initial laboratory evaluation may include various tests to exclude other entities in the differential diagnosis. DKA is present when:

- Serum glucose concentration is more than 300 mg/dL
- Serum nitroprusside test is positive at 1:2 dilutions or greater
- Blood pH is below 7.3 (although the pH may be falsely elevated by other variables)
- Serum bicarbonate concentration is below 15 mEq/L

Monitoring

Laboratory Values Initial tests specifically needed to begin monitoring the course of therapy for DKA should include:

- Blood gases
- pH
- Electrolytes
- BUN
- Glucose
- Creatinine
- Osmolality
- Ketones
- Lactate

- Calcium
- Magnesium
- Phosphate

Hourly determinations should follow for:

- pH
- PCO_2
- Na^+
- K^+
- Glucose
- Ketones

Intervals are lengthened only when stable control has been achieved. The full initial panel should be repeated every 4 to 6 hours during the first 24 hours of treatment. For patients with mild DKA, fewer laboratory tests and interventions may be needed; effective use of such a low-cost approach has been documented.

Other Key Functions

- Electrocardiogram (ECG) should be monitored and displayed continuously. A lead II strip, run and saved hourly, aids in detecting severe alteration in K^+ and Ca^{2+}.
- Urine output must be carefully followed. Patients in shock should have a bladder catheter placed.
- Neurologic status should be assessed at least hourly, and in obtunded patients, a method of quantification (such as the Glasgow Coma Scale) is helpful.

Clearly, such patients require individualized care and frequent monitoring of vitals by a nurse skilled in pediatric intensive care.

Shock Children with shock from DKA severe enough to warrant admission to the PICU should have:

- Continued aggressive fluid therapy
- Careful monitoring
- An arterial catheter to permit continuous measurement of blood pressure and to provide a means for rapid blood sampling for monitoring acid base, electrolyte, and glucose status
- A central venous pressure line to help in studying volume status
- A urinary bladder catheter to monitor ongoing losses and promptly detect renal failure from the antecedent hypoperfused state

Adequate vascular access for volume resuscitation is crucial. This requirement may be complicated by the need to have one intravenous line dedicated to an insulin infusion, another to infusions of other drugs (e.g., pressors), and so on.

Cerebral Edema

Incidence Despite improvements in management of DKA in the past 25 years, mortality because of cerebral edema remains unchanged. Estimates of the incidence of clinically apparent cerebral edema range from 0.1 to 1.0%, probably because of different interpretations of what significantly constitutes the problem. The outcome of cerebral edema is poor.

Increased Risk with Hydration It is widely believed that cerebral edema is a result of treatment of DKA, specifically rehydration. One study found that rates of hydration greater than $4 L/m^2$ carried a higher risk of cerebral edema. This association remains contested, however, and specific risk factors for cerebral edema have been elusive and controversial.

Indications for Lumbar Puncture The indications for lumbar puncture and ICP monitoring in DKA are unclear. In children, especially infants, with DKA, who have fever and clouded sensorium, concerns should always be raised about sepsis or meningoencephalitis and whether a lumbar puncture should be performed to prove the existence of infected cerebrospinal fluid (CSF) before antimicrobial therapy is initiated.

Intubation Endotracheal intubation for airway protection should be strongly considered in children in DKA in coma (Glasgow Coma Score of 7 or less). ICP monitoring need not be instituted for most children with DKA who present in coma. In most, the sensorium clears with correction of the metabolic abnormalities. If the patient's neurologic status worsens or fails to improve once hyperglycemia is corrected, CT scanning and ICP monitoring are needed.

Aggressive management of elevated ICP in a child treated for DKA may be unsuccessful, but it may offer some chance for good recovery in an as yet poorly identified subset of children.

Pulmonary Edema This unusual finding in DKA is possibly related in part to osmolality changes. The observation of increasing oxygen requirements with or without radiographic changes consistent with pulmonary edema has been reported.

Care should be taken to ensure that adequate arterial blood oxygenation continues in order to avoid further tissue injury (especially CNS) and prolonged acidosis. Low plasma oncotic pressure should be avoided, and any potential neurogenic cause for pulmonary edema should be treated promptly.

Cardiac Dysrhythmias Life-threatening disturbances in cardiac rhythm can be caused by hyperkalemia, hypokalemia, or hypocalcemia, all of which can occur in patients being treated for DKA. On admission of a child with DKA to the emergency department, ECG monitoring should be started and continued until the child is clearly responding to therapy with normalizing blood chemistries and neurologic status.

Management of Diabetic Ketoacidosis

Effective care of the critically ill child in DKA is as outlined in Table 24.3.

Diabetic Ketoacidosis versus Hypoglycemia One note of caution: A child with known diabetes who presents with obtundation may not be in DKA, but may in fact be hypoglycemic (e.g., from an overdose of insulin). Therefore, if hyperglycemia cannot be documented promptly, the child should receive intravenous dextrose at a dose of 0.5 g/kg (2 mL of 25% dextrose [D25W] in water/kilogram). D50W should always be diluted with an equal volume of water. Risk (even if the patient really is hyperglycemic) is minimal, and benefits to a potentially hypoglycemic brain may be enormous.

Table 24.3
Initial Treatment for Suspected Diabetic Ketoacidosis

Goal	Time	Approach
1. ABCs	First minutes	Intubate if patient is comatose and ensure adequate breathing and circulation
2. Differential diagnosis and begin monitoring	First minutes	Brief history Venipuncture (large bore IV) and complete blood cell count, blood urea nitrogen, glucose, electrolytes, osmolality, pH, Pco_2, Ca^{2+}, Mg^{2+}, PO_4, and spun hematocrit; Do Chemstrip test Electrocardiogram: monitor and check rhythm strip (check T-waves)
3. Volume repletion	First minutes	Assess blood pressure, heart rate, and skin perfusion Give normal saline or lactated Ringer's solution 10 mL/kg repeatedly as needed to reverse shock
4. Reverse hyperglycemia and ketosis	After Step 2 is in progress, give regular insulin of 0.1	U/kg/h intravenously
5. Fine-tune biochemistry	After Steps 2 and 3 are in progress, change volume replacement to 0.45% saline solution with 25 mEq KCl and 20 mEq K_2HPO_4/L	Adjust solution according to monitored electrocardiogram electrolytes, and pH
6. Avoid hypoglycemia	When glucose ≤300 mg/dL, add 5% dextrose to intravenous fluid	Increase to 10% dextrose if necessary

Insulin Infusion As soon as hyperglycemia and ketosis are confirmed, a continuous intravenous infusion of regular insulin is established at a rate of 0.1 U/kg/hour through a separate intravenous line. There is no established need for an initial intravenous bolus of 0.1 U/kg insulin. When the serum glucose decreases to 300 mg/dL, 5% dextrose is added to the intravenous fluids.

Bicarbonate Therapy The use of sodium bicarbonate in children with DKA remains controversial, largely because the putative benefits and risks remain unproved.

Risks versus Benefits When acidosis is severe (pH < 7.1), bicarbonate therapy has been proposed to:

- Improve myocardial function
- Reduce the potential for dysrhythmia
- Diminish insulin resistance
- Reduce the work of breathing
- Hasten recovery from coma
- Avoid the hyperchloremic state that can prolong acidosis

Stated risks include:

- Increased hemoglobin-oxygen affinity (thus risking increased tissue hypoxia)
- Paradoxically increasing CNS acidosis (by more rapid diffusion of CO_2 than HCO_3 across the blood-brain barrier)
- Reducing the ionized fraction of calcium
- Producing hypokalemia

Administration If bicarbonate is to be given, the best method of infusion is to include it in the crystalloid solutions that are given in the first few hours, at a concentration of 25 to 50 mEq/L. Rapid injection should be avoided.

Tris(hydroxymethyl)aminomethane (THAM) Tris(hydroxymethyl)aminomethane (THAM), as an alternative to sodium bicarbonate, has been offered promise in reducing brain tissue acidosis in an animal model of traumatic brain injury and to increase brain cellular lactate export in a preliminary report on a model of global brain ischemia.

Transition from Pediatric Intensive Care Unit to Ward

Switch to Subcutaneous Insulin Administration When acidosis has resolved, mental status is normal, and interest in food returns, the patient may be advanced to oral feeding and subcutaneous insulin. The proper sequence is to allow a meal or snack at an appropriate time, give regular insulin (subcutaneously) at a dose of 0.25 U/kg (or more or less as indicated by the preceding drip requirements), and discontinue the intravenous drip of insulin. Then, it is appropriate to discontinue any central venous or arterial catheters and arrange to transfer the patient out of the PICU.

REGIMEN A common initial subcutaneous regimen is obtained by first calculating the total daily dose and then splitting the total dose into two thirds to be taken in the morning before breakfast and one third in the evening before dinner. Each premeal dose is also split into two thirds intermediate-duration insulin and one third short-acting insulin. Because even the short-acting insulin preparations take at least half an hour to act, if the patient is receiving insulin infusion in the PICU, the infusion should be discontinued only half an hour after the subcutaneous injection. Also, before administering the injection, it should be verified that a meal is available to the patient within half an hour and that the patient is sufficiently alert and interested in eating.

Hyperosmolar Hyperglycemic Nonketotic Coma

Characteristic Findings Hyperosmolar hyperglycemic nonketotic coma (HHNC) is an extremely unusual occurrence in childhood and is characterized by:

- Marked hyperglycemia
- Hyperosmolality
- Dehydration
- Lowered level of consciousness in the absence of ketosis or acidosis
- Serum osmolality in excess of 350 mOsm/L

Etiology The causes of HHNC can be grouped into three broad categories: lack of water, excess of glucose, and excess of counterregulatory hormones (glucagon is elevated, but not in relation to insulin). The cause of HHNC in any child should be investigated carefully. Special attention should be given to over supply of glucose, restriction of fluid, and administration of any of the medications mentioned, either accidentally or as a manifestation of child abuse.

Diagnosis The initial differential diagnosis and laboratory screening tests are the same for HHNC and DKA. Close monitoring of osmolality, glucose, sodium, potassium, chloride, calcium, phosphate, and magnesium is continued through the first 24 hours of treatment.

Hyperosmolar Hyperglycemic Nonketotic Coma versus Diabetic Ketoacidosis The important differences in pathogenesis and treatment between these two disease entities are due to negligible ketoacid production in the HHNC. The absence of ketosis is due to a normal insulin:glucagon ratio.

Fluid Replacement Therapy Fluid replacement consists initially of boluses of 20 mL/kg of normal saline solution infused as rapidly and as frequently as is needed to reverse shock. In the absence of hyperkalemia (or peaked T waves on ECG), potassium is added to the initial intravenous fluids in a concentration of 10 to 20 mEq/L. The need for phosphate replacement is even less clear in pediatric HHNC than in DKA; hence, phosphate is best left out of intravenous fluids initially.

Insulin Insulin is used with great caution in HHNC, because serum glucose can fall precipitously. An initial continuous intravenous infusion of 0.05 U/kg/hour may be adequate and is adjusted based on closely monitored reagent-strip and laboratory blood glucose measurements. When the blood glucose reaches 300 mg/dL, 5% dextrose is added to intravenous fluids. If the blood glucose level continues to fall, the insulin drip should be reduced or stopped before hypoglycemia ensues.

Hyperglycemia in the Head-Injured Child Although hyperglycemia in the head-injured child is common, it may not be severe enough to qualify as HHNC.

Causes Serum glucose levels are elevated because of:

- Increased endogenous catecholamines and corticosteroids from the stress of injury
- Administration of pressors and inotropes (sympathomimetic agents), corticosteroids (to minimize cerebral edema), and intravenous dextrose
- Replacement solution containing 5% glucose used to counter urine losses in a patient with diabetes insipidus (1 to 2.5% dextrose in a balanced salt solution may be sufficient)

Hyperglycemia has been shown to correlate with the severity of brain injury, although there is controversy as to whether hyperglycemia really is a poor prognostic sign.

Approaches to Management One approach to hyperglycemia in the brain-injured patient is to withhold dextrose initially (from a few hours to a few days, with careful monitoring of blood glucose), under the assumption that the risks to the brain of giving glucose outweigh the benefits to the rest of the body. The other approach is to continue dextrose in the nutritional support and to use insulin when hyperglycemia is a problem.

Continuous infusion of insulin starting at 0.05 U/kg/hour provides more exact and smooth control over blood glucose than does intermittent subcutaneous insulin and may improve tissue anabolism while the potentially harmful effects of high blood glucose levels on the injured brain are avoided.

An over supply of carbohydrates can be problematic, even if blood glucose is normal. If over supply of carbohydrates allows for fat deposition, the respiratory quotient may exceed 1.0; the increase in CO_2 production necessitates an increase in minute ventilation and can make hyperventilation or weaning from mechanical ventilation difficult. The increase in CO_2 may also lead to a rise in ICP, which may be undesirable in a child with head trauma.

Hypoglycemia All mentions of blood glucose in this section refer to measurements derived from whole blood. Whole blood yields glucose values that are 10 to 15% lower than measurements obtained from serum or plasma. Glucose measurements can be lowered if the sample contains excessive numbers of leukocytes (as in leukemia) or nucleated RBCs. Bedside glucose measurements can be taken by various means, with the glucose oxidase reagent strip method demonstrating the best accuracy.

Neonatal Period

GLUCOSE LEVELS Glucose homeostasis is balanced more tenuously in neonates than in adults. The normal-term neonate, in the fed state, shows a decline in blood glucose from maternal levels to 50 mg/dL at 2 hours of age, rising to approximately 70 mg/dL by the third day of life. Blood glucose levels are normally lower in premature neonates.

- In neonates weighing less than 2500 g, hypoglycemia is said to exist when the blood glucose is less than 20 mg/dL.
- For term infants above 2500 g, hypoglycemia is defined by a blood glucose level below 30 mg/dL in the first 72 hours and below 40 mg/dL thereafter.

TRANSIENT HYPOGLYCEMIA Neonatal hypoglycemia usually is transient, occurring in the first 48 hours after birth, and the cause is usually unclear. Hypoglycemia may be asymptomatic or may produce any part of a broad spectrum of symptoms:

- Tremulousness
- Poor feeding
- Hypotonia
- Temperature instability
- Periodic breathing
- Apnea
- Cyanosis
- Convulsions
- Coma

These are nonspecific symptoms and should be ascribed to hypoglycemia only if correction of low blood glucose resolves the symptoms.

Commonly known causes of transient hypoglycemia include:

- Maternal diabetes
- Neonatal hypothermia
- Asphyxia
- Polycythemia
- Infections
- Respiratory distress syndrome (RDS)
- Adrenal hemorrhage
- Small size

Prompt recognition of hypoglycemia is aided by careful observation of newborns at risk. Hypoglycemia may be avoided by ensuring oral or intravenous (as 10% dextrose) glucose supply in the first few hours of life.

Asymptomatic transient hypoglycemia that is successfully treated early carries a good prognosis.

DEXTROSE ADMINISTRATION The preferred method of administration for neonates is as a 10 to 20% solution supplying 4 to 8 mg/kg/minute continuously after an initial bolus of 0.5 to 2.0 g of dextrose/kg in a 25% solution. Fifty percent dextrose is not used in neonates because of its extremely high osmolality (approximately 2800 mOsm/L), which may cause significant local tissue damage.

Central venous access may be necessary in order to deliver these high-osmolality solutions. An umbilical artery line also can be used, with the caveat that if the tip of the catheter is near the take-off of the superior mesenteric artery (at T11 or T12) or celiac (T10) artery from the aorta, the pancreas may receive arterial blood that is very rich in glucose. The pancreas may thus sense hyperglycemia and increase insulin release, even in the presence of systemic hypoglycemia.

PERSISTENT NEONATAL HYPOGLYCEMIA Persistent neonatal hypoglycemia reflects a more serious disorder and may be more difficult to treat. Causes include:

- Hereditary disorders of carbohydrate metabolism (glycogen storage disorders, galactosemia, hereditary fructose intolerance, or fructose-1,6-diphosphatase deficiency)
- Hereditary defects in amino acid (maple syrup urine disease, propionic acidemia, tyrosinosis, or methylmalonic aciduria)
- Insulin excess due to many causes (e.g., Beckwith-Wiedemann syndrome, erythroblastosis fetalis, trisomy 13, and the islet cell dysmaturation syndrome, which includes β-cell hyperplasia, or islet cell hyperplasia)
- Deficient human growth hormone, cortisol, or ACTH

MANAGEMENT AND TREATMENT Initial steps in managing neonates with persistent hypoglycemia are the same as those used in managing patients with transient hypoglycemia. Other treatment methods, including hydrocortisone use (5 mg/kg/day in two doses) or prednisone (1 mg/kg/day), may be of help. Diazoxide (10 to 15 mg/kg/day orally in three doses) may decrease insulin release and aid in achieving normoglycemia. Repeated random collections of blood for simultaneous insulin and glucose level testing may reveal relative hyperinsulinemia.

If the infant has hyperinsulinism and medical therapy is failing to maintain normoglycemia, laparotomy may be indicated for resection of tumor or, in the absence of tumor, for subtotal pancreatectomy. Continuous subcutaneous infusion of somatostatin (8.3 mg/kg/hour) and glucagon (5.4 mg/kg/hour) has been used successfully as a temporizing measure and offers theoretical advantages over maintaining continuous intravenous infusions.

Infancy to Adolescence

ETIOLOGY Two thirds of hypoglycemia cases (blood glucose < 45 mg/dL) in infants older than 1 month are idiopathic; within this group are included unclassified cases (20%), cases of leucine-sensitive hypoglycemia (30%), and cases of ketotic hypoglycemia (50%). The other one third of the cases of hypoglycemia are due to a wide variety of disorders (Table 24.4).

TREATMENT

Dextrose Intravenous dextrose (0.5 g/kg) can be given as a 25% solution to a child of any age; the 50% solution is best reserved for adolescents whose veins are large enough to tolerate the osmolality. The bolus of dextrose should be followed by a constant intravenous infusion of 10% dextrose.

Glucagon Given intravenously or intramuscularly (0.1 to 0.3 mg/kg, up to 1 mg maximum), this agent generates its immediate effect by glycogenolysis; therefore, it is ineffective in disorders in which glycogen is absent (starvation, ketotic hypoglycemia), glycogen storage or lysis is abnormal (the glycogeneses), or liver function is inadequate (e.g., Reye syndrome, hepatitis). Furthermore, glucagon should be accompanied by a supply of dextrose to avoid depletion of carbohydrate stores.

Other pharmacologic uses for glucagon include:

- Treating low-cardiac output states after cardiopulmonary bypass surgery or from congestive myocardial infarction
- Congestive heart failure
- Beta-adrenergic blocker toxicity

It is expensive, however, and causes hypokalemia and hyperglycemia, as well as nausea and vomiting in awake patients.

Diazoxide Unlike glucagon, diazoxide impedes the release of insulin and is useful only in hyperinsulinemic patients. Hyperinsulinism is identified by persistence of nonketotic hypoglycemia despite dextrose replacement and is documented by insulin levels.

The dosage of diazoxide is 10 mg/kg/day divided into two or three enteral doses. Because of its extremely potent hypotensive effect, even at 1 mg/kg, intravenous delivery is less desirable and dictates a slow infusion with careful monitoring of blood pressure. Hydrocortisone, 5 mg/kg/day, or its glucocorticoid equivalent may be a useful adjunct in persistent hypoglycemia. As mentioned previously, continuous infusion of glucagon and somatostatin subcutaneously may hold promise for safe and effective temporizing treatment of hypoglycemia due to hyperinsulinism.

DISORDERS OF WATER HOMEOSTASIS
Introduction

Cell structure and function are critically dependent on homeostasis of water and ion concentrations. Consequently, multiple regulatory systems with

Table 24.4
Causes of Hypoglycemia

Lack of available glucose or its precursors	Enzymatic defects	Liver disease
Inadequate caloric intake	Glycogen synthetase deficiency	Hepatitis
Low-birth-weight infants	Glycogen storage diseases	Cirrhosis
Kwashiorkor	Type I (glucose-6-phosphatase deficiency)	Fatty degeneration of the liver (Reye syndrome)
Low-phenylalanine diet		Idiopathic hypoglycemia
Starvation		Neonatal hypoglycemia
Impaired absorption or excessive loss	Type III (amylo-1,6-glucosidase or debranching enzyme deficiency)	Small-for-gestational-age infants
Chronic diarrhea		Infants of mothers with toxemia
Intestinal disaccharidase deficiency	Type IV (hepatophosphorylase deficiency)	Infants with CNS hemorrhage or infection
Monosaccharide malabsorption	Galactosemia (galactose-1-phosphate uridyltransferase deficiency)	Infants with respiratory distress syndrome
Renal glycosuria		Abrupt cessation of intravenous hypertonic glucose solutions
Increased peripheral glucose utilization	Hereditary fructose intolerance (fructose-1-phosphate aldolase deficiency)	Onset after 2 months of age
Hyperinsulinism		Leucine-sensitive hypoglycemia
Infants of diabetic mothers	Fructose-1,6-diphosphatase deficiency	Ketotic hypoglycemia
Infants with erythroblastosis	Deficiencies in hormonal regulation	Unclassified (unknown) types
Beckwith syndrome	Growth hormone deficiency	Miscellaneous
Nesidioblastosis	Adrenocortical insufficiency	Pharmacologic or toxic
β-cell hyperplasia, idiopathic	Addison's disease	Salicylate
Leucine-sensitive hypoglycemia	Congential adrenal hyperplasia	Alcohol
Islet cell adenoma	Corticotropin deficiency	Oral hypoglycemia agents (biguanides, sulfonylureas)
Subclinical diabetes mellitus	Corticotropin unresponsiveness	Insulin
Extrapancreatic tumors	Catecholamine deficiency	Unripe ackees (hypoglycin) (Jamaican vomiting sickness)
Mesenchymal tumors	Glucagon deficiency	THAM-TRIS (hydroxymethyl aminomethane)
Hepatoma	Inborn errors of amino acid metabolism	Phosphorus
Adrenocortical carcinoma	Maple syrup urine disease	Defects in regulatory function of CNS
Pseudomyxoma	Propionicacidemia	Tumors, hemorrhage, injury infection
Teratomas	Tyrosinosis	Cold
Epithelial tumors	Metylmalonic aciduria	
Congenital neuroblastoma	Isovaleric acidemia	
Wilms' tumor		
Deficiency in hepatic glucose formation and release		

Adapted from Kogut M. Hypoglycemia: pathogenesis, diagnosis, and treatment. In: Gluck L, Cone T, Dodge P, eds. Current problems in pediatrics. Chicago: Year Book, 1974:3.

CNS, central nervous system.

redundant sensing and effector arms serve to maintain this homeostasis within a narrow range.

Syndrome of Inappropriate Secretion of Antidiuretic Hormone (SIADH)

This common problem in the PICU presents as relative hypersthenuria with hyponatremia. Suggestive clinical signs include:

- Hyponatremia
- Low urinary output
- High urinary specific gravity
- High urinary sodium excretion
- A disorder of inappropriately excessive secretion of ADH, leading to decreased free water clearance

The diagnosis of SIADH is indicated, however, when serum osmolality is low (< 280 mOsm/kg) and urinary osmolality is high (> 600 mOsm/kg).

Concomitant Conditions

Clinicians should anticipate development of SIADH in a wide variety of clinical situations, which are listed in Table 24.5.

SIADH after Hypothalamic or Pituitary Surgery This situation is worthy of special mention, because if the sudden appearance of SIADH is not promptly recognized, significant morbidity can result. Transection of axons emanating from the preoptic or paraventricular neurons and terminating in the posterior pituitary prompts a characteristic triphasic time course of diabetes insipidus followed by SIADH and then again by diabetes insipidus. The first phase is due to the lack of secretion of AVP and lasts 1 to 4 days. The second is due to the unregulated release of AVP and lasts up to 10 days. The last phase occurs if insufficient neurons survive to release an adequate amount of AVP; this phase is permanent.

Daily monitoring of specific gravity, serum sodium, and fluid balance provide adequate warning of the transition from one phase to another. Daily weights also are helpful in this regard.

Conditions Involving Excessive Sodium Loss Conditions that may mimic SIADH in producing excessive urinary sodium losses in the face of hyponatremia include:

- Adrenal insufficiency
- Diuretic use
- Renal tubular dysfunction
- Hypothyroidism

Table 24.5
Disorders Associated with the Syndrome of Inappropriate Secretion of Antidiuretic Hormone

Central nervous system disorders
Infection
  Tuberculosis
  Bacterial meningitis
  Encephalitis
Trauma
Hypoxia/ischemia
Psychosis
Tumor
Guillain-Barré
Ventriculoatrial shunt block
Acute intermittent prophyria
Cavernous sinus thrombosis
Subarachnoid hemorrhage
Multiple sclerosis
Anatomical abnormalities
Vasculitis
Chest infection
  Tuberculosis
  Bacterial pneumonia
  Bacterial empyema
  Mycoplasma pneumoniae
  Viral
  Fungal
Positive pressure ventilation
Decreased left atrial pressure
  Pneumothorax
  Asthma
  Cystic fibrosis
  Mitral valve commissurotomy
  Patent ductus arteriosus ligation
Malignancy
Drugs
  Increase arginine vasopressin secretion
    Vincristine
    Cyclophosphamide
    Carbamazepine
    Morphine
    Phenothiazine
    Ara-A
  Potentiate renal effect of arginine vasopressin
    Acetaminophen
    Indomethacin
Other infections
  Bacterial lymphadenitis
  Bacterial arthritis
  Bacterial abscess
  Bacterial sepsis
  Rickettsial
Diabetic ketoacidosis
Idiopathic

Adapted from Kaplan S, Feigin R. Syndromes of inappropriate secretion of antidiuretic hormone in children. Adv Pediatr 1980;27:247.

Cerebral Salt Wasting In cerebral salt wasting, as in SIADH:

- Hyponatremia can be marked and occurs in association with normokalemia
- Urinary sodium is inappropriately high
- Vasopressin is elevated in response to volume depletion caused by diuresis
- Urinary output is not particularly low
- Volume restriction is not effective in restoring eunatremia

Instead, large amounts of salt supplementation are required to restore normal sodium concentrations.

Therapy

Fluid restriction is safest when accompanied by an understanding of the quantitative requirements for water balance. To maintain water balance, the patient should be supplied with 0.5 L/m^2 (to excrete osmotic load) plus 0.5 L/m^2 (to make up for insensible losses) minus 0.25 L/m^2 (supplied by the patient metabolism), for a total of 0.75 L/m^2. Fluid supplementation in a patient subject to maximal antidiuresis at a rate greater than 0.75 L/m^2 daily results in hyponatremia.

Symptomatic Hyponatremia A child with symptomatic hyponatremia requires more aggressive therapy. Symptoms relate to the lowering of plasma osmolality and are primarily neurologic, from malaise to obtundation, coma, and seizures. In symptomatic hyponatremic patients, 3% saline is given in an amount calculated to restore serum sodium to a conservative target of 125 mEq/L over a few hours.

$$\text{Sodium deficit (mEq)} = 0.6 \times \text{BW (in kg)} \times (125 - \text{measured Na}^+)$$

Because 3% saline contains 0.513 mEq of sodium/milliliter, the volume to infuse is easily calculated. The solution contains approximately 1000 mOsm/L and, consequently, is irritating to veins and potentially injurious to tissues into which it might extravasate. To correct the osmolar deficit rapidly, however, it must be given undiluted. Too rapid correction may be dangerous and risks the onset of pontine myelinolysis; therefore, the replacement dose should be calculated to increase the serum sodium concentration at no more than 0.6 to 1 mEq/hr. Again, sodium supplementation should be used only in an acute emergency (to avoid precipitating acute volume overload); SIADH is best treated with strict fluid restriction in most cases.

Hypovolemia and Hyponatremia Blood volume must be corrected (and the diagnosis of SIADH may be suspected unless there is some obvious reason for hypovolemia, such as hemorrhage). Fluid restriction is contraindicated, at least until an adequate blood volume is restored, preferably with normal saline solution or blood products. Long-term therapy for SIADH, including treatment with lithium, demeclocycline, and phenytoin, is generally out of place in the PICU.

Diabetes Insipidus (DI)

Classification and Pathophysiology

Diabetes insipidus (DI) is seen in a variety of rare situations in the PICU. It consists of two broad categories: vasopressin sensitive (central) and vasopressin insensitive (nephrogenic).

Diagnosis

The hallmark of diagnosis is an excessive flow of dilute urine. Urine osmolality generally is less than 200 mOsm/L, which corresponds approximately to a specific gravity of less than 1.005. However, since water reabsorption in the proximal tubule is intact, urine osmolality may reach 400 in the context of severe dehydration.

Differential Diagnosis Differential diagnosis should include:

- Nonoliguric renal failure
- Excessive fluid intake
- Osmotic diuresis

When seen in the PICU, either of the latter two disorders is likely to be the consequence of infusion of fluid that provides free water greatly in excess of ongoing losses.

Osmotic diuresis is, at times, produced deliberately by infusions of such agents as mannitol and radiographic contrast media, but it may also be produced by hyperglycemia. The key differentiating feature is that urine osmolality remains close to that of plasma.

Confirmation of Diagnosis Children with nonoliguric renal failure are usually distinguishable by the fractional excretion of sodium, defined as the ratio of sodium clearance over creatinine clearance, expressed as a percentage:

$$[(\text{Urine Na}^+) \times (\text{plasma creatinine})] \, | \, mq \, [(\text{urine creatinine}) \times (\text{plasma Na}^+)] \times 100$$

This can be remembered as the percentage of filtered sodium that is excreted and is usually less than 1%.

Given these considerations, there is seldom if ever an indication in the critically ill child to proceed through a classical diagnostic workup with water deprivation or to measure plasma levels of AVP. If, in the PICU, the patient has hypotonic polyuria with hypertonic plasma, then he or she has DI. The only remaining diagnostic test is a trial of intranasal desmopressin (DDAVP) or intravenous AVP to tell whether the patient has AVP-responsive DI.

Therapy

After intracranial suprasellar surgery, the onset of DI is anticipated. Often, however, DI is not anticipated and arises in a patient already ill from trauma, infection, or massive brain ischemia. Volume losses may be sizable in children who can ill afford any hemodynamic instability.

Replacement Fluids

Isotonic and Hypotonic Solutions For patients in shock, initial fluid replacement consists of large volumes of isotonic solutions. A dose of 20 mL/kg of body weight should be given as often and as rapidly as is necessary to reverse shock.

After shock has been treated, the fluid administered should be hypotonic. Given that patients with DI can have urine osmolality as low as 50 mOsm/kg, replacing fluid losses with fluid that has a tonicity greater than this low urine osmolality will likely lead to increasing serum hypertonicity.

Dextrose Supplementation Solutions with no more than approximately 37 mEq of sodium/liter (one fourth normal saline) avoid excessive sodium loading, but require the addition of dextrose to maintain an osmolality of infusate above 200 mOsm/L (each gram of dextrose/liter (0.1%) of infusate adds approximately 6 mOsm/L. Large volumes of an approximately correct solution can be made by adding equal volumes of 5% dextrose in water and 0.45% normal saline, yielding 2.5% dextrose in 0.2% normal saline solution.

These intravenous fluids may result in hyperglycemia when given at high rates, particularly in patients in life-threatening situations who have high levels of counterregulatory hormones (particularly cortisol and epinephrine, which lead to increased gluconeogenesis and insulin resistance). Patients given large doses of glucocorticoids (e.g., high-dose dexamethasone) during and after neurosurgery are particularly at risk. Hyperglycemia leads to osmotic diuresis if the glucose level exceeds the renal threshold of approximately 180 mg/dL. To avoid this situation, it may be necessary to reduce the dextrose load or institute a continuous infusion of insulin, with careful attention to blood glucose values.

Infusion Rates Matching intravenous infusion rates to urine output should be reassessed at hourly intervals and followed very carefully, with plasma and urine osmolalities determined every 2 to 4 hours and serum sodium concentrations determined as frequently. As in any hypernatremic state, correction should occur over approximately 48 to 72 hours. Often, appropriate fluid administration is all that is necessary for management of DI.

Aqueous Arginine Vasopressin Continuous infusion of aqueous AVP for treatment of central DI is a rational alternative to fluid management alone. DDAVP (1- desamino-8-D-arginine vasopressin) therapy, administered by intranasal or subcutaneous route, is not as safe.

ADMINISTRATION The optimum rate of infusion of AVP has not been well established, but 1.5 mU/kg/hour is used at many critical care centers. There is no shortage of alternate dosage schemes. The infusion rate can be increased (doubled every 30 minutes) or decreased, but it is likely that there is a ceiling to the effectiveness of AVP. It should rarely be necessary to infuse more than 10 mU/kg/hour (435 pg/kg/minute).

COMPLICATIONS AVP is a potent vasoconstrictor, and experimentally this effect is most extreme in severe CNS injury. Although myocardial infarction from generalized vasoconstriction is of lesser concern in children than in adults, other harmful effects may be seen from massive systemic vasoconstriction. Generalized tissue ischemia can result in profound lactic acidosis. Local effects may include actual infarction of skin over the extremities. For these reasons, extremely high rates of AVP infusion should be used only with great caution.

DISORDERS OF CALCIUM, MAGNESIUM, AND PHOSPHATE METABOLISM
Calcium

Derangements of calcium flux and concentration in the critical care setting usually are of relatively brief duration and rarely result in skeletal abnormalities, even though they can cause significant physiologic disturbances.

Hypercalcemia

Incidence Hypercalcemia is encountered less often than is hypocalcemia in the PICU because the two disorders most frequently associated with elevated Ca^{2+} concentration in adults, namely hyperparathyroidism and cancers of breast, lung, kidney, head, and neck and myeloma, are less common in children. Even more rare is the humoral hypercalcemia of malignancy that is usually associated with parathyroid hormone-related peptide. More commonly, hypercalcemia due to malignancy in childhood is caused by direct bony invasion or metastasis by tumor or tumor lysis.

Treatment

Calcium Reduction Measures for directly reducing serum Ca^{2+} concentration include:

- Hydration with saline solution (10 mL/kg/hour) with furosemide (1 mg/kg every 6 hours)
- Restriction of Ca^{2+} intake
- Avoidance of vitamin D, thiazides, and Ca^{2+}-containing antacids
- Phosphates (intravenously 0.15 to 0.30 mmol/kg over 12 hours) and etidronate (intravenously EHDP, a biphosphonate that is an effective inhibitor of osteoclastic activity, 15 to 50 mg/kg over 4 hours)
- Oral and rectal phosphates (0.5 to 1 mmol/kg/day)

In all of these methods, risks include:

- Hypocalcemia
- Metastatic calcification

- Hypotension
- Renal failure
- Heart failure

These intravenous agents may bring about the desired result quickly but may also risk precipitous hypocalcemia. Precautions for this method of therapy are:

- Prehydration
- Careful monitoring of electrolytes
- Avoidance in the face of hyperphosphatemia or renal impairment

The product of the concentrations of calcium and phosphorus ($Ca^{2+} \times$ P) (in mg/dL) should be kept below 60, and the patient should be monitored for metastatic calcification (by slit-lamp examination and soft tissue radiographs).

Excessive Bone Resorption When this process is significant (malignancy, immobility), effective inhibitors include:

- Calcitonin (4 to 8 U/kg intravenously over 24 hours)
- Mithramycin (10 to 25 g/kg intravenously for 2 to 21 days)
- Glucocorticoids (prednisone, 1 to 2 mg/kg/day intravenously divided into four doses; or hydrocortisone, 1 to 5 mg/kg four times a day)
- Indomethacin (1 mg/kg/day)

Hypocalcemia

Etiology Causes of hypocalcemia include parathyroid hormone deficiency, vitamin D deficiency, and chelation or depletion.

Parathyroid Hormone Deficiency This state can be induced by:

- Direct injury to or absence of the parathyroids (idiopathic disease, trauma, radiation, infiltration, or surgery)
- Excision, ischemia, or necrosis of the parathyroid glands after thyroid surgery
- Severe bodily injury (trauma, burns, sepsis)
- Pancreatitis
- Maternal hyperparathyroidism
- Drugs
- Severely low magnesium concentrations

Hypomagnesemia may inhibit release of parathyroid hormone as well as impair end-organ response to parathyroid hormone.

Vitamin D Deficiency Vitamin D activity may be affected by:

- Decreased uptake from the gut (dietary lack, malabsorption)
- Decreased activation (liver disease, renal disease, pseudohypoparathyroidism, rhabdomyolysis, lack of sunlight),
- Increased loss of vitamin D (nephrosis, anticonvulsant use)

In many countries, including the United States, vitamin D2 supplementation in many foodstuffs, including milk, has made nutritional rickets very rare. The inherited forms of vitamin D deficiency are similarly rare, including pseudovitamin D deficiency.

Differential Diagnosis Differential diagnosis of hypocalcemia changes with the age of the patient. Early neonatal hypocalcemia (birth to 4 or 5 days old) is most common in premature infants, those with severe neonatal cardiorespiratory distress, and those with diabetic mothers. Causes of this phenomenon are not fully elucidated but probably include prolonged suppression of the parathyroid glands by the relatively hypercalcemic fetal environment, insufficient calcium delivery in the early neonatal diet, and decreased mobilization of skeletal calcium due to elevated levels of stress hormones.

Treatment

Calcium Chloride Hypocalcemia should be treated unless it is borderline and asymptomatic depending on the underlying disorder. Patients with impending neuromuscular or cardiovascular collapse require prompt restoration of serum ionized calcium. A reasonable approach is to give, intravenously, 0.1 mL of 10% $CaCl_2$/kg over 5 to 10 minutes through a secure catheter in a large vein, if possible. Calcium salts precipitate in bicarbonate, so the two should never be given in the same line.

Because calcium infusions are associated with cardiac dysrhythmias, patients should have continuous ECG monitoring, and atropine should be readily available before a calcium bolus is infused intravenously. Once the patient is asymptomatic, intravenous boluses of calcium should be replaced, if possible, with oral supplements (or added to intravenous infusions).

Treating Concomitant Deficiencies Normocalcemia may be difficult to sustain in the presence of hypomagnesemia, hypoparathyroidism, or inadequate vitamin D. Hypomagnesemia is best treated with 0.3 to 1 mEq of magnesium chloride per kilogram over 12 to 24 hours. Magnesium sulfate is less desirable, because sulfates complex with calcium. Hypoparathyroidism, pseudohypoparathyroidism, and vitamin D deficiency are all managed by adding vitamin D in an appropriate form to Ca^{2+} supplementation.

Magnesium

Normally, total plasma magnesium concentration is 1.4 to 2.0 mEq/L (1.7 to 2.4 mg/dL). Plasma magnesium is 65% to 80% bound to proteins. Little is published about the relative value of measuring total versus ionized plasma magnesium.

Magnesium has therapeutic uses, including as an antihypertensive or anticonvulsant agent and recently as treatment for asthma (i.e., bronchodilator).

Hypermagnesemia

Incidence Hypermagnesemia is extremely uncommon. ECG changes occur with values above 5 mEq/L and symptoms generally occur with values above 10 mEq/L.

Therapy Treatment of isolated hypermagnesemia should consist simply of restricting intake and inducing diuresis. If the hypermagnesemia is producing symptoms, more aggressive treatment is warranted.

As a rapid temporizing measure, calcium may be given intravenously. Neonatologists commonly administer 100 mg of calcium gluconate/kilogram (equivalent to 30 mg of calcium chloride/kilogram) or approximately 10 mg of elemental calcium/kilogram. For children, approximately 10 mg of calcium chloride/kilogram is appropriate, followed with diuresis or, if necessary, dialysis (both peritoneal and hemodialysis are effective).

Whereas calcium partially reverses the deleterious effects of magnesium, it also reverses any therapeutic effects. This is worth bearing in mind when dealing with patients with seizures or preeclampsia; calcium reverses the anticonvulsant properties of magnesium.

Hypomagnesemia

Hypomagnesemia occurs in 11% of hospitalized patients, in comparison with the 9% with hypermagnesemia. Studies in PICUs have found 20% to 50% of patients to be hypomagnesemic, with the lowest incidence in the patient group with the poorest renal function (i.e., the lowest renal magnesium loss).

Contributing Factors Increased GI losses can be due to:

- Malabsorption states
- Laxative use
- Bowel fistulas
- Small bowel disease or resection
- Prolonged nasogastric suction

Renal losses may be due to:

- Diuretics
- Aminoglycosides
- Chemotherapeutics
- Vitamin D
- Calcium
- Digitalis
- Amphotericin B
- Insulin
- Theophylline
- Alcohol

- Transfusions
- Cardiopulmonary bypass
- Intrinsic renal disease (nephritis, nephrosclerosis, renal tubular disease, acute tubular necrosis)
- Stimulation by other disorders, such as DKA, hypophosphatemia, hypercalcemia, possibly hypokalemia, hyperparathyroidism, hyperaldosteronism, or hyperthyroidism

Excessive losses in sweat and breast milk have also been noted, and pancreatitis is believed to be associated with hypomagnesemia (which may, in turn, contribute to hypocalcemia in pancreatitis). Familial hypomagnesemia may involve both poor gut absorption and defective renal reabsorption.

Cardiovascular Manifestations   The cardiovascular manifestations of hypomagnesemia also overlap with those of hypocalcemia and hypokalemia (and may, at least in part, be due to the latter two secondary disorders). Characteristic changes include:

- Increased P-R and Q-T intervals as well as flat broad T-waves on ECG
- Ventricular tachydysrhythmias
- Increased susceptibility to digitalis toxicity

Associated Electrolyte Disturbances   Such disturbances associated with hypomagnesemia include:

- Hypokalemia
- Hyponatremia
- Hypophosphatemia
- Distal renal tubular acidosis

Because magnesium reabsorption is coupled with renal reabsorption of calcium and sodium, the increased renal losses of sodium and calcium result in increased magnesium loss.

Treatment

Role of Renal Function   If GFR is reduced, magnesium replacement may result in hypermagnesemia. Also, if the patient has not been fed for an extended period of time, tissue stores probably are depleted unless intravenous fluid contains maintenance amounts of magnesium (as do most total parenteral nutrition solutions).

Regimen of Magnesium Infusion   It may take 4 or 5 days to achieve equilibrated normomagnesemia. For patients with normal renal function and no increased losses of magnesium, supplying the normal daily magnesium requirement of 0.3 to 0.4 mEq/kg/day intravenously should suffice. Up to 1 mEq/kg/day is probably safe, if necessary, in patients with normal renal function. These intravenous infusions are best delivered in the maintenance-fluid solution rather than as a bolus. The renal threshold for excretion of magnesium is at plasma concentrations of 1.5 to 2.0 mg/dL, so that high peak concentrations due to rapid magnesium infusions can result in a relatively high degree of renal excretion, giving a poor clinical response. Again, the serum magnesium level should be followed closely, especially in patients with poor renal function.

Phosphate

Phosphorus exists in the body in the form of phosphates—the salts of phosphoric acid (H_3PO_4). In the biologic pH range, phosphates exist as HPO_4^{2-} and $H_2PO_4^{2-}$ a molar ratio of 2:1 to 6:1 (average, 4:1). The average phosphate valence, then, is approximately -1.8. Rather than report phosphates in milliequivalents or amounts of H_2PO_4 and HPO_4^{2-} in millimoles/liter, clinical laboratories in the United States report either milligrams of phosphorus/deciliter or the equivalent in inorganic (i.e., not complexed to organic molecules) phosphate, generally abbreviated as PO_4 with no stated valence. This convention is used in this chapter.

Hyperphosphatemia

Excessive serum phosphorus concentrations (PO_4) essentially are clinically silent, except insofar as they cause hypocalcemia. Rising serum PO_4 rapidly lowers Ca^{2+}. The binding of Ca^{2+} and PO_4 results in metastatic (i.e., soft tissue) calcification when the product of the concentrations (in milligrams/deciliter) of total calcium and inorganic phosphorus exceeds 60. The falling Ca^{2+} level stimulates parathyroid hormone secretion and inhibits renal formation of $1,25(OH)_2D$. Phosphaturia then follows as a result of the effects of both the increased parathyroid hormone and the hyperphosphatemia itself on reducing the maximal threshold rate. As the Ca^{2+} concentration falls, the patient may begin to exhibit signs of tetany, which may become profound.

Causes

Excessive Intake Phosphate intake must be fairly massive in order to overwhelm the normally effective renal excretory mechanism. Such intake generally results from massive intravenous infusions or from oral or rectal phosphate overuse. Other exogenous sources of phosphorus include the "white phosphorus" in incendiary bombs, which can be absorbed through skin burn wounds.

Inadequate Excretion PO_4 excretion is suboptimal when the maximal threshold rate:GFR ratio rises. Hence, any cause for a decrease in GFR (e.g., renal failure, volume depletion, myocardial failure) or an increase in maximal threshold rate (by growth hormone, vitamin D, hypoparathyroidism, pseudohypoparathyroidism) reduces phosphate excretion. The hyperphosphatemia that occurs may be sufficient to push the calcium-phosphate product well above 60 and result in metastatic calcifications. It is thought that this is the reason for the calcification of the cornea and basal ganglia seen in many patients with hypoparathyroidism or pseudohypoparathyroidism.

Intracellular Fluid to Extracellular Fluid Shifts Shifts of PO_4 from ICF to ECF are seen in a variety of clinical situations in which cell lysis is prominent, such as oncotherapy, rhabdomyolysis, and shock. For the same reason, RBC breakage during blood drawing may produce spurious hyperphosphatemia. When the cause is unclear, measurement of GFR and of daily urinary PO_4 loss may clarify the nature of the problem. (Normal phosphorus urinary excretion is < 1500 mg/day in adults.)

Treatment General maneuvers include:

- Elimination of excess intake
- Use of aluminum hydroxide antacids (1 mL/kg every 6 hours helps, even in the absence of enteral PO_4 intake)
- Restoration of plasma volume with saline solution
- Insulin and glucose administration
- Dialysis

Note that symptomatic hypocalcemia, if present, receives the highest priority for treatment.

Hypophosphatemia

Abnormally low serum PO_4 concentrations are seen in a wide variety of clinical situations and are the converses of the categories cited for hyperphosphatemia: reduced intake, increased excretion, and shifts from ECF to ICF. Some disease states, such as DKA, may involve all three mechanisms.

Diabetic Ketoacidosis Excess urinary losses of phosphate in DKA arise from a tendency of glycosuria (by competing for the PO_4 reabsorption mechanism), ketonuria, and acidosis to lower the maximal threshold rate. The problem is exacerbated by osmotic diuresis and diminished dietary intake as the child becomes ill. Insulin drives the serum PO_4 (along with glucose and potassium) into cells, further aggravating hypophosphatemia.

Other Disorders That Reduce Serum PO_4 Levels

- Renal tubular disorders (congenital, recovery from acute tubular necrosis or renal transplantation)
- Acidosis
- Pregnancy
- Heavy-metal poisoning
- Hypokalemia
- Paint and glue sniffing
- Wilson's disease
- Glycosuria (i.e., even without DKA)
- Lack of or resistance to vitamin D

- Hyperparathyroidism
- Reye's syndrome
- Increase in GFR

Consequences of Hypophosphatemia

Rickets Rickets is especially likely to develop in rapidly growing infants supported by total parenteral nutrition without adequate phosphate; however, it can also occur well into adolescence.

Reduced 2,3-DPG in Red Blood Cells The observed 2,3-DPG changes in RBC have not proven to be clinically significant, nor has phosphate replacement in DKA been well demonstrated to be of more than theoretic benefit.

ATP Depletion ATP depletion appears to be the final common pathway for many of the clinical manifestations of hypophosphatemia, including:

- Depressed leukocyte phagocytosis
- Increased RBC
- Platelet destruction
- Muscular weakness
- Respiratory failure
- Depressed myocardial function
- Rhabdomyolysis
- CNS dysfunction (from mood changes to seizures and coma)
- Liver failure

Treatment Treatment ideally begins in anticipation of, rather than in response to, a falling concentration of serum PO_4. If the serum phosphorus level is less than 1.0 mg/dL, intravenous correction is appropriate. For phosphorus values of 0.5 to 1.0 mg/dL, suggested infusion doses range from 0.05 to 0.25 mmol of PO_4/kilogram given intravenously over 4 to 12 hours. Patients with a serum phosphorus concentration below 0.5 mg/dL should receive PO_4 at 0.09 to 0.5 mmol/kg over 4 to 12 hours.

Known risks of PO_4 infusion include:

- Hyperkalemia (the potassium salt of PO_4 is usually used)
- Hypocalcemia
- Metastatic calcification
- Hypomagnesemia
- Hyperphosphatemia
- Hypotension
- Hyperosmolality
- Renal failure

The lower end of the dosage ranges should be used in the presence of hypocalcemia or renal failure, and PO_4 should not be given if hypercalcemia is present.

DISORDERS OF THE THYROID

Thyrotoxic Crisis

Clinical Presentation

Because thyrotoxicosis has a nonspecific presentation in the critically ill patient, a history is most helpful. If the patient is a neonate, a maternal history of autoimmune thyroid disease is relevant. Otherwise, a history of prior thyroid disease or a diagnosis of one of the syndromes or disorders known to be associated with thyrotoxicosis is helpful.

Causative Event Usually, some precipitating event triggers the abrupt onset of thyrotoxic crisis, such as:

- Infection
- Trauma
- Surgery
- DKA
- Radiation
- Exogenous thyroid hormone ingestion
- Toxic adenoma of the thyroid
- Haloperidol use
- Iodide ingestion

Associated Disorders The disorder in children is found in association with:

- Diabetes mellitus
- Juvenile rheumatoid arthritis
- Down syndrome
- McCune-Albright syndrome
- Addison's disease
- Myasthenia gravis
- Hashimoto's thyroiditis
- Systemic lupus erythematosus
- Chronic active hepatitis
- Nephrotic syndrome

Any child known to have an endocrinopathy or autoimmune disease should be considered at risk for thyroid disease.

Clinical Manifestations

Thyrotoxic crisis shares features with sepsis, malignant hyperthermia, anticholinergic poisoning, transfusion reaction, and adrenal crisis.

Symptoms and Signs Symptoms are generally insidious in onset and, at first, are frequently assumed to be normal signs of adolescence. Severity of symptoms is not related to the concentration of T_3 or T_4. Indeed, T_4 and T_3 levels in a thyrotoxic crisis are often in the same range as in cases of moderate thyrotoxicosis that do not even require hospitalization (as in cases of thyroid hormone overdose).

The most common reported findings in childhood thyrotoxicosis, in descending order, are:

- Goiter
- Tachycardia
- Nervousness
- Increased pulse pressure
- Proptosis
- Increased appetite
- Tremor
- Weight loss
- Heat intolerance
- Dysrhythmias
- Congestive heart failure (although high-output failure is rare except in the severely compromised neonate or the older adolescent)
- Shock
- Psychosis
- Coma
- Seizures

Physical Findings

- Fever
- Cutaneous flushing
- Diaphoresis
- Weakness
- Lethargy
- Confusion
- Extreme tachycardia
- Hepatomegaly
- Jaundice
- Nausea
- Vomiting

Untreated, the illness progresses to extreme hyperpyrexia, coma, and death.

Diagnostic Studies Serum should be sent for determination of the levels of T_4, free T_4, T_3, and free T_3, if available. For a child who is critically ill, further testing is ill advised in most cases, and treatment should begin promptly.

If the severity of illness warrants placement of a pulmonary artery catheter, confirmation of the hypermetabolic state is found in elevation of the cardiac index and oxygen consumption index. Echocardiography can provide similar information noninvasively.

Neonatal Thyrotoxicosis Although more frequently a disorder managed in the neonatal intensive care unit, symptoms may become apparent only after discharge of the newborn from the hospital. Mothers with Graves' disease may have transplacental passage of TSIs. As levels of antithyroid drugs fall in the child's bloodstream, the child becomes progressively more hyperthyroid. Symptoms may reach a crisis by 1 to 2 weeks of age, at which point the infant demonstrates the following:

- Fever
- Irritability
- Evidence of sepsis
- Failure to thrive
- Diarrhea
- Feeding intolerance
- Hepatosplenomegaly
- Thrombocytopenia
- Seizures

Given these symptoms, other diagnoses must be considered, including infection (congenital and acquired neonatal), predelivery drug abuse in the mother, and congenital heart disease (presenting as congenital heart failure).

Treatment

Therapy for the child in thyroid storm is directed at the triggering illness, the hyperdynamic cardiovascular state, the effects of the accelerated metabolic state, and the thyroid gland itself.

- Intravenous propranolol (0.01 mg/kg) is given by slow push every 10 minutes until the hyperdynamic cardiovascular state is improved or a total of 5 mg is given
- Propylthiouracil given by nasogastric tube, at 20 to 30 mg/kg/day in four divided doses, stops organification of iodide and reduces intrathyroidal and peripheral conversion of T_4 to T_3
- Sodium iodide can be infused intravenously 1 hour after administration of propylthiouracil at 1 to 2 g/day
- Glucocorticoids may reduce serum T_3 levels
- Dexamethasone, 0.1 mg/kg given every 6 hours, should be more than sufficient
- Oral radiocontrast agents sodium ipodate and iopanoic acid have been used as potent inhibitors of peripheral conversion of T_4 to T_3

Salicylates, surgery, and use of radioiodine are not part of the acute therapy for thyroid storm.

After the patient is stable, propranolol can be continued orally at 4 mg/kg/day in four divided doses, with a 10-mg dose generally being adequate (although some adolescents may require up to a 60-mg dose). Clinical improvement should be seen within 24 hours, and resolution of the crisis should be achieved within a week.

Nonthyroid Illness (Sick Euthyroid Syndrome)

In the PICU, nonthyroidal illness is the most common cause of abnormal thyroid hormone levels. Variation in the thyroid hormone levels in nonthyroidal illness typically involves depression of T_3, variably associated with depression of T_4 (typically in more severe and prolonged critical illness) without elevation of TSH. As patients recover from their critical illness, T_3 and T_4 return to the normal range, sometimes accompanied by a rise of TSH to the range found in hypothyroid patients.

In adult patients, the severity of disease and mortality correlate inversely with T_4 and T_3 levels. Of note, attempts to improve mortality rates in these patients with use of supplemental T_4 or T_3 has either failed to show benefit or has been inconclusive at best.

Factors that can affect thyroid hormone levels include the following medications:

- Glucocorticoids (decrease in T3, increase in T4)
- Propranolol (decrease in T3, increase in T4)
- Propylthiouracil (decrease in T3, increase in T4)
- Anticonvulsants (phenytoin and carbamazepine; increase hepatic metabolism and displace T4 from binding proteins)
- Dopamine (blunt TSH level)
- Somatostatin (blunt TSH level)
- Opioids (blunt TSH level)
- Dexamethasone (blunt TSH level)
- Furosemide (displace T3 and T4 from binding proteins)
- Salicylates (displace T3 and T4 from binding proteins)
- Povidone-iodine

During critical illness, there are changes both in measured peripheral thyroid hormone concentration and conversions and in thyroidal axis regulation and responses. Total T_4 and T_3 levels are often found to be low and are the result of several mechanisms.

Hypothyroidism

Hypothyroidism in PICU patients is more often a coexisting illness than a primary or life-threatening problem. Most infants with congenital hypothyroidism are identified by mandatory newborn screening in the United States. This screening, performed on a small quantity of blood dried on filter paper and sent to a reference laboratory, has documented an incidence of congenital primary hypothyroidism (due to ectopic gland or athyreosis) approaching 1 out of 3500. These infants are asymptomatic or minimally symptomatic, and the diagnosis is easily missed until permanent neurologic impairment has occurred.

Several factors in the PICU may thwart the screening programs, depending on how they are implemented. For example, hypothyroid infants who are receiving dopamine or a pharmacologic dose of dexamethasone may have a suppressed TSH response in the presence of a marginal T_4 level and therefore have normal results on neonatal screening. Blood transfusion or cardiopulmonary bypass may falsely normalize the results (a false-negative test). If possible, the patient should be screened before blood-product exposure; if this is not possible, testing should be postponed to a later date.

ENDOCRINE THERAPY OF CATABOLIC STATES

Critically ill children are at risk for the effects of prolonged catabolism. Multiple hormones (e.g., cortisol, epinephrine) are stimulated under the stress of severe illness, leading to lipolysis, muscle catabolism, and bone resorption. In addition, the nutrition of children in the PICU, even when receiving parenteral nutrition, can be insufficient and thereby accelerate the catabolism. When recovery from the disease state would require considerable anabolism (e.g., in burns), prolonged catabolism can contribute to long hospitalizations, difficulty in weaning from ventilators, and increased mortality.

CARCINOID SYNDROME

Carcinoid tumors are a group of very rare, highly differentiated neuroendocrine neoplasms that usually occur in the gut. The appendix is the most common location of carcinoid tumors in children. Their presentation is usually similar to appendicitis, and appendectomy is usually curative since the malignant potential of carcinoid tumors is very low. These tumors release a variety of hormones and mediators. The most common are serotonin, histamine, and kinins (bradykinin, kallikrein).

INBORN ERRORS OF METABOLISM

Most commonly, intensivists care for these patients in the context of an operative procedure (e.g., tracheostomy), intercurrent illness (e.g., aspiration pneumonia), or metabolic imbalance (e.g., hyperammonemic crisis) in a child with a known diagnosis. On occasion, however, an extremely sick child comes to the PICU and only later after a prolonged and extensive workup is found to have a metabolic disorder.

In this section, signs and symptoms that may alert the vigilant physician are reviewed, and a brief overview of the workup is given. The highlights of a number of conditions with special PICU-related considerations are provided.

Antenatal Diagnosis and Neonatal Screening

Some of the more commonly screened diseases include:

- Phenylketonuria
- Maple syrup urine disease
- Galactosemia
- Congenital adrenal hypoplasia

Many other tests are available (e.g., biotinidase deficiency). The particular panel used in newborns varies from state to state.

Clinical Presentation

Many metabolic illnesses present early in life, often in association with the introduction of protein to the diet (e.g., urea cycle disturbances), hypoglycemia (e.g., glutaric acidemia type II), or hypotonia (e.g., Pompe disease).

Other diseases present later in life, often with insidious signs, such as:

- Slowing or loss of developmental milestones
- Failure to thrive
- Vomiting
- Lethargy or obtundation
- A syndrome resembling Reye syndrome
- Hyperventilation or apnea
- Seizures (especially if intractable)
- Muscular abnormalities

Physical Findings

Patients may demonstrate such signs as:

- Jaundice
- Hepatomegaly (seen in many of these conditions)
- Cataracts (e.g., galactosemia)
- Macrocephaly (e.g., glutaric acidemia type I)
- Cardiomyopathy (e.g., long chain fatty acid oxidation defects)
- Urine of a characteristic odor (e.g., "mousey" in phenylketonuria) or color (e.g., black in alkaptonuria)

Family history may provide useful information, such as consanguinity, previous neonatal deaths, and a previous child with metabolic disease.

Table 24.6
Characteristic Biochemical Abnormalities of Some Inborn Errors of Metabolism

Disease	Defect
Urea cycle defects	Hyperammonemia, primary respiratory alkalosis
Organic acidemias	Hyperammonemia, metabolic acidosis with increased anion gap, neutropenia, thrombocytopenia
Amino acidopathies	Ketosis
Disorders of carbohydrate metabolism	Nonglucose reducing substances in urine, lactac acidosis, hypoglycemia

Table 24.7
Screening Workup for Metabolic Disorders

Blood
  Arterial blood gas, ammonia, and calcium
  Arterial or venous glucose, creatinine, electrolyte levels (and anion gap), blood urea nitrogen, creatinine, uric acid
  Liver function tests, particularly in the presence of hyperammonemia (e.g., prothrombin time, partial thromboplastin time, aminotransferases, albumin)
  Freeze sample for further analysis (e.g., amino acids, carnitine)
  Complete blood cell count
  Blood culture
Urine
  Urinalysis (reagent strip, including reducing substances, glucose, ketones, pH)
  Save an aliquot for further analysis (e.g., amino acids and organic acids, carbohydrates, orotic acid, glycosaminoglycans)
  Urine culture
Cerebrospinal fluid
  If obtained, hold an aliquot in the freezer for further testing (e.g., amino acids, lactate, pyruvate)

Laboratory Findings

Suggestive biochemical abnormalities are outlined in Table 24.6. Some of these presentations may be easily mistaken for sepsis in a sick infant. (Sepsis is also not uncommon in galactosemia and propionic and methylmalonic acidemia.)

Initial Approach to the Patient

Once an inborn error of metabolism is suspected, all enteral feeding stops and an intravenous glucose/electrolyte solution is administered. Laboratory tests (Table 24.7) to evaluate the presence of an inborn error of me-

Table 24.8
Common Disorders Involving Inborn Error in Metabolism

Disease	Metabolic Error	Clinical Characteristics	Comments
Glycogen storage disease I	Glucose-6-phosphatase deficiency	Massive hepatomegaly, severe lactic acidosis and hypoglycemia, short stature, bleeding diathesis, hyperuicemia, and Fanconi-like nephropathy	Treat patients as if they have a "full stomach" owing to hepatomegaly. Maintain glucose-containing infusion and monitor serum glucose and pH. Obtain preoperative bleeding time.
Glycogen storage disease II (Pompe)	Alpha-glucosidase deficiency; infantile, juvenile, and adult forms.	Hypotenoia, muscle weakness, macroglossia, cardiomyopathy, recurrent pneumonia, and hepatomegaly	Electrocardiogram reflects poor cardiac function: left axis deviation, short P-R interval, and inverted T-waves. Anesthesia induction has caused cardiac arrest and v-fib. Avoid drugs with cardiac depressant effects.
Galactosemia	Galactose-1-phosphate uridyl transferase deficiency	Failure to thrive, vomiting, dehydration, hypoglycemia, jaundice and hepatomegaly, cirrhosis, coagulopathy, predisposition to gram-negative sepsis in newborn period	Managing fluids, electrolytes, and glucose is key. Avoid lactose.
Phenylketonuria	Phenylalanine hydroxylase deficiency	Mental retardation, seizures, hypopigmentation, mousey odor, eczema	Avoid phenylalanine and aspartame
Homocystinuria	Cystathionine beta-synthase deficiency	Optic lens dislocation, mental retardation, seizures, arterial and venous thrombi and thromboemboli, osteoporosis, other skeletal abnormalities	Thrombosis (due to increased platelet adhesiveness) and abnormal vasculature can occur in any vascular bed and usually are cause of death. Preoperative evaluation of central nervous system,

continued

Table 24.8
Common Disorders Involving Inborn Error in Metabolism

Disease	Metabolic Error	Clinical Characteristics	Comments
			heart, and other organs is warranted. Avoid conditions predisposing to thrombosis and wrap legs or use pressurized boots.
Maple syrup urine disease	Defective branched chain ketoacid dehydrogenase leading to accumulation of those amino acids and their alpha-keto acids	Mental retardation, seizures, metabolic acidosis, liver failure, thromboembolism	Manage glucose and pH
Mucopoly-saccharidosis type I (Hurler syndrome)	Alpha-L-iduronidase deficiency, a lysomal enzyme disorder	Short stature, coarse facies, macroglossia, abnormal teeth, short thick neck, deposition of mucopolysaccharide in larynx and trachea leading to airway narrowing, meningeal thickening leading to hydrocephalus, corneal clouding, mental retardation, contractures with poor joint mobility, restrictive lung disease, pulmonary infections, abdominal hernias, cardiomyopathy, coronary artery disease, valvular heart disease	All organ systems affected. Children are difficult to intubate. Limited pulmonary and cardiac reserve. Congestive heart failure and pulmonary hypertension may occur. Cardiac manifestations are commonly the cause of death.
Other mucopoly-saccharidoses		Vary by type	Less extensive and severe than Hurler syndrome. Atlantoaxial instability seen in types IV, VI, and VII. Fiberoptic or lighted-stylet intubation avoids neurologic damage.

continued

Table 24.8
Common Disorders Involving Inborn Error in Metabolism

Disease	Metabolic Error	Clinical Characteristics	Comments
Urea cycle disturbances	Ornithine transcarbamylase deficiency, carbamyl phosphate synthetase deficiency	Lethargy, hypotonia, vomiting, coma (may need ventilatory support), seizures, hyperammonemia (may be associated with cerebral edema and hyperventilation), increased glutamine and alanine, increased orotic aciduria	Hyperammonemia determines the severity of symptoms. Intercurrent illness or large protein load exacerbates the disease. Treatment focus is on improving nitrogen elimination. Nitrogen-free parenteral nutrition reduces plasma nitrogen by reducing protein catabolism.
Gaucher disease (glucocere-brosidosis, glucosyl-ceramide lipidosis)	Glucocerebrosidase deficiency; a type of sphingolipidosis that is a subtype of lysosomal enzyme disorder	Type I: hepatosplenomegaly and pancytopenia, bony degeneration, vertebral fractures, aseptic necrosis of the femoral head, bone pain, pulmonary disease	Address hematologic abnormalities preoperatively. Fracture potential hinders positioning. Trismus and retroflexed head position makes intubation difficult. Increased risk for aspiration.
		Type II: rapid, devastating onset. Trismus, strabismus, retroflexion of the head, difficulty with secretions (recurrent aspirations), hepatosplenomegaly, spasticity, seizures	
		Type III: features of types I and II but slower in onset	
Lesch-Nyhan syndrome	Hypoxanthine-guanine phosphoribosyl transferase deficiency	Hyperreflexia, dystonia, chorea, athetosis, seizures, self-mutilation, aggressive behavior, subcutaneous uric acid tophi, renal calculi, nephropathy, regurgitation, vomiting, increased serum uric acid level	Sedation may be crucial; benzodiaze-pines or rectal barbiturates are good choices. Use measures to mitigate chances of aspiration. Pica-caused perioral scarring may hinder intubation. Use drugs

continued

Table 24.8
Common Disorders Involving Inborn Error in Metabolism

Disease	Metabolic Error	Clinical Characteristics	Comments
			cleared through the kidneys with caution. Avoid succinylcholine. Some patients show increased sensitivity to narcotics and abnormal sympathetic response to stress and exogenous catecholamines.
Porphyrias	Defects in porphyrin synthesis; hepatic and erythropoietic are two types	Abdominal pain, seizures, SIADH, psychosis, cranial nerve paresis, autonomic dysfunction, peripheral neuropathy, hypoventilation	Erythropoietic forms mainly expressed in childhood; hepatic types from adolescence onward. Barbiturates, ethanol, dilantin, diazepam, local anesthetics, pentazocine corticosteroids, imipramine, and tolbutamide trigger acute intermittent porphyria and are hazardous in variegate porphyria and hereditary coproporphyria.

tabolism and to rule out infection, acquired metabolic disorders (e.g., poisoning), nutritional abnormalities, and other acquired illnesses are performed during the acute phase of illness, not after treatment is under way. Eventually, the final specific laboratory test is done (e.g., muscle biopsy, fibroblast assays).

The intensivist's most important goal is to suspect and then support the child with an inborn error in metabolism (Table 24.8). The specifics of workup and management of the illness are best left to the experts. There are many excellent reviews of the decision trees involved in diagnosing these conditions.

25.

Poisoning and the Critically Ill Child

Alan D. Woolf, Ivor D. Berkowitz, Erica Liebelt, and Mark C. Rogers

INTRODUCTION

Accidental poisoning in children younger than 5 years of age accounts for 85 to 90% of pediatric poisonings. Poisoning in the child 5 years of age and older is generally considered intentional and comprises the remaining 10 to 15% of childhood poisonings. Alcohol and street drugs are popular with teenagers, and unintentional overdoses occasionally ensue. Suicide attempts or suicide gestures account for most hospital admissions of poisoned teenagers.

Table 25.1 lists the agents most frequently responsible for severe poisoning in children. Accidental intoxication in young children usually is caused by the ingestion of a single product. Conversely, suicidal adolescents frequently ingest multiple drugs, potentially making both the diagnosis and the management of intoxication in such patients more complicated and difficult.

CLINICAL APPROACH TO THE POISONED CHILD

Immediate Evaluation and Diagnosis

Emergency cardiorespiratory stabilization and basic life support must precede any diagnostic steps in the poisoned child who presents with the most life-threatening systemic manifestations of drug intoxication-respiratory failure with hypoxia, hypotension, arrhythmias, and seizures.

Table 25.1
Drugs Involved in Serious Childhood Poisonings^a

Drugs	Others
Acetaminophen	Alcohols (ethyl, isopropyl, methyl)
Antiarrhythmics	Ethylene glycol
Anticonvulsants	Caustics
Antihistamines	Herbicides
Antihypertensives	Organophosphates
Aminophylline	Other pesticides
Aspirin	Petroleum distillates
β-Blockers	
Calcium channel blockers	
Digoxin	
Hallucinogens	
Iron	
Opioids	
Oral hypoglycemic agents	
Theophylline	
Tricyclic antidepressants	

^aFrom Kilham HA. Hospital management of severe poisoning. Pediatr Clin North Am 1980;27:603.

Diagnosis

The diagnosis of poisoning may be obvious, such as when a young child is found holding an empty drug bottle or with a mouth full of pill fragments. In many cases, however, the diagnosis is difficult or is not considered, because an older patient purposefully falsifies the medical history or because the patient, due to insufficient age or confused mental status, is unable to provide accurate information.

The clinician should consider the possible diagnosis of poisoning when a child younger than 5 years old manifests the following:

- Acute symptoms of disturbed consciousness
- Abnormal behavior
- Seizures
- Coma
- An unusual odor
- Respiratory distress
- Shock
- Arrhythmias
- Metabolic acidosis
- Severe vomiting and diarrhea
- Cyanosis
- Unresponsiveness to oxygen (methemoglobinemia)
- Puzzling multisystem disorders

In adolescent and adult victims of accidental trauma, underlying drug and ethanol intoxication should be considered.

Laboratory tests may be necessary to rule out the presence of "silent" or coingested toxins present with no symptoms (e.g., acetaminophen). Local poison control centers can be of assistance in making a diagnosis in an unknown poisoning, developing a management strategy, and locating exotic antidotes.

History

During the stabilization period, the clinician should obtain the following information from parents, family members, friends, or paramedics who accompanied the patient to the hospital:

- Possible intoxicating agents
- Mode of intoxication
- Maximum potential dose
- Time since exposure
- Information about available drugs in the home or illnesses of the patient or other family members
- Initial clinical symptomatology before arrival at a facility

Poisoning as a form of child abuse should be considered if the history does not appear consistent with the physical and laboratory findings.

Physical Examination

In a patient with a questionable exposure to a toxic agent, specific physical findings may be elicited that can either suggest a diagnosis of poisoning by a particular agent or group of drugs (Table 25.2) or indicate that underlying disease rather than intoxication is the cause of the clinical problem.

Certain poisonings are associated with prominent clinical findings and can be grouped into "toxidromes" to aid diagnosis of intoxication in a patient with unknown ingestion (Table 25.3).

Laboratory Diagnosis

Simple, readily available clinical laboratory tests can play an important role in the diagnosis and management of a poisoned patient. Electrolytes, glucose, arterial blood gas, measured osmolality, and urinalysis can suggest the diagnosis of a specific intoxication, particularly in a comatose patient.

Toxicology screens generally detect narcotics, analgesics, barbiturates, some cyclic antidepressants, sedative-hypnotics, alcohols (except ethylene glycol), and drugs of abuse. In most laboratories, urine is the specimen of choice for initial qualitative screening, while quantitative levels of drugs, volatile alcohols, and confirmation of positive urine tests should be performed on blood samples.

Table 25.2
Clinical Manifestations of Poisonings[a]

Sign or Symptom	Poison
Odor	
Bitter almond	Cyanide
Acetone	Isopropyl alcohol, methanol, acetylsalicylic acid
Pungent aromatic	Ethchlorvynol
Oil of wintergreen	Methyl salicylate
Pear	Chloral hydrate
Garlic	Arsenic, phosphorus, thallium, organophosphates, selenium
Alcohol	Ethanol, methanol
Petroleum	Petroleum distillates
Skin	
Cyanosis (unresponsive to oxygen— methemoglobinemia)	Nitrates, nitrites, phenacetin, benzocaine
Red flush	Carbon monoxide, cyanide, boric acid, anticholinergics
Sweating	Amphetamines, LSD, organophosphates, cocaine, barbiturates
Dry	Anticholinergics
Bullae	Barbiturates, carbon monoxide
Jaundice	Acetaminophen, mushrooms, carbon tetrachloride, iron, phosphorus
Purpura	Aspirin, warfarin, snakebite
Temperature	
Hypothermia	Sedative hypnotics, ethanol, carbon monoxide, phenothiazines, tricyclic antidepressants (TCAs), clonidine
Hyperthermia	Anticholinergics, salicylates, phenothiazines, TCAs, cocaine, amphetamines, theophylline
Blood pressure	
Hypertension	Sympathomimetics (especially phenylpropanolamine in over-the-counter cold remedies), organophosphates, amphetamines, PCP
Hypotension	Narcotics, sedative hypnotics, TCAs, phenothiazines, clonidine, β-blockers, calcium channel blockers
Pulse rate	
Bradycardia	Digitalis, sedative hypnotics, β-blockers, ethchlorvynol, calcium channel blockers
Tachycardia	Anticholinergics, sympathomimetics, amphetamines, alcohol, aspirin, theophylline, cocaine, TCAs
Arrhythmias	Anticholinergics, TCAs, organophosphates, phenothiazines, digoxin, β-blockers, carbon monoxide, cyanide, theophylline
Mucous membranes	
Dry	Anticholinergics
Salivation	Organophosphates, carbamates
Oral lesions	Corrosives, paraquat
Lacrimation	Caustics, organophosphates, irritant gases
Respiration	
Depressed	Alcohol, narcotics, barbiturates, sedative/hypnotics
Tachypnea	Salicylates, amphetamines, carbon monoxide
Kussmaul	Methanol, ethylene glycol, salicylates
Wheezing	Organophosphates
Pneumonia	Hydrocarbons

continued

Table 25.2
Clinical Manifestations of Poisonings[a]

Sign or Symptom	Poison
Pulmonary edema	Aspiration, salicylates, narcotics, sympathomimetics
Central nervous system	
Seizures	TCAs, cocaine, phenothiazines, amphetamines, camphor, lead, salicylates, isoniazid, organophosphates, antihistamines, propoxyphene, strychnine
Pupils, miosis	Narcotics (except Dermerol and Lomotil), pheothiazines, organophosphates, diazepam, barbiturates, mushrooms (muscarine types)
Mydriasis	Anticholinergics, sympathomimetics, cocaine, TCAs, methanol, glutethimide, LSD
Blindness, optic atrophy	Methanol
Fasciculation	Organophosphates
Nystagmus	Diphenylhydantoin, barbiturates, carbamazepine, PCP, carbon monoxide, glutethimide, ethanol
Hypertonous	Anticholinergics, strychnine, phenothiazines
Myoclonus, rigidity	Anticholinergics, phenothiazines, haloperidol
Delirium/psychosis	Anticholinergics, sympathomimetics, alcohol, phenothiazines, PCP, LSD, marijuana, cocaine, heroin, methaqualone, heavy metals
Coma	Alcohols, anticholinergics, sedative hypnotics, narcotics, carbon monoxide, tricyclic antidepressants, salicylates, organophosphates, barbiturates
Weakness, paralysis	Organophosphates, carbamates, heavy metals
Gastrointestinal system	
Vomiting, diarrhea, abdominal pain	Iron, phosphorus, heavy metals, lithium, mushrooms, fluoride, organophosphates, arsenic

[a]From Guzzardi L, Bayer MJ. Emergency management of the poisoned patient. In: Bayer M, Rumack BH, Wanke LA, eds. Toxicologic emergencies. Bowie, MD: Robert J. Brady, 1984.

Because many drugs and toxins are not commonly included in toxicology screening, a negative screen does not always rule out poisoning. Each clinician should be familiar with his or her hospital's toxic screen. It is important to provide the toxicology laboratory with information about the suspected agents and clinical manifestations of the intoxication and to communicate when specific drug quantitation must be performed on an emergency basis so that prompt therapeutic interventions can be made.

TREATMENT

Decontamination

Surface Decontamination

After the patient has been stabilized, the clinician should prevent further intoxication. To halt skin contact with external poisons (e.g., organophosphate

Table 25.3
Toxidromes[a]

Drug Involved	Clinical Manifestations
Anticholinergics (atropine, scopolamine, tricyclic antidepressants, phenothiazines, antihistamines, mushrooms)	Agitation, hallucinations, coma, extrapyramidal movements, mydriasis, flushed, warm dry skin, dry mouth, tachycardia, arrhythmias, hypotension, hypertension, decreased bowel sounds, urinary retention
Cholinergics (organophosphates and carbamate insecticides)	Salivation, lacrimation, urination, defecation, nausea, and vomiting, sweating, miosis, bronchorrhea, rales and wheezes, weakness, paralysis, confusion and coma, muscle fasciculations.
Opiates	Slow respirations, bradycardia, hypotension, hypothermia, coma, miosis, pulmonary edema, seizures
Sedative/hypnotics	Coma, hypothermia, central nervous system depression, slow respirations, hypotension, tachycardia
Tricyclic Antidepressants	Coma, convulsions, arrhythmias, anticholinergic manifestations
Salicylates	Vomiting, hyperpnea, fever, lethargy, coma
Phenothiazines	Hypotension, tachycardia, torsion of head and neck, oculogyric crisis, trismus, ataxia, anticholinergic manifestations
Sympathomimetics (amphetamines, phenylpropanolamine, ephedrine, caffeine, cocaine, and aminophylline)	Tachycardia, arrhythmias, psychosis, hallucinations, delirium, nausea, vomiting, abdominal pain, piloerection
Alcohols, Glycols (methanol, ethylene glycol) also **Salicylates, Paraldehyde, Iron, Isoniazid, Phenformin**	Elevated anion gap metabolic acidosis

[a]From Motenson NC, Greensher J. The unknown poison. Pediatrics 1974;54:337.

insecticides, corrosive agents), the patient's contaminated clothing is removed and his or her skin washed with large quantities of water. Ocular exposure is halted by irrigating the patient's eyes with copious amounts of saline or water. Never apply any neutralizing chemical to the skin or instill it into the eye.

Dilution

Dilution as an initial step in gastrointestinal decontamination may result in enhanced gastrointestinal (GI) absorption of ingested poisons; therefore, this treatment is not recommended for noncaustic ingestions. Oral dilution of an ingested alkaline or weak acid caustic with milk or water may be beneficial in decreasing tissue damage if it is performed immediately after exposure.

Gastrointestinal Tract Decontamination

The physician who treats a child with a known or suspected toxic ingestion should develop a rational approach to GI decontamination that is individualized based on the following factors:

- Patient's age
- Substance ingested
- Time since ingestion
- Presence of coingestants

It is also important to understand each decontamination intervention and its limitations.

In deciding whether GI decontamination is needed, the physician must consider three factors:

1. Risk to the patient caused by the ingestion
2. Likelihood that gastric emptying will remove a clinically significant amount of the ingestion
3. Whether the benefits of removing the amount of agent outweigh the risks of gastric emptying

Emesis Syrup of Ipecac, in the dose of 10 mL for infants 6 months to 1 year of age, 15 mL for young children, and 30 mL for adolescents and adults, is the drug of choice for inducing emesis. It is highly effective, producing emesis in less than 30 minutes in at least 90% of children. Ipecac usually produces an average of three episodes of emesis within 30 to 60 minutes after administration. Administering water after the ipecac is of little benefit. The dose of ipecac may be repeated once if emesis does not occur within 30 minutes.

Syrup of Ipecac may be indicated for home use to begin treatment for potentially toxic ingestions. In the emergency department, it may play a role when gastric emptying is needed for substances that may not pass through a large lavage tube, such as plant or mushroom fragments, adherent masses of pills, or large pills or pill fragments, particularly enteric-coated and sustained release tablets.

Contraindications to the use of ipecac syrup include:

- Child younger than 6 months of age
- Nontoxic ingestion
- Lethargic or comatose patient
- Ingestion of caustic agents
- Seizures associated with the intoxication
- Compromised gag reflex
- Concomitant ingestion of sharp, solid substances
- Children with hemorrhagic diathesis

- Ingestion of a large quantity of drug that might rapidly produce seizures or coma, such as tricyclic antidepressants (TCAs) or propoxyphene
- When vomiting will delay administration of an oral antidote

There have been no reports of direct ipecac toxicity when it has been administered in the recommended doses. Ipecac toxicity after an overdose is characterized by:

- Nausea
- Vomiting
- Diarrhea
- Cardiac arrhythmias
- Hypotension
- Tremor
- Weakness
- Seizures

Chronic ipecac intoxication may result in dehydration, electrolyte abnormalities (especially hypokalemia), myopathy, and cardiomyopathy.

Gastric Lavage No controlled study has shown either emesis or lavage to be clearly superior in drug removal. When gastric emptying is indicated, gastric lavage is preferable to ipecac-induced emesis in the majority of potentially life-threatening poisonings.

After aspiration of gastric contents, with the patient lying on his or her left side, head slightly lower than feet, the physician uses the largest orogastric lavage tube that can be accommodated reasonably and safely passed (e.g., a 16 to 28 French tube in children, 36 to 40 Fr in adolescents). A smaller caliber nasogastric or feeding tube may be used for liquid toxins. Lavage is undertaken with water or 0.45% saline in aliquots of 150 to 200 mL for adolescents and 50 to 100 mL in young children until the return is clear, a total volume of 1 to 2 L in children and adolescents and 500 mL to 1 L in toddlers. In young children, a 0.45% or normal saline solution is preferable to prevent hyponatremia.

Gastric lavage is most effective when performed within 1 to 2 hours after the toxic ingestion. Because opioids, phenothiazines, and TCAs may delay gastric emptying time, however, substantial quantities of such drugs may be removed by gastric decontamination for a few hours after ingestion.

Gastric lavage is contraindicated with:

- Strong acid or alkali ingestion
- Ingestion of sharp materials or drug packets
- When the ingestion is deemed nontoxic

Activated Charcoal Activated charcoal can adsorb many different drugs effectively, thereby decreasing their systemic absorption from the gastrointestinal tract. Activated charcoal is best administered mixed with water as a slurry, in a dose of 10 times the estimated weight of the compound ingested because in vitro, optimal binding of several drugs is produced at a charcoal:drug ratio of 10:1. Clinically, when the dose of the ingested drug is unknown, a dose of 1 g/kg for children and 50 to 100 g for adults is recommended.

A single dose of activated charcoal should be administered after most suspected toxic ingestions. Activated charcoal is more effective than gastric emptying in preventing drug absorption and just as effective as gastric emptying and charcoal in a selected sample of poisoned patients. Substances poorly or not adsorbed by charcoal include:

- Iron
- Lithium
- Alcohols
- Mineral acids or bases
- Most solvents
- Most water-insoluble compounds, including hydrocarbons

A history of ingesting a substance unlikely to be adsorbed to activated charcoal should not preclude its use, however, because the history is many times incomplete or inaccurate, and coingestion of substances well adsorbed to charcoal is common. Because of prolonged absorption, activated charcoal should be administered 12 to 24 hours after ingestion of anticholinergic drugs, narcotics, and sustained release and enteric coated preparations.

Activated charcoal is generally safe and has few contraindications. The use of charcoal after ingestion of caustic substances is not indicated. Charcoal is also not recommended when the child has ingested pure petroleum distillates and other agents not well adsorbed to charcoal but that do carry a high risk of pulmonary aspiration. Therapeutic doses do not effectively adsorb either alkalis or mineral acids, and the fine black powder may interfere with the endoscopic examination of the esophagus and stomach.

Adverse effects of charcoal include:

- Nausea
- Vomiting
- Constipation
- Pulmonary aspiration

Aspiration of charcoal sometimes results in fatalities; therefore, it is necessary to stress the importance of adequate airway protection before its administration.

Cathartics These agents are administered to patients with orally induced intoxications to reduce drug absorption by shortening intestinal transit time.

Saline cathartics administered alone are not as effective as activated charcoal in reducing drug absorption. Studies suggest that a single dose of charcoal with a cathartic is warranted to evacuate the gastrointestinal tract as treatment for some specific ingestions.

Magnesium citrate is administered at a dose of 4 mL/kg with a maximum dose of 300 mL, magnesium sulfate at 250 mg/kg up to a total dose of 30 grams. Sorbitol is recommended for children ages 1 to 12 years and adolescents ages 13 to 19 years (0.5 g/kg of 70% concentration [10 to 20 mL in children, up to 50 to 100 mL in adolescents]). Children under 1 year of age are at risk for severe fluid shifts and electrolyte abnormalities. Because many charcoal preparations are premixed with sorbitol, they should not be routinely administered on a repetitive basis to children. Mineral oil or stimulant cathartics like castor oil are not recommended because of the risk of aspiration and enhanced toxin absorption.

Contraindications to the use of cathartics include:

- A dynamic ileus
- Diarrhea
- Abdominal trauma
- Intestinal obstruction
- Magnesium sulfate or citrate in patients with renal failure

No adverse effects have been reported when there are no contraindications to using appropriately dosed cathartics. Case reports have shown that cathartic-induced hypermagnesemia can occur in patients with normal renal function in accidental overdoses or after multiple doses of magnesium cathartics. Hypocalcemia, hyperphosphatemia, and hypokalemia have been reported after use of hypertonic phosphate enemas.

Young children are at particular risk after excessive sorbitol dosing for the following:

- Severe fluid and electrolyte abnormalities
- Intravascular volume depletion
- Hypernatremia
- Shock
- Acidosis

Whole Bowel Irrigation   Using isotonic polyethylene glycol electrolyte solutions (such as CoLyte® or Golytely®), the gastrointestinal tract is flushed, without causing fluid and electrolyte shifts, in order to reduce the bioavailability of the drug or toxin by decreasing the time available for drug absorption. Whole bowel irrigation (WBI) has been used successfully to treat poisoning involving:

- Iron
- Ampicillin
- Lithium
- Enteric coated salicylates

Whole bowel irrigation may be indicated for life-threatening ingestions of drugs poorly adsorbed to activated charcoal (e.g., lithium, iron, lead chips), drugs too massive for activated charcoal alone (sustained release theophylline, calcium channel blockers), or ingested drug packets or vials. The dose is 1 to 2 L/hour in adolescents and adults and 0.5 L/hour in children. WBI should be used for 4 to 6 hours or until the rectal effluent is clear.

Contraindications to WBI include ileus and abdominal perforation or obstruction. Adverse effects include rectal itching and vomiting, especially with rapid administration. WBI is not a substitute for activated charcoal, which should be administered before or during WBI solution if a charcoal-adsorbable drug is involved. The overall role of WBI in managing poisonings is still being evaluated.

Other Gastrointestinal Decontamination Modalities Sodium polystyrene sulfonate (i.e., Kayexalate®) is effective in preventing gastrointestinal absorption of lithium and increasing its elimination. Cholestyramine enhances the elimination of organochlorine pesticides, such as Lindane and Kepone.

Surgical intervention is indicated in the following situations:

- When heroin or cocaine drug packets create mechanical obstruction
- If packets containing large amounts of cocaine rupture, immediate surgical removal of the remaining drug may be warranted after appropriate medical stabilization because of the lack of an antidote and the potential life-threatening toxicity of cocaine
- After massive iron ingestion, surgical gastrotomy may be warranted if serious systemic toxicity persists or gastrointestinal bleeding occurs despite aggressive gastric emptying and WBI.

Antidotes

For most cases of intoxication, supportive care, not the administration of an antidote, is the backbone of effective therapy and care. Use of a pharmacologic antagonist or a chelating agent should be considered, however, when caring for a critically ill poisoned child. Unfortunately, however, only a small proportion of poisoned patients are amenable to such therapy.

Flumazenil is a specific receptor antagonist to the respiratory and neurologic depressant effects of benzodiazepines. Flumazenil also has been used successfully to reverse periodic apnea in a neonate associated with maternal benzodiazepine use during pregnancy.

HASTENING THE ELIMINATION OF POISONS

Methods that enhance the excretion of many poisons include diuresis, hemoperfusion, dialysis, urinary pH control, gastric suctioning, exchange transfusion, plasmapheresis, activated charcoal administration, and drug antibodies. Because the clinical superiority of some of these methods over conservative, supportive care alone is not always well established in children, it is important to weigh the risks and complications of the procedure against the potential benefits before implementation. Recommended techniques for accelerating the removal of drugs in some common poisonings are provided in Table 25.4.

Diuresis With or Without Alteration of Urine pH

A drug that is a weak acid or base will become ionized by gaining or donating a hydrogen ion. By altering the pH of the urine, the proportion of ionized or nonpolar drug can be enhanced, "trapping" this poorly resorbed compound in the tubular lumen, reducing reabsorption and enhancing excretion. At a physiologic blood pH (e.g., 7.40), most of the salicylate is in ionized form and unable to cross cell membranes where it could do harm. If the urine is alkalinized to a pH 7.5–8.0, most of the salicylate in the renal tubular lumen will be in ionized form and will be excreted, as opposed to being reabsorbed into the blood by renal tubular processes.

Diuresis is accomplished by the administration of intravenous fluids at one to three times maintenance requirements to establish a urine output of 2 to 5 mL/kg/hr. Bladder catheterization allows accurate measurement of urine output. Because some infants with salicylate intoxication may be considerably dehydrated, rapid rehydration may be necessary before diuresis can be accomplished. Diuretics such as mannitol and furosemide can be added to ensure high urine flow rates.

Alkalinization of the urine to pH 7.0 or greater is achieved by adding sodium bicarbonate in concentrations of 50 to 75 mEq/L to the intravenous fluids. Hypokalemia, whether preexistent or induced by the bicarbonate administration, may make the patient relatively resistant to attempts at producing urinary alkalinization. Aggressive potassium supplementation corrects this situation.

Use of acetazolamide, a carbonic anhydrase inhibitor, is no longer recommended because it has been found to enhance the penetration of salicylate into the central nervous system.

Complications of diuresis include:

- Fluid overload
- Cerebral edema
- Pulmonary edema
- Hyponatremia
- Water intoxication

Alkalemia and hypokalemia can complicate sodium bicarbonate use. Urine pH values and serum sodium, potassium, and acid-base parameters must be frequently monitored when these techniques are employed.

Table 25.4.
Common Intoxications and Poisonings

Poison	Clinical Features	Diagnostic Information	Elimination Method[a]	Therapy
Acetaminophen	Hepatic dysfunction > 7.5 g adults >140 mg/kg children > 250 mg/kg causes severe dysfunction	SGOT > 10,000 IU/L	E, L, C; Ch if other drugs ingested	N-Acetylcysteine • Given orally within 24 h or ingestion • Loading dose: 140 mg/kg • Maintenance: 70 mg/kg q 4 h for 17 doses. Repeat dose if vomiting occurs within 1 h • Intraduodenal administration in patients with persistent vomiting • Improves morbidity and mortality in patients with hepatic failure
Stage 1 (First 12–24 h)	Nausea, anorexia, vomiting. Central nervous system (CNS) symptoms suggest ingestion of additional drugs.			
Stage 2 (24–36 h)	Gastrointestinal (GI) symptoms resolve. Hepatic dysfunction.	↑Transaminases, bilirubin, partial thromboplastin time (PTT)		
Stage 3 (Day 3–4)	Hepatic dysfunction, nausea, vomiting, anorexia, symptoms of hepatitis. Less common: fulminant liver failure, renal failure, pancreatitis, myocardial injury			

continued

Table 25.4
Common Intoxications and Poisonings

Poison	Clinical Features	Diagnostic Information	Elimination Method[a]	Therapy
Stage 4 (7–8 d)	Recovery phase	Normal LFT, liver biopsy		
Alcohols				
Isopropyl alcohol (hair tonic, rubbing alcohol, aftershave lotions, perfumes, skin lotions, antifreeze)	Prolonged lethargy, dizziness, ataxia, confusion, coma, nystagmus vomiting, abdominal pain, hematemesis from gastritis. Severe: deep coma, hypotension, pulmonary edema, hypoventilation, respiratory arrest, hypothermia	Breath odor of isopropyl alcohol and acetone. Serum levels show mild acidosis, hypoglycemia	E, L, HD when blood level > 400–500 mg/dL	
Methanol (gas-line antifreeze, windshield washer fluid, model airplane fuel, paint remover) Exposure: oral, inhalation, skin ≤5 mL lethal to toddlers; 1 mL/kg lethal in adults	Initial: mild inebriation, drowsiness. 6–24 h after exposure: restlessness, headache, vertigo, CNS depression, nausea, vomiting, abdominal pain, photophobia, blurred vision. Severe: coma, convulsions, apnea	Kussmaul breathing, formaldehyde breath odor, hyperemia of optic disks, retinal edema, dilated pupils Metabolic acidosis, pH and base deficit	E, L, Ch recommended. HD when blood levels > 50 mg/dL, severe metabolic acidosis, and neurologic and visual symptoms	Ethanol PO or IV IV loading dose of 10% ethanol: 7.5 mL/kg (adults). 8.75 mL/kg (peds); 125 mg/kg/h maintenance. Blood alcohol determinations ensure therapeutic levels.

	Signs and symptoms	Laboratory/Diagnostic		Treatment
Ethylene Glycol (cosmetics, automobile radiator antifreeze)		Metabolic acidosis, ↑ anion gap, hypocalcemia, UA shows oxalate crystals	E, L; HD highly effective	Ethanol Loading dose: 0.6 g/kg IV (adult), 0.7 g/kg (peds) to achieve blood level of 100 mg/dL. Maintenance dose: 125 mg/kg/h
Stage 1 (30 min–12 h)	Slurred speech, ataxia, confusion, somnolence, nausea, and vomiting; coma and seizures when severe			
Stage 2 (12–18 h)	Pulmonary edema, tachypnea, tachycardia, cyanosis			
Stage 3 (1–3 d)	Renal failure, flank pain, hematuria, proteinura			
Anticholinergics	Agitation, hallucinations, coma, extrapyramidal movements, mydriasis, flushed and warm dry skin, dry mouth, tachycardia, arrhythmias, hypotension, hypertension, decreased bowel sounds, urinary retention	Hx and PE findings are diagnostic. Monitor electrolytes, blood glucose. ECG to measure AQ and QRS intervals	L, Ch	Physostigmine 2.0 mg (adults) 0.5 mg, IV, IM, SC (peds) repeat 5 min intervals until desired effect to max of 2 mg; not for use in TCA poisoning. Benzodiazepines or phenobarbital for seizures; lidocaine for ventricular dysrhythmias; magnesium sulfate for torsade de pointes.
Drugs: antihistamines, TCAs, phenothiazines, antiparkinsonian drugs, belladonna alkaloids (atropine, scopolamine) muscle relaxants antispasmodics				

continued

Table 25.4
Common Intoxications and Poisonings

Poison	Clinical Features	Diagnostic Information	Elimination Method[a]	Therapy
Plants: mushrooms, jimsonweed, deadly nightshade, bittersweet, Jerusalem cherry, black henbane				
Caustics (ammonia > 5%), powdered laundry detergent, drain openers, mildew removers, button batteries, cleaning solutions for commercial pipeline and steel storage tanks, rust, cement, toilet bowls, swimming pools, ovens	Nausea, vomiting, oropharyngeal placques, burns and swelling, dysphagia and throat pain, refusal to eat or drink, fever, respiratory distress, cardiovascular collapse, hypocalcemia (hydrofluoric acid), abdominal pain, subcutaneous emphysema, pneumothorax, pneumomediastinum, peritonitis	Physical evidence is diagnostic. Endoscopy within first 24 h to assess and stage damage. Radiography to track swallowed batteries	Extensive washing to dilute dermal or ocular exposures; fresh air for inhalations. Avoid ipecac, gastric lavage, and activated charcoal. Exothermic reaction resulting from neutralization exacerbates tissue destruction	NPO after ingestion of liquid caustics. Batteries in esophagus require surgical removal; those in stomach or intestines pass uneventfully.

Cocaine ("Crack") Nasal insufflation, IV ingestion of bags 1–3 g orally or 750–800 mg IV may be lethal	Seizures, vasoconstrictive hypertension, hyperthermia, ischemic cardiac complications, chest pain, CNS bleeding and infarction, end-organ failure, coma	UA reveals ecgonine metabolites up to 72–96 h after use. Commercial assays reveal concentrations < 200 µg/L. Toxic screen of blood and urine is recommended.	Ch for swallowed cocaine: WBI for bags in intestines	Monitor in ICU as long as patient has new-onset neurologic events, chest or abdominal pain, cardiovascular lability. Surgical intervention for bowel obstruction or ischemia. Hypertensive crisis: phentomaline (5–10 mg IV), nifedipine, nitroglycerin, verapamil (10 mg IV) Benzodiazepines for seizures
Cyanide Inhaled gas lethal within seconds; enteric or cutaneous exposure may take minutes to hours	Dizziness, headache, palpitations, tachypnea, hypertension, confusion, convulsions, nausea, vomiting, bradycardia, red reinal arteries and veins	Smell of bitter almonds, elevated anion gap metabolic acidosis, decrease/ equivalence of arterial-mixed venous oxygen content different, normal artery PO_2 and O_2 saturation, plasma lactate concentration > 10 mmol/L	L, Ch C; 100% O_2	Sodium nitrite Adults: 300 mg (10 mL of 3% solution is given 2.5 to 5.0 mL/min, followed by 12.5 g sodium thiosulfate IV as 50 mL of a 25% solution. May repeat with half of original dose if no clinical improvement
Hydrocarbons (turpentine, ine oil, gasoline, lamp oil, kerosene, lacquer thinner, charcoal lighter fluid, furniture polish)	Gasping, persistent coughing, gagging, choking, tachypnea, rales, ronchi, wheezing within 2 h of significant aspiration, followed by fever	ABG shows hypoxemia, hypercarbia. Check carboxyhemoglobin level after methylene chloride exposure.	L for camphor, pine oil, drug combinations. No gastric evacuation needed for highly viscous petroleum distillates (mineral oil, fuel oils, lubricants)	Supplemental O_2 and bronchodilators for wheezing associated with aspiration pneumonitis

continued

Table 25.4
Common Intoxications and Poisonings

Poison	Clinical Features	Diagnostic Information	Elimination Method[a]	Therapy
	(aspiration pneumonitis) lethargy, irritability, dizziness, confusion, excitement, stupor, coma, burning of mouth and oropharynx, nausea and vomiting, abdominal pain. Hematemesis with toluene, benzene, pine oil, and turpentine	CXR shows basilar infiltrates and fine perihilar densities as early as 20 min and as late as 24 h after aspiration	Ipecac-induced emesis is contraindicated when ingested substance causes mucous membrane irritation or when CNS toxicity results in loss of consciousness	
Iron First phase (1–6 h)	Nausea, vomiting, diarrhea, abdominal pain, progressing to severe hemorrhagic gastroenteritis, shock, encephalopathy	Serum iron levels (mg/dL) predict toxicity: < 100, unlikely; 100–500, mild to moderate; 500–1000, severe; > 1000, potentially lethal	No physiologic mechanism to enhance iron excretion. E, L, WBI	Deferoxamine 15 mg/kg/h IV until urine color is normal or iron level is < 100 mg/100 mL
Second phase (6–12 h)	GI and neurologic symptoms improve, deceptive quiescence	Serum glucose to monitor hyper- and hypoglycemia. ABG to assess severity of metabolic acidosis.		

Third phase (1–4 wks)	GI symptoms, return, shock, CNS depression, metabolic acidosis, liver dysfunction, renal failure	Test black stools for occult blood		
Fourth phase (4–6 wks)	Pyloric, gastric, and intestinal stenosis			
Opioids (opium, morphine, codeine, heroin, butorphanol, fentanyl, levorphanol, meperidine, methadone, propoxyphene, pentazocine, Lomotil, dextramethorphan)	Respiratory depression, miosis, impaired consciousness, hypotension, bradycardia, seizures (meperidine, propoxyphene), hypoxemia, cyanosis	CXR shows pulmonary edema, fluffy perihilar infiltrates. Qualitative detection of opioids or metabolites in urine confirms clinical diagnosis	L, once stable. Ch, C later.	Naloxone 0.1 mg/kg (neonates, children 1 mo to 5 y (<20 kg). Minimum dose in older children is 2.0 mg. If no response, 2.0 mg every 2–3 min to 10 mg. 10 mg used for acute methadone, propoxyphene, pentazocine, diphenoxylate, or codeine overdoses
Organophosphates (OP) and Carbamate Insecticides (CI) Absorbed through skin, GI tract, conjunctiva, respiratory tract.	OP: Salivation, lacrimation, urination, defecation, GI distress, muscle fasciculations, weakness, paralysis, areflexia, hypertension, tachycardia, pupillary dilation, pallor, restlessness, emotional lability, headache, tremor,	OP: RBC acetylcholinesterase and plasma pseudoacetylcholinesterase levels are diagnostic.	Wash, Ch	Atropine 2–5 mg IV (adults), 0.05 mg/kg IV (peds); repeat every 10–30 min to achieve drying of oral and bronchial secretions. Pralidoxime 20–40 mg/kg to 1 g IV over 30 min in adults. Repeat dose after 1 h if weakness persists.

continued

Table 25.4
Common Intoxications and Poisonings

Poison	Clinical Features	Diagnostic Information	Elimination Method[a]	Therapy
	drowsiness, confusion, slurred speech, ataxia, delirium, psychosis, coma, seizures, cardiorespiratory depression.			
	CI: tachycardia and hypertension followed by bradycardia			
Phencyclidine (PCP) Smoking, snorting, oral, IV	Mild to severe systolic and diastolic hypertension, nystagmus, midsize or miotic pupils, hyperactive reflexes, muscle rigidity, catalepsy, opisthotonus, dystonic reactions, facial grimacing, myoclonus, athetosis, ataxia, moderate hyperthermia, coma	Distinguish PCP from other psychedelic drug intoxications by nystagmus, ataxia, blank stare, sensory anesthesia, hypertension, absence of mydriasis.		General supportive care. Continuous monitoring, sedation when combative.
Salicylates Aspirin in antihistamines,	Tinnitus, fever, sweating, tachycardia, hyperventilation,	Plasma salicylate concentration is diagnostic. Levels	E, L, Ch, C HP, HD for severe	Sodium bicarbonate 1–2 mEq/kg IV bolus, followed by 88–100 mEq NaHCO3 in 1 L of D5 0.25% NaCl to run at 1.5 to 2

sympathomimetics, anticholinergics, narcotics, acetaminophen, over-the-counter sleep aids, sunscreens	nausea and vomiting, dehydration, restlessness, agitation, delirium, lethargy, coma, seizures	(mg/kg) predict toxicity: < 150, no toxicity; 150–300, mild to moderate; 300–500, severe; > 500, potentially lethal. Other findings: respiratory and/or metabolic acidosis; transient respiratory alkalosis; hyperglycemia, glycosuria, hypokalemia, hypernatremia, hypocalcemia.	intoxication. HD indicated with salicylate level > 100 mg/dL, renal failure, noncardiogenic pulmonary edema, persistent CNS symptoms, CHF, severe acid-base imbalances, progressive deterioration of vital signs.	times maintenance fluid rate until urine flow is good. Goal is urine pH between 7 and 8.
Theophylline	Nausea, vomiting, hematemesis (less frequent), tremor, anxiety, sinus tachycardia, widened pulse pressure	Seizures, hypotension, and ventricular dysrhythmias are predicted by theophylline level > 80–100 µg/mL. Other findings: hypokalemia, hypophosphatemia, hyperglycemia, leukocytosis, metabolic acidosis	E, L, C or WBI Clearance is longer in neonates and in patients with liver dysfunction, CHF, acute viral illnesses with high fever, coadministration with drugs such as erythromycin and cimetidine Clearance is enhanced with cigarette and marijuana smoking, phenobarbital, diphenylhydantoin.	Charcoal HP is preferred. Charcoal dose: 0.5–1.0 g/kg every 2 h until theophylline level drops two levels, then every 4 h until level is < 20 µg/mL Benzodiazepines for seizures, followed by barbiturates

continued

Table 25.4
Common Intoxications and Poisonings

Poison	Clinical Features	Diagnostic Information	Elimination Method[a]	Therapy
Tricyclic Antidepressants (TCA)	Coma, convulsions, arrhythmias, dry mucous membranes, dry and flushed skin, mydriasis, blurred vision, tachycardia, orthostatic hypertension, decreased GI motility, urinary retention, confusion, agitation, lethargy, delirium, seizures (within 2 h of ingestion), respiratory depression	Glucose, electrolytes, arterial blood gas (assess metabolic acidosis), UA; 12-lead ECG recommended for all patients	L, C, Ch	Sodium bicarbonate; Initial bolus: 1–2 mEq/kg, followed by continuous infusion with 100–150 mEq in 1 L of 5% dextrose in water titrated over 4–6 h to achieve blood pH of 7.45–7.55. Endpoint: normal ECG and clinical improvement; Other options: lidocaine; norepinephrine; cardiopulmonary bypass in severe poisoning; Continuous cardiac monitoring for 12–24 h after ingestion

[a] E, Ipecac-induced emesis; L, gastric lavage; C, cathartics; Ch, charcoal; WBI, whole bowel irrigation; HD, hemodialysis; HP, hemoperfusion.

Hemodialysis

Hemodialysis describes the movement of solutes through a semipermeable membrane along a concentration gradient. Drugs that are dialyzed effectively have a molecular structure and physical characteristics that enable rapid diffusion across the dialysis membranes.

Methanol is an ideal candidate for removal by dialysis. It is a small molecular weight (i.e., 32 daltons), poorly protein-bound, highly water soluble compound that has a low V_D of 0.6 L/kg. In addition, it is metabolized to toxic metabolites that are themselves dialyzable. In comparison, TCAs are poorly removed by dialysis. They are lipid soluble and greater than 90% protein-bound, with a large V_D of 20 l/kg.

Hemoperfusion

In this process, compounds are cleared from the blood as it comes into direct contact with an adsorbent material contained in a cartridge in an extracorporeal circuit. Charcoal can adsorb both polar and nonpolar compounds and is the adsorbent of choice for polar compounds, such as salicylates. Amberlite XAD-4 is superior to other hemoperfusion adsorbents for removing such lipid-soluble drugs as barbiturates, glutethimide, methaqualone, ethchlorvynol, meprobamate, TCAs, theophylline, and digoxin (see Table 25.4). In fact, extraction of many of these drugs from the perfusing blood is almost complete, and the clearance often equals the blood flow rate through the coil.

The gradual reduction in drug clearance during charcoal hemoperfusion necessitates changing the charcoal cartridge every 2 to 4 hours. Reduction of clearance is slower with Amberlite XAD-4 cartridges, which usually do not require changing during the course of hemoperfusion.

The volume of distribution (V_D) remains important in determining the clinical usefulness of hemoperfusion. It does not affect the clearance or extraction ratio. The rate-limiting factors in hemoperfusion are:

- Affinity of the adsorbent for the drug
- Rate of flow through the cartridge
- Rate of equilibration of the drug from peripheral tissues to blood

A double-lumen catheter placed in the subclavian or femoral vein establishes the extracorporeal circuit. Such a technique is suitable for children as small as 10 kg. The umbilical artery and vein can be used for vascular access in the newborn. For children beyond the newborn period but weighing less than 10 kg, two separate venous sites must be cannulated because the double-lumen catheters are generally too large to be placed in these infants.

The adsorptive column is flushed with saline before use to remove accumulated particles, and the circuit is primed with saline or heparinized whole blood. The amount of blood removed from the patient into the extra-corporeal circuit should not exceed 10% of the blood volume to prevent cardiovascular instability and hypotension. Clotting within the circuit is prevented with heparin. The blood is pumped in an antigravity direction at high flow rates-between 2 and 10 mL/kg—to take advantage of the extraction efficiency of the columns.

Complications during hemoperfusion include:

- Hypotension
- Thrombocytopenia
- Hypocalcemia
- Hypoglycemia
- Hypothermia

Platelet counts usually return to normal after 24 to 48 hours, and bleeding complications are uncommon. Placement of a hemodialyzer in series with the hemoperfusion circuit may minimize hypothermia and electrolyte disturbances when performing hemoperfusion in small infants. Blood glucose and calcium concentrations should be monitored during the perfusion.

Activated Charcoal "Gastrointestinal Dialysis"

Orally administered activated charcoal increases the nonrenal clearance of drugs such as phenobarbital, aminophylline, carbamazepine, salicylate, and digitoxin, even if they have been administered parenterally (see Table 25.4). This technique allows enhanced diffusion of drug from the systemic circulation across the gut mucosa into the lumen.

Activated charcoal (1 g/kg in a child, or 50 to 100 g in an adult) should be orally administered every 2 to 4 hours. Some concerns raised include the possibility of aspiration in obtunded patients unless intubated or that charcoal prepared in osmotic cathartics may produce dramatic fluid shifts in young children when given in multiple doses or in excess.

Plasmapheresis

Plasma removal by continuous centrifugation, used in drug intoxications to facilitate removal of highly protein-bound drugs (e.g., theophylline, digoxin-antibody fragment complex), has largely been replaced, when indicated, by hemoperfusion.

Exchange Transfusion

Exchange transfusion has been used as therapy in drug intoxications, especially in small infants and particularly when intoxication is complicated by intravascular hemolysis and methemoglobinemia. In addition to removing the intoxicating drug, fragmented and methemoglobin-containing cells are replaced by intact erythrocytes. In general, drug clearances are disappointing with this technique.

Immunotherapy

Antibody therapy, in which antibodies bind to drugs, reverse their toxicity, and enhance their elimination, has been used with dramatic results in children with severe digoxin intoxication unresponsive to conventional therapy.

SPECIFIC INTOXICATIONS

Table 25.4 outlines the clinical features and management strategies for specific poisons and toxic agents that are common in children.

26

Hematologic Disorders in the Pediatric Intensive Care Unit

John B. Gordon, Mark L. Bernstein, and Mark C. Rogers

The hematologic issues of most concern in the pediatric intensive care unit (PICU) are often secondary to other disease processes such as cancer, trauma, and infection. The emphasis of this chapter, however, is on specific hematologic topics not discussed elsewhere in the book.

SICKLE CELL DISEASE

Sickle cell disease (SCD) refers to those hemoglobinopathies characterized by the formation of sickled red cells in response to deoxygenation. Sickle cell anemia is the most common cause of SCD.

Inheritance Pattern

This autosomal recessive disorder is caused by the substitution of valine for glutamine at the sixth amino acid position of the β-chain of hemoglobin. The heterozygous state, hemoglobin AS (i.e., sickle cell trait), occurs in approximately 8% of American blacks, while homozygosity occurs in 0.4%. Caucasians, particularly those of Mediterranean origin, occasionally are affected. The other common causes of the SCD phenotype are hemoglobin SC and hemoglobin Sβthal.

Clinical Presentation

The most frequent clinical manifestations of SCD are:

- Vaso-occlusive events involving any vascular bed
- Splenic sequestration

- Acute aplasia
- Splenic dysfunction

These may lead to life-threatening complications requiring admission to the PICU, such as stroke and acute chest syndrome, acute anemia, and sepsis. Death from SCD occurs most often in children who are younger than 5 years of age, because of either splenic sequestration or septicemia.

A "vicious cycle" is established in which flow slows (perhaps because of hypotension or increased adherence of red cells with narrowing of the vascular lumen), causing local hypoxemia and acidosis with consequent sickling of red cells (Table 26.1). Viscosity then increases, giving rise to even slower flow with eventual sludging in the capillary bed (Fig. 26.1). There is currently no therapy that can effectively and safely inhibit gelation and subsequent sickling of red blood cells; therefore, current management of the sickle cell patient focuses on minimizing the complications of SCD.

Vaso-occlusive Crisis

Precipitating Factors

The acute vaso-occlusive crisis can be defined functionally as an ischemic insult resulting from vascular occlusion due to sickled cells. Various conditions have been associated with vaso-occlusive crises (Table 26.2). Unfortunately, no obvious precipitant can be identified in some vaso-occlusive crises; nonetheless, the first step in managing the child with SCD involves prevention of those precipitating events if possible.

Perioperative Prevention

Preventive measures include:

- Cancel elective surgery in the presence of signs and symptoms of infection
- Maintain good hydration at all times

Table 26.1
Factors that May Promote Sickling

1. Pressure related
   a. Hypotension
   b. Pulmonary hypertension
2. Resistance related
   a. Vasoconstriction
   b. Increased hemotocrit (>35%)
3. Desaturation related
   a. Hypoxemia
   b. Acidosis

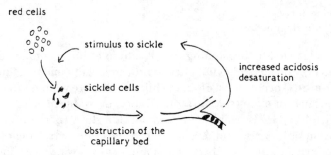

Figure 26.1. The "Vicious Cycle" of Progressive Sickling Causing Intravascular Occlusion.

Table 26.2
Clinical Precipitants of a Vaso-occlusive Crisis

1. Pressure related
   a. Hypotension
      i. Dehydration
      ii. Shock
      iii. Anesthetics
      iv. Other drugs
      v. Tourniquets
   b. Increased central venous pressure
      i. Pericardial disease
      ii. Heart failure
2. Resistance related
   a. Vasoconstriction
      i. Shock
      ii. Cold
   b. Increased viscosity (increased hematocrit)
      i. Dehydration
      ii. Transfusion (excessive)
3. Miscellaneous
   a. Infection
      i. Viral
      ii. Bacterial
   b. Overexertion
   c. Hypoxia
      i. Pneumonia
      ii. Altitude

- Prevent hypoxia both intraoperatively and postoperatively (O_2 by mask and vigorous postoperative encouragement to cough and deep breathe; perform incentive spirometry)
- Avoid other precipitating factors (e.g., hypothermia; prolonged use of tourniquets)

Preoperative Transfusion

It has become routine to reduce the risk of vaso-occlusive crisis through preoperative blood transfusions. For elective surgery, repeated simple transfusion in the clinic every 3 weeks may be used to keep the hematocrit at approximately 35% and the reticulocytes below 1%, thus inhibiting endogenous sickle erythrocyte production. Because of the shortened survival of the patient's own sickle cells, their number will gradually decrease, and that of the transfused cells, increase. After 3 to 4 months, the percentage of Hb S will be less than 20 to 30%, so that surgery may be safely undertaken. Weekly small-volume partial exchange transfusions (5 to 10 mL/kg) can lower the percentage of Hb S to less than 30% in approximately 6 weeks. In more urgent cases, large-volume partial exchange transfusion using simultaneous withdrawal and infusion of red blood cells may be employed.

Indications Various prophylactic and therapeutic indications for transfusion therapy include:

- Prophylactic
- Preoperative
    Poststroke
    Pregnancy
- Therapeutic
    Acute chest syndrome
    Stroke
    Spinal cord infarct
    Persistent priapism
    "Uncontrollable (nonresolving) crisis"
    Multiple trauma

In all circumstances, it is necessary to screen the donor blood for sickle hemoglobin. Furthermore, the risks of blood transfusion must be weighed against the benefits in every situation.

- Benefits of transfusion are an increase in the hematocrit and a decrease in the Hb S concentration, providing better oxygen delivery, and reducing the risk of vaso-occlusion.
- Risks of transfusion include infection, alloimmunization, transfusion reaction, hemochromatosis, and, rarely, death.

Partial Exchange Transfusion

In the setting of critical illness, partial exchange transfusion is superior to simple red cell transfusion, because it accomplishes the dual objectives of diminishing the risk of sickling and increasing the oxygen-carrying capacity without volume overload. In performing partial exchange transfusion, the percentage of sickle hemoglobin is reduced to less than 30%, thus diminishing the risks of vaso-occlusion and ongoing local ischemia. While a post-transfusion hematocrit of 35% will inhibit erythropoiesis, care must also be taken not to increase the total hematocrit above 35 to 40% in an effort to avoid the complications of relative hyperviscosity in this population. Two tables based on a mathematical model of blood volume and the efficiency of partial exchange transfusion are shown in Tables 26.3 and 26.4.

An alternative approach follows:

1. Preparation
   a. Decision to transfuse
   b. Insertion of venous and arterial catheters (or two large-bore venous catheters, if possible)
   c. Blood sent to laboratory for:
      Complete blood count
      Quantitative sickle cell preparation (this appears to correlate well with the quantity of Hb SS noted on electrophoresis)
      Electrolytes and calcium determination
   Cross-match with PRBC (sickle negative)

Table 26.3
Means for Calculating Volume of Transfusion with a Target Hemotocrit of 36%[a,b]

If Initial Hematocrit = 10%	Multiply Pounds by 19.2	or Kilograms by 42.2
11%	18.6%	40.9
12%	18.0	39.6
13%	17.4	38.3
14%	16.8	36.9
15%	16.2	35.6
16%	15.5	34.2
17%	14.9	32.8
18%	14.2	31.3
19%	13.6	29.9
20%	12.9	28.4
21%	12.2	26.9
22%	11.5	25.3
23%	10.8	23.8
24%	10.1	22.2
25%	9.3	20.5
26%	8.6	18.9
27%	7.8	17.2
28%	7.0	15.4
29%	6.2	13.6
30%	5.4	11.8

[a]This table assumes that the blood given has a hematocrit of 75% and that the patient's blood volume is 82.6 mL/kg.

[b]From Nagey DA, et al. Isovolumetric partial exchange transfusion in the management of sickle cell disease in pregnancy. Am J Obstet Gynecol 1983;147:693. With permission.

Table 26.4
Means for Calculating Volume of Transfusion[a,b]

Initial Hematocrit (%)	Initial % A (%)					
	0	5	10	20	30	40
10	22.4	21.0	19.5	15.6	13.5	10.3
11	24.3	22.8	21.3	18.1	14.8	11.3
12	26.2	24.6	22.9	19.5	16.0	12.3
13	28.1	26.3	24.6	21.0	17.2	13.2
14	29.9	28.1	26.2	22.4	18.4	14.1
15	31.6	29.7	27.8	23.8	19.5	15.1
16	33.4	31.4	29.4	25.1	20.7	16.0
17	35.1	33.0	30.0	26.5	21.8	16.9
18	36.7	34.6	32.4	27.8	22.9	17.8
19	38.4	36.1	33.9	29.1	24.0	18.7
20	40.0	37.7	35.3	30.4	25.1	19.5
21	41.5	39.2	36.7	31.6	26.2	20.4
22	43.1	40.6	38.1	32.9	27.3	21.2
23	44.6	42.1	39.5	34.1	28.3	22.1
24	46.1	43.5	40.9	35.3	29.4	22.9
25	47.5	44.9	42.2	36.5	30.4	23.8
26	49.0	46.3	43.5	37.7	31.4	24.6
27	50.4	47.6	44.8	38.8	32.4	25.4
28	51.8	49.0	46.1	40.0	33.4	26.2
29	53.1	50.3	47.3	41.1	34.3	27.0
30	54.5	41.6	48.6	42.2	35.3	27.8

[a]This table assumes that the transfused blood is free of sickle hemoglobin and has a hematocrit of 75%. It also assumes that the patient's blood volume is 82.6 mL/kg. The target volume is 70% A hemoglobin. Multiply the table entry by the patient's weight in kilograms.

[b]From Nagey DA, et al. Isovolumetric partial exchange transfusion in the management of sickle cell disease in pregnancy. Am J Obstet Gynecol 1983;147:693. With permission.

2. Procedure
   a. Volume of packed cells: 2 × (patient's hematocrit ÷ hematocrit of transfused unit) × 70 mL/kg × wt (kg))
   b. Rate

   Adjust intravenous line so transfusion occurs over 4 to 6 hours (obviously more difficult if more than 1000 mL is to be exchanged)

   Withdraw blood at 10- to 15-minute intervals from arterial line or large-bore venous catheter

   Balance maintained within 5% of blood volume (blood volume, 80 mL/kg)
   c. Monitoring

   Heart rate and blood pressure (continuously)

   Hematocrit (every 2 hours and at last hour)

   Electrolytes, calcium (at last hour)

d. Endpoint
    Hematocrit 33 to 37% (add FFP to remainder of PRBC if hematocrit is
    > 35%)
    %Hb S is <40% (initial screening by quantitative sickle cell preparation, fol-
    lowed by chromatography or electrophoresis)

Clinical Presentation

Manifestations of vaso-occlusive crisis include the general complaints
of fever, malaise, anorexia, and the specific complaints of pain or other
symptoms and signs related to the organ involved. Common sites of vaso-
occlusive crisis include:

- Bone
- Marrow
- Cortex (long bones)
- Dactylitis (hands and feet)
- Abdomen
- Chest
- Brain
    Myocardial infarction
    Hemorrhage
- Miscellaneous
    Penis (priapism)
    Spinal cord
    Orbit (apex syndrome)

Management Approach

The aim of therapy is to remove the precipitating cause, treat complications
of the crisis, and prevent further vaso-occlusion.
    A general approach to managing a vaso-occlusive crisis follows:

1. Diagnosis
    a. History (is it a typical crisis?)
    b. Physical examination
    c. Laboratory tests
        Complete blood count
        Quantitative sickle cell preparation
        Ancillary tests
2. Treatment
    a. Oxygen, if hypoxemic
    b. Hydration (D5–0.45% saline with KCl at 1.5 × maintenance)
    c. Antibiotics
    d. Pain control (morphine or fentanyl infusion or regional anesthesia)

Acute Chest Syndrome

Clinical Presentation

Acute chest syndrome (ACS) is characterized by fever, pleuritic chest pain, tachypnea, cough, hypoxemia, and an infiltrate on chest radiographs.

Etiology

The etiology of the syndrome is most often not identified. There are reports of bone marrow emboli, in situ thromboses, and asthma. In perhaps 25% of cases, bacterial pneumonia, often *Streptococcus pneumoniae*, is identified. One report cites 13% of patients with ACS had *Chlamydia pneumoniae* infection. A ventilation-perfusion scan may be helpful in distinguishing recent infarction from infectious etiologies.

Therapy

Therapy of the ACS follows the general principles outlined previously.

Pain Relief

Pain relief is essential to allow effective cough and pulmonary toilet. We favor continuous infusion of fentanyl (1–2 μg/kg/hour), but in the future, patient-controlled analgesia devices may supplant the fixed-rate infusions. Epidural anesthesia relieves pain and reduces splinting, allowing better breathing and coughing. It will cause a sympathectomy, which may improve regional blood flow. In any case, a properly placed (thoracic) epidural catheter with low-dose bupivacaine (1/8–1/4%) may obviate the need for exchange transfusions in ACS.

Antibiotic Therapy

We initiate antibiotic therapy (i.e., cefuroxime and erythromycin) in any febrile child under 10 years of age diagnosed with ACS, whether an organism has been identified or not. Any child who is at risk for unusual organisms (e.g., airway intubation or long hospital stay) is treated with antistaphylococcal and antipseudomonas agents (e.g., nafcillin and ceftazidime with or without an aminoglycoside such as tobramycin).

Supplemental Oxygen

Supplemental oxygen may benefit hypoxemic patients. Although supplemental oxygen will not enhance arterial oxygenation in the face of severe ventilation-perfusion mismatch, we routinely administer O_2 via mask or nasal prongs in an effort to maintain arterial PO_2 above 90 mm Hg and hemoglobin saturation above 98%. In the child with severe ACS and adult respiratory distress syndrome (ARDS), intubation is often required in addition to the exchange transfusion. Further issues in the treatment of ARDS are discussed in Chapter 4.

Exchange Transfusion

The decision to perform a partial exchange transfusion depends on the child's condition. Partial exchange transfusion of children with relatively mild signs and symptoms of ACS is recommended by many hematologists with a view to minimizing the progression of the disorder. This approach may obviate the need for intubation, because the ACS often resolves promptly after transfusion. If hypoxemia is severe (e.g., PaO_2 under 100 mm Hg with an FIO_2 of 0.6), exchange transfusion is needed. Similarly, if the patient presents with severe, advanced ACS with widespread infarction and a radiographic picture indistinguishable from ARDS, an urgent exchange transfusion is required.

Other Complications of Sickle Cell Disease

Stroke

The etiology and pathogenesis of thrombotic stroke in children with SCD are not known. Angiographic evidence suggests that vascular obstruction usually occurs in large vessels, such as the carotids or major cerebral arteries; however, there may also be a smaller subset of patients with small vessel disease. Regardless of the etiology of the lesion, progressive large-vessel occlusion eventually results in an infarct.

Diagnosis The diagnosis of stroke is made on the basis of the usual clinical signs. On admission of a child with neurologic signs suggesting stroke, computed tomography (CT) or magnetic resonance imaging (MRI) must be performed to rule out treatable lesions, such as subdural bleeding, if the child's history suggests this possibility. If there are no signs of increased intracranial pressure, a lumbar puncture should be performed to exclude the unlikely, but possible, coexistence of an infectious process.

Management and Therapy The most important intervention in the child presenting with stroke is an immediate partial exchange transfusion aimed at preventing progression of the stroke. Beyond that, therapy for the child with stroke is supportive. If a large infarct has occurred, it is necessary to observe the child for possible intracranial hypertension. Anticoagulant therapy is contraindicated. Prompt institution of physical therapy will aid in long-term management.

The natural history of untreated stroke in SCD is one of recurrent infarcts and progressive arterial occlusion that can be seen on angiograms. Chronic transfusion therapy aimed at maintaining the hematocrit above 35% and the Hb S below 30%, thus avoiding sickling episodes, is effective in preventing evolution of the vascular lesions seen on an angiogram and in preventing subsequent strokes.

Bony Crises

Bony crises may involve marrow (i.e., long bones, vertebrae) or the cortex itself. In children younger than 2 years of age, the small bones of the hands and feet are most frequently involved, giving rise to the hand-foot syndrome or dactylitis.

Clinical Manifestations Pain, fever, and leukocytosis are common. Rarely, marrow involvement will cause aplasia or embolism. Usually, however, pain is the principal problem and resolves with general supportive care. In the case of cortical involvement, pain, redness, and swelling are seen over the affected area.

Bony Crisis versus Osteomyelitis Differentiating the two conditions requires diagnostic procedures, including culture of the blood and the lesion. Examination of the fluid obtained from a needle aspirate of the affected area may reveal the causative organism. A combination of bone and marrow scanning may be helpful in distinguishing between osteomyelitis and a bony infarct. Despite the relative rarity of infection compared with a bony vaso-occlusive crisis, if redness and swelling are present, particularly over only one bone, initial therapy should include antibiotics effective against the typical organisms: Salmonella and *Staphylococcus aureus*. When culture results are available, the antibiotics can be appropriately adjusted.

Abdominal Crises

Abdominal crises arise from occlusion of mesenteric vessels or the vessels of some of the viscera (e.g., spleen, kidney). The autosplenectomy noted by age 5 years in children with sickle cell anemia presumably results from repeated infarcts.

Clinical Manifestations Abdominal crises are characterized by pain, fever, malaise, anorexia, and occasionally, nausea. Bowel sounds are absent or sparse and abdominal tenderness is common.

Differential Diagnosis The major differential diagnosis in severe abdominal crises is between vaso-occlusive crisis and a surgical condition. A good history and physical examination may obviate the need for laparotomy. If the pain is typical of previous crises, it is likely again a crisis; if not, other causes must be excluded.

Cholecystitis is probably the most common differential diagnosis. The excessive hemolysis associated with SCD results in gallstones, which can be identified on plain film radiographs or by sonogram.

Therapy Therapy of the abdominal crisis follows the general principles noted previously, with emphasis on adequate hydration as well as pain control to prevent the pulmonary atelectasis that often occurs from splinting of the abdomen. If an attack does not resolve after 3 to 6 days, a surgical condition must be suspected and more vigorously sought.

Aplasia and Sequestration Crises

In addition to the chronic moderate anemia of SCD, acute drops in hemoglobin level may result from either aplasia or, in younger children, sequestration crises. The cause of an aplastic crisis is rarely known with certainty, but it is often ascribed to minor infectious episodes, particularly with parvovirus. Resolution is usually spontaneous; however, transfusion may be needed during the acute phase.

A more dramatic and potentially fatal form of severe anemia is acute sequestration crisis (ASC), an acute drop in hemoglobin (more that 2 g/dL) associated with splenomegaly, reticulocytosis, and signs of intravascular volume depletion. Acute shock associated with a decrease in hemoglobin of more than 4 g/dL is fatal in 35% of cases. A relatively minor episode of ASC (i.e., hemoglobin level drops only 2 to 4 g/dL) must be carefully noted, because 20 to 50% of children will have a recurrence.

Presentation and Management Crises related to ASC occur in children between 10 and 27 months old and virtually never after 5 years of age, unless they have Hb SC or Hb Sβthal. The child with an ASC appears pale, is irritable, and may be in shock. Therapy consists principally of restoring circulating blood volume. Initially, lactated Ringer's solution or normal saline may be used to reverse shock; however, prompt blood transfusion is essential.

The risk of recurrence is significant, so health care services are limited, or close follow-up care of the child is impossible, splenectomy is recommended after one episode of ASC. If good health care is available and the parents can be taught how to monitor spleen size and observe the child for symptoms of sequestration, then observation, rather than splenectomy, may be appropriate. In view of the infectious risks to the young child after splenectomy—even one with impaired splenic function, as is the case in sickle cell anemia—avoiding splenectomy seems the best approach if prompt attention to crises can be provided. Transfusion therapy aids in preserving splenic function but does not appear to decrease the recurrence rate of sequestration crises.

Infection

Children with SCD are immunocompromised, principally because of decreased splenic function. The typical infections seen in children with splenic dysfunction are caused by:

- *S. pneumoniae*
- *Haemophilus influenzae*

- Neisseria meningitides
- Salmonella
- Mycoplasma

Children with SCD are particularly at risk for septic shock induced by *S. pneumoniae.*

We advocate that any child with SCD and a temperature over 38.5°C be treated with antibiotics, whether the child looks "well" or not. Any child who looks "septic" should be treated regardless of temperature.

HEMORRHAGE

History and Physical Examination

The first step in identifying the cause of bleeding is to obtain a good history and physical examination (Table 26.5).

Patient history guides the physician to an initial appreciation of whether the bleeding is isolated or part of a larger illness. It also determines the chronicity of the situation. Similarly, the physical examination should explore these two issues. Determining the clinical severity of the hemorrhage

Table 26.5
Information to Obtain During History and Physical Examination of Hemorrhage Patients

Etiologic classification of hemorrhage
1. Vessel related
   a. Trauma
   b. Surgery
   c. Vasculitis
2. Platelet related
   a. Thrombocytopenia
   b. Thrombocytopathy
3. Plasma phase related
   a. Congenital factor deficiency
   b. Liver disease
   c. Disseminated intravascular coagulation
Physical examination in assessing for shock
1. Cardiovascular
   a. Pulse
   b. Blood pressure
   c. Capillary refill
   d. Peripheral temperature
2. Respiratory
   a. Rate
   b. Effort
3. Renal: urine output
4. Cerebral: mental status

(e.g., if shock is present or imminent) requires assessment of cardiovascular, respiratory, renal, and cerebral function.

Diagnosis

After the presence of shock has been established and appropriate initial therapy has been instituted (Table 26.6), a more extensive physical examination can be performed, searching for clues to the cause of hemorrhage. In particular, purpura and petechiae may suggest platelet dysfunction or the loss of vascular integrity, whereas purpura and oozing from venous puncture sites may point to a defect in the plasma phase of coagulation.

The history and physical examination will thus suggest the likely cause (or at least the etiologic category) and will aid in identifying the severity of the hemorrhage. A few laboratory tests usually suffice to narrow the differential diagnosis to one or two possibilities (Table 26.7). When the category of illness is identified, therapy can often be initiated.

Transfusion Therapy

Therapy for the bleeding child has three phases: initial resuscitation if in shock, restoration of hematocrit to normal (or acceptable) levels, and correction (if possible) of the underlying disorder. Restoring the hematocrit requires transfusion therapy. Most blood banks now fractionate their units into PRBC, FFP, platelet concentrates, and cryoprecipitate. The various blood products and their uses are shown in Table 26.8.

Risks versus Benefits

Under usual circumstances, the specific replacement blood product is administered. However, the benefits of an increased hemoglobin level with its

Table 26.6
Initial Therapy of the Child with Significant Hemorrhage

Without shock
    Oxygen by mask
    Large-bore peripheral intravenous catheters
    Lactated Ringer's solution at twice maintenance levels
    Type and cross-match
    Draw samples for diagnostic tests
With shock
    Oxygen mask or endotracheal tube
    Large-bore peripheral intravenous catheters and/or central line
    Lactated Ringer's solution, 20 mL/kg infused over 5 min and repeated as needed
    Draw samples for diagnostic tests
    Insert urinary catheter

Table 26.7
Routine Hemostatic Tests[a]

Hemostasis	Normal Value	Normal Mechanism Measured	Abnormal Disease State
Platelet count	150,000 × 10⁶/L	Platelet production vs. destruction	Thrombocytopenia (radiation, chemotherapy, idiopathic thrombocytopenic purpura, DIC)
Template bleeding time	<9 min	Vascular integrity	Collagen vascular disease (vasculitides, endotoxemia, amyloidosis)
Prothrombin time	27–37 sec	Contact activation pathway	Factor deficiency (XII, XI, IX, VIII, X, V, II, fibrinogen); factor inhibitor (e.g., factor VIII inhibitor); heparin; coumadin (variably)
Partial thromboplastin time	10–13 sec	Tissue thromboplastin pathway	Factor deficiency (VII, X, V, II, fibrinogen); factor inhibitor (e.g., factor VII inhibitor); coumadin
Thrombin time	<4 sec more than control	Antithrombins, fibrinogen level and structure	Heparin; paraproteins; fibrin split products; hypofibrinogenemia (DIC, primary fibrinogenolysis); dysfibrinogenemia
Fibrinogen level	>180 mg/dL	Fibrinogen level and structure	Hypofibrinogenemia (DIC, primary fibrinogenolysis); dysfibrinogenemia (hepatoma)
Ethanol gelation test	Negative	Fibrin monomer production	Intravascular coagulation event
Fibrin degradation products	Absent	Fibrin/fibrinogenolysis	DIC, intravascular thrombosis; primary fibrinogenolysis

[a]From Kempin S, Gould-Rossbach P, Howland WS: Disorders of hemostatis in the critically ill cancer patient. In: Howland WS, Carlon GC, eds. Critical care of the cancer patient. Chicago: Year Book Medical Publishers, 1985:215

DIC, disseminated intravascular coagulation.

improved oxygen-carrying capacity or improved coagulation because of increased clotting factors or platelet count must be weighed against the risks of transfusing blood products. The dangers include:

- Microaggregates
- Anaphylaxis

Table 26.8
Summary of Blood Components

Components:	Red blood cells
Major indications:	Symptomatic anemia: decreased red cell mass
Action:	Restoration of blood volume, restoration of oxygen-carrying capacity
Not indicated for:	Pharmacologically treatable anemia; coagulation deficiency
Special precaution:	Must be ABO-compatible
Hazards:	Hepatitis, allergic reactions, febrile reactions, HIV
Rate of infusion:	Within 2 h; for massive loss, fast as patient can tolerate
Components:	Red blood cells, leukocytes removed
Major indications:	Febril reactions from leukocyte antibodies in patients who require red blood cells
Action:	(See under "Red blood cells" above)
Not indicated for:	Pharmacologically treatable anemia; coagulation deficiency
Special precautions:	Must be ABO-compatible
Hazards:	Hepatitis, HIV
Rate of infusion:	(See under "Red blood cells" above)
Components:	Red blood cells, washed deglycerolized
Major indications:	As above, also IgA sensitization
Action:	(See under "Red blood cells" above)
Not indicated for:	Pharmacologically treatable anemia; coagulation deficiency
Special precautions:	Must be ABO-compatible
Hazards:	Hepatitis, HIV
Rate of infusion:	(See under "Red blood cells" above)
Components:	Whole blood
Major indications:	Hypoxia with volume deficit; massive transfusion
Action:	Restoration of blood volume and oxygen-carrying capacity
Not indicated for:	Condition responsive to specific component
Special precautions:	Must be ABO-identical; labile coagulation factors deteriorate 24 h after collection
Hazards:	Hepatitis, allergic reactions, febrile reactions, circulatory overload, HIV
Rate of infusion:	Fast as patient can tolerate for massive loss
Components:	Fresh frozen plasma
Major indications:	Deficit of plasma coagulation factors
Action:	Source of labile and nonlabile plasma factors
Not indicated for:	Condition responsive to specific concentrate
Special precautions:	Must be ABO-compatible
Hazards:	Allergy, infections (hepatitis, cytomegalovirus, HIV)
Rate of infusion:	Approximately 0.5 mL/kg/min
Components:	Cryoprecipitated antihemolytic factor
Major indications:	Hemophilia A; von Willebrand disease; Hypofibrinogenemia; factor XIII deficiency
Action:	Provides factor VIII, fibrinogen
Not indicated for:	Coagulation defect undefined
Special precautions:	Rapid infusion and frequent repeat doses may be necessary
Hazards:	Hepatitis, HIV
Rate of infusion:	Approximately 10 mL/min

continued

Table 26.8
Summary of Blood Components

Components:	Platelets
Major indications:	Bleeding from thrombocytopenia or platelet function abnormality
Action:	Improves hemostasis
Not indicated for:	Plasma coagulation deficits; conditions with rapid platelet destruction
Special precautions:	Do not use microaggregate filters
Hazards:	Hepatitis, allergic reactions, febrile reactions, HIV
Rate of infusion:	One unit (from white blood cell) every 10 min (platelet packs obtained by pheresis require longer transfusion times)
Components:	Granulocytes
Major indications:	Neutropenia and infection
Action:	Provides circulating granulocytes
Not indicated for:	Infection responsive to antibiotics
Special precautions:	Do not use microaggregate filters; must be ABO-compatible
Hazards:	Hepatitis, allergic reactions, febrile reactions
Rate of infusion:	One pheresis unit over 2- to 4-h period; closely observe for reactions

HIV, human immunodeficiency virus.

- Hemolysis
- Coagulopathy
- Metabolic derangements
- Infection
- Alloimmunization
- Graft-versus-host disease (GVHD)

During massive transfusion, many blood components may be given that expose the recipient to multiple donors, thus increasing the risks of adverse reaction.

Massive Transfusion

Massive transfusion, defined as the replacement of at least one blood volume (estimated as 75 mL/kg for children younger than 1 year of age and for burned children; 70 mL/kg for all others), is most often required for:

- Orthopedic surgery
- Surgery for malignant disease
- Massive trauma
- Cardiopulmonary bypass surgery
- Extracorporeal membrane oxygenation (ECMO)

Problems associated with massive transfusion are the result of:

- Differences in transfused blood products, compared with those of the patient's unshed blood

- Abnormalities resulting from the underlying disease process
- In the case of cardiopulmonary bypass and ECMO, changes induced by the pump and/or oxygenator itself

Typing and Cross-Matching

A seriously ill, hemorrhaging patient may require large volumes of blood products, particularly PRBC, in a short time. For the trauma patient, there will be no blood already cross-matched, and the patient's blood type may not be known. Because a full cross-match takes 45 minutes to 1 hour, blood is often required before a full cross-match can be completed. Two different strategies may be used:

1. Use group O PRBCs as the initial blood for replacement. This approach is used by the Maryland Institute of Emergency Medical Services Systems (MIEMSS) in the setting of several severely traumatized patients presenting simultaneously.
2. Begin resuscitation with crystalloid solutions and plasma protein fraction before the blood type of the patient is obtained. The blood type can be determined within 5 minutes if a blood bank technician is immediately available.

No major transfusion reactions were observed after infusing type-specific blood, and no incompatibilities were noted on subsequent cross-match, even in the 8% of patients who had previously been transfused.

Complications of Red Blood Cell Transfusion

The most catastrophic complication after red blood cell transfusion is a major hemolytic transfusion reaction, which is most commonly due to an ABO mismatch. Deleterious metabolic effects include:

- Hypothermia, which may be prevented by warming the blood to above 32°C before administration
- Hyperkalemia due to the high plasma concentration of potassium in stored blood. Citrate may bind the divalent cations calcium and magnesium.
- Jaundice, most likely as a result of the large volumes of damaged red cells infused (up to 30% of the total volume), with an underperfused, somewhat poorly functional liver.
- Anaphylaxis usually occurs in IgA-deficient patients with high-titer anti-IgA antibodies and may follow infusion of red cells, plasma, platelets, intravenous immunoglobulin, or white cell concentrates.
- Few functional platelets and decreased levels of coagulation factors, especially the labile factors V and VIII, which can lead to a dilutional coagulopathy

We recommend monitoring the coagulation status during replacement and treating detected abnormalities on an individual basis, rather than using predetermined replacement protocols.

Cardiopulmonary Bypass

Cardiopulmonary bypass (CPB) demands, in essence, a massive transfusion, especially in infants and young children in whom the pump is primed with blood. Many of the problems encountered are similar to those already discussed. Of special concern, however, are citrate toxicity, microaggregates, and the coagulopathy induced by the pump.

Various causes of bleeding after CPB have been identified (Table 26.9) and a therapeutic plan to manage post-CPB bleeding has been developed (Table 26.10).

Clotting: Role of Platelets

Excessive bleeding due to defects in the normal hemostatic mechanism is a common problem in the critically ill child. Hemostasis is accomplished by

---

Table 26.9
Various Causes of Bleeding After Cardiopulmonary Bypass

Common (95 to 99%)
    Defective surgical hemostasis
    Acquired transient platelet dysfunction
Uncommon (1 to 5%)
    Drug-induced platelet dysfunction (i.e., use of aspirin)
    Thrombocytopenia (i.e., drug-induced or heparin-induced antibodies, sepsis, posttransfusion purpura, fat emboli)
    Vitamin K-dependent factor deficiencies (i.e., warfarin, liver dysfunction)
    Consumptive coagulopathy (sepsis, cardiogenic shock)
    Inherited clotting factor deficiencies or platelet dysfunction
    Doubtful significance
    Primary fibrinolysis
    Heparin (i.e., inadequate neutralization, rebound)
    Promatine excess

Table 26.10
Management of Bleeding After Cardiopulmonary Bypass

Site
    a. If localized (especially in mediastinal tubes), consider local (i.e., surgical) source
    b. Several bleeding sites, especially oozing from punctures, suggests systemic coagulopathy
Replacement
    a. Platelets: 1 unit per 3 to 5 kg body weight
    b. If still oozing, consider:
        Fresh frozen plasma 10–15 mL/kg
        Cryoprecipitate 1 unit/3 kg
        More platelets
    c. If available, consider: fresh (48-h-old) whole blood

the interaction of blood vessels, platelets, and the plasma phase of coagulation (the coagulation factors).

Defective Hemostasis

Platelet disorders leading to inadequate hemostasis can be considered in terms of insufficient numbers (i.e., thrombocytopenia) or defective action (i.e., thrombocytopathy).

Thrombocytopenia

Thrombocytopenia can result from inadequate production or accelerated loss or destruction of platelets.

- A platelet count of 50,000 to 100,000/mL is often sufficient to permit normal hemostasis during a surgical procedure
- If the count ranges from 20,000 to 50,000/mL, hemostasis is less likely to be achieved during surgery, although it may be if most of the circulating platelets are young.
- If the count is less than 20,000/mL, the risk of spontaneous bleeding becomes significant.

The causes of thrombocytopenia are numerous (Table 26.11).

Table 26.11
Etiology of Thrombocytopenia

1. Decreased production
   a. Bone marrow suppression (chemotherapy)
   b. Aplastic anemia
   c. Malignancy
   d. Congenital amegakaryocytosis
2. Accelerated destruction or loss (nonimmune)
   a. Congenital
      i. TORCH infections[a]
      ii. Giant hemangioma
   b. Acquired
      i. Hemolytic-uremic syndrome, thrombotic thrombocytopenic purpura
      ii. Infection
      iii. Disseminated intravascular coagulation
      iv. Necrotizing enterocolitis
      v. Massive transfusion
      vi. Hypersplenism
3. Accelerated destruction or loss (immune)
   a. Infection
   b. Idiopathic thrombocytopenic purpura
   c. Neonatal passive immunization
   d. Autoimmune disorders
   e. Drug-induced

[a]Toxoplasmosis, rubella, cytomegalovirus, herpes.

Thrombocytopathia

Defective platelet function is a less common cause of significant bleeding in children requiring intensive care, except for the problems seen after CPB or ECMO. There are many causes of thrombocytopathy. Of these, drug-induced defects must be emphasized, because many of the drugs implicated are administered to critically ill children (Table 26.12). Because children in PICUs are often at risk for bleeding, these drugs may aggravate the situation.

Table 26.12
Drugs that Inhibit Platelet Function After Ingestion[a]

1. Antibiotics
   a. Ampicillin
   b. Carbenicillin
   c. Cephalosporin
   d. Methicillin
   e. Penicillin G
   f. Ticarcillin
2. Antihistamines
   a. Chlorpheniramine maleate
   b. Diphenhydramine
3. Nonsteroidal antiinflammatory agents
   a. Aspirin
   b. Naproxen
   c. Phenylbutazone
   d. Sulindac
   e. Sulfinpyrazone
4. Chemotherapeutic agents
   Mithramycin
5. Ethyl alcohol
6. Glyceryl guaiacolate
7. Heparin
8. Macromolecules
   Dextran
9. Nitrofurantoin
10. Phenothiazines
    a. Chlorpromazine
    b. Promethazine
11. Pseudoephedrine hydrochloride
12. Pyrimido-pyrimidine compounds
    Dipyridamole
13. Tricyclic antidepressants
    a. Amitriptyline
    b. Desmethylipramine
    c. Imipramine
    d. Nortriptyline
14. Triprolidine
15. Vinca alkaloids
16. Valproate sodium

[a]From Nathan DG, Oski FA. Hematology of infancy and childhood. Philadelphia: WB Saunders, 1981:1306. With permission.

Diagnosis

The diagnosis of defective hemostasis resulting from platelet inadequacies is made on the basis of clinical and laboratory findings. Suggestive clinical findings include:

- Petechiae
- Purpura
- Easy bleeding and bruising
- Signs and symptoms of malignancy or renal failure

Similarly, the physical examination may differentiate between multisystem disease and a specific platelet disorder.

Laboratory investigation should include:

- Complete blood count
- Blood smear
- PT
- PTT
- FDP

Causes of Low Platelet Count

Decreased platelet number suggests a production failure or enhanced destruction. In the absence of a known underlying marrow-infiltrating disorder such as leukemia, immune destruction is most likely in the general pediatric population (e.g., out of the PICU setting). In the neonate, this is most frequently due to transplacentally transferred anti-PLA1 or anti-HLA IgG antibody (alloimmune destruction). In the older child, the autoimmune destruction is due to idiopathic thrombocytopenic purpura (ITP). In the PICU, decreased production from secondary effects of illness or medication and enhanced destruction due to consumption, often from sepsis-related DIC, are more prominent.

Platelet Transfusion

Platelet transfusion may be offered in some disorders.

Technique Platelet concentrates are prepared from whole blood (WB). A typical unit of platelets contains approximately 85% of the platelets in a unit of WB. They are administered through a platelet filter (not a microaggregate filter). As a rough guide to dosage in the setting of nonimmune thrombocytopenia, 1 unit per 5 to 7 kg body weight will result in an increase of 50,000/mL.

Complications Platelet infusion can result in GVHD, so all platelets given to immunocompromised hosts should be irradiated. Other complications include:

- Fever and chills, which can be avoided by premedication with antihistamines and acetaminophen
- Urticaria
- Anaphylaxis
- Hypotension with rapid infusion of platelets (over 20 minutes), so infusion of platelets should be over at least 20 minutes

Idiopathic Thrombocytopenic Purpura

Platelet infusion is ineffective in increasing platelet counts in children with immune-mediated thrombocytopenias, the most common of which is ITP.

Acute ITP is typically seen in children ages 2 to 6 years, during the colder months. The etiology is uncertain, although it often follows a viral infection.

Clinical Signs and Symptoms

The child usually presents with:

- Petechiae
- Oozing from mucous membranes
- Absence of fever, bone pain, lymphadenopathy, and hepatosplenomegaly, which are more common in infiltrative disorders, especially the leukemias

Therapy ITP rarely requires any therapy other than observation, let alone PICU admission. Although gingival bleeding and mild hematuria are common, serious bleeding is rare (estimated incidence of serious intracranial hemorrhage is less than 1%). Although the risk of intracranial hemorrhage is low, many hematologists still advocate the use of steroids or intravenous immunoglobulin therapy for children with acute ITP and platelet counts under 20,000/mL. Doses of 4 mg/kg raise the platelet count, and high-dose steroid administration (methylprednisolone 30 mg/kg for the first 3 days) has been shown to increase the platelet count over 150,000/mL within 3 days. Intravenous γ-globulin therapy (400 mg/kg each day for 5 days) has also been shown to cause an increase in platelet count over 150,000/μL. The advantage of steroids over IgG is principally that the former are much cheaper to administer. Again, however, whether there is a definite need for this therapy in any but the actively bleeding child is debated.

Serious bleeding, when it occurs, may require emergency splenectomy, because simple platelet infusion is ineffective in raising the count and therapy with IgG or high-dose steroids may not have a sufficiently rapid effect on the platelet count. After splenectomy, platelet survival is prolonged and hemostasis can be secured. However, splenectomy raises the long-term risks of serious infection and should not be undertaken unless absolutely essential.

Coagulation: Role of Plasma Phase

Clot Formation

The formation of a platelet plug will temporarily stop bleeding. This plug is then solidified by generation of a fibrin clot through the combined action of the coagulation factors. A cascade of coagulation protein enzymatic reactions are triggered, resulting in the generation of thrombin and a fibrin mesh network that combines with the platelets, resulting in the stable clot.

Without a system of fibrinolysis after clot formation, however, there would be no possibility of blood resuming its normal flow. Fortunately, normal plasma contains substances that inhibit the coagulation factors thrombin and factor Xa, and endothelial cells play a crucial role in the fibrinolytic process by which the body actively dissolves clots. Various clinical conditions, however, may lead to the thrombotic and hemorrhagic syndrome of disseminated intravascular coagulation (DIC) (Table 26.13).

Disseminated Intravascular Coagulation

Sepsis may lead to DIC, and a variety of organisms have been implicated. Characteristically, gram-negative infections release endotoxin that binds directly to a specific platelet receptor, causing the release reaction and furthering both pathologic thrombosis and subsequent platelet exhaustion.

Clinical Manifestations Sepsis-related DIC is a fulminant process whose predominant clinical manifestation is hemorrhage. The potential for widespread microthrombosis leading possibly to organ ischemia is dramatically evident in purpura fulminans.

- Intravascular occlusion of the terminal arterioles in the skin gives rise to sharply demarcated areas of hemorrhagic necrosis, which may coalesce if larger vessels are subsequently occluded. Digit or even limb gangrene may supervene.
- Renal damage varying from glomerular injury to cortical necrosis may occur.
- A confused state, convulsions, or coma may be furthered by microvascular occlusion in what may be an underperfused brain.
- Pulmonary injury and gastrointestinal ulceration may result from clots in small vessels.

The laboratory abnormalities characteristic of DIC (Table 26.14) reflect the combination of excess thrombosis and fibrinolysis.

Therapy The mainstay of therapy in DIC is treatment of the underlying disease. For example, in obstetric disorders, evacuation of the uterine contents removes the thrombotic stimulus and allows rapid normalization of hemostasis. Elimination of the thrombotic initiators is more difficult in sepsis or other shock states, in which there may be diffuse vascular damage.

Use of Heparin Antithrombin therapy as an adjunct to treatment of the underlying disorders has classically been heparinization. Unfortunately, the

Table 26.13
Causes of Disseminated Intravascular Coagulation (DIC)

1. Infection
   A. Gram negative
   Endotoxin
      i. Kallikren—kinins (e.g., bradykinin) (decreased blood pressure)
      ii. Activates factor XII, platelets
      iii. Endothelial damage
      iv. Activates factor VII (monocyte tissue factor production)
   B. General mechanisms
      i. Direct endothelial damage
      ii. Antigen-antibody complexes
      Platelet activation
      iii. Direct platelet activation
      iv. Venous/vascular stasis
2. Tumor
   A. Leukemia
   Acute promyelocytic leukemia
   Factor VII-like activity
   B. Solid tumors
      i. X-activating activity (especially in mucinous adenocarcinoma)
      ii. Endothelial injury and prothrombinase assembly
3. Severe head injury
   Tissue thromboplastin activity
4. Obstetric
   A. Abruption
   B. Retained dead fetus
5. Neonatal
   A. Necrotizing enterocolitis
   B. Respiratory distress syndrome
6. Hemolytic-uremic syndrome
7. Giant hemangioma
8. Miscellaneous
   A. Shock (anaphylaxis, heat stroke, etc.)
   B. Snakebite
   C. Transfusion reactions

main side effect of heparin is hemorrhage, so that heparin has been a controversial medication for use in DIC. Some respected authorities still advocate its cautious use, although some retrospective reviews suggest no benefit in either the neonate or the adult. A controlled trial in adults showed no benefit to heparinization and, in fact, demonstrated increased bleeding in those with hemorrhage shock who had been treated with heparin.

Indications for heparin in DIC follow:

- May improve outcome in purpura fulminans, in which fibrin deposition in small vessels is of major pathologic significance

Table 26.14
Laboratory Tests in DIC, Liver Disease, and Primary Fibrinolysis

Test	DIC	Liver Disease	Primary Fibrinolysis
Blood smear	Fragmented red blood cells: ↓ platelets	Targets; occasional ↓ platelets	
Platelet count	<150,000; may be <50,000	Variable; rarely <50,000	nl
aPTT (intrinsic)	Prolonged	Prolonged	Prolonged
PT (extrinsic)	Prolonged	Prolonged	Prolonged
Fibrinogen	<150 mg/dL	<150 mg/dL only if severe disease or fibrinolysis	<150 mg/dL
FDP	>40 μg/mL	Usually <40 μg/mL	>40 μg/mL
BβRP	+	+	+
FPA	+	? −	−
D-Dimer	+	? −	−
VIII $\frac{5}{32}$ C/VIII $\frac{5}{32}$ CAg or VIII $\frac{5}{32}$ C/VIII $\frac{5}{32}$ Ag	↓	?	Probably ↓
ATIII	↓	↓	? nl
Prekallikrein	↓	↓	

DIC, disseminated intravascular coagulation; +, present; −, absent; ?, uncertain; ↓, decreased; BβRP, Bβ-related peptides; FPA, fibrinopeptide A; VIII$\frac{5}{32}$ C, VIII coagulant activity; VIII$\frac{5}{32}$ CAg, VIII coagulant antigen; VIII$\frac{5}{32}$ Ag, VIII-related antigen; ATIII, antithrombin III; and nl, normal.

- Significant dermal or acral ischemia with patchy decreased skin perfusion, but without full-blown purpura fulminans
- End-organ dysfunction, such as brain, kidney, heart, or lung dysfunction, at least in part due to microthrombin
- May normalize coagulation in acute promyelocytic leukemia by interfering with the action of the tissue factor-like activity in the granules, although meticulous and aggressive replacement therapy may be equally effective in this setting

Platelet and Coagulation Factor Replacement Replacement is probably indicated in patients with DIC and significant hemorrhage, despite the risk of "feeding the fire," along with vigorous treatment of the etiologic disorder. A dose of FFP in 10 to 15 mL/kg supplies all factors in limited concentration. One unit of platelets per 5 kg body weight is estimated to raise the platelet count 50,000/mL. One unit of cryoprecipitate per 5 kg body weight will raise the fibrinogen concentration approximately 75 mg/dL. This replacement should also be undertaken in victims of snake bite, along with the administration of specific antivenom.

Hemophilia

The most common severe inherited bleeding disorders are the hemophilias. Hemophilia A, or classic hemophilia, is a deficiency of functional factor VIII:C, the coagulant portion of the factor VIII molecule. The VIII:C may be functionally absent but immunologically present (low VIII:C, higher VIII:CAg), implying production of an aberrant molecule. Alternatively, no molecule may be synthesized, with consequent low values of both VIII:C and VIII:CAg. The factor VIII-related antigen, VIII:Ag, and the platelet-aggregating activity of its multimer, the Rcof, will be normal. Similarly, in Christmas disease or hemophilia B, factor IX activity will be decreased. Cross-reacting material, representing a functionally deficient IX, may or may not be present.

Most bleeding episodes involve the muscles and joints and, more rarely, mucosal surfaces, perhaps because muscles and joints are relatively deficient in tissue factor activity and so require the augmentation pathway of VIII:C and IX for factor X activation. This bleeding rarely requires intensive care and so is not further discussed here.

Replacement Therapy Bleeding may be life-threatening because of quantitative loss. Volume loss and the oxygen-carrying capacity (red cells) should be replaced in accordance with the general principles of patient management in these situations. In addition, factor replacement therapy is required.

If the bleeding disorder is not yet specifically diagnosed but has been suspected because of excessive bleeding in relation to the extent of injury, a screening PT and PTT should be performed. An emergency factor assay can usually be performed within 1 hour and can give an idea of which factor is deficient. The level after bleeding may be lower than the patient's usual level, because of consumption of limited stores. After the deficient factor has been identified, more definitive replacement therapy can be given.

In VIII:C and IX deficiency, the PT is normal, but the PTT is prolonged, usually at least 60 seconds in patients with severe deficiencies. Both factors are contained in FFP and should be administered in a dose of at least 15 mL/kg. One unit of VIII:C activity per kilogram will raise the VIII:C level approximately 2%. FFP contains 1 unit/mL, so a large volume is required for adequate replacement. Cryoprecipitate contains 60 to 80 units of VIII:C activity per bag, and each bag is usually approximately 10 mL in volume. For major bleeding, correction to at least 70% and perhaps to 100% activity (50 units/kg) is recommended.

In factor IX-deficient patients, 1 unit of factor IX/kg will raise the activity only slightly more than 1%. Replacement to more than 80% would, therefore, require administering 80 units per kilogram body weight of lyophilized IX concentrates, which are heat-treated as are the VIII:C concentrates. Blood precautions should be observed both when drawing up the concentrate and when performing the venipuncture. The concentrate may be administered either through a filtered needle or through a filtered Soluset.

Sites of Bleeding The central nervous system and the airway are the two most common potentially lethal areas of bleeding in the hemophiliac. After all but the most minor head trauma, replacement therapy to levels of 100% activity should be given.

Head Trauma In patients with mild to moderate classic hemophilia who have suffered a relatively minor injury, DDAVP, a vasopressin analog, may be administered in a dose of 10 $\mu g/m^2$ (maximum 24 μg), diluted to a final concentration of 0.5 $\mu g/mL$ in normal saline, intravenously over 20 minutes. If brain swelling is suspected, however, DDAVP should not be used, because it may lead to water retention, although water intoxication has not been reported at this dose.

Side effects include:

- Facial flushing (possibly from prostacyclin release)
- Mild light-headedness
- Hypotension during the first hour (presumably from prostacyclin release as well), although it is rarely severe
- Headache
- Backache

A CT scan of the brain should be performed to rule out intracranial bleeding; however, a negative result should not be overly reassuring, since the bleeding may be delayed. Therefore, a repeat CT scan should be done if the patient clinically deteriorates.

Airway Bleeding Airway bleeding may follow local trauma, including prolonged dental work. Again, replacement to levels of 100% activity should be given.

Management of Inhibitors From 10 to 15% of patients with VIII:C deficiency develop anti-VIII:C antibodies or inhibitors. Management of these patients remains a clinical challenge. In patients with low-titer inhibitors (less than 5 Bethesda units), the antibody may be overwhelmed by large doses of VIII:C followed by a continuous VIII:C infusion. This therapy causes an anamnestic antibody rise in 4 to 5 days and so is reserved for life-threatening situations.

In patients with higher-titer inhibitors, IX concentrates or activated IX concentrates are given. Factor VIII:C bypassing activity is present in IX concentrates, perhaps reflecting activated factor X (Xa) activity. Activated complexes, which presumably contain more of this activity, are commercially available, although expensive (e.g., FEIBA, Autoplex). They are titered for IX levels, not for bypassing activity levels, so the dose recommended for bleeding, 80 units/kg, is empiric. The Xa may cause a low-grade state of DIC through widespread thrombin activation, so that fibrinolytic inhibitors such as tranexamic acid or ε-aminocaproic acid (Amicar) must be avoided when IX complexes are given.

An alternative approach is to use porcine factor VIII. Porcine factor VIII prepared from slaughterhouse-derived pork plasma is often active in patients with anti-human factor VIII:C inhibitors. Many of these patients have low or no anti-pork factor VIII inhibitors. Pork factor VIII:C is able to support normal hemostasis and has been used repeatedly in some patients, with no loss of efficacy. A recombinant activated factor VII is also available. It bypasses the factor VIII:C blockade and has been used in a limited number of inhibitor patients with good results.

THROMBOSIS
Deep Venous Thrombosis

Although spontaneous deep vein thrombosis (DVT) is rare in children and the incidence of pulmonary embolism or other end-organ damage such as stroke and renal vein thrombosis due to spontaneous DVT is low, the incidence of iatrogenic arterial and venous thrombosis has increased with more pervasive use of intravascular catheters for invasive monitoring or therapies in neonatal and PICUs and in cardiology. The incidence of hemodynamically significant venous thrombosis might be as high as 5 to 10%.

The factors involved in the pathogenesis of thrombosis, injury to the vessel wall, stasis of the blood, and increased coagulability, are present in children with central lines, for there is often endothelial damage from the catheter, both the underlying condition and the catheter size may contribute to decreased blood flow, and in the face of sepsis and other disorders (Table 26.15), the child may be more coagulable. Other circumstances that may predispose to thrombosis in the PICU include:

- Immobilization as occurs after head injury or orthopedic or neurologic surgery
- Deficiencies of fibrinolytic enzymes
- Other diseases similar to those leading to DVT in adults

Diagnosis
Clinical Clues

Because of its rarity, the diagnosis of DVT requires a high degree of suspicion. Certain suggestive features include:

- Family history of hypercoagulability
- Preceding history of nephrotic syndrome
- Injury leading to prolonged immobilization
- Placement of an intravascular catheter

Table 26.15
Causes of Increased Coagulability[a]

Physiological Alteration	Clinical Condition
Blood flow	
Hypovolemia	Shock, dehydration
Hyperviscosity	Polycythemia; increased protein level; increased white blood count and platelet count; sudden cardiac death
Mechanical stasis	Immobilization after surgery
Foreign bodies	Catheters, cardiac prostheses
Vessels	
Anatomic defects	Congenital heart disease; vascular anomalies
Endothelial disorders	Vasculitis; inflammation
Blood coagulation	
Increased and/or abnormal procoagulants	Cancer; pregnancy; dysfibrinogenemias; inflammatory bowel disease
Decreased anticoagulants	Antithrombin III deficiency; protein S or C deficiency
Decreased fibrinolysis	Hereditary defects
Increased platelet-vessel reactivity	Coronary artery disease; diabetes mellitus; transient ischemic attacks
Mixed or idiopathic	Hemolytic-uremic syndrome; thrombotic thrombocytopenia purpura; oral contraceptive use; nephrotic syndrome; recurrent idiopathic deep vein thrombosis

[a]Modified from Hathaway WE. Use of antiplatelet agents in pediatric hypercoagulable states. Am J Dis Child 1984;138:301–304. With permission.

Unfortunately, in some instances, the initial presentation may be a pulmonary embolus or a stroke.

Diagnostic Procedures

A variety of tests are used to confirm the diagnosis of DVT:

- Venography
- Impedance plethysmography
- Ultrasonography
- Thermography
- I-125 fibrinogen leg scanning

Venography is the "gold standard," but it is not always available, has a significant false-negative rate, and carries risks associated with the injection of radiopaque dyes. Impedance plethysmography and ultrasonography are useful for femoral and pelvic DVT but less so for calf thromboses. The I-125 fibrinogen scanning is more accurate with distal than with proximal thromboses. A combination of techniques (e.g., Doppler ultrasonography complemented by venography in uncertain cases) has been advocated by some authors as an efficient approach to the diagnosis. The ultrasonographic route would seem particularly useful in the child with suspected great vein or atrial thrombus.

Therapy

Anticoagulation or thrombolytic therapy is a clear choice if a large proximal DVT is present or if there are no factors predisposing the patient to severe hemorrhage. The decision to use these methods in a critically ill child with high risks of gastrointestinal, intracerebral, or other bleeding is more difficult.

Assessment before Treatment If therapy is to be used, initial hematologic studies should include a PT, PTT, fibrinogen concentration, and platelet count. In the case of a child presenting with a spontaneous DVT, a search for any factors contributing to a hypercoagulable state should also be undertaken (e.g., AT III, Prot C, Prot S, Plasminogen).

Antithrombotic Therapy The usual pharmacologic options includes heparin, warfarin, and thrombolytics like streptokinase, urokinase, and recombinant tPA.

Heparin Heparin is most commonly used in the therapy of distal DVT, while proximal DVT or established pulmonary embolism is treated with heparin or thrombolytics by others.

- In adults, an initial intravenous dose of 5000 units of heparin or 50 units/kg is followed by a continuous infusion rate of 15 to 25 units/kg/hour, with a goal of achieving an activated clotting time (ACT) of 150 to 190 sec.
- In newborns and older infants, higher infusion rates (e.g., 20 to 35 units/kg/hour) are sometimes needed. The risk of bleeding can be minimized by closely following the ACT or measuring the PTT regularly and keeping it in the 1.5 to 2 times control range (usually 50 to 70 seconds). After acute anticoagulation has been achieved, oral therapy with warfarin sodium is initiated if chronic anticoagulation is indicated.

Plasminogen Activators

In contrast to heparin, which acts as a cofactor with antithrombin III to prevent coagulation, the plasminogen activators, urokinase, streptokinase and tPA, increase fibrinolysis, thereby lysing the clot. In children, fibrinolytic therapy has been used in great vein and atrial thromboses, in renal vein thromboses, for occlusion of grafts, and in cases of arterial thrombosis. Its use is relatively contraindicated in patients with likely bleeding sources (e.g., intracranial bleeding, gastrointestinal hemorrhage) and during the early postoperative period. Again, as with heparin therapy, the risks of bleeding must be weighed against the risks of the thrombosis. Moreover, the effects of these agents can be fairly quickly reversed by stopping the infusion and administering FFP.

Urokinase versus Streptokinase

When comparing urokinase and streptokinase, urokinase has a lower incidence of allergic reactions but it is more expensive, making streptokinase the drug of choice.

In neonates and children, the dose range of streptokinase was 1000 to 4000 units as a loading dose followed by 1000 units/hour in three studies or 50 to 100 units/kg/hour in another. In most studies, the dose was raised by 500 to 1000 IU/kg/hour if there was no response to the initial therapy. Urokinase dosage in children is approximately 4000 IU/kg as a loading dose followed by 4000 to 6000 IU/kg/hour. The duration of therapy with these agents is usually brief (24 to 72 hours), by which time the clot will have lysed if the therapy is effective.

Fibrinogen levels and clotting functions can be used to monitor excessive plasminogen activator administration. Moreover, the addition of FFP may be necessary to replenish the stores of plasminogen needed for clot lysis. Unfortunately, both of these drugs activate both plasminogen in the circulation and that bound to fibrin, so they cause degradation of fibrinogen and other clotting factors as well as lysis of the clot.

tPA

tPA has the advantage of relatively selectively activating that plasminogen bound to fibrin, although its clear benefits over streptokinase or urokinase remain to be proved. In the case of DVT, heparin therapy may be required to prevent rethrombosis after initial clot lysis with the plasminogen activator. Subsequently, oral anticoagulation may be required.

Arterial Thrombosis

Arterial thrombosis in children and neonates is usually the result of retrograde cardiac catheterization for diagnosis of congenital heart disease or insertion of a femoral artery or umbilical artery catheter for monitoring.

Diagnosis The signs of obstructed arterial flow are clear:

- Distal extremities become pale and without a pulse
- Decreased urine output
- Signs of gut ischemia

If decreased perfusion is noted, the line should be removed if at all possible and the limb observed to establish whether the obstruction was due to thrombosis or spasm. Spasm may be relieved by injecting small amounts of lidocaine. If the signs of obstruction do not resolve within a few hours of removal of the intraarterial line, a thrombus must be considered.

Therapy The treatment regimen we use for suspected arterial thrombosis is a modification of that proposed by Lock and colleagues:

1. A period of observation of 4 hours to exclude the possibility of simple vasospasm
2. If the pulse is still absent after 4 hours, the child is heparinized with 50 U/kg of heparin; then an infusion of heparin aimed at maintaining the PTT at 1.5 to 2 times normal is continued
3. If after 24 hours there is still no pulse, streptokinase therapy is initiated 4 hours after the heparin is stopped

Younger neonates appear to be more resistant to lysis therapy, possibly because of lower plasminogen concentrations. Thus, concomitant administration of FFP or cryoprecipitate has been advocated by some, although this may not improve the fibrinolytic activity of the drug.

With either venous or arterial thrombosis, failure of medical management may lead to surgical intervention. Ligation of the inferior vena cava may be life-saving in the patient with a proximal DVT unresponsive to heparin or lysis therapy. Similarly, thrombectomy has been used in treating aortic thrombosis, although the efficacy of this approach in young infants has been limited.

With thrombosis, as with so many disorders in the PICU, prevention is more efficacious than treatment. However, with the exception of selected surgical patients and perhaps immobilized trauma patients, prophylaxis with pneumatic stockings and low-dose heparin will not prevent most thromboses seen in the PICU.

27.

Multiple Trauma

James C. Fackler, Myron Yaster, Reginald J. Davis, Vera F. Tait, J. Michael Dean, Andrew L. Goldberg, and Mark C. Rogers

Multisystem trauma accounts for 50% of deaths occurring in children older than 1 year—nearly 23,000 lives are lost per year. For each child who dies, there are four survivors who are permanently disabled. Significant head trauma is encountered in approximately 50% of children who have sustained blunt trauma. Virtually all fatalities from trauma result from significant central nervous system injury.

Discussion of head and spinal cord trauma is the focus of Chapter 14.

INITIAL ASSESSMENT

Although emphasis is placed on the "golden hour" in trauma management, the first 60 seconds of a child's presentation are paramount. The clinician must determine if the patient's airway is patent, if he or she is breathing, if respiratory efforts are adequate, if stridor or cyanosis is present, if breath sounds are symmetric, if the trachea is in the midline, if protective airway reflexes are adequate, if there is circulatory collapse, if blood loss is controlled, and if the patient is conscious.

The first 20 to 30 minutes of evaluation and resuscitation will determine survival (with minimal morbidity) in most cases. This period is divided into a primary survey with initial resuscitation; a secondary survey, which consists of a complete examination from head to toe; and finally, definitive care, which usually occurs in the pediatric intensive care unit (PICU) environment. Every institution should have a patient transfer protocol for definitive care after the initial evaluation and management (Fig. 27.1).

Primary Survey

Airway

Three goals of airway management are: to relieve anatomic obstruction, to promote adequate gas exchange, and to prevent the aspiration of gastric contents. Airway obstruction most commonly occurs because the tongue or pharyngeal soft tissues collapse into the airway. Other causes include foreign materials (e.g., vomitus, blood, large food pieces), severe maxillofacial injury, and injuries to the larynx or chest.

After relieving anatomic airway obstruction, the clinician must assess gas exchange (see Chapter 1).

Intubation

Indications Endotracheal tube placement is required for:

- Delivery of high concentrations of oxygen
- Use of positive end-expiratory pressure (PEEP)
- Internal stabilization of a flail chest
- Controlling ventilation
- Patients with: burns of the face and neck, hemodynamic instability, need for sedation for diagnostic study, or a serious central nervous system (CNS) injury

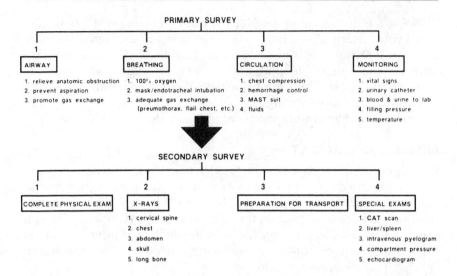

Figure 27.1. Protocol for the Resuscitation, Assessment, and Diagnosis of the Critically Injured Child. This protocol is composed of a primary and secondary survey. The primary survey is composed of the initial resuscitation, whereas the secondary survey is composed of a complete physical examination, X-ray and other diagnostic studies, and preparation for transport.

Approach Oral endotracheal intubation is preferred in all initial situations. Nasal intubation attempts often lead to bleeding, which may obstruct visualization and delay the airway placement.

As with all trauma victims, techniques to minimize regurgitation of stomach contents are imperative (see Chapter 2).

Normal Airway

Neuromuscular Blockade If the patient's airway is normal and intubation is required, the clinician commonly performs rapid neuromuscular blockade with succinylcholine (1.5 to 2.0 mg/kg) (see Chapter 2). Succinylcholine use is controversial in patients with open globe injuries and increased intracranial pressure; however, proper airway management must always take precedence in a balance of risks and benefits.

Contraindications to the use of succinylcholine include:

- Extensive burns
- Crush injuries
- Various neuromuscular diseases

Within several hours of these injuries, succinylcholine can be administered safely for the purpose of securing an airway.

Rapid Sequence Intubation The technique, patient response, and options after failure of intubation are discussed in Chapter 2.

Complicated Airway The clinician should anticipate complicated tracheal intubation when the patient's midface, mandible, neck, or larynx is injured, because bone fragments, hematoma, or edema can cause complete airway obstruction. In the presence of maxillofacial or airway injury, the clinician should never risk sudden airway obstruction with paralyzing or hypnotic agents or pass an endotracheal (or any) tube blindly. Blind nasal intubation using an endotracheal tube or even a nasogastric tube can lead to intubation of the nasal sinuses or the cranium or cause further dislodgement of bone and tissue. Blunt injuries of the neck can fracture and disrupt the airway and usually are associated with cervical spine injury. These are best managed through tracheostomy under local anesthesia or needle cricothyroidotomy (see Chapter 2).

Patients having neck, serious head, or deceleration injuries should be assumed to have cervical spine injury. The primary goal of initial management is to prevent further injury by reducing external compression and preventing further displacement of the injured elements. Tracheal intubation in patients with cervical spine injury is described in Chapter 2.

Breathing Once a patent airway is established, the next step in evaluation is establishing the adequacy of breathing or ventilation. If apnea is present or if hypoventilation is noted, the clinician should institute artificial ventilation immediately with 100% oxygen. In most situations, ventilation is begun at rates of approximately 10 to 15 breaths/minute and tidal volumes of 10 to 15 mL/kg. Minute ventilations of 150 mL/kg/minute will usually provide arterial carbon dioxide pressures of approximately 40 mm Hg. If poor ventilation results from abnormal chest wall dynamics, either internally from a pneumothorax or externally from a flailing chest wall, each of these conditions must be rapidly evaluated and treated.

Pneumothorax Because of either lack of movement of the chest wall or absence of breath sounds, needle aspiration should be carried out immediately and followed by intercostal chest tube placement if pneumothorax is verified. There may not be time to obtain a chest radiograph if the child's ventilatory function is deteriorating.

Flailing Chest Wall Positive pressure ventilation will stabilize the chest wall and achieve adequate ventilation. In spite of an adequate airway and effective ventilation, there may still be hypoxia and arterial desaturation due to pathologic right-to-left shunting through damaged pulmonary tissue, or secondary to aspiration, pneumonia, or lung contusion. Although these latter problems require subsequent evaluation and treatment, the initial approach is always the same; namely, to ensure the airway and maintain adequate ventilation with 100% oxygen.

Circulation

Hemorrhagic Shock Patient survival, as well as morbidity (Table 27.1), is directly related to the speed with which shock is corrected. The prompt correction of hypovolemia is a crucial factor in the prevention of posttraumatic

Table 27.1
Advanced Trauma Life Support Classification of Shock

Class I
  15% acute blood volume loss or less
  Blood pressure normal
  Pulse increased 10–20%
  No change in capillary refill
Class II
  20–25% loss of blood volume
  Tachycardia >150 beats/min
  Tachypnea 35–40 breaths/min
  Capillary refill prolonged
  Systolic blood pressure decreased
  Pulse pressure decreased
  Orthostatic hypotension >10–15 torr
  Urine output >1 mL/kg/h
Class III
  30–35% blood volume loss
  All of the above signs
  Urine output <1 mL/kg/h
  Lethargic, clammy, vomiting
Class IV
  40–50% blood volume loss
  Nonpalpable pulses
  Obtunded

sequelae (e.g., acute renal failure, development of respiratory failure). Although easily recognized with external hemorrhage, fractures of the long bones or pelvis produce hidden blood loss that may reach 1000 to 2000 mL in 70-kg patients.

The basic steps in the management of hemorrhagic shock are:

- Control of active hemorrhage
- Institution of intravenous lines
- Aggressive crystalloid and blood replacement

Control of obvious external hemorrhage is of paramount importance; in most situations, direct pressure over the site of hemorrhage is successful.

Massive abdominal hemorrhage or hemorrhage after fracture of the long bones of the lower extremities can be controlled with military anti-shock trousers (MAST) (see subsequent section).

In extreme situations, massive abdominal hemorrhage may be controlled by thoracotomy and cross-clamping the descending aorta. This technique, however, does not always achieve complete hemostasis, and abdominal control of the bleeding must be accomplished rapidly to prevent abdominal visceral ischemia.

When a MAST is unavailable or control of hemorrhage requires immediate surgery, catecholamines such as epinephrine or norepinephrine are used to support the patient en route to the operating room. Both epinephrine and norepinephrine may cause irreversible mucosal ischemia, and they should be used only as a temporary means.

Blood Volume

Estimating Volume Blood volume estimates are based on the patient's optimal weight. Through age 14 years, the percentage range is 6.5 to 8.0% of the total body weight (e.g., 65 to 80 mL/kg optimal body weight). In newborns, this estimation approaches 9 to 10% of the optimal body weight. Volume deficit is best evaluated by examination.

Heart Rate as a Monitor The most sensitive monitor of cardiac output and reserve in a child is the heart rate; thus, the adequacy of circulation is assessed primarily by noting the quality, rate, and regularity of the pulse and secondarily assessed by obtaining the blood pressure. Young children vasoconstrict rapidly and may maintain a normal central blood pressure even though they have lost as much as 25% of their circulating blood volume. Heart rate elevation, therefore, is a much earlier sign of hypovolemia.

Fluid Replacement The definitive therapy of blood loss and extracellular fluid loss is the administration of intravenous fluids and blood.

Vascular Access The simplest, safest, and most rapid means of obtaining venous access is by percutaneous peripheral vein cannulation. Because of the smaller size of veins in children and veins usually collapse when a child is in shock, initial cannulation may require cutdown; the brachial vein of the upper extremity or, when MAST are not in use, the saphenous vein of the lower extremity are usually easiest to access. Alternatively, central venous cannulation is useful. Favored entry sites include the internal and external jugular and subclavian veins. Speed is essential, but sterile technique and proper positioning must not be neglected.

Types of Fluid Although different types of fluids can be used for resuscitation after trauma, there is no substitute for blood, particularly in class III and IV patients. The debate concerning the use of colloids and crystalloids has raged for decades. Initially, 20 to 30 mL/kg of lactated Ringer's is given as quickly as possible. If systemic arterial blood pressure does not return to normal levels after fluid challenge, additional volume and blood are infused and titrated against urine output, skin perfusion, heart rate, and blood pressure.

If systemic arterial blood pressure and central venous pressure cannot be maintained with 50 mL/kg of balanced salt solution and blood, MAST are applied. The most frequent error made in the immediate therapy of the trauma patient is slow or inadequate administration of fluid and blood.

Whole Blood Blood must be used for class III or IV patients (blood loss in excess of 30% of the effective circulating volume). Fresh whole blood is the ideal and preferred blood product because of its ease of administration, the presence of clotting factors, cost effectiveness, and because it most closely duplicates what is being lost. Unfortunately, fresh whole blood is rarely, if ever, available.

Packed Red Blood Cells Most often, packed red blood cells (PRBC) are available. A unit of PRBC has an average hematocrit of 65 to 75%. Unfortunately, the increased hematocrit and high viscosity obtained by packing blood makes its administration difficult. It is recommended to "reconstitute" packed or red blood cells with normal saline, 5% albumin, or, if coagulopathy is documented, fresh frozen plasma.

Cross Matching In the emergent resuscitative phase of therapy in class III and class IV patients, time may not allow a full type and cross match to be accomplished before transfusion. It is best to obtain at least an ABO-Rh type-specific blood with or without a partial cross match. The immediate phase cross match will fail to detect only a few unexpected antibodies outside the ABO system, most of which are clinically insignificant.

Hemostasis With the exception of factor V and factor VIII, all plasma coagulation factors are relatively stable in banked blood. With massive hemorrhage and transfusion (more than 15 units of stored blood in adults) or more than two blood volumes in a child), hemostatic defects occur. The hemostatic defects are related to the numbers and function of platelet and circulating protein coagulation factors (see Chapter 26). Frequent monitoring of coagulation screening tests and platelet counts are necessary as well as aggressive correction of hypovolemia to avoid the coagulation defects associated with prolonged shock.

Military Antishock Trousers MAST are invaluable for transport and emergency resuscitation when abdominal or lower extremity hemorrhage or shock is present. These pneumatic garments are available for children older than 4 years of age. They are particularly useful in the stabilization of pelvic, hip, and long bone fractures of the lower extremity and as a means to tamponade lacerated arterial and venous injuries in these organs. MAST function by autotransfusion or by increasing peripheral vascular resistance.

Contraindications to the use of the MAST suit include the setting of pulmonary edema and respiratory distress, and after abdominal trauma when the viscera are protruding.

Monitoring

Urinary Catheter

Urine production may cease after hemorrhagic shock; urine output of 0.5 to 1.0 mL/kg/hour is the goal of fluid therapy. In addition to measuring urine production, the bladder catheter facilitates the diagnosis of urinary tract injury and rhabdomyolysis.

- Microscopic or gross hematuria strongly suggests urinary tract injury. Because the insertion of the urethral catheter itself can cause hematuria, the clinician ideally should examine a spontaneously voided specimen.
- Rhabdomyolysis results in myoglobin release and myoglobinuria and is common after crush injuries and electrical burns.

Prompt diagnosis is essential because renal failure (i.e., acute tubular necrosis); electrolyte abnormalities involving potassium, phosphorus, and calcium; and cardiac dysrhythmias may rapidly lead to death. Rhabdomyolysis is diagnosed by gross pigmentation of the urine and must be differentiated from other urinary pigments such as hemoglobin, porphyria, and blood.

Blood Pressure and Filling Pressures

Arterial blood pressure may be normal with as much as a 15 to 25% loss of total blood volume. Intra-arterial pressure monitoring is the method of choice in seriously injured patients.

   Estimating Intravascular Volume When blood loss is significant or massive amounts of fluids and blood are required, estimation of intravascular volume through central venous pressure (CVP) or pulmonary capillary wedge pressure (PCWP) monitor is essential. In children with normal hearts, right heart filling pressures are adequate. The clinician should place a flow-directed balloon-tipped pulmonary artery catheter if:

- Circulatory instability persists
- Significant lung disease is present
- Cardiac output determinations are necessary

Gauging Fluid Administration

Fluids are infused on the basis of the pressure response to a fluid challenge, not the pressures initially measured. When the CVP is less than 8 cm H_2O, or the PCWP is less than 12 mm Hg, 10 to 20 mL/kg of balanced salt solution is infused over 10 minutes. If at any time during the infusion:

- CVP increases by more than 5 cm H_2O or
- PCWP increases by more than 7 mm Hg

the infusion is immediately discontinued.
   After the infusion, if:

- CVP has increased by less than 5 cm H_2O but more than 2 cm H_2O, or
- PCWP has increased by less than 7 mm Hg but more than 3 mm Hg

the patient is observed for a 10-minute interval.
   If, during the interval of observation:

- CVP exceeds 2 cm H_2O above the starting value, or
- PCWP exceeds 3 mm Hg above the starting value

the patient is monitored, but no additional fluid is administered. If, on the other hand, CVP or PCWP falls below 2 cm H_2O or 3 mm Hg, respectively, the fluid challenge is resumed. Fluids are administered until either the hemodynamic signs of shock are corrected or the "5–2" or "7–3" rule is violated.

Environment

In the ABCs of resuscitation, consider "D" diagnosis and "E" the environment. A child must be completely undressed for proper evaluation and resuscitation. Naked children placed in a cold environment (even room temperature), however, rapidly lose heat because of their large body surface area relative to their body mass. Additionally, the younger the child, the less subcutaneous tissue available for heat insulation.

Children may be warmed in three ways: with external heating lamps, by warming intravenous fluids and blood, and by wrapping all exposed body parts in plastic bags. The last technique prevents evaporative heat loss and is quite effective at heat conservation.

As a last step in the primary survey, the clinician performs a rapid neurologic evaluation. The Glasgow Coma Scale score should be estimated (see Table 27.2). A more extensive neurologic examination is not pertinent at this time.

Secondary Survey

Physical Examination

A complete physical examination and reassessment, including the child's back, and should take place approximately 15 to 20 minutes into the period of primary resuscitation. The order of physical examination of the child's body may vary, but injuries should be evaluated in descending order of urgency. Finding one injury, even if severe, should not stop the remainder of the evaluation. Evaluation should always be gentle, with particular attention to manipulation of the spinal axis. Vital signs should be obtained repeatedly.

Head and Neck Start with the child's eyes, face, and scalp. Localized hematomas and ecchymoses, especially those located in the periorbital region and behind the pinna of the ear, should be carefully sought because they indicate basilar skull fractures. Similarly, the tympanic membrane and nose should be examined for blood and cerebrospinal fluid (CSF) as evidence of either basal skull fracture or meningeal tear.

After the patient's cervical spine is stabilized, the clinician should examine the neck for subcutaneous emphysema, hematoma, or localized pain. The cervical spine is palpated as is the trachea to ensure that the tra-

Table 27.2
Glasgow Coma Score

Activity	Best Response	Score
Eye opening	Spontaneous	4
	To verbal stimuli	3
	To pain	2
	None	1
Verbal	Oriented	5
	Confused	4
	Inappropriate words	3
	Nonspecific sounds	2
	None	1
Motor	Follows commands	6
	Localizes pain	5
	Withdraws in response to pain	4
	Flexion in response to pain	3
	Extension in response to pain	2
	None	1

Modified Coma Score for Infants

Activity	Best Response	Score
Eye opening	Spontaneous	4
	To speech	3
	To pain	2
	None	1
Verbal	Coos and babbles	5
	Irritable cries	4
	Cries to pain	3
	Moans to pain	2
	None	1
Motor	Normal spontaneous movements	6
	Withdraws to touch	5
	Withdraws to pain	4
	Abnormal flexion	3
	Abnormal extension	2
	None	1

chea is in a midline position. Spinal cord injury may also be suspected in patients with unexplained, refractory shock, especially in the presence of good peripheral perfusion.

Chest In addition to adequacy and rate of ventilation, any asymmetry or painful chest should be observed with particular attention to the presence of a flail segment. Blood pressure should be redetermined.

Abdomen and Pelvis Examination of the patient's abdomen is begun and repeated at 15- to 20-minute intervals. A specific diagnosis of intra-abdominal injury is not necessary at this point, but the physician needs to decide whether surgical intervention is urgent or emergent.

A rapidly expanding abdominal girth indicates ongoing bleeding and is an urgent indication for further diagnostic studies, possibly including peritoneal lavage or computed tomography (CT) scan on the way to the operating room or PICU. An oralgastric tube should be passed in all patients with abdominal trauma.

The back is part of the abdominal examination, and the patient should be turned for proper evaluation. The bony prominences of the pelvis need to be palpated for tenderness and instability. The perineum needs to be carefully examined for laceration, hematoma, or active bleeding. If a pelvic fracture is suspected or seen on a radiograph, a rectal examination should be carried out to evaluate the possibility of bone fragment injury to pelvic structures.

Occasionally, examination of other body areas may also suggest an abdominal injury. Shoulder pain, in particular, is often seen and suggests diaphragmatic irritation. Possible causes are free air in the abdomen or splenic injury (particularly with left upper quadrant pain). Although genitourinary tract injury is common, most of these injuries are subtle.

Extremities The clinician looks for signs of abrasion, contusion, or hematoma formation. Bony instability is noted, and a neurovascular examination is performed to assess the presence of compromised blood flow and development of a compartment syndrome. Inadequate concern about the neurovascular supply to an extremity or lack of recognition of such an injury leads to unnecessary morbidity. Blood vessels in injured limbs are vulnerable to compression or laceration and can continue to bleed, exacerbating hypovolemic shock and bleeding into an intact fascial compartment, causing the compartment syndrome. Additionally, motion around the injury site causes unnecessary pain to the patient.

Neurologic Examination

A thorough stepwise examination includes assessment of the cranial nerves and peripheral motor and sensory evaluation. The high incidence of head injury, as well as the devastating problems that may follow, requires maximal diagnostic and therapeutic interventions by the physician. The Glasgow Coma Scale is a standardized examination and should be documented for all head-injured patients (Table 27.2).

The parameters of the neurologic examination detail the patient's responses to verbal and auditory input and to a variety of peripheral sensory stimuli. The coma scale is useful in all patients so that repeated examinations, which form the foundation for appropriate management, will be the same even if performed by different examiners.

History of Injury

In addition to a history of the onset of the injury, a careful medical history is obtained because childhood illnesses and systemic diseases may complicate the ultimate management of this acute episode. Appropriate consultants in medical and surgical specialties should be called early during resuscitation.

At this stage in preparation for transfer to either the PICU or the operating room, the primary resuscitating physician must maintain a high index of suspicion and awareness of early signs of deterioration or development of new complications. The physician must be responsible for the comprehensive care of the child so that the patient is broken down into organ systems with the overall picture lost in consequence.

Definitive Care

At this stage, the child should be either hemodynamically stable with a controlled airway or rapidly on the way to the operating room because of instability. In the former situation, appropriate specialized radiologic studies, including CT or radionuclide scanning, are appropriate before the child is taken to the PICU. In preparing the child for transport, the clinician must control the airway and should monitor the circulatory system constantly.

CHEST TRAUMA IN INFANTS AND CHILDREN
Evaluation

Virtually all chest injuries can be diagnosed during the initial primary assessment and during the secondary survey of the chest after careful physical examination and the use of chest radiographs and the electrocardiogram (ECG). Injuries that are immediately life-threatening and present during the initial assessment period include:

- Airway obstruction
- Open pneumothorax
- Flail chest
- Tension pneumothorax
- Massive hemothorax
- Cardiac tamponade

Injuries that are potentially life-threatening and often are present when the chest radiograph and electrocardiograph are obtained include:

- Tracheobronchial tears
- Pulmonary contusion
- Myocardial contusion
- Ruptured diaphragm
- Esophageal rupture
- Partial aortic transection

Open Pneumothorax

Massive blunt trauma to the child's thorax may cause a loss of a portion of the chest wall or may be the result of a penetrating injury. The initial treatment is simple and direct. The defect in the chest wall is covered with a sterile-occlusive dressing, which converts the open pneumothorax to a closed pneumothorax. The dressing is taped securely in place and a chest tube is placed in the pleural space and connected to suction; this then becomes the management of a tension pneumothorax with or without an association hemothorax.

Flail Chest

Flail chest is characterized by a chest wall segment that has lost continuity with the thorax and moves paradoxically with changes in intrathoracic pressure.

Definitive treatment of the flail chest takes place in the PICU by controlled ventilation (i.e., PEEP). The inflated lung acts as a splint, stabilizes rib fractures, and decreases pain associated with the chest wall injury. Analgesics should also be administered because of the pain associated with chest wall movement. Often, the severity of the underlying injury to the lung is more of a determinant in recovery than is the chest wall injury itself.

Cardiac Tamponade

Cardiac tamponade is rarely associated with blunt trauma in children. It may result from stab or gunshot wounds to the heart or from penetration of a fractured rib into the heart. Most children with pericardial tamponade will ultimately require surgical exploration.

The classic clinical presentation of "paradoxical pulse" and severe hypotension with distended neck veins is seen in children and adults. If the physical findings and signs suggest tamponade, a definitive diagnosis is made by pericardiocentesis using a large (i.e., 14-gauge) plastic over-the-needle catheter that can also be used to continue temporizing initial treatment by pericardiocentesis. This is best performed by the left subxiphoid route with the needle aimed at the left shoulder at an angle of 45°.

The ECG can be monitored by attaching an alligator clip to the V5 electrode. The QRS complex will change dramatically when the epicardium is touched.

Secondary Survey of Thoracic Injuries

The most common occult and potentially serious injuries to the chest and its contents are subsequently addressed in order of frequency.

Pulmonary Contusion

Strong suggestive signs of pulmonary parenchymal injury in a child are:

- Hemoptysis or suctioning blood from the endotracheal tube
- Subcutaneous emphysema in the base of the neck
- Persistent air leak after placement of a chest tube for pneumothorax

Pulmonary contusion from blunt injuries to the chest is common and frequently is associated with both localized pulmonary edema and atelectasis. Patients present with respiratory distress, particularly hypoxemia, due to the right-to-left shunting through the contused, atelectatic, and underventilated pulmonary parenchyma. Radiographic evidence of pulmonary contusion includes early consolidation of lung parenchyma that may be focal and tends to resolve over 2 to 6 days. Overhydration of such patients must be carefully avoided.

Pulmonary Laceration

Tears into the pulmonary parenchyma may result from blunt trauma due to fractured ribs or compression of the chest wall even without fractures with impingement into the parenchyma. A laceration obviously can occur from any type of penetrating injury. Minor peripheral parenchymal lacerations rarely cause major problems and usually are successfully treated by chest tube insertion for the associated pneumothorax and reexpansion of the lung against the chest wall. Major hemorrhage is rarely associated with peripheral parenchymal injuries, and therefore, reexpansion of the lung with a chest catheter is adequate treatment.

Pulmonary Hematoma

Both a parenchymal contusion and parenchymal laceration may be associated with contained bleeding or hematoma in the lung tissue, resulting from blunt as well as penetrating trauma. Although radiographic findings of pulmonary hematomas may be dramatic, hematomas usually resolve in a few days when they are treated expectantly.

Abscess formation resulting from secondary infection is uncommon in children; nevertheless, because of the potential seriousness of this complication, prophylactic antibiotics are usually indicated.

Tracheobronchial Tears

Penetrating injuries to the trachea or major bronchi are usually obvious, but blunt injuries are both more frequent and more difficult to diagnose. If there is subcutaneous emphysema in the cervical area, this diagnosis should be suspected immediately.

The most common injuries to the tracheobronchial tree are suggested by noisy breathing, which indicates partial airway obstruction. When such signs are present or when an injury is suspected, early bronchoscopy to visualize the trachea and major bronchi is mandatory to confirm a presumptive diagnosis.

If there is a persistent large air leak after placement of a chest tube for pneumothorax, a significant tear of a major bronchus probably is present. Under such circumstances, a second chest tube and even a third may be necessary to control the leak and the child should undergo endoscopy and eventual thoracotomy to control the air leak and to repair the bronchial tear.

Indications for early thoracotomy are:

• Continued extensive air leak
• Compression of the tracheobronchial tree
• Expanding hematoma in the mediastinum and neck

Respiratory management of these patients may be extraordinarily difficult because positive pressure ventilation will primarily ventilate the path of least resistance, namely, the fistula. Often, spontaneous ventilation, even when the patient is intubated, is useful. A double-lumen endotracheal tube can isolate the fistula and allow one-lung ventilation in older patients but is impractical for children. High-frequency ventilation has resulted uniformly in improvement of arterial blood gas levels, even when pulmonary air leak is associated with failure of conventional mechanical ventilation.

Myocardial Contusion

The diagnosis of a myocardial contusion is made on the basis of dysrhythmias or routine ECGs in a clinical situation where blunt trauma to the anterior chest wall has occurred. Because children with myocardial contusion are at risk from sudden dysrhythmias, they require admission to a critical care unit and constant cardiac monitoring.

Rupture of the Diaphragm

Traumatic rupture of the diaphragm is not uncommon in children and results from compression forces over the lower chest and upper abdomen. Rupture is more common on the left side, possibly because the right diaphragm is buttressed by the liver. Small areas of diaphragmatic tear may not cause immediate symptoms, but eventually they will result in progressive herniation through the diaphragmatic defect. These injuries frequently are missed initially because the radiographic findings may be interpreted as an elevated diaphragm or atelectasis or pleural fluid in the lower chest.

Rupture of the lung should be suspected when the left diaphragm is not clearly visualized on the initial chest radiograph or when there is a hemopneumothorax that does not clear completely with placement of a chest tube. Rupture of the diaphragm may be found at the time of abdominal exploration for severe intra-abdominal injury. The treatment for a tear of the diaphragm is urgent operative repair.

Impending Thoracic-Aortic Disruption

Impending or partial aortic disruption as well as a tear of the great vessels is extremely uncommon in children because rarely are such severe forces brought to bear on the chest and mediastinal structures in this age group. Tears of the thoracic aorta are fatal in 80 to 90% of adults. An expanding mediastinal hematoma may indicate the need for an emergency aortogram.

Emergency Room Thoracotomy in Children

Emergency room thoracotomy is rarely needed in adults and is probably never indicated in children except when cardiopulmonary arrest does not respond to external cardiac massage and good ventilatory support. Emergency room thoracotomy is rarely, if ever, successful. Even urgent thoracotomy in an operating room environment is rarely indicated, but may be necessary for:

- Massive, progressive hemothorax with continuing blood loss more than 100 mL/hour through a chest tube
- Major cardiac wounds, which often present with hemopericardium
- Impending disruption of the thoracic aorta
- Rupture of the tracheobronchial tree with uncontrolled air leak

POSTTRAUMATIC RESPIRATORY FAILURE

After trauma and injury, a variety of events can occur initially that immediately causes respiratory failure. In contrast, acute respiratory distress syndrome (ARDS) may develop approximately 12 to 24 hours after the injury.

Many therapeutic maneuvers required to treat an injured patient may aggravate the pathophysiologic responses of the lung:

- Infusion of saline, plasma, and blood products used to restore the effective circulating volume may enhance fluid leakage into the alveoli
- High concentrations of oxygen used in treating ARDS may produce oxygen toxicity and collapse of the most severely ventilation-perfusion mismatched alveoli via resorption of oxygen (i.e., "resorption atelectasis")
- Mechanical ventilation may result in barotrauma and further exacerbate the disease process

ABDOMINAL TRAUMA IN INFANTS AND CHILDREN

The basic principle of evaluating a child with a possible abdominal injury is the surgical determination of whether operative intervention is necessary for an acute abdomen injury or control of hemorrhage. The extent of intraabdominal injury is often difficult to determine because of an inadequate history or a presumed inconsequential injury and the frequent absence of obvious clinical signs of internal injury. The frequent presence of abdominal injury in the unconscious child makes evaluation even more difficult. Most deaths related to intra-abdominal injuries are caused by early hemorrhage or later peritonitis. During the initial abdominal examination, therefore, priority is given to whether intraabdominal hemorrhage is the most immediate threat to life.

Penetrating Wounds

Penetrating wounds usually are caused by gunshot and stabbing, which may cause injury to any (or all) of the abdominal viscera and vessels. For practical purposes, all penetrating wounds of the abdomen require operative intervention, preceded by the initial ABCs of management in hemodynamic resuscitation. Penetrating injuries result either in bleeding or perforation of hollow viscera, and therefore, frequently give early evidence of peritoneal irritation or hemorrhagic shock. If there are not such internal injuries, the initial findings may be occult, but, nevertheless, exploration at an appropriate time and on an urgent schedule is indicated.

Occasionally, penetrating wounds result in evisceration of abdominal contents. The organs should not be replaced into the abdomen nor be allowed to twist and to kink. Rather, the abdominal contents should be covered with moist, sterile dressings until operative repair can take place.

Blunt Trauma

Blunt injuries account for at least 90% of major abdominal injuries in children.

Hemorrhage

Hemorrhage due to blunt trauma to the spleen or liver or disruption of major vessels is the main focus of attention, because it is the most immediate threat to life. In this situation, use of MAST are lifesaving. A frequent error in early management of the trauma patient is the ill-timed removal of MAST. Massive hemorrhage may occur immediately or evolve slowly because of general hypotension, which, to some extent, decreases further blood loss.

Solid Organ Injury

The most commonly injured solid organs are the spleen and liver. The organs may be so severely injured with massive damage that immediate exploration is indicated as soon as the ABCs have been managed.

The pancreas and the duodenum may also be injured, usually by high-speed deceleration, as occurs when a child crashes against the handlebars of a bicycle or as a result of blunt trauma from child abuse.

The hollow viscera may also be lacerated by deceleration injuries and torn at their sites of attachment, that is, at the ligament of Treitz and the ileocecal valve area.

Other structures subject to injury include the kidneys, ureter, bladder, and mesentery. Concomitant injuries may involve the ribs, pelvis, and spine.

Secondary Survey

Abdominal examination may be difficult because a child is often apprehensive or unwilling and unable to cooperate if semicomatose or unconscious. Relatively trivial, or apparently insignificant, trauma may be responsible for major intestinal or pancreatic injuries and injuries to the liver and spleen. Careful assessment of the abdomen may reveal significant abdominal pathology.

Diagnostic Study

Laboratory Findings After the physical examination, appropriate laboratory studies are done:

- Serum amylase level, which, when elevated, indicates pancreatic injury, bowel ischemia, or transection of the proximal intestine
- Type and crossmatch
- Complete blood count
- Prothrombin time (PT)
- Partial thromboplastin time (PTT)
- Urinalysis, which may demonstrate hematuria or myoglobinuria

Imaging The most accurate diagnostic tools (aside from serial physical examination) are:

- Radionuclide scans
- CT scans with contrast enhancement
- Intravenous pyelogram (IVP) with cystogram and urethrogram
- Peritoneal lavage

Plain films of the abdomen are seldom helpful.

Computed Tomography Computed tomography scanning documents the extent of solid organ injury, images the pancreas and kidney, and demonstrates the presence of free blood, fluid, and air in the abdomen. In many centers, the abdominal CT scan has replaced the IVP for the evaluation of renal trauma. Problems with CT scanning include:

- Radiation exposure
- Transport of the seriously injured patient from the PICU
- Difficulty in patient monitoring while he or she is in the scanner

Intravenous Pyelogram Because of the risk of potentially serious reaction to contrast media in children with renal trauma, unnecessary radiation exposure, and delay in the diagnosis of other injuries, use of the IVP is recommended when:

- Urinalysis demonstrates gross hematuria with physical evidence of renal injury
- There is an unstable clinical course with blood loss
- Renal artery injury is suspected

Peritoneal Lavage In most centers where radionuclide scanning or CT are used to evaluate abdominal trauma, peritoneal lavage is rarely used. It is still a useful test for assessing intraabdominal bleeding, however, and for judging the need for surgical exploration of the abdomen.

Because lavage irritates the peritoneum for 24 to 48 hours, it may obscure subsequent abdominal evaluation and is, therefore, not performed early in the clinical course of the patient. Peritoneal lavage is performed by inserting a pediatric-sized peritoneal dialysis catheter under direct vision through the lower abdominal midline with infusion of 10 mL/kg of crystalloid solution into the abdominal cavity. A simple peritoneal tap is no longer considered adequate for the evaluation of intra-abdominal bleeding.

Management

The diagnosis of specific intra-abdominal injuries is often difficult on initial examination, and an aggressive diagnostic approach based on an established protocol is mandatory. Meticulous physical examination, repeated as often as necessary with the maintenance of a high index of suspicion for abdominal injury, is the basic guideline for successful treatment of blunt trauma to the abdomen.

If the abdominal injuries result in significant blood losses that prevent successful reestablishment or maintenance of vital functions and specifically indicate marked hypovolemia, then the child should be taken immediately to the operating room for urgent laparotomy and resuscitation. Serious injuries to the spleen and liver frequently are self-limiting, and the child may only need volume replacement with crystalloid or blood and may not require operative intervention. Such nonoperative treatment of proven injuries to the liver and spleen should be carried out in tertiary care facilities by pediatric specialists in an intensive care environment. It should never be attempted in community hospital environments because of the possibility of rapid deterioration.

CHILD ABUSE

Deliberate versus Accidental Injury

Deliberately inflicted and accidental trauma may produce similar types of injury. Clues obtained from the history and the physical examination may help in their differentiation.

History

- Story related by the parents that varies with the clinical findings
- Parents appear inappropriately concerned about the severity of their child's injury
- Parents appear reluctant to give information or are inconsistent about the dates of the injury
- History of low birth weight or complicated neonatal course associated with maternal illness or separation
- Infrequent visiting patterns in the neonatal intensive care unit

Physical Examination

- Signs of general neglect, such as poor skin hygiene, malnutrition, or failure to thrive
- Evidence of old healed lesions, such as burns (e.g., cigarettes, forced contact with heating devices), scalds (e.g., forced immersion, particularly of the buttocks and perineum), abrasions, and soft tissue swellings
- Evidence of sexual abuse, such as condylomata, perianal and genital hematoma, venereal disease (oral and genital), pain in anogenital area, and pregnancy

Dating the Injury

The physical examination should document growth parameters and include description of soft tissue injuries and photographs of all injuries. Retinal hemorrhages are said to be diagnostic of the shaken baby syndrome. Estimation of the age of cutaneous contusions on an abused child is usually more often requested of the pediatrician and the intensivist than the pathologist.

The contusions should be enumerated, and their pattern, shape, color, location, and size measured and catalogued. Wilson's summary (Table 27.3) has been an invaluable aid. Color photographs are essential in further documenting the nature of these lesions.

Table 27.3
Relationship Between Color and Age of Contusions[a]

Color	Age
Reddish-blue or purple	Immediate/<1 day
Blue-purple	1–5 days
Green	5–7 days
Yellow	7–10 days
Brown	10–14 days
Resolution	2–4 weeks

[a]Modified from Wilson EF. Estimation of the age of cutaneous contusion in child abuse. Pediatrics 1977;60:750. With permission.

Laboratory Investigation

Tests that may be essential in documenting and discerning the etiology of the child's problem include:

- Hematocrit, platelet count, and coagulation profile rule out a bleeding diathesis
- Electrolytes, blood urea nitrogen, liver function tests, and blood for toxicology to establish or rule out causes of coma, such as Reye syndrome, renal failure, and poisoning
- Urinalysis for toxicology and evidence of renal trauma
- Oral, genital, and anal cultures for evidence of venereal disease

Radiography

Radiographic assessment is mandatory. Studies to be obtained include posteroanterior and lateral skull and chest radiographs (i.e., for rib fractures), complete skeletal survey, including hands, long bones, fingers, and toes; and, when applicable, a CT scan.

Radiographic manifestation of child abuse reveals new and old injuries. Common findings include:

- Subperiosteal hemorrhages
- Epiphyseal separations
- Periosteal shearings
- Metaphyseal fragmentations
- Previously healed periosteal calcifications
- Shearing of the metaphysis

Computed Tomography Scanning

The CT scan is particularly important in assessing the child with an altered level of consciousness. This examination can reveal evidence of structural intracranial damage, such as:

- Intracranial hemorrhage
- Subdural or epidural hematoma
- Contusions
- Cerebral edema in the absence of major known trauma, such as occurs in motor vehicular injury

28.

Burns, Inhalational Injury, and Electrical Injury

Ellen A. Spurrier, Robert M. Spear, and Andrew M. Munster

Nearly 5,000 children die each year from burns, and many more are left scarred and disabled. Adequate fluid resuscitation, effective treatment of complications, and improved surgical techniques have increased survival over recent decades.

PATHOPHYSIOLOGY OF THERMAL INJURY

All tissues and organ systems demonstrate pathophysiologic changes as a result of thermal injury. These changes are summarized in Table 28.1.

ESTIMATION OF BURN SIZE AND DEPTH

Burn Size

Burn size is expressed as a percentage of the total body surface area (BSA). The contribution made by specific parts of the body to the total BSA changes, depending on the age of the child, until adult proportions are reached at 15 years of age. This percentage may be estimated by the "rule of nines" in children over age 15 years (Fig. 28.1) but requires a more exact measurement in younger children (Fig. 28.2). The size of one side of the child's hand, approximately equal to 1% of the BSA, may be useful in estimating the size of small burns.

Burn Depth

Burn depth traditionally has been classified in terms of degrees, first through fourth. A more useful classification has been favored by most clinicianssuperficial, superficial partial-thickness, deep partial-thickness, and full-thickness injury. The descriptions overlap, and both are outlined subsequently.

The size and depth of a burn should be estimated at regular intervals during the child's hospital course to assess possible extension of injury and healing. Clinicians with less than extensive experience in burn care should not make a definite diagnosis of the depth of a burn in the first few days, especially in smaller children, because the daily change in the appearance of the burn can be quite surprising.

First-degree Burn

This superficial injury is characterized by erythema and pain and perhaps minor blistering. Sunburn is an example. Tissue loss is restricted to epithelial cells. No treatment is required except for pain relief. Very rarely, an extensive first-degree burn may require intravenous fluid therapy.

Second-degree Burn

Tissue death occurs through the epidermis and into a variable portion of the dermis in the second-degree burn.

Table 28.1
Summary of Systems Affected by Thermal Injury

Integument
    Coagulation necrosis, cell death
    Edema
Cardiovascular
    Decreased cardiac output
    Lower central venous pressure and pulmonary capillary wedge pressure
    Hypertension
Pulmonary
    Increase in pulmonary arterial pressure
    Increase in lung lymph flow
    Pulmonary edema
Renal
    Decreased renal blood flow
    Increased glomerular filtration rate
    Hypermetabolic state
    Hyperdynamic circulation
Hepatic
    Clinical jaundice
    Conjugated hyperbilirubinemia
Hematologic
    Thrombocytopenia followed by thrombocytosis
    Increase in levels of fibrinogen and factors V and VII
    Elevated fibrin-fibrinogen split product levels
    Congenital coagulation disorders
    Disseminated intravascular coagulation
    Sepsis
    Hypofibrinogenemia
    Prolongation of prothrombin time and partial thromboplastin time
    Decrease in red cell mass
    Low hemoglobin
    Refractory anemia
Central nervous system
    Encephalopathy caused by hypoxia, hypovolemia, hyponatremia, sepsis, cortical vein
        thrombosis, and gliosis secondary to "water shed" infarct
Gastrointestinal
    Curling's ulcer
    Gastric mucosal abnormalities
    Acalculous cholecystitis
    Superior mesenteric artery syndrome
    Alterations in intestinal permeability
Metabolic
    Skeletal muscle breakdown
    Increased oxygen consumption
    Lipolysis
    Hepatic gluconeogenesis
Immunity and infection
    Immunocompromise
    Infection

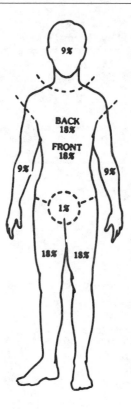

Figure 28.1. An estimate of the percentage of total body surface skin that is burned can be obtained by use of the "rule of nines" whereby the total surface area of skin is divided into areas equaling 9% of the total. (From Demling RH. Fluid and electrolyte management. Crit Care Clin 1985;1:34.)

Superficial Partial-Thickness Damage

The extent of damage to the dermis is slight in superficial partial-thickness damage. Healing takes place with little or no scarring. If the patient is black, pigment will return to the injured area. Clinically, a superficial partial-thickness burn is moist, red, and tender. Within a few days, the color becomes pale as the superficial eschar develops, but very often, viable dermal papillae can be seen through the thin eschar as tiny red dots separated by intervals of no more than 1 mm.

Deep Partial-Thickness Damage

Tissue necrosis occurs through most of the dermis, with preservation of the deepest portion of the dermal papillae and the skin appendages, in deep

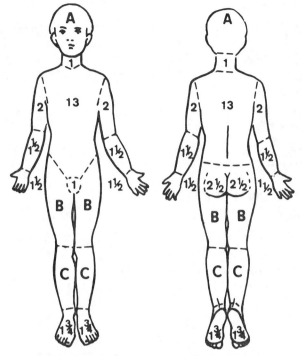

PERCENTAGE OF SURFACE AREA OF HEAD AND LEGS AT VARIOUS AGES.

	AGE IN YEARS				
AREA IN DIAGRAM	0	1	5	10	15
A = ½ of head	9½	8½	6½	5½	4½
B = ½ of one thigh	2¾	3¼	4	4¼	4½
C = ½ of one lower leg	2½	2½	2¾	3	3¼

Figure 28.2. This chart of body areas, together with the table showing the percentage of surface area of the head and legs at various ages, can be used to estimate the surface area burned in a child. (From Solomon JR. Pediatric burns. Crit Care Clin 1985;1:161.)

partial-thickness damage. Healing will still occur, but it will take up to 6 weeks and may be accompanied by scarring. If there is infection or nutritional inadequacy, bacterial invasion may convert this to a full-thickness burn.

Clinically, a deep partial-thickness burn is also moist and tender, but the developing eschar is whiter and appears thicker. Dermal papillae or "skin buds" either are not visible through the layer or, if visible, are separated by 2 to 3 mm.

Third-degree Burn

In this full-thickness injury, the necrotic area extends through all layers of the skin into the hypodermic fat. This type of burn may heal by contracture if it is very small, but surgical closure usually is indicated. The appearance of such a burn varies from dry and charred to red and nonblanching with pressure. It is not sensitive to touch.

Fourth-degree Burn

Fourth-degree burn implies deep injury to bone, joint, or muscle, usually occurring secondary to high-voltage electrical injury.

CLASSIFICATION OF BURNS

Minor Burn

The total surface area involved is less than 5%. No significant involvement of hands, feet, face, or perineum is present. No full-thickness component and no other complications are present. These children may be treated as outpatients if social circumstances permit.

Moderate Burn

A moderate burn is characterized by involvement of 5 to 15% of BSA or by the presence of any full-thickness component. Involvement of the hands, feet, face, or perineum or the presence of any complicating factor, such as chemical or electrical injury, also constitutes moderate burn. These patients should be admitted to the hospital.

Severe Burn

Severe burns are characterized by a total burn size greater than 15% of BSA, by a full-thickness component in excess of 5% of BSA, or by the presence of smoke inhalation or carbon monoxide poisoning. The child should be admitted to a special burn treatment facility or pediatric intensive care unit (PICU) after he or she is stabilized.

EPIDEMIOLOGY AND PREVENTION

Burns are a leading cause of death due to injury in young children (1–4 years) in the United States, second only to motor vehicle accidents. Burns are the third leading cause of injury-associated death in children overall (0–19 years), following motor vehicle accidents and drowning. Mortality associated with burn injury has declined over the past 10 years. It appears that young children, including infants, survive burn injury at least as well as young adults.

INITIAL CARE

Initial care of the burn victim as recommended by the Committee on Trauma of the American College of Surgeons involves:

- Assessment for airway compromise
- Stopping the burning process
- Beginning fluid resuscitation

Evaluation of Injury

Assessment of the degree of injury includes estimation of size and depth of burn as described previously. A brief history of the mechanism of injury may provide clues to associated trauma or inhalation injury. Exposure to fire in an enclosed space increases the likelihood of significant smoke inhalation. Explosions often propel the victim a distance, resulting in fractures, internal injuries, head trauma, flail chest, and pulmonary contusion. The patient's medical history should be ascertained as well.

Management Steps

Steps in the initial management of burn victims follow:

- Remove all of the patient's clothing; synthetic fibers may melt into hot plastic residue that continues to burn the patient
- Flush sites of chemical burns with copious amounts of water for 20 to 30 minutes
- Initiate early tracheal intubation in patients whose history or physical examination suggests thermal injury to the airway
- Place a large-bore intravenous catheter in a peripheral vein, through burn tissue if necessary, in patients with burns greater than 20% of BSA who require replacement of intravascular volume. In adolescents and adults, placement in an upper extremity is desirable because of a high incidence of phlebitis in saphenous veins.
- Begin an infusion of lactated Ringer's solution
- Place a bladder catheter to quantitate urine flow as a guide to fluid requirements in patients who are treated with intravenous fluid
- Place a nasogastric tube in patients with burns of significant magnitude
- Weigh the patient to allow calculation of estimated fluid needs
- Collect blood samples for complete blood count (CBC), type and crossmatch, carboxyhemoglobin, coagulation, and blood chemistry profiles. An arterial blood gas measurement may also be appropriate

Circumferential extremity burns require special care to prevent distal limb ischemia.

- Remove all jewelry and assess for cyanosis, impaired capillary refill, or neurologic signs (e.g., paresthesias or deep pain)

- Doppler assessment of pulses is useful
- Escharotomy may be necessary if circulatory insufficiency is present

Analgesia and Wound Care

Narcotic analgesics should be given only after assurance that restlessness and anxiety are caused by pain rather than by hypoxia or hypovolemic shock. Initial wound care should be limited to application of a clean dry dressing to decrease pain in partial-thickness burns. Blisters should be left intact. Antiseptic solutions are contraindicated, and applying cold water to relieve pain should be avoided in patients with extensive burns.

Tetanus Prophylaxis

Children more than 7 years of age who have completed their immunization series (i.e., three or more doses) should receive intramuscular adult type tetanus and diphtheria toxoids if it has been more than 5 years since their last dose. Younger children who have not completed three doses should receive diphtheria and tetanus toxoids or diphteria and tetanus toxoids and pertussis vaccine if appropriate. Any patient whose immunization series is uncertain or is less than three doses should receive the age-appropriate toxoid and tetanus immune globulin.

TRANSPORTING THE BURNED CHILD

Initial stabilization of the burned child may be carried out in the emergency department or PICU. After the airway is secured and fluid resuscitation and other appropriate measures have been undertaken to ensure tissue perfusion and oxygenation, the clinician should consider should referring the child to a regional burn center. An accurate and complete record of care delivered and patient data should accompany the patient.

In accordance with the recommendations of the American Burn Association, patients with the following injuries usually require referral to a burn center:

- Partial-thickness and third-degree burns involving more than 10% of the total BSA in patients under 10 years or over 50 years of age
- Partial-thickness and third-degree burns exceeding 20% of the BSA in other age groups
- Partial-thickness and third-degree burns involving the face, eyes, ears, hands, feet, genitalia, perineum, and major joints
- Third-degree burns larger than 5% of the BSA in any age group
- Electrical burns, including lightning injury (i.e., significant volumes of tissue beneath the surface may be injured and result in acute renal failure and other complications)
- Chemical burns

- Burns associated with significant fractures or other major injury in which the burn injury poses the greatest risk of morbidity or mortality
- Burn injury with inhalation injury
- Lesser burns in patients with significant preexisting disease

INTRAVENOUS FLUID THERAPY

The necessity of restoring intravascular volume with salt-containing fluids has led to improved survival of burn patients.

Urine Output

The most useful index of adequate intravascular replacement is urine output. A urine output of 0.5 to 1.0 mL/kg/hr is optimal. With rare exceptions, a urine output below 0.5 mL/kg/hr indicates insufficient intravascular volume.

Diuretics are rarely indicated in burn patients, and induced diuresis obscures the most useful gauge of intravascular volume. Diuretics may be necessary for some patients (i.e., those with electrical injury, soft tissue injury, muscle burn) with pigmenturia that does not clear with vigorous hydration. Other indices ordinarily useful in assessing volume status have limitations when applied to the burn patient.

Relation to Burn Size

As a practical guide:

- Children with burns exceeding 15% of BSA require intravenous resuscitation
- If the burn size exceeds 30% of BSA, placement of a central venous catheter is recommended
- If the burn is over 50% of BSA, two central venous catheters may be required

In children with burns greater than 30% of BSA, in whom the need for prolonged intravenous therapy can be anticipated, we place the initial intravenous catheter through a burned area while it is still relatively sterile, preserving unburned sites for later use. In smaller burns, the intravenous catheter should be placed in an unburned site.

Sterile technique in placing central catheters is of utmost importance because of the high incidence of infectious complications, including bacterial endocarditis, when using central venous and pulmonary artery catheters in burn patients.

Fluid Formulae

Crystalloid resuscitation provides the principal element necessary to restore circulating plasma volume, namely, the sodium ion. Investigations regarding the use of hypertonic saline solutions for burn resuscitation in hopes of decreasing fluid administration and tissue edema have yielded conflicting results. The most popular formula for estimating fluid requirements is the Parkland formula, a pure crystalloid formula that may be supplemented with colloid during the second 24 ours. We use the Parkland formula as follows.

First 24 hours: Lactated Ringer's solution, 4 mL/kg/BSA burned (in percent). In infants, maintenance fluid volume (1500 mL/m^2/day) given as lactated Ringer's solution must be added to the Parkland formula. One-half of this volume is given in the initial 8 hours postburn, and the other half is given during the next 16 hours. The rate of resuscitation should be adjusted to maintain a urine output of 0.5 to 1.0 mL/kg/hr.

Second 24 hours: Maintenance fluid (1500 mL/m^2/day) is begun with glucose-containing hypotonic fluid. Colloid may be used to improve urinary output and treat hypoalbuminemia. Following the second postburn day, the clinician should choose intravenous fluid that will maintain normal sodium, phosphate, calcium, and potassium homeostasis. Because of the intense adrenal response to burn stress, potassium wasting in the urine is common and may reach 200 mEq/L.

AIRWAY MANAGEMENT

Need for Intubation

Burn patients may require tracheal intubation for:

- Central nervous system dysfunction
- Inhalation injury to the lung
- Pneumonia
- Sepsis
- Surgical procedure with general anesthesia

Children with evidence of thermal injury to the airway should undergo tracheal intubation early, before edema progresses to airway obstruction and intubation becomes difficult or impossible.

Intubating the Child with Thermal Injury

Burns of the face, lips, pharynx, and hypopharynx can lead to massive edema, making visualization of the larynx extremely difficult or impossible. Tracheal intubation before the onset of edema allows a standard approach, namely, the use of intravenous anesthetics and a muscle relaxant. A "rapid sequence" technique with cricoid pressure is suggested, because aspiration of gastric contents is a significant risk.

The strategy for securing an airway in the child who has developed signs of upper airway obstruction is similar to that employed in other diseases in which upper airway anatomy is distorted (e.g., epiglottitis [see Chapter 2]). In these situations, muscle relaxants or sedation is contraindicated before successful tracheal intubation. With continuous monitoring and attention to cardiorespiratory status, the child should be transported to the operating room for intubation. Using a flexible fiberoptic bronchoscope as a guide for the tracheal tube may be successful. Tracheotomy should be avoided when possible in the burned patient, particularly when the tracheotomy would be placed through burned tissue.

Abnormal Response to Succinylcholine

Burn-injured patients develop abnormal responses to muscle relaxants that are frequently used to facilitate tracheal intubation and/or maintain neuromuscular blockade. Succinylcholine is contraindicated in burn patients beginning approximately 48 hours after injury. Hyperkalemia leading to cardiac arrest is a potential complication of succinylcholine use in the postburn period. Succinylcholine may be an appropriate drug for tracheal intubation during initial resuscitation, as its rapid onset and resolution are useful in the setting of a full stomach or questionable airway. The period of risk for succinylcholine-induced hyperkalemia begins 5 to 15 days postburn and lasts for 3 to 16 months.

Relative resistance to nondepolarizing muscle relaxants in seriously burned patients has been reported. The exact mechanism of this unusual response to depolarizing relaxants is unknown but would appear to be secondary to altered pharmacodynamics in patients with thermal injury.

WOUND MANAGEMENT

The burn wound should be cleansed gently with saline, and blisters should be debrided. This may be done in the hydrotherapy tub or in bed. Following a brief period of drying, a suitable topical agent should be applied to the wound, and the wound dressed. Escharotomy or fasciotomy may become necessary within hours of admission to relieve peripheral vascular or nerve compression. Occasionally, thoracic escharotomy is necessary to facilitate chest expansion.

Medications

It is our practice to administer penicillin to patients with major burns as antistreptococcal prophylaxis for 3 days. Penicillin may be given intravenously in doses appropriate for age. Intramuscular or subcutaneous medication should not be given in the early stages of burn therapy until complete cardiovascular stability has been established.

Topical Chemotherapy

The most commonly available agents and their advantages and disadvantages are outlined in Table 28.2. Topical therapy is applied twice daily following

Table 28.2
Commonly Used Topical Antibacterial Agents

Name	Advantages and Disadvantages	Side Effects	Dressing Orders
Silver sulfadiazine (Silvadene)	Broad antibacterial action; painless; fair penetration of eschar	Sulfonamide sensitivity (rash); absorption into fetal circulation is unknown; contraindicated in pregnancy; occasional leukopenia (reversible on discontinuation)	Apply twice daily; cover with a light layer of dressings on extremities; leave face and chest open
Mafenide (Sulfamylon)	Excellent antibacterial action, particularly against Gram-positives and *Clostridia*, also Gram-negatives; rapid eschar penetration	Painful; sulfonamide sensitivity (rash); carbonic anhydrase inhibition leading to acidosis	Apply twice daily; leave face, chest, and abdomen open; one light layer of dressings elsewhere
Aqueous silver nitrate solution	Universal antibacterial action; poor penetration of eschar	Leaking of chloride into the dressings with potential hypochloremic alkalosis; strong staining of tissues	Apply twice daily; dress with a light layer of gauze dressings
Iodophors (e.g., Efodine)	Universal antibacterial action; poor penetration of eschar	Strong staining of tissues; iodine absorption Rapid development of resistance; conjunctivitis if contacts the conjunctiva	Apply twice daily; dress with a light layer of gauze dressings
Topical bacitracin cream	Limited antibacterial action; poor eschar penetration; cosmetically acceptable, easy to apply; transparent		Should only be applied to small areas of cosmetic importance, e.g., second-degree burns of the face; leave open; apply twice daily

cleansing and debridement of the burn wound in a hydrotherapy tub or in bed. Light sterile dressings are applied following use of the topical cream. If silver nitrate solution is used, bulky dressings are necessary.

Biologic Dressings

Allograft, amnion, and artificial dressings are useful when the eschar has separated completely and the wound is clean and awaiting surgical closure. They are also useful for the protection of donor sites after surgery and on fresh partial-thickness burns for pain relief, provided the area involved is not large enough to need thorough protection from infection, which biologic dressings do not provide. Of the materials available, allograft is preferred by most burn surgeons, with fresh, fresh frozen, and lyophilized being the order of priority.

Surgery

Indications

Surgery for wound closure is required for areas of full-thickness injury and for areas of deep partial-thickness burn that would heal with delay and scarring. In patients with burns of life-threatening size, there is urgency in performing surgery and covering the wound before substantial colonization takes place.

Wound Coverage

The principal form of wound coverage is autografting, which creates a donor site. During the last decade, the following technique for culturing autologous and allogenic epithelium for burn wound coverage has been developed. Grafting may be performed to a clean burn bed from which all eschar has separated or to a surgically excised burn bed. The practice of early surgical excision and closure is becoming increasingly popular. Ideally, the wound is excised and closed as soon as the child is stable enough for a major general anesthetic, often within the first 2 to 3 days of admission.

NUTRITION

Appropriate nutrition has a major impact on the recovery of burn victims. In addition to meeting the patient's requirements for macronutrients and micronutrients, the composition, timing, and route of feeding may influence metabolic rate, immune function, and rate of infection. Nutritional support, therefore, may affect length of hospital stay and mortality in patients with serious burns.

Formulae for Determining Energy Needs

Formulae in current use are summarized in Table 28.3. The lower range of target calories recommended by Wolfe or the Recommended Dietary

Table 28.3
Formulae for Determining Energy Needs of Pediatric Burn Patients

	Age (y)	Daily Requirement
Wolfe	All	Basal metabolic rate × 2
Hildreth and Carvajal	All	1800 kcal/m^2 + 2200 kcal/m^2 body surface burned
Recommended daily allowance (RDA)	0–0.5	kg weight × 115 kcal
	0.5–1.0	kg weight × 105 kcal
	1–3	kg weight × 100 kcal
	4–10	kg weight × 85 kcal
	M: 11–14	kg weight × 60 kcal
	F: 11–14	kg weight × 48 kcal
Curreri Junior	0–1	Basal cal + 15 kcal/% burn
	1–3	Basal cal + 25 kcal/% burn
	3–15	Basal cal + 40 kcal/% burn

Allowance provides a reasonable starting point for pediatric burn patients. Current recommendations for patients with burns of more than 10% of BSA are 20% total kilocalories provided from protein, nonprotein kcal:/nitrogen ratio 100:1 or 2.5 g/kg/day amino acids.

Route of Feeding

Enteral feeding appears to have benefits over the parenteral route in preventing hypermetabolism and catabolism and intestinal translocation of viable organisms. Very early (i.e., 4 hours postinjury) institution of enteral nutrition may lead to early achievement of positive nitrogen balance.

PAIN MANAGEMENT

Pain associated with burn injuries may vary from continuous background pain of moderate intensity to excruciating pain associated with therapeutic procedures such as debridement, physical therapy, and burn dressing change. Pain relief guidelines follow.

Mild to Moderate Pain

Nonopioid analgesics such as acetaminophen may be useful for suppressing mild background pain. Moderate pain may be responsive to orally administered opioids (e.g., oxycodone, morphine) or in the instance of continuous pain, methadone or sustained-release preparations of morphine. Most children find the oral route of administration acceptable.

Severe Pain

Intravenous morphine is widely administered when pain is severe. Initial dosage of 0.1 to 0.2 mg/kg is recommended with the caveat that the effective dose will vary from patient to patient. Frequent small doses (0.02–0.04 mg/kg) may be administered every 5 to 10 minutes to achieve adequate analgesia without rigid adherence to a standard dosage.

Tolerance can be anticipated when opioids are administered over an extended time, and doses may be adjusted upward. Respiratory depression due to opioid administration is unusual during painful procedures but may be reversed with naloxone should it occur.

Short Duration of Pain Control

Fentanyl may be useful for a particularly painful intervention of short duration. Ketamine has been used successfully in alleviating pain associated with short procedures in burn units. The popularity of ketamine stems from its properties of:

• Profound analgesia
• Respiratory and cardiovascular stimulation
• Relative preservation of airway reflexes

Side effects include:

• Hypertension
• Delirium
• Hallucinations
• Aspiration of gastric contents
• Laryngospasm

Anticholinergics (i.e., glycopyrolate, atropine) need to be administered with ketamine.

Patient-Controlled Analgesia

Patient-controlled analgesia (PCA) has been shown to be safe and effective in managing postoperative pain in children and adolescents, and a preliminary report suggests efficacy in burn patients.

PSYCHOSOCIAL ASPECTS OF BURN THERAPY
Need for Support

The care of the severely burned child is an exceedingly stressful experience for the child, family, and staff. Fear, pain, abandonment, and disfigurement contribute to the child's emotional difficulties following injury. There is evidence that the approach taken by burn nurses to aversive procedures such as burn dressing change influences the child's emotional response to those events and hospitalization in general.

Family members of a burned child are also vulnerable to emotional problems. They often feel guilt, and concerns regarding the child's survival, finances, and disruption of the home may be overwhelming. The patient and family are in need of psychologic support from the outset and may require years of care.

Child Abuse

Evidence of child abuse should be sought at admission of a burned child. Specific patterns of burn injury that strongly suggest inflicted injury are:

- Isolated burns of the buttocks
- Symmetrically scalded hands or feet of full-thickness depth (i.e., indicating forcible immersion in hot liquid)

SMOKE INHALATION INJURY

Inhalation injury accounts for a large percentage (i.e., 50–80%) of the mortality associated with major burns. Victims of smoke inhalation may succumb to asphyxia, thermal injury of the airway, carbon monoxide and cyanide toxicities, or pulmonary injury.

Asphyxia

Asphyxia probably accounts for death in most fire victims who die before reaching the hospital. In an enclosed space, fire rapidly consumes the available oxygen, with ambient oxygen concentration falling to 5% in some circumstances. The cardiodepressant effects of inhaled toxic fumes may further diminish oxygen delivery to the brain and other vital organs. Hypoxia interferes with mental and physical capacities and, consequently, with the ability of a victim to escape from a burning environment.

Thermal Injury of the Airway

Direct thermal injury to the lungs may occur when steam is inhaled, because it has 4000 times the heat-carrying capacity of dry air. Thermal injury from smoke inhalation, usually limited to the supraglottic airway, may cause life-threatening airway edema very rapidly; therefore, a high index of suspicion and early recognition are paramount.

Clues to significant thermal inhalation injury include:

- History of enclosed-space fire
- An unconscious victim
- Respiratory distress
- Burns to lips and nose

- Stridor and hoarseness
- Soot in the mouth or nose

These findings should prompt an examination of the mucosal surfaces of the mouth and pharynx for evidence of erythema or blisters. If this examination is positive or if there is evidence of evolving airway obstruction, tracheal intubation should be performed.

Fiberoptic examination may allow a more thorough inspection of the supraglottic airway for burns and perhaps facilitate intubation. Special considerations regarding tracheal intubation of burned patients were described previously and in Chapter 2.

Carbon Monoxide Poisoning

Carbon monoxide (CO) intoxication accounts for nearly half of the fatal poisonings in the United States, with 3,500 people dying each year from exposure to it. The higher metabolic rate of the child results in more rapid uptake of CO, putting the pediatric patient at significant risk from CO exposure.

Diagnosis

The diagnosis of CO poisoning is made from a history of exposure, physical signs and symptoms, and laboratory data, including measurement of CO hemoglobin concentration. A CO hemoglobin value within normal limits does not rule out recent CO poisoning, however. If significant time has elapsed

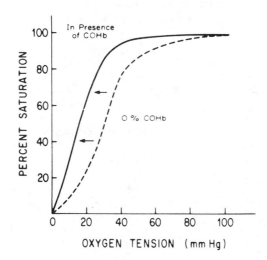

Figure 28.3. Oxygen Saturation in Carbon Monoxide Poisoning. (From Zimmerman SS, Truxal B. Carbon Monoxide poisoning. Pediatrics 1981;68:218, reproduced by permission of Pediatrics.)

since exposure to CO or if supplemental oxygen has been given, the CO hemoglobin values may have declined by the time the first blood sample was analyzed for CO hemoglobin concentration.

Clinicians may be misled and rule out CO poisoning when a normal oxygen saturation is reported, because oxygen saturation usually is estimated on the basis of measured partial pressures of oxygen. The partial pressure of oxygen is frequently normal in CO poisoning (or greater than normal if oxygen is administered), although the oxygen saturation of hemoglobin is low. In the presence of a significant CO hemoglobin concentration, oximetry is required to measure the actual oxygen saturation of hemoglobin. Pulse oximetry also is inaccurate in carbon monoxide poisoning because CO hemoglobin absorbs light at the wavelengths used by this device. To the pulse oximeter, CO hemoglobin looks like oxygen hemoglobin, and therefore, a patient with high CO hemoglobin levels and low SaO_2 will have a normal saturation measured by pulse oximetry.

Organ System Responses to Carbon Monoxide Poisoning

Carbon monoxide poisoning affects most organ systems to varying degrees (Table 28.4).

Signs, Symptoms, and Presentation

The signs and symptoms of CO poisoning in the pediatric patient may be subtle and nonspecific, making the diagnosis of CO poisoning difficult when a typical history of exposure is lacking. Symptoms associated with varying concentrations of carboxyhemoglobin are presented in Table 28.5.

Therapy

The mainstays in the critical care of the child poisoned with CO are oxygen therapy, supportive care, and specific treatment of complications:

- The comatose or hypercapnic child should be intubated.
- Cerebral edema, if present, should be treated with hyperventilation, hyperosmolar agents (e.g., mannitol), diuretics, and fluid restriction. Steroids, contraindicated in major burns, are frequently used, although evidence of efficacy is lacking.
- Mild acidosis should not be corrected pharmacologically, because acidosis results in a rightward shift of the oxyhemoglobin dissociation curve, facilitating release of oxygen to tissues.

Oxygen Therapy

Oxygen (100%) by a tight-fitting, nonrebreathing mask should be given as soon as CO poisoning is suspected and should be maintained until the CO hemoglobin concentration falls below 5%. It is inappropriate to

Table 28.4
Organ System Responses to Carbon Monoxide (CO) Poisoning

Cardiovascular
  Elevation of heart rate
  Cardiac output increase as CO hemoglobin concentration exceeds 30%
  S-T segment and T-wave abnormalities
  Atrial fibrillation
  Intraventricular block
  Extrasystoles
  Ischemia
  Infarction
Pulmonary
  Edema, possibly caused by tissue hypoxia, toxic effects of CO on alveolar membranes,
    myocardial damage leading to left ventricle failure, aspiration after loss of
    consciousness, concomitant smoke inhalation, neurogenic pulmonary edema
Neurologic
  Headache
  Lethargy
  Delirium
  Depression
  Irritability
  Akinetic mutism
  Amnesia
  Dysphasia
  Unilateral/bilateral pyramidal signs
  Extrapyramidal signs
  Hemiplegia
  Cortical blindness
  Delayed neurologic changes
  Disorientation
  Slurred speech
  Dizziness
  Weakness
  Seizures
  Decreased level of consciousness
  Facial spasms and trismus
  Cerebral edema
  Sequelae including memory impairment, personality alterations, and signs of parietal
    lobe dysfunction
Muscular and renal
  Muscle necrosis leading to myoglobinuria and subsequent acute renal failure
Cutaneous
  Erythema
  Edema
  Blistering
  Skin necrosis
Ophthalmologic
  Blindness
  Visual field deficits secondary to cortical lesions
  Retinal venous congestions
  Retinal papilledema
  Retinal hemorrhages
  Red retinal veins

continued

Table 28.4
Organ System Responses to Carbon Monoxide (CO) Poisoning

Auditory
  Hearing loss
  Tinnitus
  Nystagmus
  Ataxia
Miscellaneous
  Hyperamylasemia
  Hyperuricemia
  Hepatic and intestinal injury
  Neurologic and sequelae in unborn child of CO-poisoned mother

Table 28.5
Symptoms Associated with Varying Concentrations of Carbon Monoxide (CO) Hemoglobin

CO in Atmosphere (%)	CO Hemoglobin in Blood (%)	Physiologic and Subjective Symptoms
0.007	10	Shortness of breath on vigorous exertion; possible tightness across the forehead; dilation of cutaneous blood vessels
0.012	20	Shortness of breath on moderate exertion; occasional headache with throbbing in temples
0.022	30	Decided headache; irritable; easily fatigued; judgment disturbed; possible dizziness; dimness of vision
0.035	40–50	Headache; confusion; collapse; fainting on exertion
0.080	60–70	Unconsciousness; intermittent convulsion; respiratory failure; death if exposure is prolonged
0.195	80	Rapidly fatal

withhold oxygen therapy until laboratory confirmation of CO poisoning is obtained.

Oxygen is critical in eliminating CO by mass action, significantly reducing the half-life of CO. The half-life of CO is 5 to 6 hours when breathing 21% oxygen, one and one-half hours when breathing of 100% oxygen, and less than 30 minutes when breathing 100% oxygen at 2.5 atmospheres absolute pressure (ATA) (Table 28.6).

Table 28.6
Body Oxygen Levels on Room Air, 100% Oxygen at 1 ATA, and 100% Oxygen at 2 ATA[a]

Body Site	Breathing Room Air	100% Oxygen at 1 ATA	100% Oxygen at 2 ATA
Inspired PO_2	147 torr	760 torr	1520 torr
Alveolar PO_2	105 torr	660+ torr	1400+ torr
Arterial PO_2	80–100 torr	500+ torr	1200+ torr
Hemoglobin oxygen	19.1 mL O_2/100 mL	20.1 mL O_2/100 mL	20.1 mL O_2/100 mL
Dissolved oxygen	+0.3 mL O_2/100 mL	+2.3 mL O_2/100 mL	+4.3 mL O_2/100 mL
Total blood oxygen	19.4 mL O_2/100 mL	22.1 mL O_2/100 mL	24.1 mL O_2/100 mL
Tissue PO_2	40 to 50 torr	50 to 100 torr	300 to 400 torr
Tissue O_2	0.10 mL O_2/100 mL	0.15 to 0.3 mL O_2/100 mL	0.9 to 1.2 mL O_2/100 mL

[a]Assuming normal lungs and circulation and a hemoglobin level of 15 g/dL.

Hyperbaric Oxygen Therapy

Hyperbaric oxygen allows adequate tissue oxygenation by means of oxygen dissolved in plasma rather than oxygen carried by hemoglobin. The dissolved oxygen content alone approaches the amount necessary to supply oxygen requirements (see Table 28.6). See Chapter 6 for more information on hyperbaric oxygen therapy.

Hyperbaric oxygen is considered the mainstay of therapy for a patient with a CO hemoglobin concentration above 25% and signs and symptoms of CO poisoning. Meyers et al. recommend 46 minutes of 100% O_2 at 3 ATA, followed by 2 ATA for 2 hours or until the CO hemoglobin level falls below 10%. Patients who remain unconscious are given a second treatment 6 hours later. At this time, the benefit of hyperbaric oxygen versus 100% oxygen in CO poisoning remains unknown, although some authors believe that hyperbaric oxygen therapy may lead to a reduction in sequelae and may be useful in the therapy of recurrent symptoms in CO poisoning.

Prognosis

Larkin et al. found acidosis on admission to be a poor prognostic sign in CO poisoning. Yet Strohl et al. reported that three patients with acidosis, including one patient with a pH of 6.34 recovered without neurologic sequelae. Bour and Ledingham found that reversal of coma within the first 48 hours was associated with recovery. Correlation between level of consciousness on admission and development of neuropsychiatric sequelae has been identified. Long-term follow-up is necessary to identify and treat the sequelae of CO poisoning.

Cyanide Toxicity

Hydrogen cyanide is present in smoke generated by the combustion of many materials present in the household. Blood cyanide levels in the lethal range have been detected in victims of house fires and air crashes. Cyanide poisoning from smoke rarely occurs in the absence of CO toxicity, and the two may act synergistically to inhibit oxidative metabolism. The treatment of cyanide poisoning in the setting of smoke inhalation is difficult because a rapid diagnostic test is not usually available and the antidotes may have adverse effects.

Pulmonary Inhalation Injury

Smoke is composed of many respiratory irritants produced during combustion of structural materials and home furnishings. It is the effect of these chemicals rather than heat that account for the lung pathology produced by smoke inhalation.

Characteristic pathophysiologic changes include:

- Mucosal erythema, edema, and areas of mucosal sloughing in the tracheobronchial tree and pulmonary parenchyma
- Increased pulmonary capillary permeability
- Increased lung lymph flow
- Higher extravascular lung water content
- Decreased ciliary function
- Destruction of pulmonary macrophages
- Altered surfactant production

Clinical Features

The clinical correlates of this widespread pathophysiology include:

- Increased airway resistance
- Airway plugging
- Bronchorrhea
- Interstitial edema
- Atelectasis
- Decreased pulmonary compliance
- Bronchitis
- Pneumonia
- Respiratory failure

Victims most severely affected develop respiratory insufficiency early, with prominent bronchospasm and lung consolidation. The development of pulmonary edema characterizes a second phase, with onset 6 to 72 hours from injury. Almost all children surviving beyond day 3 develop bronchopneumonia.

Diagnosis

Patients with pulmonary injury resulting from smoke inhalation may be asymptomatic and have a normal chest radiograph or minor abnormality on presentation. Often, inhalation injury must be diagnosed on the basis of a history of smoke exposure in a closed environment. Arterial blood gases may be normal for 12 to 24 hours, and the earliest abnormality is often a decreased ratio of arterial PO_2 to percentage of inspired oxygen.

Therapy

The treatment of smoke inhalation respiratory injury is supportive.

- Humidified oxygen
- Aggressive pulmonary toilet
- Mechanical ventilation and positive end-expiratory pressure in cases of severe injury

Fluid therapy in patients with inhalational injury traditionally has been parsimonious, because of fears of inducing or exacerbating pulmonary edema. Little modification of traditional burn resuscitation formulae seems indicated, although urine output in the low-normal range (0.5 mL/kg/hr) is acceptable.

Antibiotics are indicated for documented or suspected infection. Pathogens causing pneumonia include *Staphylococcus aureus* in the initial days postburn and Gram-negative organisms, particularly the *Pseudomonas* species, subsequently. Corticosteroid usage is controversial in inhalational injury. Infectious complications are more frequent in patients treated with steroids.

ELECTRICAL INJURY

Electrical injury encompasses several different types of injury, including the severe surface and deep tissue injury associated with heat production as current flows through tissues. High-voltage injury, including lightning injury, results in the most significant damage and is discussed subsequently. Electrical injury also involves pathophysiologic changes that occur as low-voltage electrical current flows through vital structures such as the heart and the central nervous system. Multisystem dysfunction with a variety of complications is common in severe electrical injury.

Pathophysiology

Electrical injury is primarily a burn resulting from heat produced as current flows through the resistance of tissues. In limbs of smaller cross-sectional area, the tissue damage is greater because current density is higher and is concentrated in a smaller area; therefore, the heat per unit volume of tissue is greater. In the past, emphasis on varying tissue resistances underscored the belief that once skin resistance was overcome, current traveled preferentially through tissues of low resistance. In high-tension electrical injury, however, this is not the case.

Types of Electrical Injury

The amount of tissue damage in electrical injury depends on several factors, including voltage. By definition, high-tension electrical injury occurs when voltage is greater than 1000 V.

Three types of injury are found in high-tension electrical injury.

Surface Burns

This injury results from ignition of clothing or from the heat of the current traveling close to the skin. These burns are frequently full-thickness, because the dazed or unconscious patient is unable to escape from the environment.

Entry/Exit Wounds

The entry wound usually is charred and depressed, with swelling proximal to the wound. At the site of grounding, a collection of energy results in extensive tissue necrosis as the current explodes through the skin, creating an exit wound that is usually charred, dry, and circumscribed.

Arc Burns

Arc burns are produced by a current that travels external to the body, as an electric arc forms between two objects of opposite charge (usually a highly charged source and the ground). The arc contains electrons and ionized particles and takes a fusiform course from one pole to the other, with burns occurring when the arc strikes the patient. The temperature of such arcs may reach 3000°C.

Type of Current

At low voltages, alternating current is more dangerous than direct current because of its ability to "freeze" the extremity to the source of electricity. The slowly alternating current of household sources (60 Hz) results in tetanic muscle contractions. If a hand makes contact with the source, the victim may be unable to release the grasp, because the forearm flexors are more powerful than the extensors. Resistance and heat production are increased until carbonization of tissue occurs and the point of contact is broken. At high frequencies, alternating and direct current have a similar effect because the sensitivity of the individual muscle fiber to electrical stimulus is exceeded.

Clinical and Pathologic Findings

The hallmark of electrical injury is a deep burn, frequently involving muscle and other structures. This type of injury necessitates a different therapeutic approach than is used with surface burns, as clinical course, complications, and sequelae are unique to this type of thermal injury.

Cardiorespiratory Findings

Cardiac arrest is common in electrical injuries and is precipitated by a variety of mechanisms:

- The conducting system of the heart is particularly sensitive to the common frequency of 60 Hz, with ventricular fibrillation caused by current passing through the chest at 100 mA, such as between an arm and a leg or between both arms.
- Asphyxiation can result from tetanic spasm of the respiratory muscles at a current density of 30 mA.
- Respiratory arrest without cardiac arrest may result from electrical injury and rapidly leads to cardiac arrest if artificial ventilation is not instituted.
- Death can result from cardiac arrest in electrical injury without demonstrable surface injury.
- Transient arrhythmias occur in 30% of patients.
- Cardiac rupture has been reported.

Neurologic Findings

Frequent neurologic complications are:

- Loss of consciousness
- Seizures
- Deafness
- Mood disturbances
- Peripheral nerve injury, secondary to vascular injury or thermal injury or by a direct effect of the electrical current

Following electrical injury, peripheral nerve injury is usually transient, unless the injury is a direct result of the burn.

Renal Findings

Acute renal failure is more common in electrical than surface burns, occurring, in part, from the massive release of myoglobin from damaged muscle. Renal injury can also result from direct damage by the electrical current.

Vascular Findings

Vascular complications include delayed hemorrhage from underlying vessels and thrombosis resulting from progressive tissue edema.

Gastrointestinal Findings

Gastrointestinal complications include gastroduodenal ulcerations, ileus, and late development of cholelithiasis.

Treatment

Cardiopulmonary Resuscitation

Prompt cardiopulmonary resuscitation results in a favorable prognosis in patients suffering cardiac arrest from electrical injury. Vigorous and prolonged resuscitation of such victims is indicated.

Fluid Administration

Fluid therapy is similar to that for burn injury, although larger volumes usually are necessary for a given percentage of surface burn, because of the large "hidden" component of electrical injury. Fluid administration is adjusted to maintain a liberal urine output (i.e., 2 mL/kg/hr) until gross clearing of myoglobinuria occurs. Mannitol and sodium bicarbonate are advocated by some to prevent acute tubular necrosis from pigment precipitation in the renal tubules. Intravenous fluids are adjusted following gross clearing of pigmenturia to maintain a urine output of 0.5 to 1.5 mL/kg/hr.

Fasciotomy

Indications for immediate surgical decompression include:

• Extensive limb burns
• Marked limb edema
• Decreased distal nerve function
• Absent pulses
• Persistent severe pain

Lightning

Lightning is a fascinating, albeit uncommon form of high-voltage electrical injury. Only 150—300 people die each year in the United States secondary to lightning strike. Nearly two thirds of people struck by lightning survive. The injury incurred from lightning is often devastating, because temperatures of 60,000°F and current exceeding 1 million V are generated. As with other high-voltage injury, survival depends, in part, on rapid cardiopulmonary resuscitation, as apnea rather than cardiac standstill is the primary event that ultimately leads to arrhythmia and death.

29.

Pain, Sedation, and Postoperative Anesthetic Management in the Pediatric Intensive Care Unit

Myron Yaster, Jolene D. Bean, Scott R. Schulman, and Mark C. Rogers

INTRODUCTION

In the intensive care unit, pain and sedation management often is ignored and relegated to the lowest rank of therapeutic priorities because of the fear that critically ill patients can neither tolerate potent analgesic drugs nor their side effects. Unfortunately, in its extremes, this policy has resulted in children being paralyzed with muscle relaxants without the concomitant use of analgesics, hypnotics, or amnestics despite the fact that muscle relaxants have absolutely no sedative or analgesic properties.

PAIN ASSESSMENT

Pain intensity or severity can be measured in children as young as 3 years of age by using either the "Oucher" scale (developed by Dr. J. Beyer), which is a two part scale with a vertical numerical scale (0–100) on one side and six photographs of a young child on the other (Fig. 29.1).

In infants and critically ill patients who are unable to communicate, pain has been assessed by measuring physiologic and behavioral responses to nociceptive stimuli:

- Blood pressure
- Heart rate changes
- Levels of adrenal stress hormones
- Facial expression
- Body movements
- Presence of tears
- Intensity and quality of crying

We use the behavioral scoring system developed by Hannallah et al. (Table 29.1) to assess postoperative pain. Defining the location of pain accurately is readily accomplished by using either dolls or action figures or by using drawings of body outlines, both front and back.

NONOPIOID (OR "WEAKER") ANALGESICS

The "weaker" or "milder" analgesics, of which acetaminophen (i.e., Tylenol) and salicylate (i.e., aspirin) are the classic examples, comprise a heterogenous group of nonsteroidal anti-inflammatory drugs (NSAID). These agents are administered enterally via the oral or, on occasion, the rectal route, and are particularly useful for inflammatory, bony, or rheumatic pain. Ketorolac can be administered parenterally (0.5 mg/kg 6 times/hour; maximum dose 30 mg).

This family of drugs is the most preferred group of analgesics prescribed by pediatricians because they are relatively safe, have few cardiopulmonary side effects, and are nonaddictive. The nonopioid analgesics often are administered in combination with more potent agents, such as

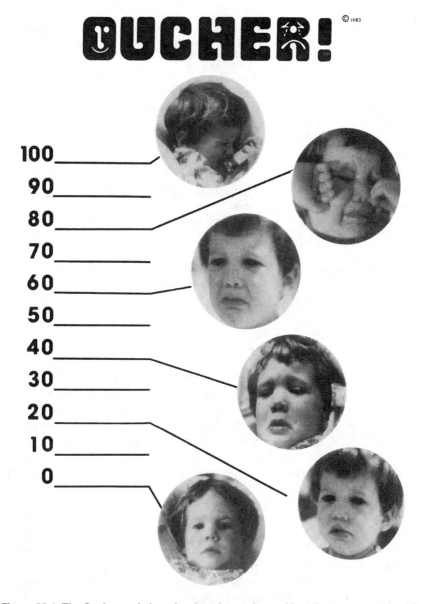

Figure 29.1. The Oucher scale is a visual analog scale used in pain assessment in children. Note that the higher the score, the greater the child's pain. (Developed and copyrighted by Judith E. Beyer, R.N., Ph.D. For more information, contact Dr. Beyer at the University of Colorado Health Sciences Center School of Nursing, Denver, CO. The Oucher scale is reprinted with permission from its author.)

Table 29.1
Objective Pain Score[a]

Blood pressure (systolic)	≤10% of control	0
	11–20% of control	1
	>21% of control	2
Crying?	Not crying	0
	Crying but responds to TLC	1
	Crying but does not respond to TLC	2
Movement	None	0
	Restless	1
	Thrashing	2
Agitation	Patient asleep or calm	0
	Mild	1
	Hysterical	2
Verbal evaluation or body language	Asleep or states no pain (preverbal child—no special posture)	0
	Mild pain or cannot localize (preverbal child—flexing extremities)	1
	Moderate pain and can localize (preverbal child—holding location of pain)	2

[a]A score ≥6 signifies significant pain and should be treated with a potent analgesic.

codeine because, regardless of dose, they reach a "ceiling effect" above which pain cannot be relieved.

There is little information in the pediatric literature on the use of the newer NSAIDs, such as ibuprofen, naprosyn, tolectin, indomethacin, or ketorolac. Furthermore, because of its possible role in the production of Reye syndrome, aspirin has been largely abandoned in pediatric practice as well. Fortunately, acetaminophen is equally effective and potent as aspirin in the treatment of pain. When administered in normal doses ($10–15$ mg/kg^{-1}), it has few serious side effects. Acute overdosage or poisoning may produce fulminant hepatic failure and death.

OPIOIDS

Opioid Receptors

The opioids most commonly used in the management of pain are μ-agonists (Table 29.2). Mixed agonist-antagonist drugs act as agonists or partial agonists at one receptor and antagonists at another receptor. Mixed (opioid) agonist-antagonist drugs include pentazocine, butorphanol, nalorphine, and nalbuphine. Most of these drugs are agonists or partial agonists at the κ- and σ-receptors and antagonists at the μ-receptor.

The μ-receptor and its subspecies and the κ-receptor produce analgesia, respiratory depression, euphoria, and physical dependence. The κ-re-

Table 29.2
Commonly Used μ-Agonist Drugs

Agonist	Equipotent IV Dose (mg/kg)	Duration (h)	Bioavailability (%)	Comments
Morphine	0.1	3–4	20–40	Seizures in newborns; also in all patients at high doses Histamine release, vasodilation→→avoid in asthmatics and in circulatory compromise MS-contin 8–12 h duration
Meperidine	1.0	3–4	40–60	Catastrophic interactions with MAO inhibitors Tachycardia; negative inotrope Metabolite produces seizures; not recommended for chronic use
Methadone	0.1	6–24	70–100	Can be given IV even though the package insert says s.c. or IM
Fentanyl	0.001	0.5–1.0		Bradycardia; minimal hemodynamic alterations Chest, wall rigidity (>5 μg/kg rapid IV bolus); Rx naloxone or a succinylcholine, pancuronium
Codeine	1.2	3–4	40–70	PO only Prescribe with acetaminophen
Hydromorphone (Dilaudid)	0.015–0.02	3–4	40–60	< Central nervous system depression than morphine < Itching, nausea than morphine Can be used in IV and epidural patient-controlled analgesia
Oxycodone (component opioid in Tylox)	0.1	3–4	50–70	Excellent oral bioavailability, much less nausea and vomiting than codeine and is preferred; often prescribed combined with acetaminophen (Tylox)

ceptor, located primarily in the spinal cord, produces spinal analgesia, miosis, and sedation with minimal associated respiratory depression.

Morphine

Pharmacologic Effects Morphine (from Morpheus, the Greek god of sleep) is the standard for analgesia against which all other opioids are compared. When small doses, 0.1 mg/kg^{-1} (intravenous, intramuscular), are administered to otherwise unmedicated patients in pain, analgesia usually occurs without loss of consciousness. The range of physiologic effects of morphine and all other narcotics at equipotent doses is detailed in Table 29.3.

Table 29.3
Physiologic Effects of Opioids by Organ System

Central Nervous System	Respiratory System	Cardiovascular System	Gastrointestinal System	Urinary System
Analgesia	Antitussive	Bradycardia (fentanyl, morphine)	Decreased motility and peristalsis (treatment for diarrhea, constipation common)	Increased tone in ureters, bladder, and detrusor muscles of the bladder
Sedation	Decreased minute ventilation, respiratory rate, and tidal volume	Tachycardia (meperidine)	Increased sphincter tone: sphincter of Oddi, ileocolic	
Nausea and vomiting	Depressed ventilatory response to carbon dioxide and oxygen	Histamine release, venodilation (morphine)		
Miosis		Minimal effects on cardiac output, except meperidine		
Seizures				
Dysphoria				
Euphoria				
Psychotomimetic behaviors, excitation				

The elimination half-life of morphine in adults and older children is 3 to 4 hours and is consistent with its duration of analgesic action. The $t1/2\beta$ is more than twice as long in newborns younger than 1 week of age than in older children and adults, and is even longer in premature infants. Clearance is similarly decreased in the newborn compared to the older child and adult; therefore, infants younger than 1 month of age will attain higher serum levels that will decline more slowly than older children and adults. This may also account for the increased respiratory depression associated with morphine in this age group.

Clinical signs that predict impending respiratory depression include somnolence, small pupils, and small tidal volumes. Aside from newborns, patients at particular risk include those with:

- Altered mental status
- Hemodynamic instability
- History of apnea or disordered control of ventilation
- Hepatic or renal disease
- Known airway problem

Suggested Dosage The "unit" dose of intravenously administered morphine (0.1 mg/kg) is modified based on patient age and disease state (see Table 29.2). To minimize the complications associated with intravenous morphine (or any opioid) administration, we recommend titration of the dose at the bedside until the desired level of analgesia is achieved. Use of continuous infusion regimens of morphine (0.02 to 0.03 mg/kg/hour) and patient-controlled analgesia help to maximize pain-free periods. Longer acting agonists, such as methadone, may be used.

Because of limited bioavailability of oral morphine, the clinician needs to multiply the intravenous dose by three to five times when converting intravenous morphine requirements to oral maintenance. Oral morphine is available as a liquid, tablet, and sustained release preparations (MS-contin). MS-contin cannot be crushed and given via a feeding tube.

Fentanyl(s)

Because of its rapid onset and brief duration of action, fentanyl has become a favored analgesic for:

- Bone marrow aspirations
- Fracture reductions
- Suturing lacerations
- Endoscopy
- Dental procedures

Fentanyl is approximately 100 times more potent than morphine (the equianalgesic dose is 0.001 mg/kg^{-1}, see Table 29.2). Sufentanil, a potent fentanyl derivative, is approximately 10 times more potent than fentanyl. It is most commonly used as the principal component of cardiac anesthesia and is administered in doses of 1 to 30 µg/kg. Alfentanil is approximately 5 to 10 times less potent than fentanyl and has an extremely short duration of action, usually less than 15 to 20 minutes.

Pharmacologic Effects Fentanyl's ability to block nociceptive stimuli with concomitant hemodynamic stability is excellent and makes it the drug of choice for trauma, cardiac, or intensive care unit patients. Fentanyl also prevents the biochemical and endocrine stress (catabolic) response to painful stimuli that may be so detrimental in the seriously ill patient. Rapid infusions of fentanyl (0.005 mg/kg^{-1} or greater) is associated with chest wall rigidity, which may make ventilation difficult or impossible. Chest wall rigidity can be treated with either muscle relaxants, such as succinylcholine or pancuronium, or with naloxone.

Suggested Dosage To provide analgesia for short procedures, 2 to 3 µg/kg is delivered intravenously. The dosage is reduced if any sedative (e.g., midazolam or chloral hydrate) is administered concomitantly.

To provide virtually complete anesthesia in the ICU or operating room, the dosage is 10 to 50 µg/kg. The lower dose is often used to provide anesthesia for intubation, particularly in the newborn and in head trauma, cardiac, and hemodynamically unstable patients.

To provide analgesia and sedation in intubated and mechanically ventilated patients, particularly those receiving ECMO, a loading dose of 10 µg/kg is followed by continuous infusion (2 to 5 µg/kg/hour). Rapid tolerance develops and an increasing dose of fentanyl is required to provide satisfactory analgesia and sedation.

Meperidine (Demerol)

This synthetic narcotic is most commonly used in children as either a premedicant for anesthesia (or sedation) or as a treatment for postoperative pain. It is ten times less potent than morphine and has pharmacokinetic properties that are similar.

Pharmacologic Effects Meperidine is a narcotic agonist that can produce analgesia, sedation, euphoria, dysphoria, miosis, and respiratory depression. At equianalgesic doses (see Table 29.2), there is little quantitative difference between meperidine and morphine in producing these effects. Meperidine is unique in its ability to prevent or stop shivering associated with:

- Amphotericin administration
- Blood product (particularly platelet) transfusions
- General anesthesia
- Hypothermic

Like morphine, meperidine may produce nausea, vomiting, or both. Meperidine differs from morphine in that large doses (toxic levels) may produce slow waves on the electroencephalogram. Additionally, high levels of meperidine's principal metabolite, normeperidine, may produce tremors, muscle twitches, hyperactive reflexes, and convulsions. Indeed, because of the accumulation of this metabolite, the prolonged use of meperidine should be discouraged, if not avoided completely.

Suggested Dosage Meperidine is effective when administered orally or parenterally. We prefer its use as an oral narcotic preparation (see Tables 29.2 and 29.4).

When administered intravenously (1 mg/kg^{-1}) for pain control, meperidine offers few advantages over morphine and must be given cautiously and by titration at the bedside. A much smaller intravenous dose (0.25 to 0.5 mg/kg) effectively prevents or stops shivering. Based on meperidine's plasma half-life of elimination, the frequency of administration ranges between 3 and 4 hours.

Methadone

Noted for its slow elimination, long duration of effective analgesia, and high oral bioavailability, methadone is being used increasingly for postoperative pain relief and for the treatment of intractable pain.

Berde and colleagues recommend an intravenous loading dose of 0.1 to 0.2 mg/kg^{-1}, and then titrating in 0.05 mg/kg^{-1} increments every 10 to 15 minutes until analgesia is achieved. Supplemental methadone can be administered in 0.05 to 0.1 mg/ kg^{-1}-increments administered by slow intravenous infusion every 4 to 12 hours as needed.

We also use methadone and sustained-relief morphine (MS-contin) to wean patients who have become opioid dependent after prolonged analgesic therapy. When used to treat dependence and withdrawal symptoms, clonidine, an α2-agonist can be administered concomitantly in doses of 2 to 5 µg/kg to reduce withdrawal symptomatology significantly.

Hydromorphone

Although hydromorphone is effective when administered intravenously, subcutaneously, epidurally, or orally, intravenous administration is used most commonly in the intensive care unit. After a loading dose of 0.005 to 0.015 mg/kg, a continuous infusion ranging between 0.003 to 0.005 mg/kg/hour is started. Supplemental boluses of 0.003 to 0.005 mg/kg are administered either by the nurse or by the patient as needed.

Patient-Controlled Analgesia

Demand analgesia or patient-controlled analgesia (PCA) devices are microprocessor driven pumps with a button that the patient presses to self-administer a small dose of opioid. This type of treatment is particularly suitable for:

Table 29.4
Commonly Used Sedatives

Drug	Route of Administration	Dose (mg/kg)	Comments
Diazepam (Valium)	PO	0.2–0.5	Sedation, anxiolysis, and amnesia
	IV	0.05–0.2	No analgesic properties
	IM	NR	Painful on injection, poorly absorbed after IM injection
Midazolam (Versed)	PO	0.5	See diazepam
	IV	0.05–0.1	3–4 times more potent than diazepam
	IM	0.05–0.15	Painless on injection, well absorbed after IM injection or PO or PR
	PR	0.3–1.0	IV preparation can be given PO, bitter;
	IN	0.3–0.5	disguise with concentrated grape-
	PR	0.5–0.75	flavored Kool-aid
Pentobarbital	PO	2–4	Hypnotic
(Nembutal)	IM	2–4	No analgesic properties
	PR	2–4	Maximum dose 150 mg
Droperidol (Inapsine)	IM	0.01–0.075	Sedation, occasionally dysphoria
	IV		Antiemetic
			α and dopaminergic blocker
Promethazine	IM	0.5–1.0	Sedation
(Phenergan)			Antiemetic
Chloral hydrate	PO	25–100	Hypnotic, no analgesic properties
	PR		Maximum dose 2.0 g
			Minimal respiratory depression
Hydroxyzine	IM	0.5–1.0	Sedation
(Vistaril)			Antiemetic
Meperidine	PO	1–2	This drug combination, developed at
(Demerol)			The Children's Hospital of
+			Philadelphia is effective PO or IM
Diazepam (Valium)	IM	0.2	Must be given at least 30 min before
+			the procedure
Atropine		0.02	
Midazolam (Versed)	IV	0.05–0.1	Primarily used to minimize procedure-related pain, this combination can rapidly produce apnea and hypoxemia
+			
Fentanyl		0.001–0.002	Titrate midazolam 0.05 mg/kg slowly, the peak effect occurs 4–5 min after administration
Meperidine	IM	2	The classic "Lytic cocktail" is associated with respiratory depression, hypotension, and hypothermia
(Demerol)			
+			
Promethazine		1	Dose should be reduced by 2/3 in
(Phenergan)			cyanotic heart disease
+			
Chlorpromazine		1	No longer recommended, mentioned
(Thorazine)			only for historical importance
+			

continued

Table 29.4
Commonly Used Sedatives

Drug	Route of Administration	Dose (mg/kg)	Comments
Ketamine	IV	0.025–2.0	Potent analgesic, amnestic; transient hypnotic effect; "dissociative anesthetic," heralded by nystagmus; hallucinogen
	IM	3–10	Useful in rapid sequence intubations
	PO	6–8	to induce unconsciousness, particularly asthma
			Releases endogenous catecholamines, effective in asthma and ? hypotension
			OK in congenital heart disease, including right-to-left shunt, e.g., tetrology of Fallot
			Potent sialogogue, always give with atropine (0.02 mg/kg) or glycopyrrolate (0.01 mg/kg)
			Nightmares (5–10% of patients) can be prevented or treated with benzodiazepines
			Contraindicated with elevated intracranial pressure or with preexisting psychosis
			Protective airway reflexes are blunted. Endotracheal intubation ensures airway protection. NPO status 8 h preadministration.

- Adolescent patients
- Patients in acute pain (individuals with cancer or sickle cell anemia in vaso-occlusive crisis)
- Postoperative patients

Patient-controlled analgesia requires a patient with enough intelligence and manual dexterity and strength to operate the pump.

Intrathecal/Epidural Opioid Analgesia

Because of high concentrations of opioid receptors in the spinal cord, it is possible to achieve analgesia, in both acute and chronic pain, with small doses of opioids administered in either the subarachnoid or epidural spaces. CSF opioid levels, particularly for morphine, are several thousand times greater than those achieved by the parenteral route (see below). It is these high levels that produce the profound and prolonged analgesia that accompanies intrathecal/epidural opioid administration.

Opioid Antagonists

Naloxone is a pure opioid antagonist that antagonizes the effects of pure agonist drugs (e.g., morphine) and the effects of mixed agonist-antagonist drugs (e.g., butorphanol). It is extremely potent and nonselective in its opioid reversal effects. Naloxene not only antagonizes the sedation, respiratory depression, and gastrointestinal effects of the opioid agonists, but also reverses analgesia as well.

Occasionally, a life-threatening "overshoot" phenomenon may occur, with the development of tachypnea, tachycardia, hypertension, nausea and vomiting, and sudden death.

KETAMINE

Pharmacologic Effects

This sedative, amnestic, and analgesic is particularly useful in treating procedure-related pain (e.g., catheterization, tracheal intubation, chest tube insertion, lumbar puncture, fracture reduction, dressing changes in burn patients, and others) and in inducing anesthesia in patients with congenital heart disease, particularly those with right-to-left shunts. In critically ill patients and in patients with asthma, it produces anesthetic effects with minimal perturbations of the cardiovascular or respiratory systems. Despite its many useful properties, many adverse side effects are associated with its use (see Table 29.4).

Dosage and Route of Administration

Ketamine is effective whether administered intravenously, intramuscularly, or enterally (oral, rectal, or transmucosal). When administered in small doses (0.25 to 0.5 mg/kg intravenously, 2 to 3 mg/kg intramuscularly, or 4 to 8 mg/kg enterally), ketamine provides adequate sedation and analgesia for short painful procedures. The dosage should be reduced in the presence of hypovolemia or catecholamine exhaustion.

Regardless of how it is administered, or for what purpose, we strongly recommend concomitant administration of a benzodiazepine (midazolam, 0.05 mg/kg intravenously, 0.1 mg/kg intramuscularly) and an antisialagogue (atropine, 0.02 mg/kg intravenously or intramuscularly) to reduce the incidence of emergence delirium, nightmares, and increased salivation, respectively, that are associated with ketamine use.

LOCAL ANESTHETICS

In the intensive care unit, local anesthetics provide continuous postoperative and posttraumatic pain relief using indwelling catheters placed in either the epidural, pleural, or other spaces. To be used safely, a working knowledge of the differences in how local anesthetics are metabolized in infants and children is necessary.

Pharmacologic Action

The local anesthetics are tertiary amines and are of two types: either "esters" (e.g., tetracaine [Pontocaine], pro-caine [Novocain], chloroprocaine [Nesacaine], cocaine) or "amides" (lidocaine [Xylocaine], prilocaine, bupivacaine [Marcaine, Sensorcaine]) (Table 29.5).

Toxicity

At recommended clinical dosages (see Table 29.5), local anesthetic plasma levels usually remain well below recognized toxic concentrations. Toxic effects occur and depend on the rapidity of rise and the total plasma concentration achieved following drug administration.

Mild side effects that occur at low plasma concentrations include:

- Tinnitus
- Light-headedness
- Visual and auditory disturbances
- Restlessness
- Muscular twitching

Table 29.5
Local Anesthetics

Drug (Concentration)	Maximum Dose of Local Anesthetic (mg/kg)[a]		
	Caudal/Lumbar Epidural	Peripheral Nerve	Duration of Action
Lidocaine (Xylocaine) (0.5–2.0%)	5–7[b]	5–7[b]	Intermediate
Bupivacaine (Marcaine) (0.25–0.50%)	2–3[b]	2–3[b]	Long
Tetracaine (Pontocaine) (0.1–0.2%)	2	2	Long
Procaine (Novocain) (0.5–10%)	10–15[b]	10–15[b]	Short
Cocaine (4–10%)	NR[c]	1–2[d]	Intermediate
Prilocaine (Citanest) (1–2%)	NR[c]	5–7[b,e]	Intermediate

[a]These are suggested safe upper limits for local anesthetic administration. Accidental intravenous or intra-arterial injection of even a fraction of these amounts may result in systemic toxicity.

[b]The higher dose is recommended only with the concomitant use of epinephrine 1#200,000.

[c]NR, not recommended.

[d]For topical use only, maximum adult dose is 200 mg.

[e]Maximum dose 600 mg, is not recommended in children younger than 6 months of age.

Severe side effects that occur as plasma levels rise include:

- Seizures
- Arrhythmias
- Coma
- Cardiovascular collapse
- Respiratory arrest

The treatment of toxic responses to local anesthetics is the same as for any emergency: maintaining a patent airway, ensuring adequate breathing, and supporting circulation (ABC's).

Local anesthetic allergy is rare and is often mistakenly attributed to adverse experiences occurring during dental anesthesia. Tachycardia and a sense of flushing and dizziness following nerve root infiltration with procaine and epinephrine is usually caused by direct intravascular injection of epinephrine and does not mean that the patient is allergic to local anesthetics.

Regional Anesthetic Techniques

Many critically ill and injured patients can benefit from regional anesthetic use even when other analgesic therapies may be harmful or ineffective.

Subcutaneous Injection

Subcutaneous infiltration of the skin with a local anesthetic solution, particularly lidocaine, is common practice in pediatric patients before the performance of many painful medical and surgical procedures.

Eutectic Mixture of Local Anesthetics Cream

Eutectic mixture of local anesthetics (EMLA) cream, a topical emulsion composed of prilocaine and lidocaine, produces complete anesthesia of intact skin following application. Unfortunately, for best effect, EMLA cream must be applied and covered with an occlusive dressing (such as Saran wrap) for 60 minutes before a procedure is performed. This limits its use unless the site is prepared well in advance of anticipated use. Furthermore, if the procedure is a venipuncture, multiple sites must be prepared, in case the clinician's initial attempt is unsuccessful.

Epidural Anesthesia/Analgesia

The administration of local anesthetics, opioids, and α2-agonists to the epidural space, at any level, provides remarkably effective analgesia with minimal side effects. Local anesthetic administration is noted for its versatility and safety.

Application and Effects   Depending on the agent and concentration of agent used, sensory, motor, and/or sympathetic nerves can be blocked. When entering the epidural space (Fig. 29.2), at the level of the sacrococcygeal ligament, a "caudal" block is produced. When entering at the lumbar or thoracic level, a "lumbar" or "thoracic" epidural is produced. Caudal epidural blockade is easier to perform than a lumbar epidural and has a lower risk of accidental dural puncture. On the other hand, larger volumes of local anesthetic are required to produce blockade, and the risk of infection, particularly with indwelling catheters, may be greater.

Prevention of infection is paramount. Experience with intravenous therapy suggests that the epidural solutions and the delivery tubing proximal to the catheter should be changed every 24 to 48 hours. How long catheters can be left in place is unknown. We routinely remove them within 5 days of insertion.

Because epidural catheters may be kept in place for many days at a time, they must be fastened securely both at the skin and at the connection (usually a Touhy-Borst "O" ring) to the infusion pump. Indeed, accidental withdrawal of the catheter or disconnection is the most common cause of failure when using this analgesic technique.

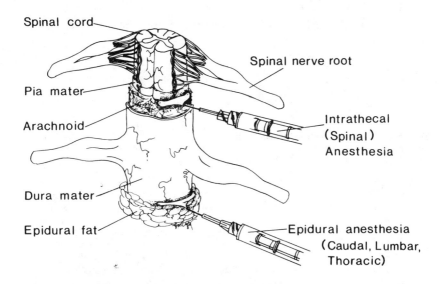

Figure 29.2. The relationship between the spinal cord and its coverings, namely the pia mater, arachnoid, and dura mater are demonstrated. In an intrathecal or "spinal" injection, the needle passes through the dura and arachnoid into the subarachnoid space, which contains cerebrospinal fluid. In an epidural injection, the needle passes through the ligamentum flavum but remains above the dura mater.

Local Anesthetic Dosage

Bupivacaine and lidocaine are the most commonly used local anesthetic agents used in epidural analgesia. There are multiple dosage schemes based on patient age, height, weight, and level of analgesia required.

Spinal opiates produce analgesia without altering autonomic or neuromuscular function. Additionally, both light touch and proprioception are preserved. Unlike local anesthetics, spinal opioids allow patients to ambulate without orthostatic hypotension.

In clinical practice, when local anesthetics are used, assessment of the height of neural blockade is tested by the ability of the patient to perceive whether a pinprick to the skin is sharp or dull (Table 29.6).

Complications

Aside from the potential of local anesthetic accumulation following continuous infusion or by a direct intravascular local anesthetic injection, urinary retention and infection at the sight of injection are among the few complications that have been reported with this technique to date. Hypotension, a common side effect of high epidural blockade in adults, is almost unheard of in children younger than 8 year of age, even when high thoracic blockade is achieved. Epidural insertion is contraindicated in patients with a coagulation disorder and if there is an infection at the site of insertion.

Common side effects associated with the use of intrathecal/epidural narcotics include:

- Facial or segmental pruritus
- Urinary retention

Table 29.6
Assessment of Dermatomal Blockade

Landmark	Segmental Level	Significance
Pinky, ring finger	C8	All cardioaccelerator fibers (T1–T4) are blocked Potential for diaphragmatic paralysis (C3–C5) and apnea is great
Nipple line	T4	Possibility of cardioaccelerator blockade Effective analgesia for upper abdominal procedures
Tip of the xyphoid	T6	Splanchnic (T5–L1) innervation blocked
Umbilicus	T10	Sympathetic blockade of lower extremities, uterus, bladder, ureters
Inguinal ligament	T12	
Outer aspect of foot	S1	L5–S1 nerve roots are the most difficult nerves to block with an epidural approach

- Nausea and vomiting
- Respiratory depression

These side effects occur with greater frequency when opioids are administered intrathecally as opposed to epidurally. Except for urinary retention, reversal of adverse side effects, with maintenance of adequate analgesia, can be achieved through the use of a low-dose (0.001 to 0.002 mg/kg^{-1}) naloxone infusion. Pruritus and nausea can also be treated with intravenous diphenhydramine (Benadryl), 0.5 to 1.0 mg/kg.

Although rare, respiratory depression is a major risk when using intrathecal/epidural opioids. Regardless of the opioid and route of administration, a regular system of monitoring for respiratory depression is required. In addition to clinical observation of signs that predict impending respiratory depression (e.g., somnolence, small pupils, small tidal volumes), we also recommend using oxyhemoglobin saturation monitoring, particularly in the first 24 hours of instituting this therapy.

SEDATION AND SLEEP IN THE INTENSIVE CARE UNIT

Anxiety, fear, and lack of sleep increase the perception pain and, if left untreated, can lead to psychosis in critically ill patients. "Intensive care unit-induced psychosis," which typically occurs 3 to 5 days after admission to the intensive care unit, is caused by a combination of such factors as the patient's premorbid personality (attitude toward illness, age, and defense mechanisms), psychologic disturbances, and the environment (frightening atmosphere, lack of sleep, unusual and disturbing sounds, lack of windows, deprivation of day-night cycles, and others).

Factors that prevent sleep in critically ill patients include:

- Constant light
- Noise
- Rounds
- Visitors
- Anxious family
- Pain
- Procedures
- Blood letting
- Endotracheal intubation
- Fear of machines in the intensive care unit
- Concerns resulting from misinterpretation of staff conversations

Although there are some situations in which sedation, anxiolysis, and sleep are undesirable, patients will benefit by the promotion of sleep and by the relief of anxiety in most cases.

Benzodiazepines

Pharmacologic Effects

The benzodiazepines (e.g., diazepam [Valium], midazolam [Versed], triazolam [Halcion], and lorazepam [Ativan]) are extremely potent amnestics, anticonvulsants, sedatives, hypnotics, and skeletal muscle relaxants. They are effective whether given parenterally or enterally and work by augmenting γ-aminobutyric acid (GABA) and glycine transmission. GABA is the major inhibitory neurotransmitter within the brain whereas glycine is an inhibitory neurotransmitter in the spinal cord and brain stem. Binding of benzodiazepines to GABA receptors produces sedation, anxiolysis, muscle relaxation, and anticonvulsant activity. Their antagonists, such as flumazenil, have the clinical effect of reversing benzodiazepine-induced sedation and respiratory depression.

Benzodiazepines markedly impair the acquisition of new information ("anterograde amnesia") whereas stored information ("retrograde amnesia") is unaffected. In fact, this latter attribute is often used by the intensivist when treating critically ill children.

Midazolam

Midazolam is a water-soluble benzodiazepine that is four times more potent than diazepam and is well absorbed via intramuscular, oral, rectal, or transmucosal routes of administration (see Table 29.4). Unlike diazepam, midazolam can be administered intravenously and painlessly and rarely causes thrombophlebitis. At physiologic pH, midazolam becomes highly lipophilic and rapidly crosses the blood-brain barrier to gain access to the benzodiazepine receptors in the central nervous system, which explains its rapid onset, short duration of action following a single parenteral dose, and by minimal accumulation following repeated or continuous infusion dosing. Midazolam can be used to induce general anesthesia when it is administered intravenously.

Dependence and withdrawal symptoms may occur with cessation of prolonged (> 1 week) continuous sedation with midazolam or an opioid. Benzodiazepine-induced withdrawal symptoms are similar to withdrawal symptoms of opioids and alcohol. Clonidine, 3 to 5 μg/kg, administered by transdermal patch may be helpful in treating many of the withdrawal symptoms. Alternatively, patients should be gradually tapered from their drugs rather than being abruptly cut off ("cold turkey").

Diazepam

Diazepam has been largely replaced in clinical practice by midazolam. The solvent vehicle for parenteral administration contains several organic solvents, such as propylene glycol and sodium benzoate, that are dangerous in the newborn, and its poor water solubility makes absorption from an intramuscular site erratic and incomplete. The oral or intravenous route of administration is preferred, although even the intravenous route is problematic because diazepam is painful when administered intravenously and causes thrombophlebitis.

Administered orally or intravenously, diazepam rapidly allays anxiety and apprehension and can be used as an anticonvulsant to stop seizure activity temporarily. The oral dose is two to three times the intravenous dose and takes 30 to 90 minutes to produce similar hypnotic effects.

Barbiturates

Barbiturates have been supplanted for the most part by the benzodiazepines for the treatment of insomnia both in and out of the intensive care unit. These drugs globally depress the central nervous system to various degrees, and produce effects ranging from sleep and sedation (low doses) to general anesthesia (high doses). Caution must be exercised when using barbiturates in patients with pain because, in small doses, they increase the perception of pain and cause excitement rather than sedation ("antanalgesic"). When barbiturates are given in doses sufficient to produce general anesthesia, pain perception, in addition to consciousness, is obliterated.

Infrequently, barbiturates produce an idiosyncratic, hyperkinetic reaction in children characterized by agitation, incoherence, disorientation, and tantrums. All but methohexital are potent anticonvulsants and can be used acutely and chronically for this purpose.

Also, barbiturates must be given with great caution in hemodynamically unstable patients, because all barbiturates directly depress the myocardium and the arterial vascular tree and cause significant hypotension.

Chloral Hydrate

Chloral hydrate, the "gold standard" hypnotic in pediatric practice, is a short-acting (6 to 8 hours), relatively safe, short-term agent, that is useful in treating insomnia and for producing immobility for painless procedures, such as computerized tomography or magnetic resonance imaging.

In therapeutic doses (see Table 29.4), chloral hydrate has little, if any, effect on respiration or blood pressure. Toxic doses, however, produce apnea and hypotension. Unfortunately, like barbiturates, chloral hydrate has absolutely no analgesic properties, and excitement and delirium may be initiated if it is given to patients in pain.

Chloral hydrate is irritating to the skin and mucous membranes, and gastric necrosis has been reported following toxic doses. Because it has a ghastly taste and often causes nausea and vomiting when given orally, chloral hydrate often is administered rectally.

POSTANESTHETIC MANAGEMENT

Many patients admitted to the pediatric intensive care unit are surgical patients admitted for continuous perioperative monitoring and support.

ANESTHETIC RISK

Contributing Factors

Perioperative mortality has improved significantly and the risk of an anesthetic-related death in a healthy patient is now less than 1:10,000. Factors that increase anesthetic risk include the need for emergency surgery, the presence of organ system failure, anemia, and extremes of age. Risk, however, is not only limited by the patient's medical condition; the type of surgery significantly affects perioperative mortality and morbidity. The risk of anesthesia and surgery can never be reduced to zero. Factors such as loss of a patient's airway, inability to ventilate and oxygenate, uncontrolled blood loss, anesthetic drug overdosage, equipment failure, and physician error all contribute to this.

Preoperative Risk Assessment

The physical status score (Table 29.7) consolidates the accumulated data of a history and physical examination and defines the estimated perioperative risk. A thorough history of the present illness; past medical and family medical and anesthetic histories; and a summary of significant physical findings should be made available to the anesthesiologist prior to surgery (Table 29.8).

In general, disease states that compromise the cardiovascular and respiratory systems or alter the function of the autonomic nervous system place patients at increased risk (Table 29.9). Specific situations that increase pe-

Table 29.7
ASA Physical Status Classifications

Class 1
No organic, physiologic, biochemical, or psychiatric disturbance
The pathologic process for which operation is to be performed is localized and not a
   systemic disturbance
Class 2
Mild-to-moderate systemic disturbance caused by the condition to be treated surgically or
   by other pathophysiologic processes
Class 3
Severe systemic disturbance or disease from whatever cause
Class 4
Severe systemic disorder that is already life-threatening and not always correctable by the
   operative procedure
Class 5
The moribund patient who has little chance of survival but is submitted to operation in
   desperation

Table 29.8
Details of Components of Anesthetic History

Preoperative evaluation
  I. General information
    A. Name
    B. Age
    C. Preoperative diagnosis
    D. Surgeon
    E. Proposed operation
    F. Time, quantity, description of last oral intake
  II. History of present illness
  III. Medical history
    A. Surgery
    B. Anesthesia: date, type, complications
    C. Allergy/drug reaction
    D. Medications, street drug use = alter anesthetic plan
    E. Recent immunizations = possible postoperative febrile course
  IV. Family history
    A. Anesthetic complications, especially the possibility of malignant hyperthermia
    B. Inheritable diseases, to include the possibility of pseudocholinesterese deficiency
  V. Review of systems
    A. Central nervous system (CNS)
      1. Seizures = influence choice of anesthetic agents
      2. Retardation
      3. Apnea = influence time of extubation
    B. Respiratory
      1. Nasal obstruction secondary to secretions or adrenal hypertrophy
      2. Loose teeth = aspiration
      3. Asthma/bronchiolitis = possibility of wheezing on induction
      4. Frequent or current pneumonia
    C. Cardiovascular
      1. Arrhythmias = anesthetic and muscle relaxant exacerbation
      2. Congenital heart disease = complication, anesthetic inductions
      3. Acquired heart disease (drugs, trauma) = heart failure
    D. Gastrointestinal
      1. Hepatitis/jaundice = altered drug metabolism
      2. Intestinal obstruction = regurgitation and aspiration
      3. Gastrointestinal reflux = intubations problems with aspiration
    E. Renal
      1. Electrolyte abnormalities
      2. Renal failure
      3. Dialysis data, if appropriate
    F. Endocrine
      1. Diabetes mellitus = fluid and electrolyte management; coma
      2. History of steroid use = adrenal suppression and shock
      3. Abnormalities of electrolytes, such as calcium
    G. Hematologic
      1. History of bleeding and/or bruising
      2. Hemoglobin; hematocrit; sickle preparation in black patient
      3. Oncology patients: note drug therapies and side effects

continued

Table 29.8
Details of Components of Anesthetic History

    H. Musculoskeletal
        1. Severe kyphoscoliosis = intubation and ventilation problems
        2. Marked short stature = intubation difficulties
  VI. Special anesthetic problems of acute injuries and illnesses
    A. Burns = muscle relaxant interactions and electrolytes
    B. Musculoskeletal trauma = muscle relaxant interactions involving electrolytes and
       bone displacements
    C. Spinal cord injury = muscle relaxant interactions
    D. Head trauma = anesthetic induction and increased intracranial pressure;
       possibility of basilar skull fracture and placement of oral rather than nasal tubes
    E. Eye injury with open globe = vitreous extrusion during anesthetic induction
    F. Drug overdose = anesthetic interactions

patients at increased risk (Table 29.9). Specific situations that increase perioperative risk include:

- Disease or drug interaction that affects the bioavailability and excretion of pharmacologic agents used in the OR
- History of allergic and/or anaphylactic responses by the patient or family member to particular drugs or products (latex)
- Preoperative anemia, because anemia results in a reduction in oxygen-carrying capacity and may be exacerbated by routine blood loss that occurs even with minor procedures
- Family history of disease associated with increased anesthetic mortality and morbidity (malignant hyperthermia, familial periodic paralysis, porphyria, and pseudocholinesterase deficiency) and those in which the airway is difficult to manage (Pierre Robin, the Hunter-Hurler, the Goldenhar, or the Treacher Collins syndromes, and diastrophic dwarfism) (see Table 29.9)
- Hemangioma, lymphangioma, or tumors or masses that encroach on the airway require special care during instrumentation of the airway
- Association of Trisomy 21 (Down syndrome) and subluxation of the C1-C2 vertebrae.
- Various myopathies predispose patients to prolonged postoperative muscle weakness
- Prematurity is associated with greater incidence of airway-related postoperative complications, e.g., apnea, periodic breathing, atelectasis, stridor, and cyanosis.
- History of obstructive sleep apnea. Planned tonsillectomy and adenoidectomy warrant intensive care unit admission after anesthesia.

POSTOPERATIVE FAILURE TO AWAKEN

A wide spectrum of postoperative complications following anesthesia and surgery (Table 29.10) may result in failure to awaken.

Table 29.9
Conditions and Syndromes that Affect the Perioperative Course

Name	Description	Anesthetic Implications
Acrocephalopolysyndactyly	See Carpenter's syndrome	
Acrocephalosyndactyly	See Apert's syndrome	
Adrenogenital syndrome	Inability to synthesize hydrocortisone; virilization of female	All need hydrocortisone, even if not salt-losing; check electrolytes preoperatively
Albers-Schöunberg disease (marble-stone disease)	Brittle bones; pathologic fractures, anemia from marrow sclerosis; hepatosplenomegaly	Care in positioning and use of restraints
Albright-Butler syndrome	Renal tubular acidosis, hypokalemia, renal calculi	Renal impairment; correct electrolytes to within normal limits.
Albright's hereditary osteodystrophy	Ectopic bone formation, mental retardation Hypocalcemia: possible electrocardiogram (ECG) conduction defects, neuromuscular problems, convulsions	Check electrolytes, monitor ECG; altered response to muscle relaxants; risk of fat embolism; after osteotomy, fracture, or minor trauma
Alport's syndrome	Nephritis and nerve deafness; renal pathology variable; renal failure in second to third decade	Altered renal excretion
Amyotonia congenita (infantile muscular atrophy)	Degeneration of motor neurons	Administration of succinylcholine results in hyperkalemia and cardiac arrest; use minimal doses of thiopental and curare; avoid respiratory depressants
Analbuminemia	Low level of serum albumin (4–100 mg/dL)	Sensitive to drugs that bind to protein (e.g., thiopental, curare, pancuronium)
Andersen's disease (glycogen storage disease type IV)	Deficiency of glucosyltransferase (brancher enzyme); early severe hepatic cirrhosis; liver failure; splenomegaly; hemmorrhagic tendency Severe midfacial hypoplasia, relative mandibular prognathism; abnormal structure and angle of mandible (triangular facies), kyphoscoliosis	Check coagulation factors preoperatively; treat excessive bleeding with fresh frozen plasma; possibility of hypoglycemia under anesthesia Possible airway problems, and intubation may be difficult; assess respiratory status

continued

Table 29.9
Conditions and Syndromes that Affect the Perioperative Course

Name	Description	Anesthetic Implications
Angioedema	Episodic brawny edema of extremities, face, trunk airway, and abdominal viscera; usually for 24–72 h (4 h to 1 wk); onset in childhood differentiates this from idiopathic form; etiology: abnormal levels of C1 and C4 esterase inhibitor accumulation of vasoactive substances, increased vascular permeability, edema; usually painless: may have prodromal focal tingling or "tightness"; often induced by trauma or vibration; may have bouts of abdominal pain, diarrhea; hemoconcentration, resulting in hypotension, shock, pharyngeal edema (usually develops slowly); most deaths from laryngeal edema; mortality rate up to 33%; long-term treatment is with antifibrinolytic and hormonal agents; note the adverse side effects of long-term use of ∈-aminoca proic (EACA)	Check results of complement assay, hematocrit, fluid status, treatment history, previous drug reactions; observe for voice change or dysphasia; prophylaxis (especially in cases for dental or oropharyngeal manipulation): EACA for 2–3 d and/or fresh frozen plasma for 1 d, preoperatively; continue EACA IV, preoperatively and postoperatively; danazol (androgen) may be useful; acute attack: give epinephrine, steroids, antihistamine; possibly fresh frozen plasma; if pharyngeal edema is imminent or develops, perform endotracheal or nasotracheal intubation (leave in place for 24–72 h); if this is impossible, perform tracheotomy; anesthesia: regional when possible; otherwise, use extreme care when instrumenting airway; preoperatively and postoperatively, monitor vital signs closely; If CHD is present, use antibiotic prophylaxis preoperatively; intubation may be difficult
Apert's syndrome (arocephalosyndactyly)	Hypoplastic maxilla and exophthalmos; cranio synostosis, possibly with increased intracranial pressure (ICP), mental retardation, and syndactyly; congenital heart disease (CHD) may be present	
Beckwith's syndrome (Beckwith-Wiedemann syndrome; "infantile gigantism")	Birth weight >4000 g; macroglossia and exophthalmos; visceromegaly and umbilical hernia are common; persistent severe neonatal hypoglycemia caused by herinsulinism (see also neonatal hypoglycemia)	Airway problems caused by large tongue; monitor blood glucose carefully and treat hypoglycemia

Syndrome	Description	Considerations
Behçet's syndrome	Gross ulceration of mouth (usually first sign; may extend to esophagus) and genital area; uveitis, iritis, conjunctivitis, skin lesions, nonerosive arthritis; may have vasculitis and myocardial and CNS involvement; risk of sepsis at sites of skin punctures, etc.	Use sterile technique; may have history of steroid therapy; nutritional status may be poor; intubation may be difficult because of scarring in pharynx
Carpenter's syndrome (acrocephalopolysyndactyly)	Mental retardation, oxycephaly, peculiar facies, syndactly, deformed extremities, CHD, hypogenitalism	If CHD is present, use antibiotic prophylaxis preoperatively; hypoplastic mandible may make intubation difficult
Central core disease	Muscular dystrophy; hypotonia, without muscle wasting; increased risk of malignant hyperpyrexia	Preoperatively, assess respiratory status carefully; sensitive to thiopental and respiratory depressants: avoid muscle relaxants (postoperative ventilation may be required); high risk for malignant hyperpyrexia
Chediak-Higashi syndrome	Partial albinism, immunodeficiency, hepatosplenomegaly, recurrent infections	Use reverse isolation; supplemental steroid therapy; thrombocytopenia—may require platelet
Cherubism	Fibrous dysplasia of mandibles and maxilae, with intraoral masses, may cause respiratory distress	Intubation may be difficult; if there is acute respiratory distress, tracheotomy may be required
Collagen disease: dermatomyositis; polyarteritis nodosa; rheumatoid arthritis; systemic lupus of erythematosus	Systemic connective tissue diseases with variable systemic involvement; osteoporosis, fatty infiltration of muscle, anemia, pulmonary infiltration, or fibrosis	Temporomandibular or cricoarytenoid arthritis may cause airway and intubation difficulties; risk of fat embolism after osteotomy, fracture, or minor trauma; supplement steroid therapy
Crouzon's disease	Craniosynostosis, hypertelorism, parrot-beak nose, hypoplastic maxilla	Intubation may be difficult
Duchenne's muscular dystrophy	Progressive pseudohypertrophy of muscles, with cardiac muscle involvement in many cases; most die in second decade	Narrow margin of safety with anesthetic agents; high risk of malignant hyperthermia (MH) susceptibility; avoid muscle relaxants
Gorlin-Chaudhry-Moss syndrome	Craniofacial dysostosis, patent ductus arteriosus (PDA), hypertrichosis, hypoplasia of labia majora, dental and eye anomalies; normal intelligence	Assymetry of head—difficult airway Problems associated with PDA

continued

Table 29.9
Conditions and Syndromes that Affect the Perioperative Course

Name	Description	Anesthetic Implications
Gorlin-Goltz syndrome (basal cell nevus syndrome)	Multiple nevoid basal cell carcinomas, hypertelorism, mandibular prognathism, multiple jaw cysts and fibrosarcomas, kyphoscoliosis, incomplete segmentation of cervical and thoracic vertebrae; congenital hydrocephalus, mental retardation, etc.	Extreme care in positioning and intubating—cervical movement may be limited; increased ICP may be unrecognized
Guillain-Barré syndrome (acute idiopathic polyneuritis)	Acute polyneuropathy: progressive peripheral neuritis, usually involving cranial nerves; bulbar palsy, with hypoventilation and hypoventilation and hypotension; may require tracheotomy and intermittent positive-pressure ventilation (IPPV)	Try not to use succinylcholine for at least 3 mo after onset of polyneuritis; if needed, use pretreatment with nondepolarizing drugs
Holt-Oram syndrome (heart-hand syndrome)	Upper limb abnormalities: usually atrial septal defect, possibility of sudden death from pulmonary embolus, coronary occlusion	Antibiotic prophylaxis preoperatively; problems of cardiac defect; no other anesthetic problem
Homocystinuria	Thromboembolic phenomena caused by intimal thickening; extopia lentis, osteoporosis kyphoscoliosis; angiography may precipitate thrombosis, especially cerebral	Give fluids to maintain urine output; give dextran 40, to reduce viscosity and platelet adhesiveness and increase peripheral perfusion
I cell disease (mucolipidosis)	Mental retardation, Hurler-type bone changes, severe joint limitation, chronic pulmonary disease; valvar insufficiency common; death in early childhood (most by 1 y of age)	Antibiotic prophylaxis and chest physiotherapy preoperatively; give large dose of atropine preoperatively; upper airway obstruction and difficult intubation, due to infiltration of lymphoid tissue and larynx and profuse thick secretions; give adequate fluids preoperatively and humidify anesthetic gases Intubation and airway maintenance difficult—limited jaw movement, stiffness of neck and rib cage

Klippel-Feil syndrome	Congenital fusion of two or more cervical vertebrae causing neck rigidity	Intubation may be difficult; should be performed with the patient awake; if possible; otherwise, inhalation induction without muscle relaxant should be performed; do not extubate until patient is fully awake.
Maple syrup urine disease (branched-chain ketonuria)	Inability to metabolize leucine, isoleucine, and valine; severe neurologic damage and respiratory disturbances; episodes of hypoglycemia; treated by diet only, from birth; many die within 2 mo; acute, life-threatening episodes may require peritoneal dialysis or exchange transfusion	Check acid-base balance and plasma amino acids preoperatively; check serum glucose preoperatively, perioperatively, and postoperatively; state glucose infusion (at least 10–15 mg/kg/min) preoperatively and continue until diet is reestablished
Marfan's syndrome (arachnodactyly)	Connective tissue disorder; dilation and possible dissection of aortic root, resulting in aortic insufficiency; aortic, thoracic, or abdominal aneurysm; kyphoscoliosis, pectus excavatum; lung cysts; joint instability and dislocation	Antibiotic prophylaxis preoperatively; intubation may be difficult; position carefully to avoid dislocations; avoid hypertension due to aortic dissection; controlled ventilation may result in pneumothorax
Myasthenia congenita	Similar to myasthenia gravis in adults	Do not use respiratory depressants or muscle relaxants; IPPV may be required postoperatively; possibility of cholinergic crisis with anticholinesterase therapy
Myositis ossificans (Fibrodysplasia ossificans progressiva)	Bony infiltration of tendons, fascia, aponeuroses, and muscle; thoracic involvement greatly reduces thoracic compliance; progressive respiratory failure	Check respiratory function and history of steroid therapy; airway and intubation problems if neck is rigid and mouth is fixed
Myotonia congenita	Decreased ability to relax muscles after contraction; diffuse hypertrophy of muscle	Do not use muscle relaxants or respiratory depressants; MH susceptible
		Check respiratory function; do not use succinylcholine (which causes myotonia in 50%); nondepolarizing drugs do not produce good relaxation; neostigmine induces myotonia; halothane may cause shivering and myotonia postoperatively; extremely sensitive to respiratory depressants—use regional or inhalational agents, with IPPV postoperatively, if necessary; monitor ECG carefully; anticipate postoperative pulmonary complications

continued

Table 29.9
Conditions and Syndromes that Affect the Perioperative Course

Name	Description	Anesthetic Implications
Osteogenesis imperfecta	Pathologic fractures, blue sclera, deafness; kyphoscoliosis; fragility of vessels; dentin deficiency results in carious, fragile teeth	Use extreme care in positioning and intubating; teeth are easily broken; hypothermic response to atropine
Phenylketonuria	Phenylalanine hydroxylase deficiency; vomiting, CNS irritability, mental retardation, hypertonia, and convulsions; phenylalanine-deficient diet must be maintained	Induction and maintenance by inhalation technique; control ventilation; give 10% dextrose infusion (tendency to hypoglycemia); hypersensitive to narcotics and other CNS depressants; do not use ketamine or enflurane; monitor body temperature carefully; if epileptic, continue drugs
Pierre Robin syndrome	Cleft palate, micrognathia, glossoptosis; CHD in some; neonates: respiratory obstruction may occur; maintain airway and require tongue suture, intubation, or tracheotomy	Intubation may be difficult; use awake technique; patient should be fully awake before extubation
Progeria (Hutchinson-Gilford syndrome)	Premature aging starts at 6 mo to 3 y; cardiac disease—ischemia, hypertension, cardiomegaly; death from coronary artery disease may occur before 10 y of age	Anesthesia as for adults with myocardial ischemia
Prune belly syndrome	Agenesis of abdominal musculature, with renal anomalies (respiration requires use of accessory muscles); poor cough mechanism, respiratory infections; may have renal insufficiency	Check renal status; treat as for full stomach; minimize use of muscle relaxants
Riley-Day syndrome (familial dysautonomia)	Deficiency of dopamine β-hydroxylase; hypertensive and hypotensive attacks, emotional lability, absent lacrimation, abnormal sweating, insensitivity to pain, and poor sucking and swallowing; recurrent aspiration pneumonia and chronic lung disease	Labile blood pressure hypersensitive to adrenergic and cholinergic drugs; respiratory center insensitive to CO_2—IPPV is necessary; beware of aspiration potential during postoperative period (see text)

Scleroderma	Diffuse cutaneous stiffening; may have hemifacial atrophy; plastic surgery is required for contractures and constrictions; may have cardiac fibrosis or corpulmonale	Scarring of face and mouth—difficult airway and intubation; chest restriction—poor compliance; diffuse pulmonary fibrosis—hypoxia, venous access limited; check history of steroid therapy
Treacher Collins syndrome (mandibulofacial dysostosis)	Micrognathia, aplastic zygomatic arches, microstomia, choanal atresia; CHD may be present	Possible airway and intubation difficulties (less severe than with Pierre Robin deformity)
von Hippel-Lindau disease	Retinal angiomas and cerebellar hemangioblastomas; pheochromocytoma in some; may have pulmonary, pancreatic, hepatic, adrenal, or renal cysts; paroxysmal hypertension, caused by cerebellar tumor or pheochromocytoma	Assess renal and hepatic function and investigate for pheochromocytoma (urinary vanillyl mandelic acid [VMA]); hypertensive crises may occur
von Recklinghausen's disease (neurofibromatosis)	Café-au-lait spots; tumors, all parts of the CNS (and may be in larynx and right ventricular outflow tract): peripheral tumors associated with nerve trunks; kyphoscoliosis in 50%; may have "honeycomb (cystic) lung"; pheochromocytoma and renal artery dysplasia (hypertension) are common	All these patients should be investigated for pheochromocytoma (urinary VMA); test response to neuromuscular drugs—effects of depolarizing and nondepolarizing muscle relaxants may be prolonged; check pulmonary and renal function; if kidneys are affected, treat with drugs excreted by kidneys
von Willebrand disease (pseudohemophilia)	Prolonged bleeding time (decreased factor VIII activity, resulting in defective platelet adhesiveness) and capillary abnormality	Bleeding can be controlled by transfusions of fresh blood or fresh frozen plasma and/or cryoprecipitate; do not use salicylates
Werdnig-Hoffman disease (infantile muscular atrophy)	Earlier onset and more severe than Welander's muscular atrophy; feeding difficulties: aspiration of stomach contents; chronic respiratory problems; most die before puberty	Minimal anesthesia is required; do not use muscle relaxants or respiratory depressant drugs; and weaning from this may be difficult; ventilatory support may be required

Table 29.10
Etiology of Postoperative Failure to Awaken

I. Residual anesthetic effect
II. Neuromuscular blockade
III. Metabolic and electrolyte disorders
   A. Hypernatremia or hyponatremia
   B. Diabetic ketoacidosis
   C. Severe hypokalemia
   D. Hypercarbia
IV. Central nervous system event
   A. Postictal
   B. Pneumocephalus
   C. Embolic event
      1. Air embolism
      2. Cardioarterial thromboembolism
   D. Hypoxic central nervous system injury
   E. Intracranial mass lesion and/or intracranial hypertension

Residual Anesthetic Effect

When large doses of opioids are given for relatively short procedures or when a sedative agent has been administered concomitantly, persistent opioid effect renders the patient apneic and unresponsive. If the patient fails to initiate respiratory efforts while artificially ventilated, an adequate arterial carbon dioxide pressure ($PaCO_2$) must be ensured.

Neuromuscular Blockade

Neuromuscular blocking agents are used to:

- Facilitate intubation
- Provide surgically indicated muscle relaxation
- Reduce the requirement for volatile agents, the therapeutic index of which is reduced in infancy and childhood.

Residual neuromuscular blockade can render the patient unable to breathe or to demonstrate a motor response to stimulation despite autonomic and ocular must be considered.

Succinylcholine

Action This depolarizing agent causes muscular fasciculations, which increase intragastric, intraocular, and intracranial pressure. They may also be associated with the development of the myalgias. Interestingly, children under the age of 4 years may not fasciculate. The disappearance of muscle fasciculation heralds the onset of a brief period of profound neuromuscular paralysis.

Succinylcholine is unique in that it produces muscle paralysis virtually instantaneously whether it is administered intravenously (1 to 2 mg/kg) or intramuscularly (4 to 5 mg/kg). Typically, a paralyzing dose of succinylcholine produces paralysis within 1 minute of administration. This makes it the most ideal agent, despite its many known side effects, for rapid sequence intubations when the risk of pulmonary aspiration of stomach contents is high.

The neuromuscular blockade following succinylcholine can be prolonged if the patient has an abnormal, genetically derived variant of pseudocholinesterase (Table 29.11).

Side Effects

Changes in Cardiac Rhythm and Function A negative inotropic and chronotropic effect follows an initial dose of succinylcholine. In children, in whom the parasympathetic tone predominates, severe bradycardia and even sinus arrest may occur.

The bradycardia occurs with greater frequency and severity following a second dose of succinylcholine in older children and adults. It can be effectively blocked by pretreatment with atropine (0.02 mg/kg, minimum dose 0.15 mg) or glycopyrrolate (0.01 mg/kg). Succinylcholine, under stable anesthetic conditions, lowers the threshold of ventricular stimulation by catecholamines. Other autonomic stimuli, such as hypoxia, hypercarbia, endotracheal intubation, and surgical stress, are additive to this effect of succinylcholine and commonly yield a wide variety of ventricular dysrhythmias.

Increased Potassium A rise in potassium (0.5 mEq/L) generally accompanies succinylcholine administration, even in normal patients. In the presence of crush injuries, burns, paralysis, neuromuscular disease, or preexisting hyperkalemia, the succinylcholine-induced rise in potassium may be catastrophic and must be avoided.

Increased Intraocular Pressure Intramuscular or intravenous administration of succinylcholine may increase intraocular pressure, which results

Table 29.11
Factors Prolonging Neuromuscular Blockade

Depolarizing Blockade	Nondepolarizing Blockade
Deficient pseudocholinesterase	Hypothermia
Genetically derived abnormal variant	Respiratory acidosis
Pregnancy	Hypermagnesemia
Anticholinesterase-containing medication	Hypokalemia
	Antibiotic administration
Hepatic dysfunction	Aminoglycosides
Hypermagnesemia	Tetracyclines
	Lincomycins
	Polymyxins

in extrusion of the vitreous and permanent loss of vision in patients with open globe injuries. This effect is not eliminated by pretreatment with small doses of nondepolarizing muscle relaxants.

Nondepolarizing Neuromuscular Blockade Nondepolarizing agents include pancuronium, d-tubocurare, rocuronium, mivacarium, atracurium, and vecuronium (Table 29.12).

Assessing Blockade The twitch response of the adductor pollicis and flexor digitorum muscles to specific types of electrical stimulation using a peripheral nerve stimulator give clues to the presence or absence of blockade. Nondepolarizing neuromuscular blockade is characterized by:

- Decreased contraction to a single impulse
- Unsustained response to tetanic stimulation of 50 Hz at 2.5 sec
- Diminution of the fourth twitch response compared with the first twitch response, of greater than 70% after four 2-Hz stimuli (train of four)
- Facilitation of the contractile response following tetanic stimulation
- Antagonism by acetylcholinesterase inhibitors

Abolition of the fourth twitch response of the train of four correlates with a 75% reduction in standard twitch tension.

Reversing Blockade Antagonism to persistent nondepolarizing neuromuscular blockade usually can be achieved after a twitch response becomes apparent. Intravenous agents commonly used include:

- Neostigmine (0.07 mg/kg)
- Edrophonium (1 mg/kg)
- Pyridostigmine (0.2 mg/kg)

Table 29.12
Neuromuscular Blocking Agents

Agents	Intubation Dose (mg/kg)	Maintenance Dose (mg/kg)	Estimated Duration of Action (min)
Nondepolarizing			
Pancuronium (Pavulon)	0.06–0.1	0.04–0.06	45–60
Rocuronium (Zemuron)	0.6–1.2	0.3–0.6	30–60
d-Tubocurarine (curare)	0.5–0.6	0.3–0.4	45–50
Mivacurium (Mivacron)	0.2–0.4	0.1–0.2	10–15
Atracurium (Tracrium)	0.4–0.5	0.08–0.10	20–35
Vecuronium[a] (Norcuron)	0.08–0.1	0.01–0.015	25–30
Depolarizing			
Succinylcholine	1.0–2.0	Not generally given	5–7

[a]Infants 7 wks to 1 y are more sensitive to vecuronium than are others and require approximately 1½ times as long to recover.

- Atropine (0.02 mg/kg)
- Glycopyrrolate (0.01 mg/kg)

The effect of edrophonium is prompt, reaching a maximum within 1 minute after intravenous administration. Neostigmine and pyridostigmine have a slower onset of action beginning 3 minutes after injection and achieving their maximal effect at 10 to 15 minutes.

Failure of Reversal Recurrence of or failure to reverse blockade is often attributable to the presence of:

- Hypokalemia
- Respiratory acidosis
- Hypermagnesemia
- Hypothermia
- Administration of many antibiotics

Metabolic and Electrolyte Disorders

Other causes of failure to awaken include disorders in fluid and electrolyte homeostasis:

- Hypernatremia or hyponatremia
- Diabetic ketoacidosis
- Hyperosmolar nonketotic coma
- Hypoglycemia
- Hypokalemia (muscular weakness mimics neuromuscular blockade)
- Profound hypercarbia ($PaCO_2$ levels > 80 to 90 mm Hg)

In hypercarbia, sufficient fresh gas flow to prevent rebreathing must be ensured. Rapid normalization of the hypercarbic state occasionally results in arrhythmias in elderly patients suffering from myocardial impairment. This complication is exceedingly rare in pediatric patients. Rapid assessment of the major cations, glucose, PaO_2, and $PaCO_2$ should be obtained, however, in the case of an unarousable postoperative patient.

Central Nervous System Events

A wide variety of perioperative central nervous system events may alter the postoperative state of consciousness. In the presence of a positive history of a seizure disorder, head trauma, or intracranial surgery, the possibility exists that a seizure occurred during surgery and was masked by the use of neuromuscular blocking agents. The patient is then comatose because he or she is postictal. Transient paresis may become apparent as the patient awakens. The clinical course and electroencephalographic data are the major diagnostic aids.

Pneumocephalus

Pneumocephalus may occur in the course of a craniotomy or with a malfunctioning ventricular drain, particularly if nitrous oxide is used during anesthesia. Pneumocephalus has been documented to produce a state of unarousability, particularly when tension results in brain stem traction. It generally resolves over the subsequent 24 to 72 hours, usually without residual. Skull films permit the diagnosis of intracranial air. A computerized axial tomography (CAT) scan may be necessary to allow exclusion of tension pneumocephalus.

Systemic Air Embolism

All patients undergoing open-heart surgery with extracorporeal circulation and patients with known intracardiac shunts, regardless of the predominant flow direction, are at increased risk. Because of the high incidence (10 to 20%) of a probe patent foramen ovale in the pediatric population, great care to avoid intravascular air injection must be taken in every child. Air embolism affects primarily the myocardium and the central nervous system (CNS), resulting in an acute anoxic event.

Ventricular electrical instability and electrocardiographic changes consistent with an ischemic insult are the most frequently encountered myocardial effects. Neurologic deficits, depend on the location of the occluded vessel(s) and the extent of embolization. Cardioarterial thromboembolism most frequently occurs in the presence of damaged or prosthetic valves, aneurysmal dilatation, and atrial fibrillation. Most of these thrombi lodge distally at the bifurcation of the major vessels supplying the extremities, kidneys, or splanchnic bed. Approximately 20 to 25%, however, do lodge in the cerebral circulation, most commonly at the middle cerebral artery, resulting in an altered state of consciousness, seizures, and variable focal deficits. Fat emboli result primarily from bone trauma and are generally filtered by the pulmonary circulation. In the presence of an intracardiac septal defect or a massive embolic load, right ventricular failure and/or systemic embolization involving the myocardium, brain, and kidneys may occur.

Intracranial Mass Lesion, Hemorrhage, or Global Brain Edema

Surgical candidates with intracranial hypertension of whatever etiology are at significant risk of developing intracranial pressure elevations resulting in herniation or cerebral hypoperfusion during transport to the operating room, induction of anesthesia, and endotracheal intubation. Patients suspected of having intracranial hypertension require appropriate intracranial pressure and systemic arterial pressure monitoring prior to these maneuvers whenever clinically feasible. Continuous recording of mean systemic arterial pressure and intracranial pressure affords the best opportunity to ensure an adequate cerebral perfusion pressure by aggressively treating intracranial pressure elevation and maintaining systemic arterial and cerebral perfusion pressures.

Hypoxic Brain Injury

Despite many safeguards, hypoxic brain injury secondary to hypoxic gas mixtures, inappropriate ventilation, or inadequate cerebral perfusion warrants diagnostic consideration in any patient who fails to awaken. In the absence of residual anesthetics, careful serial neurologic examinations, CAT scan, and evoked potentials may support the diagnosis. In the absence of clear-cut evidence of such an event, the diagnosis remains one of exclusion.

APPENDIX

Guide to Physiologic Assessment and Formulary

Mark A. Helfaer and Steve Davis

VASOACTIVE DRIPS

The following are guidelines for the emergency administration of these drugs—more individualized regimens may be prepared in advance with commonly available drug administration computer programs. For any given drug a solution may be prepared as listed below or as follows:

(Weight in kg) $\times$ 60 $\times$ (desired total volume) = μg in the desired volume

An equivalent formula is

6 $\times$ (weight in kg) = mg to be placed in 100 mL total volume

The infusion rate in mL/h = μg/kg/min.

PEDIATRIC DOSING

A modification of the formula above can be used:

[(μg/kg/min) $\times$ 60 min $\times$ kg $\times$ 100 mL]/1000 μg/mg = the number of milligrams to be placed in 100 mL total volume so that mL/h = μg/kg/min

This reduces to

(μg/kg/min) $\times$ 6 $\times$ kg = number of mg placed in 100 mL

Example: for epinephrine,

1 mL/h = 0.1 μg/kg/min:
  = 0.1 μg/kg/min $\times$ 6 $\times$ kg
  = 0.6 $\times$ kg = number of mg placed in 100 mL so that 1 mL/h
  = 0.1 μg/kg/min.

FLUID AND ELECTROLYTES

Maintenance:

4 mL/kg/h for first 10 kg
plus 2 mL/kg h for each kg > 10 kg ≤ 20 kg
plus 1 mL/kg for each kg > 20 kg

Deficit:

Hr NPO × hourly maintenance
Replace 1/2 the deficit in the 1st hour
Replace 1/4 the deficit in the 2nd hour
Replace 1/4 the deficit in the 3rd hour

HEMATOLOGY

Blood volume

Adults: 65 mL/kg × wt
Newborns: 85 mL/kg × wt
Prematures: 95 mL/kg × wt
Acceptable blood loss (ABL)

[(Hct starting − Hct acceptable)/average hematocrit] × blood volume

Example:

Adult 60 kg, Hct = 35; acceptable Hct = 25
BV = 60 × 65 = 3900 mL
ABL = [(35 − 25)/30] × 3900 = 1300 mL

This is an estimate; if blood loss is significant, a hemoglobin or hematocrit should be obtained and changes in heart rate, blood pressure, and perfusion should be determined.

PULMONARY

Lung zones

Zone 1: PA > Pa > Pv (ventilation, no perfusion)
Zone 2: Pa > PA > Pv (perfusion, pressure gradient related to alveolar not pulmonary venous pressure)
Zone 3: Pa > Pv > PA (perfusion, pressure gradient = Pa − Pv)

Poiseuille's law:

$$\Delta P :: \dot{V}^2 \times L \times N / \pi R^4, \text{ laminar flow}$$
$$\Delta P :: \dot{V}^2 \times L \times d / \pi R^5, \text{ turbulent flow}$$

Alveolar air equation:

$$PAO_2 = (P_B - 47) \times F_1O_2 - PaCO_2/0.8$$

Lung volumes:

Dead space, $V_D/V_T = (PaCO_2 - \bar{P}eCO_2)/PaCO_2 - 0.3$
Laplace's law, $P = 2T/R$
$(A - a) \ O_2$ gradient $= PAO_2 - PaO_2$; nl 10–20

where

T,	tension;
PA,	alveolar pressure;
Pa,	pulmonary artery pressure;
Pv,	pulmonary venous pressure;
μ,	viscosity;
R,	radius;
V,	flow rate;
N,	viscosity;
$\bar{P}eCO_2$,	PCO_2 of mixed expired air.

CARDIAC

Causes of Tachycardia

1. Inadequate anesthesia
2. Hypovolemia
3. Vasodilation (isoflurane)
4. Malignant hyperthermia
5. Hyperthyroidism
6. Pheochromocytoma
7. Fever, sepsis
8. Acidosis, hypercarbia, mild hypoxemia
9. Drug effect (atropine, pancuronium)

Causes of Bradycardia

1. Severe hypoxemia
2. β-Blockers
3. Sick sinus syndrome
4. Volatile anesthetic overdose
5. Vagal reflex (oculocardiac, peritoneal traction)
6. Intracranial hypertension

Causes of Hypertension:

1. Inadequate anesthesia
2. Acidosis, hypercarbia, mild hypoxemia
3. Hyperthyroidism
4. Pheochromocytoma

Causes of Hypotension:

1. Hypovolemia
2. Anesthetic overdose
3. Vasculogenic (sepsis sympathectomy)
4. Cardiogenic

5. Malignant hyperthermia
6. Intracranial hypertension

5. Tension pneumothorax
6. Pericardial tamponade
7. Pulmonary embolus
8. Anaphylaxis, anaphylactoid reaction
9. Acidosis
10. Vasodilation

O_2 extraction $= \dot{V}O_2/\dot{D}O_2 = (C_aO_2 - C_VO_2)/C_aO_2$; normal, 0.25

$\dot{D}O_2 =$ oxygen delivery $= CaO_2 \times$ (CO in LPM) $\times$ 10; normal, 1000 mL/min

$\dot{V}O_2 =$ oxygen consumption $= (CaO_2 - C_VO_2) \times$ (CO in LPM) $\times$ 10; normal, 250 mL/min

$CaO_2 =$ arterial O_2 content (mL O_2/100 mL blood)

$C_vO_2 =$ mixed venous O_2 content (blood drawn from pulmonary artery; mL O_2/100 mL blood)

$C_cO_2 =$ calculated pulmonary capillary O_2 content (assume blood in equilibrium with alveolar O_2; use alveolar in air equation to calculate alveolar PaO_2

Oxygen content

(1.36 mL O_2)/g Hgb $\times$ Hgb(g/100 mL blood) $\times$ (% sat) + (0.003 mL O_2/100 mL blood/mm Hg) $\times$ PaO_2

Shunt equation

$(C_cO_2 - C_aO_2)/C_cO_2 - C_vO_2)$

Formula	*Normal Value*
SV = CO/HR $\times$ 1000	60–90 mL/beat
LVSWI = 1.36 $\times$ {[($\overline{MAP} - \overline{PCWP}$) $\times$ SI]/100}	45–60 g-m/m^2/beat
RVSWI = 1.36 $\times$ {[($\overline{PAP} - \overline{CVP}$) $\times$ SI]/100}	5–10 g-m/m^2/beat
SVR = [($\overline{MAP} - \overline{CVP}$) $\times$ 80]/CO	900–1500 dynes-sec/cm^{-5}
PVR = [($\overline{PAP} - \overline{PCWP}$) $\times$ 80]/CO	300–800 dynes-sec/cm^{-5}

SV, stroke volume; CO, cardiac output; HR, heart rate; BSA, body surface area; LVSWI, left ventricular stroke work index; MAP, mean arterial pressure; PCWP, mean pulmonary capillary wedge pressure; RVSWI, right ventricular stroke work index; PAP, mean pulmonary artery pressure; CVP, mean central venous pressure; SVR, systemic vascular resistance; PVR, pulmonary vascular resistance; SI, stroke index.

NEUROLOGIC PHYSIOLOGY

CPP = MABP − DSP (ICP, ITP, CVP)

where

CPP,　　cerebral perfusion pressure;
MABP,　mean arterial blood pressure;
DSP,　　downstream pressure;
ICP,　　intracranial pressure;
CVP,　　cerebral venous pressure;
ITP,　　intrathoracic pressure.

RENAL PHYSIOLOGY

Causes of oliguria

1. Prerenal (dehydration) decreased intravascular volume
2. Renal (renal failure)
3. Obstructive (Foley kinked)
4. SIADH

Causes of polyuria

1. Diabetes mellitus
2. Diabetes insipidus
3. Osmotic diuresis (mannitol)
4. Hypervolemia

Creatinine clearance (adult)

$$Ccr \ (mL/min) = [(140 - age) \times weight \ in \ kg \times 2)]/72 \times serum \ creatinine \ (mg/dL)$$

Ccr (mL/min)

80–120	Normal
40–80	Mild renal impairment
<40	Moderate to severe renal impairment

GENERAL ANESTHESIA

Endotracheal tubes

Inside diameter = [Age (years) $\times$ 16]/4, (up to age 8)

Cuffed tubes for those older than 8 years of age

Full E cylinders

| Gas | Pressure (psi) | Volume (L) |
| O_2 | 2200 | 625 |

The following is a compendium of drugs used in the pediatric intensive care unit. The dosages and indications are intended to be helpful suggestions. Some of these are controversial, however, and should be applied with appropriate caution. Sedatives, hypnotics, and analgesics are indicated by an asterisk (*).

Drug/Dose	Pharmacokinetics and Pharmacotherapeutics	Metabolism	Side Effects/Interactions	Pharmacology
*Acetaminophen • 5–15 mg/kg/dose 4–6 times/d PO, PR • Adult dose: 300–1000 mg q 4 h • Maximum adult dose: 4000 mg/d	• $t_{1/2}$ = 2 h • 0% protein bound (nontoxic) • Effective concentrations: 10–29 µg/mL • Peaks 30–60 min	• 3% urinary excretion with mostly hepatic microsomal metabolism	• Well tolerated in usual therapeutic dosages with few, if any, side effects; contraindicated in G6PD deficiency • Rash, drug fever, hematologic disturbances • Hepatic necrosis after 150–250 mg/kg • 90% of patients will have severe hepatic damage if 4 h after ingestion the level is >300 µg/mL • If the concentration 4 h after ingestion is <120 µg/mL or 12 h after ingestion level is <30 µg/mL, then little hepatic damage will occur	• Antipyretic and analgesic • Little anti-inflammatory action

continued

Drug/Dose	Pharmacokinetics and Pharmacotherapeutics	Metabolism	Side Effects/Interactions	Pharmacology
Acetazolamide (Diamox) • Diuretic and urine alkalinization 5 mg/kg dose PO, IV, IM, QD • Glaucoma: 20–40 mg/kg/d ÷ q 6 h • Elevated ICP: 25 mg/kg/d, increased by 25 mg/kg/d; maximum: 100 mg/kg/d, TID, PO, IV; maximum: 2000 mg/d • Seizures: 8–30 mg/kg/d, q 6–12 h	• $t_{1/2}$ = 4–10 h	• Renal excretion complete within 24 h	• Toxic ingestions are treated with stomach evacuation, charcoal administration, and acetylcysteine • Causes an alkaline urine because of bicarbonate sodium and potassium wasting • Systemic metabolic acidosis drowsiness, paresthesias • Treatment for absence of seizures limited by development of tolerance	• Reversible inhibition of carbonic anhydrase found in RBC, renal cortex, gastric mucosa, pancreas, eye, and CNS • Inhibits the following reaction: $H_2O + H_2CO_3$; subsequently dissociates into HCO_3 and H^+ • Decreases the rate of CSF production
Acetylcysteine (Mucomyst)	• $t_{1/2}$ = 2.1 h	• Excreted in urine	• Inhalation: bronchial pain (use with caution	• Liquifies mucus and DNA by opening disulfide

• Acetaminophen toxicity enteral load: 140 mg/kg PO, diluted 1:4 in carbonated beverage NG, then 70 mg/kg q 4 h × 17 doses PO, NG IV load: 150 mg/kg in 200 mL D5W over 15 min, then 50 mg/kg in 500 mL D5W over 4 h, then 100 mg/kg in 1000 mL D5SW over 16 h • Nebulized: 3–5 mL of 20% solution diluted with equal volume of water TID to QID		in asthmatics), bronchospasm • Stomatitis rhinorrhea, bronchorrhea, nausea, vomiting, hemoptysis • If charcoal used, give IV	bonds • For use in acetaminophen toxicity (>150 mg/kg) administered within 24 h of ingestion • Replenishes hepatic stores of glutathione
Acyclovir • HSV in newborns: 10 mg/kg/dose q 8 h IV • In children <12 years old: 250 mg/m^2/dose q 8 h IV • In adults: 5 mg/kg/dose q 8 h IV given over 1 h	• 15% protein bound • $t_{1/2}$ = 2.5 h (3.8 h in neonates) • 75% urinary excretion	• Resistance • Few side effects • Renal dysfunction • CNS effects	• Synthetic purine nucleoside analog • Activity against HSV 1 greater than HSV 11 • Interacts with viral thymidine kinase

continued

Drug/Dose	Pharmacokinetics and Pharmacotherapeutics	Metabolism	Side Effects/Interactions	Pharmacology
Adenosine • 50 µg/kg IV push, may increase by 50 µg/kg q 2 min to a max 0.25 mg/kg, max dose 12 mg • 3–6 mg IV may repeat 6–12 mg			• Contraindicated in 2nd- and 3rd-degree AV block unless pacemaker in place • Dyspnea, chest comfort hypotension, flushing headache	• Prolongs PR for supraventricular tachycardia
Albuterol (Proventil) • 2–90 µg inhalations q 4–6 h • Nebulized: 2.5–5 mg in 3 mL NS; 0.01–0.05 mL/kg q 4 h (0.5% solution)		• Hepatic COMT • Hepatic MAO	• Tachycardia, nausea, vomiting, hypertension tremor headache	• β_2 Agonist—relaxes bronchial uterine, skeletal, vascular smooth muscle • Activation of adenylate cyclase • Increased 3',5'-monophosphate
Allopurinol (Zyloprim) • 10 mg/kg/d ÷ TID • <6 y old: 150 mg/d PO ÷ TID • 6–10 y old: 300 mg/d PO ÷ TID • Adults 300 mg/d PO ÷ TID	• $t_{1/2}$ = 2–3 h (alloxanthine: $t_{1/2}$ = 18–30 h) • 0% protein bounded	• 20% excreted in feces • 30% excreted unchanged in urine	• Enhances theophylline toxicity • Rash • Hematologic abnormalities, hepatomegaly, nausea, vomiting, neuritis bone marrow suppression	• For use in hyperuricemic states (gout, antineoplastic therapy) • Inhibits xanthine oxidase • Slightly alkaline urine enhances uric acid clearance

Drug/Dosing	Pharmacokinetics/Levels	Adverse Effects	Notes
Aluminum hydroxide (Amphojel, AlternaGel) • Hyperphosphatemia: 50–150 mg/kg/d, q 4–6 h PO • GI prophylaxis: 1 mL/kg (320 mg/5 mL) q 1–2 h	• Aluminum is eliminated in urine	• Constipation • Hypophosphatemia • Hyperaluminumemia • Delay gastric emptying • Bioavailability affected with hypotension, bradycardia • Interferences with absorption of some PO medications including digoxin, iron, indomethacin	• Enhances mucus secretion • Alkalinization of GI contents
Amikacin sulfate (Amikin) • 2.5 mg/kg/dose; frequency of dose depends on age/maturity • <7 d (<28 wk: q 24 h; 28–34 wk: q 18 h; term: q 12 h) • >7 d (<28 wk: q 18 h; 28–34 wk: q 12 h; term: q 8 h)	• 4% plasma bound • $t_{1/2}$ = 2–3 h • Levels: 20–30 µg/mL (peak), trough 5–10 <7 d q 12 <28 wk q 24 28–34 wk q 18 h >34 wk q 12 h Children and adults q 8 h • 98% urinary excretion; peritoneal and hemodialysis effective	• Cochlear and vestibular toxicity occurs with high peaks in the absence of low troughs • Renal cortex toxicity • Can exacerbate neuromuscular blockade • Bone marrow suppression; eosinophilia	• Inhibits protein synthesis at the 30S mRNA • For use in Gram-negative infections • Polar cations, so poor levels attained in the CSF
Aminocaproic acid (Amicar) • 100 mg/kg (or 3 g/m² × 1 h), then 1 g/m²/h IV	• Therapeutic levels, 13 mg/dL	• Rapid administration associated with hypotension, bradycardia • Dizziness, tinnitis	• Antidote for an overdose of fibrinolytic agents • Prevents hyperfibrinolysis activators

continued

Drug/Dose	Pharmacokinetics and Pharmacotherapeutics	Metabolism	Side Effects/Interactions	Pharmacology
• Maximum: 18 g/m²/d • PO: 100 mg/kg/dose, q 6–8 h • Adults: 5 g PO, IV then 1 g/h • Maximum: 30 g/24 h • ECMO: 100–200 mg/kg load, 20–30 mg/kg/h			• Headache, rash • Nasal congestion	
Aminophylline • (1/2 dose if patient on already) • Load: 3–8 mg/kg/ 20 min • Maintenance: Neonates: 0.2 mg/ kg/h 1 mo–1 y: 0.2–0.9 mg/kg/h 1–9 y: 0.8 mg/kg/h Adults: 0.5 mg/kg/h	• Peak 1 h after dose • Trough before next dose or at steady state • Therapeutic range 10–20 mg/dL		• Tachycardia, nausea, vomiting, seizures; low therapeutic to toxic ratio; second-line agent for bronchospasm	• Inhibition of cyclic nucleotide phosphodiesterase • Diaphragmatic inotropic • Pulmonary vasodilator

continued

Amiodarone (Cordarone) • Adult load: 150 mg over 10 min 360 mg over next 6 h 540 mg over remaining 18 h • Maintenance: Adult 720 mg/d infusion • Maximum dose: 15 mg/kg/d for 3–4 wk PO	• $t_{1/2}$ = 25 d • 96% protein bound • Levels: 0.5–2.5 mg/mL	• 0% urinary excretion; metabolized in liver	• Corneal microdeposits • Peripheral neuropathy • Thyroid dysfunction • Levels >2.5 µg/mL • ? increases digoxin and quinidine levels • Pulmonary disturbances	• Increases ventricular fibrillation threshold • Slows repolarization • Suppresses ventricular tachycardia • Slows AV conduction
Amphotericin B • Test dose: 0.1 mg/kg/dose up to 1 mg/dose IV in D5W (followed by initial dose) • Initial dose 0.25 mg/kg • Increased to 1 mg/kg/d over 4 d • Maximum dose: 1.5 mg/kg/d, infused over 6 h	• 90% protein bound • $t_{1/2}$ = 15 d	• Small urinary excretion; bile excretion; hemodialysis ineffective	• ? Candida resistance • Fever and chills, hypotension, dyspnea, vomiting • Hydrocortisone (0.7 mg/kg), meperidine, and diphenhydramine can ameliorate symptoms • Renal toxicity, thrombocytopenia convulsions, anemia, anaphylaxis, electrolyte disturbances	• Binds to the steroid moiety on fungal cell membranes • Poor penetration into CSF

Drug/Dose	Pharmacokinetics and Pharmacotherapeutics	Metabolism	Side Effects/Interactions	Pharmacology
Ampicillin • Neonates <7 d old: 50–100 mg/kg/d, q 12 h IM, IV • neonates <7 d old: 100–100 mg/kg/d, q 8 h IM, IV • Children: 50–400 mg/kg/d, q 4–6 h depending on severity of infection			• See penicillin	• See penicillin
Amrinone (Inocor) • Load: 0.75 mg/kg/3 min • Maintenance: 5–10 μg/kg/min • Maximum: 10 mg/kg/d	• Duration of action, 4–6 h • 35–49% protein bound • $t_{1/2}$ = 4 h	• 25% excreted in urine	• Relaxes vascular and tracheal smooth muscle • Increase HR and SV • Decrease SVR, LVEDP • GI intolerance • Thrombocytopenia at levels	• Positive inotrope • Inhibits cyclic nucleotide phosphodiesterase
* Aspirin • 10–15 mg/kg/dose q 4 h up to antirheumatic 100 mg/kg/d, q 4 h; max dose 4 g/d	• $t_{1/2}$ = 15 min (salicylate: $t_{1/2}$ = 2–3 h)	• Excreted in urine	• Irreversible platelet dysfunction • Acute renal failure • Vasomotor rhinitis and angioneurotic edema and bronchospasm in susceptible individuals • Respiratory alkalosis and metabolic acidosis	• Inhibits cyclo-oxygenase • Inhibits the conversion of arachidonic acid to PGG_2

Drug/Dose	Pharmacokinetics	Metabolism/Elimination	Side Effects	Comments
Atenolol (Tenormin) • 1 mg/kg PO q 24 h • Maximum: 100 mg/d	• $t_{1/2}$ = 6.3 h • <5% protein bound • Lasts 45–60 min	• 85% urinary	• See propranolol	• β-Blocker, β_1 selective • See propranolol
Atracurium • Intubation: 0.6 mg/kg IV	• Lasts 45–60 min; $t_{1/2}$ = 45 • $t_{1/2}$ = 20 min	• Ester hydrolysis • Hoffman degradation	• Hypotension (2° to histamine release)	• Nondepolarizing neuromuscular blocker • Minimal ganglionic blockade • Causes histamine release
Atropine • 0.01–0.04 mg/kg IV/IM; min dose 0.15 mg • 15 mg; max 2 mg • Bronchospasm—0.05 mg/kg nebulized; min 0.25 mg, max 1 mg			• Tachycardia, dilated pupils, dry mouth, urinary retention	
Bretylium (Bretylol) • Arrest dose: 5–10 mg/kg q 15–30 min • Maximum: 30 mg/kg • Chronic: 5–10 mg/kg IV over 10–30 min q 6 h IV; may be given undiluted IM	• 0–8% protein bound • $t_{1/2}$ = 9 h	• 77% urinary excretion	• Postural hypotension • Hypotension • Nausea • Tricyclics may inhibit uptake of drug to site of action preventing hypotensive but not antidysrhythmic effect	• Inhibits the release of norepinephrine from the nerve terminals, although it may release norepinephrine • Inhibits uptake of adrenergic nerve terminals • Increases duration of action potention

continued

Drug/Dose	Pharmacokinetics and Pharmacotherapeutics	Metabolism	Side Effects/Interactions	Pharmacology
				• Increases refractory period • Increases PR and QT intervals
Calcium • Chloride salt (27% elemental calcium) • Arrest and hyperkalemia: 20 mg/kg/dose IV q 10 min • Gluconate salt (10% elemental calcium) • Arrest and hyperkalemina: 80 mg/kg/dose IV q 10 min • Tetany adult: 5–20 mL 10% calcium gluconate by slow IV		• Urinary excretion	• Subcutaneous injection (infiltrate) can cause slough • Vasodilation upon rapid injection • Bradycardia, arrhythmias	• Affects cardiac contractility by its effect on the plateau phase of the action potential • Hypercalcemia: weakness, lethargy, and coma • Hypocalcemia: seizures
Captopril (Capoten) • Neonates: 0.01–0.05 mg/kg/dose up to	• $t_{1/2} = 2$ h	• 50% urinary excretion • 30% protein bound	• Rare side effects • Rashes, hypotension • Rare potassium	• Inhibits the conversion of inactive angiotensin I to angiotensin II

0.5 mg/kg/dose q 6–24 h • Infants: 0.15–0.3 mg/kg/dose to max. of 6 mg/kg/d ÷ QD to QID • Children: 0.5 mg/kg/dose to max. of 6 mg/kg/d			retention • Reduction of adolesterone production • Coronary and cerebral blood flow preserved • Pulmonary artery pressure decreased • Increased renin production • Useful in the treatment of CHF
• Adults: 25–50 mg PO BID to TID; increase weekly by 25 mg/dose in up to a maximum of 450 mg/d			
Carbamazepine (Tegretol) • Children >6 y: 5 mg/kg/d increase q 5–7 d to 10 mg/kg/d 6–12 y: 10 mg/kg/d ÷ BID increase to 20 mg/kg/d <12 y: 200 mg/d increase by 200 mg/kg/d q wk • Maximum: 1200 mg/day	• 75% protein-bound hepatic oxidative enzymes • Levels: 6–12 mg/L • $t_{1/2}$ = 10–20 h	• Reduces levels of ADH • Clonidine may inhibit antiseizure activity • Coma, convulsions, respiratory depression, ataxia, diplopia, nausea, vomiting, aplastic anemia, leukopenia, thrombocytopenia, agranulocytosis, dermatitis, lymphadenopathy, splenomegaly	• For generalized tonicoclonic, simple, complex, and partial seizures • Facilitate inhibitory inputs • ? Partial adenosine agonist

continued

Drug/Dose	Pharmacokinetics and Pharmacotherapeutics	Metabolism	Side Effects/Interactions	Pharmacology
Cefamandole (Mandol) • 50–150 mg/kg/d, q 4–8 h IM or IV • Maximum dose: 12 g/d	• 75% protein bound • $t_{1/2}$ = 1.8 h	• 96% urinary excretion	• See comments on cephalosporins	• Second-generation cephalosporin • See comments on cephalosporins
Cefazolin (Ancef, Kefzol) • 25–100 mg/kg/d, q 6–8 h IV • Maximum dose: 12 g/d	• $t_{1/2}$ = 0.8 h	• 80% urinary excretion	• Development of resistance • See comments on cephalosporins	• First-generation cephalosporin • Inhibition of cell wall synthesis • Activity against, *Escherichia coli, Klebsiella* spp. • See comments on cephalosporins
Cefoperazone (Cefobid) • 25–100 mg/kg/d, q 12 h IM, IV • Maximum dose: 12 g/d	• 90% protein bound • $t_{1/2}$ = 2 h	• Predominantly excreted in bile (75%)	• Hypoprothrombinemia causes bleeding • Diarrhea • See comments on cephalosporins	• Third-generation cephalosporin • Activity against *Pseudomonas aeruginosa* • Good for biliary infections • See comment on cephalosporins
Cefotaxime (Claforan) • 0–1 wk: 50–100 mg/ kg/d, q 12 h IM, IV • 1–4 wk: 75–150 mg/ kg/d, q 8 h IM, IV	• $t_{1/2}$ = 1 h	• See comments on cephalosporins	• See comments on cephalosporins	• Third-generation cephalosporin • Good CSF penetration • See comments on cephalosporins

- >4 wk: 50–180 mg/kg/d, q 4–6 h IM, IV
- Maximum: 12 g/d

Cefoxitin (Mefoxin)
- 80–160 mg/kg/d, q 4–6 h IM, IV
- Maximum 12 g/d

- $t_{1/2}$ = 0.65 h
- 73% protein bound

- See comments on cephalosporins
- 78% urinary excretion

- See comment on cephalosporins
- Best Gram-negative coverage of the second generation
- Good for mixed anaerobic and aerobic infections (e.g., pelvic inflammatory disease and lung abscess)

Ceftazidime (Fortraz)
- Neonate: 60 mg/kg/d, q 12 h IV
- Children: 90–150 mg/kg/d, q 8 h IV
- Maximum: 6 g/d

- $t_{1/2}$ = 1.5 h
- 17% protein bound

- See comments on cephalosporins
- 84% urinary excretion

- See comments on cephalosporins

- Third-generation cephalosporin
- Good activity against *Pseudomonas* spp.
- See comments on cephalosporins

Ceftizoxime (Ceftizox)
- 150–200 mg/kg/d, q 6–8 h IV, IM
- Maximum: 12 g/d

- $t_{1/2}$ = 1.8 h
- 28% protein bound

- 93% excreted in urine

- See comments on cephalosporins

- Third-generation cephalosporin
- Good CSF penetration
- See comments on cephalosporins

continued

Drug/Dose	Pharmacokinetics and Pharmacotherapeutics	Metabolism	Side Effects/Interactions	Pharmacology
Cefriaxone (Rocephin) • Infant and child: 50 mg/kg/d QD IM, IV • Meningitis: 75 mg/kg/dose × 1, then 100 mg/kg/d q 12 h IV • Maximum dose: 4 g/d	• $t_{1/2} = 8$ h	• 60% urinary excretion • 40% urinary excretion	• See comments on cephalosporins	• Third-generation cephalosporin • See comments on cephalosporins
Cefuroxime (Zinacef) • Neonates: 50–100 mg/kg/d, q 6–8 h IM, IV • Children: 50–100 mg/kg/d, q 6–8 h IM, IV • Maximum: 9 kg/d	• $t_{1/2} = 1.7$ h	• See comments on cephalosporins • 96% urinary excretion	• See comments on cephalosporins	
Cephalothin (Keflin) • 80–160 mg/kg/d, q 4–6 h IV, IM • Maximum dose: 12 g/d	• $t_{1/2} = 30–40$ min • 71% protein bound	• See comments on cephalosporins	• See comments on cephalosporins • Positive Coombs test result	• First-generation cephalosporin • The most resistant first-generation cephalosporin to β-lactamase, producing staphylococcal infections

Drug/Dose	Pharmacokinetics	Adverse Effects/Cautions	Comments
Charcoal (activated) • 1 g/kg PO or NG in 70% sorbitol solution	• Not absorbed	• Should not be given simultaneously with ipecac • If depressed mental status, secure the airway first • Diarrhea can cause electrolyte disturbances	• See comments on cephalosporin • Absorbs drugs and is lost in the feces • Especially useful in drugs with enterohepatic circulation; theophylline, phenobarbital, tricyclics, digoxin, Tegretol
*Chloral hydrate (Noctec, Aquachloral) • 25–75 mg/kg/dose PO PR • Maximum: 2 g rectally	• $t_{1/2}$ = 4–12 h • Reduced in liver	• Little effect on respiration or blood pressure at therapeutic levels • Gastric necrosis after PO • Hypotension and apnea in combination with furosemide and porphyrias	• Little analgesic effect • For sedation
Chloramphenicol (Chloromycetin) • Loading: 20 mg/kg/d IV, PO • Maintenance dose in infant <7 d old: 10 mg/kg/d, q	• Ester hydrolysis in many organs • 20–50% excreted by kidney • Mostly hepatic metabolism • levels: 15–20 mg/L • $t_{1/2}$ = 4 h • Hemodialysis ineffective • 53% protein bound	• Resistance • Rash, bone marrow toxicity • Pancytopenia (reversible and irreversible) • Nausea, vomiting	• 50S ribosomal binding, inhibiting protein synthesis • Activity against *Chlamydia*, *Mycoplasma*, rickettsial, and Gram-negative organisms

continued

Drug/Dose	Pharmacokinetics and Pharmacotherapeutics	Metabolism	Side Effects/Interactions	Pharmacology
12–24 h IV • 1–3 wk: 20 mg/kg/d, q 8–12 h IV • 3–5 wk: 30 mg/kg/d, q 6–12 h IV • >5 wk: 50–100 mg/kg/d, q 6 h IV • Maximum dose: 2 g/d			• Gray baby syndrome in neonates	• 45–99% of plasma concentrations in CSF • Irreversibly inhibits hepatic cytochrome P-450
Chlorothiazide (Diuril) • <6 mo: 20–30 mg/kg/d, q 12 h PO • >6 mo: 20 mg/kg/d, q 12 h PO • Maximum dose: 2 g/d	• $t_{1/2}$ = 1.5 h • Duration of action: 6–12 h • 95% protein bound	• Secreted by proximal tubule • 92% urinary excretion	• Urate crystal formation • Decreases renal excretion of calcium • CNS depression • Use with caution in hepatic and renal dysfunction • Hyperglycemia by diminished insulin secretion, enhanced glycogenolysis, and diminished gluconeogenesis • Increased serum triglycerides and cholesterol	• Acts directly on the distal tubule to increase sodium chloride and water loss • Some carbonic anhydrase inhibition, which causes wasting • May decrease urine volume in DI

Cholestyramine (Questran, Cumid)	Not absorbed from GI tract	• GI discomfort	• Decreases cholesterol and LDL by binding bile acids
• 80 mg/kg TID PO		• Elevated liver function tests	• Good for pruritus caused by bile salts
• Maximum: 4 g/ d TID PO		• Hyperchloremic acidosis	
		• Diarrhea can cause vitamin loss (A, D, E, K)	
		• Absorbs other oral medications given within 1 h	
Cimetidine (Tagamet)	• 19% protein bound	• Rare and minor reactions	• Reversible competitive antagonists at the histamine-2 receptor
• 5–10 mg/kg q 6 h PO or IV	• $t_{1/2}$ = 2 h	• Does not cross the normal blood-brain barrier	• Decreases volume and acidity of gastric secretion
• Maximum dose: 2400 mg/d	• Levels 0.78–3.9 µg/mL	• Compared with ranitidine, cimetidine binds P-450; increases the concentration of estradiol in males; binds to androgen receptors	• Enhances cell-mediated immune response (not ranitidine)
	• 62% urinary excretion	• Rapid IV administration may result in bradycardia	• Mostly, ranitidine has supplanted cimetidine
		• Headache, dizziness, nausea, myalgia, rashes	

continued

Drug/Dose	Pharmacokinetics and Pharmacotherapeutics	Metabolism	Side Effects/Interactions	Pharmacology
Clindamycin (Cleodin) • 15–40 mg/kg/d, q 6–8 h IM, IV • Maximum: 4.8 g/d	• $t_{1/2}$ = 2.7 h • 90% protein bound	• 10% excreted in urine, mostly hepatic metabolism	• Resistance • Antibiotic-associated colitis can occur with oral or parenteral administration • Rashes, reversible transaminitis • Potentiation of neuromuscular blockers	• Binds to the 50S subunit of the ribosome supressing protein synthesis • Excellent anaerobic activity • Poor CSF penetration • Accumulates in PMNs and macrophages
*Clonazepam (Klonopin): • Initial 0.01–0.03 mg/ kg/d, q 8 h PO • Increments: not >0.5 mg q 3 d • Maximum: 0.2 mg/ kg/d, q 8 h	• 85% protein bound • $t_{1/2}$ = 23 h • levels: 5–7 ng/mL	• <1% renal excretion • See diazepam	• See diazepam	• See diazepam • For absence and myoclonic seizures
Clonidine (Catapres) • Adults: 0.2–0.8 mg/d, q BID PO • Children: 5–25 µg/kg/d q 6	• $t_{1/2}$ = 9 h • Levels: 1.5–2 ng/mL	• 50% metabolized in liver • 50% excreted in urine	• Sedation drowsiness • Increased potency of anesthetics • Nausea • Fluid retention • Sudden withdrawal associated with hypertensive crisis • Respiratory depression at toxic doses	• α_2 Agonist • Reduces SVR, SV, and HR • Intrathecal analgesic

Drug/Dose				
*Codeine • 0.5–1.0 mg/kg/dose q 4–6 h • Maximum: 60 mg/dose • PO: sulfate and phosphate salt • s.c. and IV: phosphate salt only	• Lasts 2.5–3 h	• Metabolized in the liver; inactive metabolites excreted in urine	• Active orally • See morphine	• See morphine • Should be used with acetominophen for synergistic analgesia
Cromolyn (Intal) • Inhalation: 20 mg q 6 h for >5 hr old • Nebulization: 1 ampule (2 mL) q 6–8 h (for >2 yr old) • Aerosol: 2 puffs (800 µg/spray) QID		• 50% excreted in bile • 50% excreted in urine	• Rare side effects	• Inhibits the release of histamines and leukotrienes • Not for acute asthma
Cyclosporin (Sandimmune) • 5–10 mg/kg IV over 2–6 h QD (PO dose 3 times IV dose)	• $t_{1/2}$ = 14 h • 95% protein bound • Levels: 100–400 ng/mL	• 4% urinary excretion	• Nephrotoxicity at levels of >400 ng/mL • Slow IV infusions necessary • Hepatotoxicity • Increased susceptibility to infection and ? lymphomas	• Suppressed T cell–mediated immunity by blocking interleukin II • ? role in diabetes mellitus treatment

continued

Drug/Dose	Pharmacokinetics and Pharmacotherapeutics	Metabolism	Side Effects/Interactions	Pharmacology
Dantrolene (Dantrium) • Spasticity in children: 0.5 mg/kg BID, then TID after 1 d, increase by 0.5 mg/kg/d up to 3 mg/kg QID • Adult: 25 mg PO QD, then 25 mg PO BID to QID, increased by 25-mg increments up to 100 mg PO QID • Malignant hyperthermia: 1 mg/ kg IV; repeat PRN up to maximum of 10 mg/kg, then PO 1–2 mg/kg QID	• $t_{1/2}$ = 9 h	• Urinary excretion • Hepatic metabolism	• Hepatotoxicity, especially fulminant hepatitis • CNS changes • Enhances the action of neuromuscular blocker	• Decreases calcium release from the sarcoplasmic reticulum • Does not alter neuromuscular transmission • Relaxes muscle contractions associated with upper and motor lesions
Deferoxamine (Desferal) • Iron overdose • IM challenge: 1 g IM; vin rose color to urine indicates significant ingestion; then 500 mg q 4 h × 2		• Metabolized by plasma enzymes, then excreted in urine	• Pruritus, wheals, rash, anaphylaxis • Dysuria GI discomfort • Tachycardia	• Chelates iron • Iron levels >500 µg/dL require chelation therapy

- IV (in shock states): 15 mg/kg/h until level of <300 μg/dL, no more than 6 g/d; continue therapy 24 h after patient has produced normal color and quantity of urine
- Chronic overdose in transfusions: 2.0 g/unit of blood, not given in the same IV as the transfusion

Desmopression (DDAVP):
- 0.3–0.4 μg/kg/d IV over 15–30 min, q BID
- Intransal: 10 times the above dose
- Maximum adult dose: 40 μg/d
- Minimum dose: 2–5 μg

- $t_{1/2}$ (α) = 8 min
- $t_{1/2}$ (β) = 75 min

- Hypertension
- Dose must be titrated to the minimum quantity to obtain desired end point
- Tachyphylaxis
- Headache, nausea
- Hyponatremia

- Smooth muscle constriction
- Analog of ADH
- Increases factor VIII activity in von Willebrand's disease type 1 and hemophilia

continued

Drug/Dose	Pharmacokinetics and Pharmacotherapeutics	Metabolism	Side Effects/Interactions	Pharmacology
Dexamethasone (Decadron) • For ICP elevation, load 0.5–1.5 mg/kg IV, IM • Maintenance: 0.2–0.5 mg/kg/d, q 6 h • Airway edema: 0.25–0.5 mg/kg/dose q 6 h	• $t_{1/2}$ = 3 h	• 2.6% urinary excretion; see hydrocortisone	• See hydrocortisone	• See hydrocortisone • Compared with Hydrocortisone: 25 × the anti-inflammatory action • No sodium-retaining activity
Digoxin • Digitalizing dose in premature: 20 µg/kg PO; maintenance: 5 µg/kg day PO • Full-term: 30 µg/kg PO; maintenance: 8–10 µg/kg/d PO • Children: 30–40 µg/kg PO; maintenance: 8–12 µg/kg/d PO q 12 h • Digitalization: give half the dose, then a quarter of the dose q 8 h × 2	• 25% protein bound • $t_{1/2}$ = 39 h • Level >0.8 ng/mL • Toxic >1.7 ng/mL (10% likely) • >3.3 ng/mg (90% likely)	• Eliminated by kidney	• Nausea, diarrhea and vomiting; change in mental status • Virtually any dysrhythmia • Toxicity is exacerbated by hypokalemia, any drug that can change potassium equilibrium can cause digitalis toxicity (i.e., diuretics, amphotericin B, succinylcholine)	• Directly inhibits Na, K-ATPase increasing intracellular calcium and increases slow inward current • Positive inotrope • Negative chronotrope • Prolonged refractory period in the atria

• IV or IM dose equals PO dose in those younger than 10, but is 75% of the PO dose in those older than 10 y old				
Diltiazem • Adults: 30 mg PO QID up to 60 mg TID to QID PO	• $t_{1/2}$ = 3.2 h • 78% protein bound	• 4% urinary excretion	• Excessive vasodilation • Negative inotrope • Depression of sinus node rate • AV conduction disturbances • Use with caution in conjunction with β-adrenergic blockers	• Calcium channel blocker • Activity on smooth muscle (especially vascular) and cardiac muscle
Dimercaprol (British antilewisite) • Lead poisoning: 4 mg/kg q 4 h × 48 h IM, then 4 mg/kg q 6 h × 48 h	• Lasts 4 h	• Hepatic metabolism and urinary excretion	• Fever, pain at injection site • Hypertension; tachycardia • Nausea; headache; burning sensations; pain in throat, chest, and hands; conjunctivitis • Contraindicated in organic mercury poisoning, G6PD deficiency, and hepatic insufficiency (except as a result of metal poisoning)	• Forms sulfhydryl bonds • Lead levels of 50–60 μg/dL should warrant chelation • Alkaline urine ensures excretion of chelated metal • For lead, arsenic, gold, and mercury poisoning • Calcium EDTA should be given at a separate site

continued

Drug/Dose	Pharmacokinetics and Pharmacotherapeutics	Metabolism	Side Effects/Interactions	Pharmacology
Diphenhydramine (Benadryl) • Sedation and antihistamine: 5 mg/kg/d, q 6 h; maximum: 50 mg/dose • For dystonic reactions: 1–2 mg/kg IV; maximum dose: 300 mg/d	• 78% protein bound • $t_{1/2}$ = 4 h • Toxic, >100 ng/mL	• Hepatic metabolism	• Dizziness, tinnitus, diplopia, nausea, vomiting, anorexia • Anticholinergic effects: dry mouth and throat, urinary retention, tachycardia, changes in mental status • Paradoxical excitation in infants	• Used for sedation • Histamine-1 receptor antagonist • Central antitussive
Disopyramide (Norpace) • <1 y: 10–30 mg/kg/d, q 6 h PO • 1–4 y old: 10–20 mg/kg/d, q 6 h PO • 4–12 y old: 10–15 mg/kg/d, q 6 h PO • 12–18 y old: 6–15 mg/kg/d, q 6 h PO • Adults: 400–800 mg/d, QID PO	• 28–68% protein • $t_{1/2}$ = 6 h • Level >3 µg/mL	• 55% urinary excretion	• Cholinergic blockade (10% as potent as atropine; see atropine) • Reduces CO directly and increases SVR • Hypoglycemia • Prolongs PR interval • Apnea	• Type I antiarrhythmic slows sinus rate • Decreases slope of phase 4 depolarization in Purkinje fibers • Prolongs action potential • Increases refractory period • Increases QRS and QI_c complex • Oral treatment of ventricular dysrhythmias

Drug / Dose	Kinetics	Metabolism / Excretion	Adverse Effects / Notes	Mechanism
Dobutamine (Dobutrex) • 2 μ/kg/min • Titrate to effect; maximum: 40 μg/kg/min	• $t_{1/2} = 2.5$ min		• Metabolized in liver • Positive dromotrophy inotrophy • No effect on dopaminergic receptors • Tachycardia, especially when >20 μg/kg/min • Dysrhythmias • Contraindicated in IHSS	• β_1 Activity increases inotropy • Some α_1 agonism at high doses • Lower LVEDP • Reduction in myocardial oxygen demand while increasing oxygen supply
Dopamine (Intropin, Depastat) • 2–5 μg/kg/min titrated up from lower dose	• $t_{1/2} = 3$ min	• MAO and COMT	• No CNS effect because it does not cross the blood-brain barrier • Tricyclics and MAO inhibitors exaggerate the action • Higher rates cause α_1 effects and vascular insufficiency (20 μg/kg/min)	• Metabolic precursor of norepinephrine • β_1 Agonism direct • Releases norepinephrine • Dopaminergic agonism at 2–5 μg/kg/min causes increased blood flow to renal and mesenteric vasculature
Doxycycline (Vibramycin) • Initial: 4.4 mg/kg/d, q 12 h PO, IV up to 200 mg/d • Maintenance: 2.2 mg/kg/d, q 12–24 h PO, IV up to 100 mg/d	• $t_{1/2} = 16$ h	• Excreted in feces; unaffected in renal dysfunction	• Resistance • Hepatic toxicity • ? Renal toxicity • Brown discoloration of teeth and bones in those <7 y old • Thrombophlebitis • Hematologic abnormalities	• 30S subunit of the ribosome inhibiting protein synthesis • Some CSF penetration

continued

Drug/Dose	Pharmacokinetics and Pharmacotherapeutics	Metabolism	Side Effects/Interactions	Pharmacology
• Adult maximum: 300 mg/d, infuse over 1–4 h, not >5 mg/mL			• Antibiotic-associated colitis • Pseudotumor cerebri	
*Droperidol • Adults: for nausea or sedation: 625–1.25 mg IV • Children: 0.1–0.15 mg/kg/dose for premedication, smaller doses for nausea/vomiting	• $t_{1/2} = 2.2$ h	• Hepatic	• Potential for hypotension secondary to α-blockade (modest) • Extrapyramidal reactions	• Butyrophenone • Antiemetic properties • Sedation • Used with narcotics, notably fentanyl, to produce sedation or as part of a neurolept anesthesia technique
Edrophonium (Tensilon) • Test for myasthenia gravis: 0.2 mg/kg/dose IV; range: 0.1–10 mg • For SVT: 0.1–0.2 mg/kg/dose IV • Give 20% of dose slowly • For reversal of neuromuscular blockade: 1 mg/kg	• $t_{1/2} = 1.8$ h		• See neostigmine	• Works faster than any other reversal agent • See neostigmine

IV given after atropine 0.02 mg/kg/IV	• $t_{1/2}$ = 20–60 min	• Rapid administration causes hypocalcemic seizures • Nephrotoxic • Thrombophlebitis • Rapid IV administration in patients with cerebral edema may increase intracranial pressure	• Chelates divalent and trivalent metals • Adequate urine output must be maintained
EDTA • 1–1.5 g/m² d, q 4–12 h IM, IV • Maximum: 75 mg/kg/d IM, q BID to TID • IM is preferable to IV	• Excreted in urine		
Epinephrine • 0.1–0.2 mg/kg IV		• α and β adrenergic stimulation direct and indirect	
Epinephrine (Adrenalin) • Bolus: 5–20 μg/kg IV • Drip: 0.05 μg/kg/min IV titrated up • 10-fold the dose by ETT • In CPR, escalation to 10-fold dosing may be helpful	• Hepatic COMT and MAO	• Increases coagulation; increases total leukocyte counts; decreases eosinophils transient hyperkalemia, hyperglycemia, fear, anxiety, tension, dizziness, palpitations, tachydysrhythmias, pallor, cerebral hemorrhage	• α effects (hypertension) and β effects (tachycardia); activation of adenylate cyclase increases 3',5'-monophosphate • $β_2$ Agonist relaxes uterine and bronchial smooth muscle • Positive inotrope, chronotrope, and

continued

Drug/Dose	Pharmacokinetics and Pharmacotherapeutics	Metabolism	Side Effects/Interactions	Pharmacology
Epinephrine (racemic) (Vaponefrine, Micronefrin, Asthmanefrin solution 2.25%) • 0.05 mL/kg/dose diluted to 3 mL NS • Maximum: 1.5 mL		• Hepatic COMT and MAO	• High doses can cause vascular insufficiency	dromotrope • For use in croup (also postextubation croup) • Risk of rebound
Erythromycin • 10–20 mg/kg/d, q 6 h IV • 30–50 mg/kg/d, QID PO • PO: stearate estolate ethylsuccinate • IV: lactobionate gluceptate • Adult maximum: 8 g/d PO	• $t_{1/2}$ = 1.6 h • Levels: 0.3–1.9 μg/ mL PO, up to 10 μg/ mL IV	• 12–15% excreted in urine, demethylation in liver not removed by dialysis	• Rare side effects • Fever, eosinophilia, rashes • Hepatitis • Thrombophlebitis • Increases levels of theophylline • Common–nausea, vomitus, abdominal pain	• Macrolide antibiotic • Activity against Gram-positive organisms, *Mycoplasma, Legionella,* and *Chlamydia* spp. pertussis • Binds to 50S subunit of the ribosome • Poor CSF penetration
Esmolol • Load: 500 μg/kg/ min × 5 min • Infusion: 25–100 μg/ kg/min titrated to effect	• $t_{1/2}$ = 8 min	• Metabolized by red cell esterases	• See propranolol	• Relatively selective β_1-antagonist • See propranolol

Drug/Dose	Pharmacokinetics	Metabolism/Excretion	Side Effects/Toxicity	Notes
Ethosuximide (Zarontin) • Maintenance: 20–40 mg/kg/d 8–12 h • Maximum: 1.5 g/d	• Not bound to proteins • $t_{1/2}$ = 30–50 h • Levels: 40–100 µg/mL	• 25% excreted in urine • 75% hepatic microsomal enzymes	• GI: nausea, vomiting • SLE pancytopenia, dermatitis aplastic anemia, ataxia	
FK506 (Tacrolimus) • Children 0.1–0.5 mg/kg/d ÷ q 12 • 0.15–0.3 mg/kg/d ÷ q 12		• Hepatic metabolism • Renal excretion	• Interacts with antacids, cyclosporin • Hypertension • Renal toxicity	• Inhabits T-lymphocyte activation • Trough 10–20 mg/mL
Famotidine (Pepcid): • Adults: 20 mg q 12 h IV			• Side effects rare • Headaches, dizziness, constipation, diarrhea drowsiness	• H_2 blocker
*Fentanyl (Sublimaze) • 1–2 µg/kg/dose IV q 10 min	• $t_{1/2}$ = 3.7 h • 80% protein bound	• Termination of action by redistribution metabolized in liver	• Muscle rigidity due to dopaminergic transmission in the striatum • See morphine • Levels >1 ng/mL associated with respiration depression	• µ-Agonist more specific than morphine • See morphine
Flecainide (Tambocor) • Children 3–6 mg/kg/24 h ÷ q 8–12 PO • Adults: 100 mg PO q	• $t_{1/2}$ = 7–24 h • Trough level <0.7–1 mg/mL	• Urinary excretion	• Worsens ventricular function • Sinus bradycardia • Wider QRS, prolonged PR	• Depresses fast sodium channels • Decreases Vmax action potential in most cardiac tissue

continued

Drug/Dose	Pharmacokinetics and Pharmacotherapeutics	Metabolism	Side Effects/Interactions	Pharmacology
12 h; increase dose by 50 mg q 12 h every 4 d to maximum of 400 mg/d			• Dizziness, blurred vision, nausea, dyspnea	• Suppresses PVCs
Furosemide (Lasix) • 2 mg/kg/dose q 6–8 h PO; maximum: 600 mg/d • 1 mg/kg/dose q 6–12 h IV, IM; maximum: 6 mg/kg/single dose	• 98% protein bound • $t_{1/2} = 92$ min • toxicity: $>25\mu g/mL$	• 67% excreted in urine	• Enhances calcium excretion • Increases excretion of titratable acid and ammonia • Enhances renal blood flow • Increased pulmonary venous capacitance decreasing LV filling pressures • Metabolic alkalosis • Hyperuricemia • Deafness • Nephrotoxicity (increased in the presence of cephalosporins and renal-toxic drugs)	• Acts on the thick ascending loop of Henle by inhibiting electrolyte reabsorption • Mild carbonic anhydrase inhibition • Redistributes renal blood flow from medulla to cortex

Drug / Dose	Pharmacokinetics	Effects	Mechanism / Comments
Gentamicin • 2.5 mg/kg/dose IV or IM; frequency of dose depends on age/maturity • <7 d (<28 wk: q 24 h; 28–34 wk; q 18 h; term: q 12 h) • >7 d (<28 wk: q 18 h; 28–34 wk: q 12 h; term: q 8 h) • Children: q 8 h	• $t_{1/2}$ = 2–3 h • levels: 6–10 mg/L (peak) • <2 mg/L (trough) • >90% urinary excretion • <10% protein bound	• Cochlear and vestibular toxicity occurs with high peak in the absence of low troughs • Renal cortex toxicity • Can exacerbate neuromuscular blockade	• Inhibits protein synthesis at the 30S mRNA • For use with Gram-negative infections • Polar cations, so poor levels attained in CSF
Glucagon • 0.1 mg/kg/ up to 1 mg IM, SC (1 mg = 1 unit)	• $t_{1/2}$ = 3–6 min • Degraded in liver, kidney, and plasma	• Acts only on liver glycogen stores converting them to glucose • Increases serum glucose	• Stimulates adenylate cyclase • Positive inotrope and chronotrope • Treats insulin-induced hypoglycemia • Relaxes the intestinal tract
Glycopyrrolate (Robinul) • 0.015 mg/kg/dose q 4–8 h IV, IM		• See atropine	• Muscarinic blocker with minimal associated tachycardia or mental status changes • See atropine

continued

Drug/Dose	Pharmacokinetics and Pharmacotherapeutics	Metabolism	Side Effects/Interactions	Pharmacology
*Haloperidol (Haldol) • Age 3–12 y; sedation: 0.5–1 mg PO; psychosis: 0.05–0.15 mg/kg/d, q BID to TID PO • Age >12 y; agitation: 2–5 mg IM, PO	• $t_{1/2}$ = 17.9 h • Level: 1 ng/mL	• No urinary excretion • 92% protein bound • Hepatic microsomal metabolism	• Extrapyramidal side effects; see promethazine • Toxic levels of 15 ng/mL • Sedation • Hypotension • Lower seizure threshold	• Dopaminergic blocker • α_1-Blocker
Heparin • (120 international units = 1 mg) • Bolus: 50–100 units/kg q 4 h IV up to 500 units/kg/d continuous heparinization • Initial: 50 units/kg IV: maintenance: 10–25 units/kg/h	• 99% Protein bound • $t_{1/2}$ = 26 + (0.323 × dose in IV/kg/min)	• Metabolized in liver by heparinase • Metabolites excreted in urine	• Lines flushed with heparinized saline have higher fatty acid concentrations that inhibit binding of lipophilic drugs, thus interfering with quantification of some drugs (digoxin, propranolol, phenytoin) • Chills, fever, anaphylactic, shock, hemorrhage, osteoporosis, thrombocytopenia	• Reduces serum triglycerides by releasing tissue lipoprotein lipase • Antithrombin III and heparin cofactor II form complexes with thrombin • Heparin accelerates the velocity of this reaction, also inactivates factor X • Reversal with protamine 1 mg for every 100 units heparin • Adjust dose after clotting time (20–30 min) or PTT 1.5–2.5 times control
Hydralazine (Apresoline)	• $t_{1/2}$ = 1 h • Duration of action:	• Metabolized in liver: fast and slow acetylators	• Tachycardia, increased contractility and renin	• Directly relaxes arterial vascular smooth muscle

• Acute 0.1–0.5 mg/ kg/dose IM, IV • Chronic: 0.75–3 mg/ kg/d, q 6–12 PO	2–4 h have different bioavailabilities after oral but not parenteral administration	activity, fluid retention • Increased coronary, renal and cerebral blood flow • Postural hypotension, (uncommon) headache • Lupuslike syndrome in slow acetylators in summer, 2 mo after administration	by activation of guanylate cyclase and accumulation of GMP
Hydrocortisone (SoluCortef) • Loading: 4–8 mg/ kg/dose, maximum: 250 mg; maintenance: 8 mg/kg/d, q 6 h IV	• $t_{1/2} = 1.5$ h • Physiologic level: 16 µg/dL at 8 AM and 4 µg/dL at 4 PM • 90% protein bound • 70% hepatic metabolism; some kidney metabolism	• Cushing's habitus, psychiatric changes, cataracts, osetoporosis, myopathy, susceptibility to disease, hyperglycemia, peptic ulcers, sodium, retention, suppression of adrenal pituitary axis (adrenal axis able to mount stress response 9–10 d after 1 mo of 2 mg/kg/d prednisone) • Abrupt withdrawal: fever, myalgias and arthralgias, pseudotumor cerebri	• Physiologically 20 mg/d secreted • Steroids interacts with receptor proteins in cytoplasm • Block the effect of MIF on macrophages

continued

Drug/Dose	Pharmacokinetics and Pharmacotherapeutics	Metabolism	Side Effects/Interactions	Pharmacology
Imipenem-cilastatin (Primaxin) • 50 mg/kg/d, q 6–8 h IV • Maximum dose: 4 g/d	• $t_{1/2}$ = 1 h	• Metabolized in renal brush border by dehydropeptidase • 70% excreted in urine	• Nausea, vomiting, pruritus • ? Penicillin allergies • Seizures at high doses in those with CNS lesions	• β-Lactam ring resistant to β-Lactamase • Good anaerobic and aerobic activity, including *Listeria, Pseudomonas* spp. • Cilastatin inhibits dehydropeptidase
Indomethacin (Indocin) • Ductus closure: 3 doses separated by 12–24 h First dose: 0.2 mg/kg • Second and third doses depend on age: • <48 h: 0.1 mg/kg • 2–7 d: 0.2 mg/kg • >7 d: 0.25 mg/kg • Anti-inflammatory (>14 y old): 1–3 mg/kg/d, q TID or QID; maximum dose: 100 mg/d	• 90% protein bound • $t_{1/2}$ = 2.4 h • Levels: 0.3–3 µg/mL	• 15% urinary excretion	• GI side effects • Hematopoietic side effects • Renal dysfunction • Platelet dysfunction • Cross-reactions between aspirin and indomethacin	• Inhibits cyclo-oxygenase • Anti-inflammatory, analgesic and antipyretic • Antipyretic effects in Hodgkin's disease

Insulin
- Regular IV onset ½–1 h: lasts 5–8 h
- Semi-lente SC onset ½–1 h: lasts 12–16 h
- NPH SC onset 1–2 h: lasts 18–24 h
- In diabetic ketoacidosis: 0.1 unit/kg IV regular insulin, bolus IV followed by 0.1 unit/kg/h regular insulin
- Hyperkalemia: 0.15 unit/kg/h IV of regular insulin with 0.5 g/kg of glucose

- Kidney metabolism
- Liver metabolism

- Allergic reactions: rash
- Hypoglycemia
- Insulin binds to plastic IV administration materials

- Stimulates transport of metabolites (especially glucose) and ions (especially potassium and magnesium) through membranes
- Stimulates glycogen and fat synthesis
- Inhibits glycogenolysis and lipolysis

Isoetharine (Bronkosol)
- 1–2 puffs q 3 h
- Nebulization: 0.25–0.5 mL 1% solution diluted to 2 mL in NS q 4 h

- Nausea, tachycardia, hypertension, anxiety, headache
- See isoproterenol

- β₂ Agonist
- See isoproterenol

continued

Drug/Dose	Pharmacokinetics and Pharmacotherapeutics	Metabolism	Side Effects/Interactions	Pharmacology
Isoniazid (INH) • Treatment in children: 10–20 mg/kg/d, q 12–24 h PO; maximum dose: 500 mg/d • Adults: 5 mg/kg/d QD; maximum dose: 300 mg/d	• 0% protein bound • $t_{1/2}$ = 1.1–3.1 h	• Slow and rapid (hepatic) acetylators affect the plasma concentrations; 75–90% excreted in urine	• Resistance • Most common to least common: rash, jaundice, peripheral neuritis • Other: hematologic vasculitis, arthritis, seizures, CNS effects • Peripheral neuritis (very common especially if pyridoxine not administered • Decreases metabolism of phenytoin • Severe hepatic injury rare in <20 y olds	• Mechanism of action unknown, but tubercle bacilli take up the drug preferentially • CSF concentrations similar to plasma concentrations
Isoproterenol (Isuprel) • 0.05 µg/kg/min IV • Increase q 4 min by 0.05 µg/kg/min and titrate to effect and side effect		• Hepatic COMT • Poor substrate for MAO	• Palpitation, tachycardia, flushing of skin, angina, nausea, tachyarrhythmias	• Practically no α effects, some β_1 effects • Lowers SVR by β_2 agonism • See epinephrine • Inhibits antigen-induced release of histamine • Relaxes bronchial smooth muscle by β_2 agonism

Kanamycin
- Bacterial overgrowth in adults: 50–100 mg/kg/d, q 6 h PO; maximum dose: 12 g/d
- In infants and children: 15–30 mg/kg/d, q 8–12 h IM, IV: maximum dose: 1.5 g/d IV

- $t_{1/2}$ = 2.1 h
- Levels: peak 25–30 mg/L through <6 mg/L

- Partly absorbed PO
- 97% eliminated in urine
- 0% protein bound

- See gentamicin
- Main use is as an oral adjunct to treating hepatic coma
- Also used for "bowel prep" before surgery

*Ketamine
- Intubation: 1–2 mg/kg IV, 6–13 mg/kg/ IM
- Sedation: one-sixth of the above doses (should be given with atropine)

- 45–50% protein bound
- $t_{1/2}$ (α) = 7–17 min
- $t_{1/2}$ (β) = 2–3 h

- ? Hepatic metabolism

- See gentamicin
- Drug-induced malabsorption
- Administer over 30 min

- Releases endogenous catecholamines, increasing BP and HR
- Direct myocardial depressant
- In the absence of benzodiazepines, emergent psychosis possible
- Increases cerebral blood flow and metabolism, and increases intraocular and intracranial pressures

- Site of actions (?): cortex and limbic systems
- Reduces polysynaptic spinal reflexes
- Provides cardiovascular stability

continued

Drug/Dose	Pharmacokinetics and Pharmacotherapeutics	Metabolism	Side Effects/Interactions	Pharmacology
Ketoconazole (Nizord) • Children >2 y old: 3.3–6.6 mg/kg/QD PO • Maximum: 400 mg/d QD PO	• 90% protein bound • $t_{1/2}$ = 1.5–4 h (higher doses are associated with longer $t_{1/2}$)	• Hepatic metabolism	• May lower seizure threshold • Stimulates salivary secretions (atropine should be given concomitantly) • Reduction of gastric activity (e.g., H_2 blockers) decrease absorption • Nausea, vomiting, thrombocytopenia • Transaminitis to hepatic toxicity • ? Antagonism with amphotericin B	• Useful for many nonmeningeal fungal infections • Minimal CSF penetration
*Ketorolac (Toradol) • 1.0 mg/kg IV load; 0.5 mg/kg IV q 6 h; max. 60 mg	• $t_{1/2}$ (α) = 3–9 h	• Renal excretion • May be given PO or IM	• ? Enhances actions of nondepolarizing muscle relaxants	• Platelet dysfunction
Labetalol (Trandate) • Adults: 5–10 mg IV bolus, titrated to effect	• $t_{1/2}$ = 5 h	• 5% excreted unchanged in urine; the remainder is metabolized in the liver	• α or β activity ratio: 1:3 to 1:7 • Rashes • See propranolol	• Selective α_1 antagonism • Nonselective β antagonism • Inhibits reuptake of norepinephrine into nerve terminals

Drug/Dosage	Kinetics	Metabolism	Adverse Effects	Comments/Mechanism
Lactulose (Cephulac) • Infant: 2.5–10 mL/d, q TID to QID PO • Children: 40–90 mL/d, q TID to QID • Adults: 30–45 mL/dose, PO, BID to QID	• Latency of 1–7 d to reduce serum ammonia levels	• Minimal absorption; metabolized by gut flora to monosaccharides and lactate	• Diarrhea with electrolyte and water disturbance	• Semisynthetic nonabsorbable disaccharide • Osmotic laxative • Adjust to effect: 2–3 soft stools/d with a fecal pH of 5–5.5
Lidocaine • 1–1.5 mg/kg IV or intratracheal IV/drip of 20–50 μg/kg/min	• 70% plasma bound to α_1-glycoprotein • levels: 1.5–6 mg/L • $t_{1/2}$ = 100 min • toxicity: >7 mg/L	• Hepatic de-ethylation	• Can suppress a diseased SA node • Agitation (5 μg/mL) • Hearing disturbances • Convulsions (>7 μg/mL)	• Blocks some stimulation of laryngoscopy and tracheal intubation • Decreases slope of phase 4 depolarization of Purkinje fibers • Increases diastolic electrical threshold by increasing potassium conductance without changing resting Vmax • Treats ventricular dysrhythmias
*Lorazepam (Ativan): • 0.03–0.1 mg/kg/dose PO, IV, IM	• $t_{1/2}$ = 10–20 h	• Diazepam is metabolized to lorazepam • See diazepam	• See diazepam	• See diazepam
Mannitol • Diuretic: 0.2 g/kg IV • Cerebral edema: 0.25 g/kg IV		• Not metabolized • Filtered and excreted in urine unchanged	• Fluid overload by expansion of the extracellular space, especially in heart failure and anuria	• Osmotically active agent • ? Free radical scavenger

continued

Drug/Dose	Pharmacokinetics and Pharmacotherapeutics	Metabolism	Side Effects/Interactions	Pharmacology
*Meperidine (Demerol) • PO, IM, IV, SC: 1–1.5 mg/kg/dose q 3 h • Maximum: 100 mg q 3 h	• $t_{1/2}$ = 3 h • 60% protein bound	• Metabolized in the liver to form normeperidine	• Can accumulate and raise the serum osmolarity to dangerous levels >340 mOsm/kg • See morphine • CNS convulsant side effects, blocked by naloxone, are medicated by normeperidine • Neonates do not clear the drug well	• See morphine • Interacts with the κ receptors more than does morphine • Unique among the opioids because of its local anesthetic effects and its effect in increasing heart rate
Metaproterenol (Metaprel, Alupent) • Nebulized: 0.2–0.3 mL 5% solution in 2.5 mL NS • Aerosol: 1–3 puffs q 3 h (650 µg/puff) • Oral: 1.3–2.6 mg/kg/d q TID to QID		• Not metabolized by COMT; excreted in urine conjugated with glucuronic acid	• See isoproterenol	• β_2 Agonist selective with relatively less β_1 than isoproterenol • See isoproterenol

Drug/Dosage	Pharmacokinetics	Side Effects	Comments
*Methadone (Dolphine) • 0.7 mg/kg/d, divided q 4–6 h PO or SC	• $t_{1/2}$ = 1–1.5 d • Level: 35 µg/mL	• Constipation, sedation miosis, biliary spasm • 90% protein bound • Biotransformed in the liver	• Antitussive • Less respiratory depression • Overall abuse potential comparable to that of morphine
Methylene blue • As an aid in identifying urinary structures 1 mg/kg IV • To aid in treating drug-related methemoglobin, 1 mg/kg slowly over 15 min—used in cyanide poisoning, e.g., sodium nitroprusside toxicity, but better alternatives are sodium or amyl nitrate		• Interferes with pulse oximetry resulting in artifactual low SaO_2	• Excreted and concentrated in urine, aids in identifying urinary structures • Converts methemoglobin to hemoglobin
Methylprednisolone (Medrol, SoluMedrol) • Anti-inflammatory: 0.4–1.6 mg/kg/d, q 6–12 h IV	• $t_{1/2}$ = 12–36 h	• See hydrocortisone	• See hydrocortisone • 5 times the anti-inflammatory and half the sodium-retaining potency of hydrocortisone

continued

Drug/Dose	Pharmacokinetics and Pharmacotherapeutics	Metabolism	Side Effects/Interactions	Pharmacology
• Asthma load: 1–2 mg/kg/dose; maintenance: 0.5–4 mg/kg/dose q 4–6 h IV maximum: 250 mg/dose q 4 h				• Dosages are controversial
Metoprolol (Lopressor) • Adults: 5 mg IV, q 2 min × 3, then after 15 min 50 mg PO q 6 h, then after 2 days 100 mg PO BID • Maximum: 450 mg/d PO	• $t_{1/2}$ = 3 h	• 10% excreted in urine • 90% hydroxylated in the liver (slow hydroxylations have higher plasma levels)	• Reduction in FEV_1 in asthmatics • See propranolol	• Selective β_1 antagonist • See propranolol
Metronidazole (Flagyl) • Anaerobic infections load: 15 mg/kg IV, then 7.5 mg/kg/dose q 6 h • Maximum: 4 g/d (less frequent in neonate)	• 10% protein bound • Levels: 3–6 μg/mL • $t_{1/2}$ = 8–10 h	• <10% urinary excretion	• Disulfiramlike effects with alcohol • GI (nausea, diarrhea, etc.) • Neurotoxicity (especially CNS) • Thrombophlebitis • Red urine • Metallic taste	• Good CSF penetration • Activity against *Trichomonas, Giardia,* and amebae
Miconazole (Monistat) • >1 y: 15–40 mg/kg/ d, q 8 h	• $t_{1/2}$ = 24 h • 90% protein bound	• Hepatic metabolism	• Frequent adverse effects include: nausea, vomiting, anemia,	• No good indications as a first drug: because of toxicity

Drug/Dose	Half-life	Metabolism/Excretion	Toxicity	Comments
• Adult maximum: 1200 mg/dose q 8 h			thrombocytosis, hyponatremia, anaphylactoid reactions, CNS toxicity • Cardiorespiratory arrest when given faster than 2 h: diluted more than 200 mL arthralgias (adult dose) • Inhibits metabolism of phenytoin and warfarin	• Poor CSF penetration • Used only when first-line drugs not tolerated • Available as a 2% cream or lotion
*Midazolam (Versed) • 0.05–0.2 mg/kg IM, IV	• $t_{1/2}$ (α) = 1 h	• Hepatic metabolism	• See diazepam	• Water soluble • See diazepam
Milrinone (primacor) • Loading 50 μg/kg/10 min • Maintenance infusion 0.375–0.75 μg/kg/min	• $t_{1/2}$ (β) 2 h		• Ectopy • Hypotension	• Phosphodiesterase III inhibitor • Increases cardiac performance without increasing oxygen demand • Vasodilator
Minoxidil (Loniten) • Adults: 5 mg qd, increased up to 20 mg BID PO	• $t_{1/2}$ = 3.1 h	• 12% urinary excretion	• Prompt withdrawal causes hypertension • Toxicity: fluid retention and hypertrichosis • Reflex tachycardia	• Direct vascular smooth muscle relaxation similar to that produced by hydralazine

continued

Drug/Dose	Pharmacokinetics and Pharmacotherapeutics	Metabolism	Side Effects/Interactions	Pharmacology
*Morphine sulfate • 0.1–0.2 mg/kg/dose SC, IV, or IM	• $t_{1/2}$ = 2.5–3 h	• 33% protein bound • Hepatic conjugation	• Sedation, nausea, vomiting, respiratory depression, miosis, constipation, biliary spasm, muscular rigidity in high doses • Suppresses the cough reflex, vasodilation • Histamine release causing hypotension and bronchospasm • Withdrawal symptoms after prolonged use • May exacerbate spinal cord and brain injury by direct effects and by increasing P_aCO_2 and increasing ICP	• μ and κ agonist, little effect on σ • μ: supraspinal, analgesia, respiratory depression, euphoria, physical dependence • κ: spinal analgesia, sedation miosis • σ: dysphoric hallucinations
Nafcillin (Staphcillin) • Newborn (<7 d old: 40 mg/kg/d, q 12 h IV, IM • Newborn >7 d old: 60 mg/kg/d, q 6–8 h • Children: 100–200 mg/kg/d, q 4 h IV • Adults: 4–12 g/d, q 4 h IV	• 90% protein bound • $t_{1/2}$ = 1 h	• 27% urinary excretion (higher in extrahepatic biliary obstruction)	• See penicillin	• See penicillin • Resistant to penicillinase • Active against staphylococcal infections • Good bile and spinal fluid concentrations

Drug/Dose	Metabolism/Kinetics	Adverse effects	Comments
*Naloxone (Narcan) • 5–10 µg/kg/dose IM or IV q 3–5 min, titrated to effect may be given via endotracheal tube	• $t_{1/2}$ = 45–60 min	• Hepatic	• Can acutely precipitate a withdrawl syndrome • Can acutely cause loss of analgesia • Narcotic can outlast naloxone	• µ Receptor antagonist • ? Effect in reversal of shock and ameliorating the damage associated with CNS trauma (in large doses) • Some antagonism to κ and σ receptors
Neomycin • Acute hepatic encephalopathy: 2.5–7 g/m²/d, q 6 h PO × 5–7 d • Chronic: 2.5 g/m²/d • Bowel preparation: 90 mg/kg/d, q 4 h	• 0% protein bound	• Poorly absorbed PO • 97% eliminated in feces	• See gentamicin • Drug-induced malabsorption	• See gentamicin • Main use is as an oral adjunct to treating hepatic coma • Also used for "bowel prep" before surgery
Neostigmine • 0.06–0.07 mg/kg IV • Maximum: 3 mg	• Lasts 3–4 h	• Metabolized by plasma esterases and excreted in urine	• Salivation, lacrimation, diarrhea, vomiting, bradycardia, bronchiolar and ureteral contractions • Inhibits the action of cholinesterase	• Inhibits acetylcholinesterase • To be given with an anticholinergic (muscarinic) such as atropine
Nifedipine • 0.15–0.5 mg/kg/dose q 6–8 h PO or sublingual	• 98% protein bound • $t_{1/2}$ = 3.5 h	• 0% urinary excretion; metabolites excreted in urine	• Hypotension, tachycardia, headaches, dizziness, palpitations	• Calcium entry blocker • More potent vasodilator than verapamil and diltiazem

continued

Drug/Dose	Pharmacokinetics and Pharmacotherapeutics	Metabolism	Side Effects/Interactions	Pharmacology
• Maximum: 30 mg/dose (or 180 mg/d)				• Arterial dilator causes reflex changes to increase HR and CO slightly
Nitroglycerin • Drip: 0.1 µg/kg/min, titrated up to effect	• $t_{1/2}$ = 1–3 min • Levels: 1.2–11 ng/mL	• Hepatic reductive hydrolysis	• Venodilation reduces LVEDP and RVEDP • Headache, postural hypotension • Few side effects • Absorbed onto the plastic of many IV administration sets	• Increases cGMP in smooth muscle • Improves both myocardial oxygen supply and demand • Less effective hypotensive agent than nitroprusside
Nitroprusside (Nipride, Nitropress) • 0.5–8 µg/kg/min IV	• Toxic level of >10 mg/mL • Toxicity: >8 µg/kg/min • Onset 30 sec	• Cyanide ion is formed in the RBCs and then reduced in the liver to thiocyanate which is excreted in the urine with a $t_{1/2}$ = 3–4 d	• Hypotension, sweating, headache • Reflex tachycardia • Methemoglobinemia • Acute withdrawal can cause hypertensive crisis • Cyanide toxicity with metabolic acidosis	• Decreases both preload and afterload • Direct vascular smooth muscle vasodilator (arterioles and venules)
Norepinephrine (Levarterenol) • Test dose: 0.1–0.2 µg/kg • Infusion: 0.05 µg/kg/min, titrated up		• Metabolized in the liver	• Hypertension • α agonism can cause vascular insufficiency • Cardiac arrhythmias • Reflex bradycardia	• β_1 agonism • Little β_2 agonism • α agonist

Drug / Dose	Pharmacokinetics	Elimination	Adverse Effects	Notes
Pancuronium • Intubation: 0.1–0.15 mg/kg IV or 0.2 mg/kg IM	• Lasts 1 h	• Renal with some hepatic	• Tachycardia	• Accentuated by respiratory acidosis, myasthenic syndromes, metabolic alkalosis, local anesthetics, many antibiotics, magnesium, hypothermia, dantrolene, furosemide, nitroglycerin
Penicillin G (potassium or sodium) • <7 d parenteral 50,000–150,000 units/kg/d, q 12 h • >7 d 75,000–250,000 units/kg/d, q 6–8 h • Children: 40,000–300,000 units/kg/d, q 4–6 h	• 65% protein bound • $t_{1/2}$ = 30 min • $t_{1/2}$ (<1 wk) = 3 h	• 60–90% renal excretion • 10% by filtration • 90% by tubular secretion	• Resistance • From most to least likely: rash, fever, bronchospasm, vasculitis, serum sickness, exfoliative dermatitis, Stevens-Johnson syndrome, anaphylaxis	• Interferes with cell wall synthesis • 1 mg = 1600 units • Potassium: 1,000,000 units = 1.68 mEq • Sodium: 1,000,000 units = 1.68 mEq • Activity against Gram-positive cocci, anaerobes, some Gram-negatives • 5% of plasma concentrations found in CSF in meningitis • Probenecid blocks tubular secretion

continued

Drug/Dose	Pharmacokinetics and Pharmacotherapeutics	Metabolism	Side Effects/Interactions	Pharmacology
Pentamidine isethionate (Pentam) • 4 mg/kg/dose QD, IM or IV × 12–14 d • IM preferable to IV • Maximum total dose: 56 mg/kg		• Slowly excreted unchanged in urine $t_{1/2} = 6$ h	• Protect from light to avoid hepatotoxic compounds • IM better than IV • Breathlessness, tachycardia, dizziness, fainting, headache, vomiting, hypotension, histamine release, disruption of glucose homeostasis, renal dysfunction	• Little CNS penetration • Second-line drug after TMP-SMX for *Pneumocystis carinii* • Antiprotozoan activity
*Pentobarbital (Nembutal) • Sedation: 2–6 mg/kg/dose PO • IV coma induction: 10 mg/kg, then 1–4 mg/kg/h	• Toxic levels:1 mg/L • $t_{1/2} = 15$–48 h	• Hepatic cytochrome P-450; termination of action by redistribution	• Apnea • Hypotension • Decreases cardiac output, renal plasma flow, CBF, ICP • Increase in SVR • Contraindicated in porphyrias • Intra-arterial injection can cause loss of limb	• Antianalgesic in subanesthetic doses • Site of action: reticular activating system • Suppresses polysynaptic responses • Inhibits synapses that are GABA-ergic • Enhances GABA-induced increases in chloride conductance • Autonomic ganglionic blocker

*Phenobarbital (Luminal)
- Sedation: 2–3 mg/kg/dose PO, IM, IV q 8 h
- Seizure control: 15–25 mg/kg/dose IV
- Maximum: 600 mg/d
- Chronic: 4–6 mg/kg/d PO q 12 h

- $t_{1/2}$ = 80–120 h
- Levels: 15–40 mg/L

- See pentobarbital

- See pentobarbital

- See pentobarbital

Phentolamine (Regitine)
- In diagnosis of pheochromocytoma: 10 μg/kg/min IV, titrated up
- For pheochromocytoma: 1–5 mg IV, PRN elevated blood
- Blood pressure—may use as a continuous infusion in a dilute concentration for extravasation of vasoconstrictor: 10 mg in 10 mL infiltrated in affected site

- 10% excreted in urine

- Muscarinic agonist: salivation, lacrimation, diarrhea
- Tachycardias and GI side effect
- Orthostatic hypotension
- Tachycardia
- Vasodilation
- Nasal congestion

- α_1 and α_2 blocker
- Cardiac stimulation as well as vasodilation
- α-Adrenergic receptor blocker
- halflife of <20 min given IV
- Used in patients with pheochromoc;toma

continued

Drug/Dose	Pharmacokinetics and Pharmacotherapeutics	Metabolism	Side Effects/Interactions	Pharmacology
Phenylephrine (Neo-Synephrine) • Hypotension: 1 µg/kg IV, repeat and titrate PRN, then start with 0.01 µg/kg/min IV, drip and increase • SVT: 5 µg/kg/dose IV, titrated to effect	• Duration of action: <20 min	• Hepatic	• Decreases CO • Increases SVR, venous pressure, pulmonary artery pressure • Bradycardia (reflex)	• α_1 stimulation • May release norepinephrine • α agonism may cause vascular insufficiency in high doses
Phenytoin (Dilantin) • Seizures: 15–20 mg/kg IV • Antiarrhythmic: 2–4 mg/kg IV; maximum: 500 mg not given faster than 1 mg/kg/min • Maintenance: 4–7 mg/kg/d, q BID, IV, PO	• 90% protein bound • $t_{1/2} = 6$–24 h • Levels: 10–20 µg/mL	• Hepatic microsomal enzymes	• Cardiac arrhythmias • Hypotension megaloblastic anemia, gingival hyperplasia nystagmus, ataxia diplopia, vertigo, inhibition of ADH release, neutropenia leukopenia, dermatitis, lymphadenopathy, hypoprothrombinemia	• For treatment of all seizures except absence • Stabilizes neural membranes • Below toxic levels, there are no CNS effects • Follow QT_c interval on ECG while loading
Physostigmine (Antilirium) • Children <5 y old: 0.5 mg IV q 5 min; maximum: 2.0 mg	• Lasts 2 h	• Plasma esterases	• Atropine will reverse toxic side effects of physostigmine—salivation, lacrimation, seizures	• Inhibits the action of cholinesterase • Physostigmine crosses the blood-brain barrier

- >5 y old: 1–2 mg IV: maximum: 4 mg/30 min

Piperacillin (Pipracil)
- 75–300 mg/kg/d, q 4–6 h
- Maximum: 24 g/d

- 16–48% protein bound
- $t_{1/2} = 0.93$ h

- 71% urinary excretion

- See penicillin
- Activity against *Klebsiella* and *Pseudomonas* spp.
- Sodium: 2 mEq/g

Pitocin
- For controlling postpartum uterine hemorrhage: 10 units in 1000 mL crystalloid at 2–4 mL/min after the placenta has been delivered

- Uterine concentration may be profound
- Fetal distress if excessive uterine contraction
- Rapid administration may result in hypotension

- When used postpartum, uterine contraction decreases blood loss
- Used to induce labor

Prazosin (Minipress)
- Adults: initially 1 mg BID to TID PO, then increased
- Maximum: 40 mg/d (rarely >10 mg/d)

- $t_{1/2} = 3.1$ h

- <1% urinary excretion
- 95% protein bound

- Hypotension, especially with first dose

- α_1 antagonist
- Decrease in SVR and MAP without change in HR

Pendnisoline:
- Anti-inflammatory and asthma: 0.5–2 mg/kg/d q 6 h

- $t_{1/2} = 2.2$ h
- 90–95% protein bound

- Converted in liver to methylprednisolone
- 15% urinary excretion

- Supersensitivity to catecholamines
- Requires 3 wk for full hypertensive effect

- See hydrocortisone
- 4 times the anti-inflammatory effects and 0.8 times the sodium-

continued

Drug/Dose	Pharmacokinetics and Pharmacotherapeutics	Metabolism	Side Effects/Interactions	Pharmacology
• Physiologic replacement: 4–5 mg/m² /d, q BID			• Change in mental status • Contraindicated in depressed patients, peptic ulcer disease • See hydrocortisone	retaining effects of hydrocortisone
Primidone (Mysoline): • Initial dose for 8 y old: 125 mg/d QD; • For >8 y old: 250 mg/d QD; • Maintenance: 10–25 mg/kg/d, q BID to TID • Maximum: 200 mg/d	• Therapeutic levels: 8–12 mg/L of primidone or 15–40 mg/L of phenobarbital	• Converted to phenobarbital and PEMA	• See pentobarbital	• See pentobarbital
Procainamide (Pronestyl) • IM: 20–30 mg/kg/d, q 4–6 h (adults: 1 g/ dose × 1 • Then 250 mg q 3 h; maximum: 4 g/d) • IV load: 2 mg/kg/ dose over 5 min, repeated q 10–30 min (adult IV load: 100 mg over 2–4 min q 5 min, titrated to control of	• $t_{1/2}$ = 3 h • 16% protein bound • Levels: 3–15 µg/mL	• 67% urinary excretion; hepatic metabolism forms N-acetylprocainamide (fast and slow acetylators metabolize a different percentage of the drug)	• Hypotension, especially when dose is >600 mg • Toxicity: >14 µg/mL • Less vagolytic side effects than quinidine • Discontinuation—same criteria as in quinidine • GI disturbances, CNS disturbances, agranulocytosis, SLE syndrome	• Used for PVCs, also moderate activity on atrial flutter/ fibrillation • Decreases automaticity, Vmax, action potential amplitude • Prolonged action potential and effective refractory period • Prolongs QRS, QT • Usually digitalization should start before quinidine initiation

Drug (dose)	Pharmacokinetics	Metabolism	Side Effects	Comments
dysrhythmia; maintenance: 20–80 µg/kg/min; adult maximum: 8 g/d)				
Promethazine (Phenergan, Provigan) • Antihistamine: 0.1 mg/kg/dose q 6 h; maximum: 12.5 mg QID • Nausea and vomiting: 0.25–0.5 mg/kg/dose IM, PO, IV, PR • Sedative: 0.5–1 mg/kg/dose; maximum: 50 mg IM, IV	• $t_{1/2}$ = 20–40 h	• Hepatic microsomes, oxidation and glucuronidation	• Anticholinergic side effects: tachycardia, dry mouth, change in mental status • CV system: orthostatic hypotension by α blockade • CNS extrapyramidal signs: parkinsonism, acute dystonia, neuroleptic malignant syndrome, akathisia, dive dyskinesia, and perioral tremor • Blood dyscrasias • May decrease seizure threshold	• Phenothiazine • Antihistaminic properties • Central dopaminergic blocker including the CTZ • Blocks reuptake of amines • Prolongs barbiturate sleeping time
Propafenone • Adults: 150 mg PO q 8 h; increase to 675 mg/d over 3–4 d; maximum 905 mg/d	• 97% bound to alpha-1 acid glycoprotein • $t_{1/2}$ = 5–6 h fast metabolizers; 17 h slow metabolizers	• Extensive first pass metabolism	• Granulocytopenia • SLE-like syndrome	• AV conduction block • Bundle branch block used for JET

continued

Drug/Dose	Pharmacokinetics and Pharmacotherapeutics	Metabolism	Side Effects/Interactions	Pharmacology
Propranolol (Inderal) • Arrhythmias: 0.01 mg/kg/dose IV, titrated up 5 mg to effect • Tetralogy spells: 0.15–0.25 mg/kg/dose q 6 h PO; maximum single dose: 10 mg IV • Thyrotoxicosis for neonatal: 2 mg/kg/d PO, q 6 h; for adults: 1–3 mg/dose IV over 10 min, then 10–40 mg PO q 6 h • Hypertension: 0.5–1 mg/kg/d, q 6–12 h PO; in adults, increase 10–20 mg/dose q 3 d; maximum dose: 480 mg PO	• 93% protein bound • $t_{1/2}$ = 4 h • Level: 20 ng/mL	• Hepatic metabolism	• Bronchospasm • Withdrawal phenomenon • Augments, the hypoglycemic actions of insulin by reducing the compensatory effect of sympathetic adrenal activation • Bradycardia • Nausea, vomiting	• Nonspecific β antagonist • Local anesthetic effect • Decreases inward sodium currents, so reduces the height and rate of rise of depolarization • Decreases HR, CO • Blocks renin release from juxtaglomerular sites • Decreases spontaneous firing in atria and ectopic sites • Increases AV conduction time

Prostaglandin E_1 (PGE_1) (alprostadil) (Prostin VR) • Initial: 0.05 µg/kg/min IV, titrated up to 0.4 µg/kg/min	• 95% inactivated through one pass in the lungs	• Apnea, seizures, fever, flushing, bradycardia, hypotension, diarrhea • Decreases platelet aggregation	• Stimulates smooth muscle in low doses but relaxes at higher doses • Activates adenylate cyclase • Pulmonary and ductal tissue relaxation • New synthetic analog used for treatment of peptic ulcer disease caused by nonsteroidal anti-inflammatory drugs
Protamine sulfate • Must be titrated to effect (e.g., against ACT) • Maximum dose: 50 mg		• Dyspnea, flushing, bradycardia, hypotension avoided by central venous administration of <20 mg/min in adults • ? Histamine release • Hypersensitivity, especially to fish-allergic individuals	• Combines with heparin ionically • 1 mg protamine antagonizes 100 units of heparin
Quinidine • PO is preferable to IM which is preferable to IV	• 90% protein bound • $t_{1/2} = 6.2$ h • Effective levels: 2–6 mg/L	• Metabolized in the liver • 20% excreted in the urine • At 6 µg/mL, 10% of patients will demonstrate toxic effects	• Decrease action potential, Vmax automaticity • Prolongs action potential and refractory

continued

Drug/Dose	Pharmacokinetics and Pharmacotherapeutics	Metabolism	Side Effects/Interactions	Pharmacology
• Test dose: 2 mg/kg PO in children: 15–60 mg/kg/d, q 6 h PO • Adults: 200–400 mg/ dose q 4–6 h IV; 200–300 mg/dose q 6–8 h PO, titrated to effect (ECG changes)			• At 14 µg/mL, 50% of patients will demonstrate toxic effects • Syncope, sudden death • Paradoxical increased ventricular rate when treating atrial fibrillation, so often AV block is indicated before initiating therapy • Hypotension, tachycardia, tinnitus, hearing loss, GI disturbances, fever, anaphylaxis, thrombocytopenia	• Prolongs QRS, QT_c • Activity for atrial fibrillation and flutter, APCs, VPC, and reentry tachycardias • Some activity as an antimalacide, antipyretic, and oxytocic • Vagolytic and α-blocking properties • Can increase digoxin levels if given concomitantly
Ranitidine • Children: 2–4 mg/ kg/d, q 12 h PO; 1–3 mg/kg/d, q 6–8 h IV • Adults: 150 mg PO, BID; 50 mg IV, IM q 6–8h	• 15% protein bound • $t_{1/2} = 2$ h • Ineffective level: 100 ng/mL (50% inhibition of gastric secretion	• 69% urinary excretion • Ranitidine has poor penetration across the blood-brain barrier	• Rare and minor side effects • Ranitidine crosses the blood-brain barrier and binds less avidly to the hepatic P-450 system so that there are many fewer CNS and hepatic (i.e., drug interaction) side effects than with cimetidine	• Histamine-2 blocker inhibits gastric secretion, reducing gastric volume and increasing gastric pH

Ribavirin (Varazole)
- Aerosol (20 mg/mL sterile water)
- 12–18 h/d
- Small hepatic blood flow reductions causing accumulation of drugs that are metabolized in the liver
- For RSV treatment

Scopolamine
- IV/IM 0.2–0.4 mg transdermal patch delivers 0.5 mg over 72 h for the treatment of nausea
- Can interfere with respirator function
- Delirium, agitation
- Mydriasis/blurry vision
- Dry mouth
- Drowsiness
- Anticholinergic, muscarinic receptor blocker
- Crosses blood brain barrier
- Sedation, amnesia
- Antisialogogue

Spironolactone (Aldactone)
- Children: 3.3 mg/kg/d, q QID to BID, PO
- Adults: 15–200 mg/d, q QID to BID, PO 100–400 mg/d for primary aldosteronism (especially in preparation for surgery)
- Highly protein bound
- Metabolized in liver
- Hypercalcemia (especially in renal failure)
- Gynecomastia
- GI disturbances
- Rash
- May potentiate ganglionic blocking agents
- Antagonist of aldosterone
- Increases urinary Na/K ratio
- Sites of action include salivary glands, colon, and nephron
- Increases renal calcium excretion

continued

Drug/Dose	Pharmacokinetics and Pharmacotherapeutics	Metabolism	Side Effects/Interactions	Pharmacology
Succinylcholine • Intubation: 1–1.5 mg/kg IV or 4 mg/kg IM	• Duration <10 min • Onset 30–60 sec	• Plasma pseudocholin esterase	• Hyperkalemia associated with burns, trauma, and nerve damage, > 24 h after injury • Increases intraocular and intracranial ? pressures	• Atypical or absent pseudocholinesterase documented by a high dibucaine number associated with prolongation of action • Must have airway
Sucralfate (Carafate) • Adults: 1 g PO QID • Children: 40–80 mg/kg/24 h ÷ q 6 h PO	• Last 6 h	• Poorly absorbed systemically	• Rare side effects • Constipation • Dry mouth In uremic patients, increases serum aluminum and decreases serum phosphate levels	• Sulfated sucrose and aluminum compound polymerizing below a pH of 4 • Adheres to ulcer craters for 6 h • More adherent to duodenal than to gastric ulcers • No acid-neutralizing action and requires an acid environment to work, so antacids should be withheld 30 min before its administration

Drug/Dosage	Pharmacokinetics	Toxicity/Side Effects	Mechanism/Notes
Terbutaline (Brethine, Bricanyl) • SC: 0.005–0.01 mg/kg/dose; maximum: 0.25 mg q 15–20 min ×2 • Inhalation: 2 inhalations q 4 h	• Not metabolized by COMT	• See metaproterenol	• See metaproterenol
Tetracycline • 25–50 mg/kg/d, q 6 h PO • 10–20 mg/kg/d, q 12 h IV • 15–25 mg/kg/d, q 8 h IM • Maximum: 2 g/d	• 65% protein bound • $t_{1/2}$ = 10.6 h	• Resistance • Hepatic toxicity • ? Renal toxicity • Brown discoloration of teeth and bones in <7 y old • Thrombophlebitis • Hematologic abnormalities • Antibiotic-associated colitis • Pseudotumor cerebri	• 30S subunit of the ribosome—inhibiting protein synthesis • Some CSF penetration
*Thiopental • 1–6 mg/kg IV	• $t_{1/2}$ (α) = 3 min • $t_{1/2}$ (β) = 9 h • Termination of action is by redistribution • $t_{1/2}$ (α) is 3 min, then metabolism by P-450 in the liver ($t_{1/2}$ (β) is 9 h	• Hypotension: direct myocardial depression, ganglionic blockade • Not to be used in porphyrias • Histamine release: hypotension, bronchospasm	• Potentiates both GABA and non-GABA-induced chloride-conductance • Decreases calcium release of neurotransmitters • Decreases cerebral metabolic rate and cerebral blood flow and

continued

Drug/Dose	Pharmacokinetics and Pharmacotherapeutics	Metabolism	Side Effects/Interactions	Pharmacology
Ticarcillin • Neonates of <2 kg and of age 0–7 d: 150 mg/kg/d, q 8 h IV • >7 d: 225 mg/kg/d, q 8 h IV • >2 kg: 225–300 mg/kg/d, q 8 h IV • Children: 200–300 mg/kg/d q 4–6 h IV	• 65% protein bound • $t_{1/2}$ = 1.3 h	• 92% urinary excretion	• Intraarterial injection can cause loss of limbs • See pentobarbital • See penicillin • Decreased platelet aggregation, bleeding • With clavulanic acid = Timatin expands activity to include β lactomase producers	volume, thus decreasing intracranial hypertension • See pentobarbital • See penicillin • Each gram contains 5 mEq sodium • Enhanced activity against *Pseudomonas* spp.
Tobramycin (Nebcin) • 2.5 mg/kg/dose IV, IM; frequency of dose depends on age/maturity • At <7 d (<28 wk: q 24 h; 28–34 wk: q 18 h; term q 12 h) • At >7 d (<28 wk: q 18 h; 28–34 wk: q 12 h; term: q 8 h) • Children: q 8 h	• Levels peak 6–10 mg/L trough <2 mg/L • <10% protein bound • $t_{1/2}$ = 2.2 h; a long terminal half-life (β) $t_{1/2}$ = 100 h) due to tissue binding	• 90% urinary excretion	• See gentamicin	• See gentamicin • Enhanced activity against enterococci and mycobacteria

Drug	Half-life	Elimination	Adverse effects	Comments
Trimethaphan (Arfonad) • 50–150 µg/kg/min • As a hypertensive agent: infusion 1 mg/mL titrate to effect starting at 0.5 mg/min (rate of 30 mL/h at above concentration)		• Predominantly excreted by kidney	• Histamine release • Mydriasis and cycloplegia, constipation, xerostomia, anhidrosis, urinary retention • Potentiates action of other antihypertensives, e.g., sodium nitroprusside • Urinary retention • ? Respiratory depression	• Relatively short half-life, 15 min • Ganglionic blockade, vasodilation and hypotension, decreased cardiac output • Blocks postsynaptic blockade of acetylcholine in ganglia • Can be used to treat autonomic hyperreflexia
Trimethoprim-sulfamethoxazole (TMP-SMX) (Bactrim, Septra) • Severe infections and *Pneumocystis carinii* pneumonia; TMP dose: 20 mg/kg/d, q 6–8 h PO, IV • *Pneumocystis* prophylaxis: 10 mg/kg/d, q 12 h PO, IV	• TMP: $t_{1/2} = 11$ h • SMX: $t_{1/2} = 10$ h	• 60% TMP and 25–50% SMX excreted in urine	• Resistance • Blood dyscrasias (especially megaloblastic anemia); ashes common, renal toxicity • Hemolysis in G6PD patients	• Inhibits folic acid metabolism in bacteria (especially dihydrofolate reductase) • TMP has good CSF penetration
d-Tubocuraine • Intubation • In newborn: 0.2 mg/kg • In >6 wk old: 0.6 mg/kg IV	• 60 min	• 40–60% eliminated by kidney • Remainder; hepatic	• Hypotension	• Histamine release • Ganglionic blockade • Myocardial depression • See pancuronium (except nitroglycerin) precautions

continued

Drug/Dose	Pharmacokinetics and Pharmacotherapeutics	Metabolism	Side Effects/Interactions	Pharmacology
Valproic acid (Depakene, Depakote) • Initial: 10–15 mg/kg/d, q BID • Maintenance: 30–60 mg/kg/d, QD to TID (increase by weekly intervals)	• 90% protein bound • Levels: 50–100 µg/mL	• <3% excreted in urine	• Minimum sedation • Nausea, vomiting • Fulminant hepatitis • Phenobarbital levels increase 40% in the presence of valproic acid • Pancreatitis • Platelet dysfunction	• Antiseizure activity for all types of seizures (? use in partial seizure)
Vancomycin (Vancocin) • Neonates <7 d old: 10 mg/kg (<1000 g: q 24 h; 1–2 kg; q 18 h; > 2 kg: q 12 h • >7 d: 10 mg/kg (<1000 g: q 18 h; 1–2 kg: q 12 h; >2 kg q 8 h) • Children for CNS infections: 45 mg/kg/d, q 8 h IV; • For other infections: 30–40 mg/kg/d, q 8 h IV; maximum: 2 g/d; • For antibiotic-associated colitis: 2g/1.73 m² /d, q 6 h PO	• 55% protein bound • $t_{1/2}$ (α) = 5.6 h • Levels: 10–25 mg/L • Peak 25–40 mg/L • Trough <10 mg/L	• 90% urinary excretion	• Ototoxicity (especially at levels of >30 µg/mL) nephrotoxocity phlebitis • Red man syndrome associated with rapid IV infusion	• Gram-positive activity • Cell wall synthesis inhibition

Drug / Dose	Pharmacokinetics	Side effects	Notes
Vasopression (Pitressin) • 0.5 mU/kg/h or 22 pg/kg/min, titrated up to maximum of 10 mU/kg/h	• $t_{1/2}$ = 17–35 min	• Vasoconstriction at high doses, causing tissue ischemia, especially myocardial ischemia	• No histamine release, no ganglionic blockade, no effect on muscarinic cardiac receptors
Vecuronium • Intubation: 0.07–0.1 mg/kg IV	• 60 min duration • Onset 3 min • 10% dependent on renal function; remainder metabolized by the liver	• Void of cardiovascular effects	
Verapamil (Isoptin, Calan) • 1–15 y of age: 0.1–0.3 mg/kg IV, maximum: 5 mg • Adult: 5–10 q 30 min, administer over 2–3 min	• $t_{1/2}$ = 5 h • Level: 100 ng/mL • 90% protein bound • <3% urinary excretion	• Cardiovascular collapse when given in conjunction with a β blocker • Hypotension • Bradydysrhythmias • Controversial indications for infants <6 mo old	• Negative: dromotropy, chronotropy, inotropy • Calcium channel blocker • Vascular smooth muscle relaxation
Vidarabine (ara-A, Vira A) • HSV encephalitis: 15 mg/kg/d IV given over 12–24 h	• Dependent on renal function for elimination	• Few side effects • Nausea, vomiting, diarrhea, rash, weakness, thrombophlebitis • CNS manifestations at high doses (20 mg/kg)	• Inhibits viral DNA polymerase, especially HSV • No activity against other DNA viruses (adenoviruses, papoviruses, or RNA viruses)

continued

Drug/Dose	Pharmacokinetics and Pharmacotherapeutics	Metabolism	Side Effects/Interactions	Pharmacology
Zidovudine • Oral; neonates: 2 mg/kg/dose q 6 h in newborn of mothers who are HIV positive • 4–12 y 90–180 mg/m² /dose q 6 h more 200 q 6 h IV; 100 mg/m² /dose q 6 h • Adults (symptomatic) • 200 mg q 4 h PO chemoprophylaxis p̄ occupational exposure 200 mg PO TID in combination with lamivudine 150 mg BID and Indinavir 800 mg TID	• t$_{1/2}$ 1 h	• Bone marrow suppression, lactic acidosis	• Inhibit HIV reverse transcriptase	

ACh, acetylcholine; ACT, activated clotting time; ADH, antidiuretic hormone; APC, atrial premature contraction; ATPase, adenosine triphosphate; AV, atrioventricular; BP, blood pressure; cGMP, cyclic guanosine monophosphate; CBF, cerebral blood flow; CHF, congestive heart failure, CNS, central nervous system; CO, cardiac output; COMT, catechol-o-methyl transferase; CSF, cerebrospinal fluid; CTZ, chemoreceptor trigger zone; CV, cardiovascular; DI, diabetes insipidus; D5W, 5% dextrose in water; DNA, deoxyribonucleic acid; DT, diphtheria toxoid; ECG, electrocardiogram; FEV, forced expiratory volume, GABA, γ-aminobutyric acid; G6PD, glucose-6-phosphate dehydrogenase; GI, gastrointestinal; GMP, guanosine monophosphate; HR, heart rate, HSV, herpes simplex virus; ICP, intracranial pressure; IHSS, idiopathic hypertrophic subaortic stenosis; INH, isoniazid; LDL, low-density lipoprotein; LV, left ventricle; LVEDP, left ventricular end-diastolic pressure; LVSW, left ventricular stroke work; MAO, monoamine oxidase; MAP, mean arterial pressure; MIF, migration inhibitory factor; mRNA, messenger ribonucleic acid; NG, nasogastric; NPH, a type of insulin; NS, normal saline, PEMA, phenylethylmalonamide; PGG$_2$, prostaglandin G$_2$, PMNs, polymorphonuclear leukocytes; PTT, partial thromboplastin time; PVC, premature ventricular contraction; RBC, red blood cell; RSV, respiratory syncytial virus; RVEDP, right ventricular end-diastolic pressure; SA, sinoatrial; SLE, systemic lupus erythematosus; SV, stroke volume; SVR, supraventricular rhythm; SVT, supraventricular tachycardia; TMP-SMX, trimethoprim-sulfamethoxazole; Vmax, maximum velocity of cardiac contraction; and VPC, ventricular premature contractions.

^aComments on cephalosporins: (a) mechanism of action-inhibition of cell wall synthesis; (b) first-generation drugs (cephalothin, cefazolin)—good activity against Gram-positives, modest activity against Gram-negative; second-generation drugs (cefoxitin, cefuroxime)—increased activity against Gram-negatives; and third-generation drugs (cefotaxine, ceftazidime)—good activity against Gram-negatives at the expense of Gram-positive coverage; (c) adverse reactions: 20% of patients reacting to penicillin will cross-react with cephalosporins, decreasing the likelihood of rash, fever, bronchospasm, vasculitis, serum sickness, exfoliative dermatitis, Stevens-Johnson syndrome, anaphylaxis, nausea, vomiting, eosinophilia, interstitial nephritis and other reactions, such as phlebitis, bone marrow depression, hepatisis; (d) virtually all of the cephalosporins (except cefoperazone) are excreted in the urine, and doses must be adjusted in renal failure; virtually are all removed by dialysis in variable amounts.

INDEX

Page references in *italics* denote figures; those followed by "t" denote tables

Computed tomography—*Continued*
　for head trauma, 782
　for hepatic complications after liver
　　　transplantation, 634
　herpes simplex virus encephalitis diagno-
　　　sis, 551
　pancreatic abscess, 607–608
　sickle cell disease, 764
　of spinal cord injuries, 441–442
　subdural empyema, 558
　viral encephalitis diagnosis, 548
Concussion, 411
Conditional variables, of mechanical venti-
　　　lation, 168–169
Congenital adrenal hyperplasia, 686
Congenital heart disease, myocardial is-
　　　chemia and, 202
Congestive heart failure, 232–234, 233t
Continuous arteriovenous hemofiltration,
　　　665–666
Continuous positive airway pressure
　complications of, 189t
　description of, 175
　positive end expiratory pressure and,
　　　comparison between, 175
　pulmonary edema caused by weaning
　　　from, 219
　for unilateral diaphragmatic paralysis,
　　　138
　work of breathing effects, 112
Continuous venovenous hemofiltration,
　　　664–665
Controlled positive pressure ventilation,
　　　114
Contusion, of brain, 412
Convulsions, 521
Cordarone (*see* Amiodarone)
Coronary arteries
　anomalous origin, from the pulmonary
　　　artery
　　clinical presentation, 203
　　description of, 202–203
　　diagnosis of, 203
　　differential diagnosis, 203–204
　　natural history of, 203
　　therapy, 204
　　variants of, 202
　in Kawasaki disease, 207
Cortical lesions, 127t
Corticosteroids
　clinical uses
　　acute respiratory distress syndrome,
　　　117–118
　　bacterial meningitis, 535–536
　　brain abscess, 556
　　bronchiolitis, 81
　　fulminant hepatic failure, 612, *613*

fulminant meningococcemia, 512
　Guillain-Barré syndrome, 136
　immunosuppression, 635
　intracranial pressure, 435, 621, 622t
　myasthenia gravis, 141
complications of, 635
side effects of, 638t
synthetic, 691–692
Corticotropin releasing hormone
　primary adrenal insufficiency, 687–688
　secondary adrenal insufficiency, 689
　tertiary adrenal insufficiency, 686–687
CPB (*see* Cardiopulmonary bypass)
CPPV (*see* Controlled positive pressure ven-
　　　tilation)
Creatinine clearance, 874
CRH (*see* Corticotropin releasing hormone)
Cricoid pressure
　description of, 6
　for positive pressure ventilation, 53
Cricothyrotomy
　advantages of, 11
　indications, 11
　technique, 11–13, *12, 13t*
Critical illness syndromes
　fat oxidation disorders, 382
　hepatic encephalopathy, 386
　intracranial pressure increases, 382–386
　organic acidemias, 381
　urea cycle disorders, 381
Cromolyn sodium
　properties of, 893t
　for status asthmaticus, 94t
Crouzon's disease, effect on anesthesia,
　　　859t
Cryptococcal meningitis, 491
Cryptosporidium, 598
CSF (*see* Cerebrospinal fluid)
CT (*see* Computed tomography)
Cumid (*see* Cholestyramine)
Curare (*see* d-Tubocurarine)
Cushing's syndrome
　anesthesia, intubation, and the perioper-
　　　ative period, 691
　clinical presentation, 691
　diagnosis, 691
　etiology, 691
CVP (*see* Central venous pressure)
CVVH (*see* Continuous venovenous he-
　　　mofiltration)
Cyanide inhalational injury, 830
Cyanosis
　definition of, 219
　diagnostic approaches
　　imaging studies, 231–232
　　laboratory tests, 230–231
　　physical signs, 229–230

Hemorrhage—*Continued*
  platelet disorders
    defective hemostasis, 774
    idiopathic thrombocytopenic purpura,
        777
    low platelet count, 776
    platelet transfusion, 776–777
    thrombocytopathia, 775, 775t
    thrombocytopenia, 774, 774t
  routine hemostatic tests, 769t
  in "shaken baby" syndrome, 429
  subarachnoid, 417–418
  transfusion therapy, 770t
    cardiopulmonary bypass, 773, 773t
    complications, 772
Hemorrhage
  massive transfusion, 771–772
  risk versus benefit, 768–769, 771
  typing and cross-matching, 772
Hemorrhagic shock, 545, 791–792
Hemostasis
  perioperative, 260–261
  platelet disorders and, 774
Heparin
  clinical uses
    cardiopulmonary bypass, 260
    deep venous thrombosis, 785
    disseminated intravascular coagula-
        tion, 778–780
    fulminant meningococcemia, 512
  properties of, 906t
Hepatic encephalopathy
  ammonia level, 617–618
  neurotransmission alterations, 618
  staging system, 618–619
  treatment, 619
Hepatic failure
  ascites, 614–615
  cerebral edema
    elevated intracranial pressure and
      barbiturate use, 621
      carbon dioxide levels, maintenance
          of, 620–621, 621t
      clinical signs, 620
      fluid levels, 621
      hypothermia, 621
      steroid therapy, 621, 622t
      treatment, 620
    etiology, 619–620
  fulminant hepatic failure
    etiology, 609
    hepatitis non-A, non-B, 609
    laboratory findings, 611
    mortality rates, 611
    Reye syndrome, 609–611, *610*
    therapy
      encephalopathy, 612

  fluids and electrolytes, 612
    monitoring, 612
    steroid therapy, 612, *613*
  toxic hepatitis, 609
  gastrointestinal bleeding
    coagulopathy, 613
    portal hypertension, 614
    stress gastritis, 613–614
  hepatic encephalopathy
    ammonia level, 617–618
    neurotransmission alterations, 618
    staging system, 618–619
    treatment, 619
  hepatorenal syndrome, *616*
    diagnosis, 615
    management, 616–617
    infection, 617
  liver transplantation, 622
  management techniques, 622
  respiratory failure, 615
Hepatitis non-A, non-B, 609
Hepatorenal syndrome
  clinical presentation of, 682
  definition of, 681
  diagnostic findings, 682
  differential diagnosis, 682–683
  hepatic failure and, *616*
    diagnosis, 615
    management, 616–617
  pathophysiology of, 681
  therapy, 683
Herpes simplex virus
  encephalitis
    clinical manifestations, 549–551
    diagnosis
      cerebrospinal fluid analysis, 550
      computed tomography and elec-
          troencephalogram, 548
      infants and children, 550
      neonates, 549
    etiology, 541
      infants and children, 549–551
      neonates, 549
    infants and children, 549–551
    isolation and identification,
        545–546
    pathogenesis, 549
    therapy
      infants and children, 551
      neonates, 549
  neonatal
    clinical features of, 507t, 507–508
    epidemiology of, 506–507
    infection routes, 506–507
    precaution, 508
    therapy, 508
  therapy, 648